BEGINNING CHILD PSYCHIATRY

BEGINNING CHILD PSYCHIATRY

by

PAUL L. ADAMS, M.D.

Kempner Professor of Child Psychiatry
University of Texas Medical Branch
*   at Galveston*

and

IVAN FRAS, M.D.

Clinical Professor of Psychiatry
State University of New York
Upstate Medical Center, Syracuse,
*   and Clinical Campus, Binghamton*

BRUNNER/MAZEL *Publishers* • New York

DSM-III-R classifications and related material are reprinted with permission from the *Diagnostic and Statistical Manual of Mental Disorders, Third Edition, Revised.* Copyright 1987 American Psychiatric Association.

Library of Congress Cataloging-in-Publication Data

Adams, Paul L., 1924–
    Beginning child psychiatry.

    Includes bibliographies and index.
    1. Child psychiatry.   I. Fras, Ivan, 1936–
II. Title.   [DNLM: 1. Child Psychiatry.   2. Mental
Disorders—in infancy & childhood.   WS 350 A215b]
RJ499.A323   1988   618.92'89   87-32587
ISBN 0-87630-493-5

Copyright © 1988 by Paul L. Adams and Ivan Fras

Published by
BRUNNER/MAZEL, INC.
19 Union Square
New York, New York 10003

MANUFACTURED IN THE UNITED STATES OF AMERICA

10   9   8   7   6   5   4   3   2   1

Contents

PART III
CHILD AS FAMILY MEMBER

PART IV
CRISIS NOW

PART V
CHILD PSYCHIATRY, SIMILAR BUT DIFFERENT

Preface

This is a book for serious beginners (i.e., students and practitioners–generalists) in child psychiatry. Since the specialty itself is so new, we are all beginners in a beginning field, and therefore the volume addresses a large number of health professionals. Only since 1959 have specialists in child psychiatry been given certification through the American Board of Medical Specialties; only since 1985 has the specialty been accorded representation in the House of Delegates of the American Medical Association. Hence, child psychiatry is both old and new as a specialized medical field. Nonetheless, it is a medical discipline with particularly close ties to sister disciplines in medicine, law, and other mental health clinical fields. We describe this more fully in Chapter 37, and encourage a multidiscipline perspective.

The historical roots of child psychiatry go back as far as recorded history's respect for a child as a person in his or her own right. Respect for children is not dazzling even today. But in history we can trace our lineage through medicine and pediatrics, law, educational theories and practice, movements for social reform and revolution, the profession of social work, and the profession of child psychology (See Appendix, "Selected Chronology for Child Psychiatry to 1970.") It may seem expansionistic and grabbing that we appropriate all these separate disciplines from behavioral sciences and biomedical sciences into our terrain, but we cite those fields not because we wish to take them over but only to acknowledge their great worth to us in child psychiatry.

Our desire has been to present an updated view of what can be said about the field of child psychiatry as a growing body of knowledge, skills, and attitudes concerning the mental disorders of children. In that spirit, we have not hesitated to show preference, always, for whatever we have found practical and clinically useful. Nor have we been shy in encouraging the reader to think ahead, be imaginative and speculative, to take risks, to go beyond the materials laid out in each of the chapters, to do *Further Reading* and to dive into our *Questions for Study and Action*, at the end of each chapter. Our view is that a young science permits, and needs, our imagination so that we can ask interesting questions of both nature and society.

The reader may ask why we have constructed the book into Part I devoted to the skills of a clinician working with children, Part II assigned to disorders shown by children—disorders of behavior, feeling and cognition, as well as being victimized—and Part V concerned with the field as a profession, with Part III on the child in the family and Part IV dealing with crises in child psychiatry. Our

ix

answer is that we strive, first and foremost, to examine clinical issues throughout the book: the physical examination, the history, the interview and mental status examination, the diagnostic workup, the diagnosis, the differential diagnosis, etiology and pathogenesis whenever something of substance is known, and treatment planning. If we can encourage students and practitioners to do good clinical work with disordered children by our approach, we will have succeeded in reaching one of the vital goals of the book.

In each chapter we have adhered rather closely to nosologic changes made in the 1987 publication, DSM-III-R. We gratefully acknowledge the American Psychiatric Association's permission to paraphrase, cite, and refer to DSM-III-R. In a few parts of the text we have given attention to some categories of childhood psychopathology (such as Firesetting) that have earned a place in child psychiatry but have not been recognized by framers of the Diagnostic and Statistical Manual of Mental Disorders (DSM). Always, our interest has been to describe the major dimensions of the clinical field, and when we take exception to DSM we try to say why we have dealt differently with the topic under discussion.

Our goal has been to arouse interest in clinical child psychiatry and, with that objective in mind, we have not hesitated to take an approach that differs from some of the multiauthored textbooks and compendiums of child psychiatry that seem to prevail in our field. The two of us discovered that we had sufficiently divergent writing styles and have felt lucky that only two versions had to be brought into a single voice.

It is our good fortune to acknowledge our students both at the State University of New York at Binghamton and University of Texas Medical Branch at Galveston. Moreover, we thank Leslie F. Major, M.D., and Robert M. Rose, M.D., department chairs at our medical schools, for encouragement and support.

Paul L. Adams   *Ivan Fras*
Galveston, Texas   *Binghamton, New York*

BEGINNING CHILD PSYCHIATRY

I

INTRODUCTION TO CLINICAL WORK WITH CHILDREN

The two chapters of this first Part are devoted to clinical work with children. In Chapter 1, we look at the child's problems and complaints about the child that may be given by a parent. We discuss how to take the story from parents or child; what to observe about the child; how to carry out a diagnostic workup; how to proceed with a differential diagnosis and formulate a treatment plan.

In Chapter 2, we consider the array of treatments for children as we give a brief survey of the repertoire that will be called out on the succeeding pages of this text. Only for convenience in discussing them do we divide them into pharmacotherapies, psychotherapies, and environmental interventions, for in real practice a multimodal treatment regimen is used of necessity.

1

Clinical Skills

L ike all medical diagnostic exercises, the child psychiatric examination consists of three parts: the history, the examination, and specialized tests ("laboratory tests") and consultations. Remaining after that are differential diagnosis and, finally, treatment planning.

We shall present a descriptive overview of the first three components—with enough detail to enable the nonspecialist clinician to do the history and the basic examination, but with only general guidelines for tests (which are specialized procedures), for consultation requests, for differential diagnosis, and for treatment planning.

Our strong recommendation for improving your clinical skills of history taking, examination, and diagnostic workup is to videotape several of your interviews and study your performance on tape.

THE HISTORY

What clinicians seek is a format for history taking that is comprehensive enough to include all the ingredients necessary but at the same time to cut out any "unnecessary baggage." The history is, in most cases, taken from the parents first, with the mother being the main, and usually best, historian. We recommend seeing the parents at least once or twice before the child is examined.

Occasionally, the history can be taken over again, or supplemented, from the child. This is sometimes done as part of the examination of the child and may be left to the examiner's discretion. A history from the child's perspective is often more illuminating and candid than the one derived from the parents.

The parts of the history are as follows:

THE PRESENTING COMPLAINTS

These form the backbone of the child psychiatric history and are of greater importance than their counterpart in general (adult) psychiatry. For example, it is necessary to ask the following questions:

- What concerns you about your child?
- When did these problems start?
- Are they getting worse?
- Have these problems been noticed in school as well as at home?
- What makes them better? What makes them worse?
- How have these problems affected the child's life with you, the parents? with siblings, peers, teachers?
- Has the child's school performance suffered?

More questions like these may be asked, according to the particular situation, to pin down exactly what it is for which help is sought. The manifest and latent complaints need to be elicited.

THE CHILD'S DEVELOPMENT

Table 1–1 displays in outline form what parents can be asked about the child's history. This information is a *must*. Its detail and depth will vary with the medical sophistication of the examiner and with the peculiarities of the case.

Before proceeding with the child's development proper, the clinician will make sure (s)he has not missed any pertinent data in the obstetrical history:

- *Prenatal factors*—Inquiry is directed to physical and emotional circumstances of the pregnancy, including any obstetrical and general medical abnormalities. Of particular importance usually are toxic factors (alcohol, drugs, tobacco) and any threats to the pregnancy (threatened abortion or abnormal bleeding generally, kidney problems, etc.). This may be the point at which to inquire whether the child was wanted and planned for or an accident of fate.
- *Perinatal factors*—These include difficult birth, difficulty breathing, or other problems on the part of the child, particularly "cord around the neck," low Apgar score, other information about hypoxia such as spending time in the incubator, "requiring extra oxygen," crying "weakly" or not at all at birth, and so on. Prematurity, unusual birth weight, prolonged jaundice, and other medical and congenital abnormalities also belong here.

Table 1-1
Child Psychiatric History Outline

Age:	
Presenting problem:	Description—with descriptive quotes whenever possible Duration How started (including precipitating events or factors, if any)
Past history of any other or similar problems:	
Family history of similar problems:	
Developmental history:	Pregnancy Delivery First few days, then weeks—feeding, sleeping patterns and general temperamental characteristics of infant Basic landmarks Infant and child's attitude to parents Reactions to frustration
School experiences:	
Relationship to peers:	
Relationship to adults:	

Review of specifics:	Fears and phobias
	Scary dreams and night terrors/nightmares
	Depression
	Oppositional behavior—unresponsive to discipline
	Aggressive and destructive behavior and temper tantrums
	Cruelty
	Enuresis and/or encopresis
	Firesetting
	Specific somatic symptoms
	  tics
	  movement disorders
	  hair pulling
	  self-mutilation
	  overt and excessive masturbation

Many mothers will volunteer information about obstetrical difficulties; yet, to be on the safe side, the clinician can use the following reminders:

1. Early development—first days and weeks

This is where the astute examiner can learn a great deal about the child's constitutional-temperamental endowment. Clues abound, and the following are examples of questions to ask:

- How did the baby feed and sleep the first few days, the first few weeks?
- Was (s)he an "easy" baby, or difficult, i.e., slept fitfully, at odd times, not enough, gave mother no peace, generally cranky, difficult to settle down, stubborn?

- Did (s)he have colic, "milk allergy," "food allergy," with frequent changes of formula, finally settling on some special milk or non-milk preparation? Did (s)he spit up food?
- What was the caregiver's emotional view of the baby—"cuddly," "easy to please," or "always tense," "jumped at any sound or motion," "could not tolerate car rides," "slept all day and screamed all night"?

2. Development in the first 1–2 years

For this we ask the questions about early developmental milestones: When did (s)he start to crawl, sit up, walk, and talk? The crucial items here are not, however, the numerical answers to the above, but the descriptions of the quality of those items, since they continue the inquiry into the constitutional factors. Again, some representative questions are:

- Was the child "into everything" as soon as (s)he could move around? Did (s)he climb upon furniture, get into all the cupboards? Was the child accident-prone? Was "nothing safe" from him (more often than her)?
- If the child did not start talking within this time period, was it due to stubbornness or being "spoken for" by others?
- What was the emotional atmosphere with mother/father?
- Did the child have temper tantrums or similar reactions when not getting his/her way? Could this have been a "difficult child" (Thomas, Chess & Birch, 1968)—with nonadaptability, tendency to withdraw from new stimuli, and intense negative reactions?

Development from ages 2–5

There will be some repetition in the points inquired into, such as temper tantrums, which occur typically at this age. In addition, this phase contains the beginnings of neurotic disorders: separation anxiety, phobias, and nightmares.

The clinician has here another opportunity to check on the parent-child relationship and may ask:

- How did the parents take care of the normal fears of this age? Were they overconcerned?
- How did toilet training go? Was it permissive, or was the child toilet trained by them?

The first-grade school years—ages 5–7

The beginning of school is an important event for all children. The examiner has a great deal to inquire into, such as:

- How was the beginning of school?
- Was there separation anxiety beyond the first 1–2 weeks?

- How did the child get along socially and academically?
- If the patient is now beyond first grade, did the previous teacher report short attention span, distractibility, talking out of turn, not getting along with peers, daydreaming, rushing through assignments?
- Has the child ever been referred to the school psychologist, the school social worker, the speech therapist, the special reading teacher?

These and similar questions will give the inquisitive examiner something like "half a diagnosis" of Attention-Deficit Hyperactivity Disorder and put that clinician on the road to diagnosing developmental disabilities. By this time, it is likely that the developmental history will have caught up to the age of the child's presenting complaint.

THE FAMILY HISTORY (F.H.)

This is an area that is frequently passed by or forgotten in the interview, yet it can lead the perceptive clinician towards the diagnosis. As a rule, it will rarely be redundant to ask: "Is there anybody in the immediate or extended family who has had this, or a similar, condition?"

We should be specific and systematic in our inquiries into the family history; the parents cannot be expected to give on their own the following pertinent information:

1. *Family history of learning disability*—Has any member of the family ever had difficulties in school, especially learning disabilities, needed special help, not been able to read, not been able to do math? "Any member" includes the parents themselves, the grandparents, and various "outlying" members such as cousins. Often, learning disabilities are still present in these relatives (e.g., "Uncle Bob could never really read fast; he works well with his hands, but his wife has to read him the instructions").

2. Similarly, a family *history of hyperactivity* can be elicited. Here, too, one of the parents will often admit that he or she had been specifically diagnosed as such, or else had been a "live wire," "always on the go," and so forth.

3. A related area is *trouble with the law*—Who are the "black sheep" of the family (why are these so often mother's younger brothers?)? Are there any sociopathic relatives, difficulties getting along with authority figures, barroom fights and brawls?

4. Is there a history of *bedwetting* by parents and grandparents, when enuresis is among the child's presenting complaints?

5. Is there a history of *depression* or suicide in either parent's family?

6. Is there a general family history of *psychiatric illness?* (Not only severe illness with proven heritability, such as schizophrenia and depression, should be elicited here. Other psychiatric disorders are equally important to the child, as they are transmitted both genetically and by learning: phobias, obsessive-compulsive disorders, and paranoid disorders or attitudes.)

Many *constitutional-temperamental* traits, without specific diagnoses, are inherited: stubbornness, hyperactivity, being easily angered and having a "hot temper," or the opposite traits. They are of clinical importance, and "the difficult child" as described by Thomas and Chess is a useful concept to bear in mind (Thomas, Chess, & Birch, 1968).

"WHAT HAS BEEN DONE ABOUT THE PROBLEM?"

This question can be included in the "Presenting Complaint" part of the history taking or tackled separately, depending on the style of the examiner. In this part of the history, the clinician inquires both into treatment done by professionals and into the measures undertaken by the parents themselves. When asking, "What have you done about the problem?" the clinician will also want to know which measures were of help, and which were not.

THE MEDICAL HISTORY

This can be elicited and recorded as part of the developmental history or done separately. We look for "major items" here, such as pain, trauma, immobilization, and medical problems involving separation from the parents (e.g., hospitalization). Have there been any severe injuries? accidents? Are the child's immunizations all up to date (neglect or abuse)?

THE CHILD PSYCHIATRIC EXAMINATION

OBSERVATIONS OF NONVERBAL BEHAVIOR

The cornerstone of the examination is *observation*. Young physicians learn to inspect their patient closely, to become astute observers, which is also vital in child psychiatry. The overriding need for being an excellent observer is dictated in part by the limits of the child's communication in the first and second interviews. Many children are quite verbal, but what they choose to say, how much, and what they mean by their statements must be judged in conjunction with their observed actions. Children must be seen *and* heard if they are to be understood.

The need for astute observation is great when the child does not talk, but the most verbal child must be observed just as carefully. The fleeting glance, the glazed eye, the facial mannerism may tell us more than all the verbose child says to us.

What we look for when we observe may be put in the form of the following checklist:

- Right- or left-handed, clumsy or graceful, act his/her age?
- Good-looking or ugly or funny-looking or plain?
- Physical appearance, dress, and hygiene?
- Activity level: high, low, or normal?
- Attention span/distractibility?
- Attitude: aggressive or shy, fearful or "counterphobic" (overdoing something that might otherwise invoke fear)? stubborn, oppositional, or too pliable, too anxious to please?
- Feeling tone: some anxiety can be expected, but absence of anxiety is not abnormal either. Excessive anxiety can be observed easily, especially if the patient clings to the parent, and later perhaps to a toy, averts his/her gaze away from the other person. Outright *fear* should be noted. *Depression* can also be sensed by the examiner; it can take the form of not liking any activity, manifesting a sad expression, easy crying or becoming tearful, very brief responses, psychomotor slowing, and so on.
- Choice of play or play material: interest in toys appropriate for the opposite sex (especially when a boy consistently and persistently chooses a girl's playthings)? Predilection for aggressive play to the exclusion of anything else? Listlessness, disinterest in toys? Does the play go anywhere?
- Habits, mannerisms: tics, overt masturbation, or preoccupation with certain body parts?
- While all of the above are being observed, the examiner should construct an informal "neurological backdrop" in his mind: Does the child move normally? How skillful or clumsy is the child? In other words, how are the child's gross and fine motor coordination overall?
- How does the child end a session? handle transitions?

THE SPECIAL NEUROLOGICAL EXAMINATION

This examination, an extension of observed nonverbal behavior, assesses the status of the child's neuromuscular function as an expression of central integration in the brainstem. It therefore comprises clinical signs of any impaired nuclei of several cranial nerves in the brainstem, the afferent and efferent pathways in the spinal cord, and the vestibular and cerebellar connections to the brainstem.

Synonyms for these signs are "soft," "minor," and "nonfocal" neurological signs. The reason for the first two, perhaps unflattering, names was that in the past they were not considered to produce any "hard" evidence (according to some, no evidence at all) of neurological lesions. Recently, however, their status has risen because they do show some correlation with developmental lag and possibly with response to stimulant medications by children with Attention–Deficit Hyperactivity Disorder.

The most important point to remember is that there is good correlation and interexaminer reliability for the clinical significance of these signs among examiners who have trained and worked together, but not usually otherwise. Widely accepted criteria for how the tests are to be performed and what will constitute positive (pathological) findings are still lacking. Therefore, several basic schemata exist, with hundreds of modifications by individual practitioners. The following protocol is one that we have found useful in practice, as have other psychiatrists and neurologists.

I. Upper extremities

1. *Choreoathetoid movements*
    Technique: The child is asked to hold her or his arms outstretched, in front, fingers spread.
    Positive: Presence of movements (overall impression or 10 or more twitches in 30 seconds).

2. *Finger-thumb opposition*
    Technique: With both arms outstretched, the child is asked to touch, on one hand only, the thumb with each of his fingers. The child can either be left to choose his/her own style, in which case overall dexterity/clumsiness is noted, or be asked to do it in certain sequences. At the same time, the examiner watches the other, uninvolved hand, for "mirror" or synkinetic movements.
    Positive: Clumsiness, missing of sequences, and synkinetic movements. (Some idea of handedness can be obtained if the choice of which hand he wants to use first is granted to the child.)

3. *Diadochokinesis or alternate-motion-rate (AMR) or (alternating) pronation-supination*
    Two basic techniques can be used:
    Technique (a): The child is standing with one elbow flexed 90° and hand pointing forward, and is asked to pronate/supinate the extended hand five times.
    Positive: Movement of the elbow of 4 or more inches during test, or clumsiness and synkinesis of the other hand.
    Technique (b): The child, seated, taps the table with the palm and dorsum of the hand in rapid succession.
    Positive: Fewer than 10 taps in 10 seconds. Synkinesis should also be watched for.

4. *Finger-nose pointing test*
    Technique: The child either has to touch the tip of his/her nose with the tip of the index finger after fully extending that arm, or has to touch the tip of the examiner's index finger and then the tip of his own nose, with the examiner changing the location of his/her (the examiner's) index finger.
    Positive: Tremor or past-pointing. This test is rarely positive without a

definite central nervous system lesion, and therefore of little significance in Attention–Deficit Hyperactivity Disorder and similar disorders, but is useful as a screening device for more serious pathology.

II. *Lower extremities*

1. *Straight-line walking*

   Technique: The child is simply asked to walk on a real or imaginary line, "as if on a tightrope," if possible walking heel to toe.

   Positive: Failure to approximate heel and toe for at least 5 consecutive steps, or failure to walk along the line (broad base).

2. *Gait*

   Technique: Simple walking for 70 feet or more.

   Positive: Base of 10 inches or more, or clumsiness.

3. *Hopping on one foot*

   Technique: The child hops on one foot for about 20 feet.

   Positive: Clumsiness or failure to hop at least 5 consecutive times.

III. *Balance*

1. *Standing on one foot, eyes open (Denckla test)*

   Technique: The patient is asked to stand on one foot, without touching anything and with eyes open, for as long as he/she can.

   Positive: Less than 10 seconds for 8–12 years old, less than 5–10 seconds for younger ages.

2. *The Romberg test*

   Technique: The child is instructed to stand with feet together, arms extended forward, and eyes closed.

   Positive: Swaying back and forth motion (or side to side) exceeding 1–2 inches in both directions.

IV. *Eyes*

1. *Visual tracking movements*

   Technique: An object is moved from side to side at first and then up and down while the child focuses on it.

   Positive: Coarse tracking movements or discontinuity in tracking.

2. *Nystagmus*

   Technique: The child is asked to track to extreme lateral gaze.

   Positive: Presence of nystagmus before extreme lateral gaze is accomplished.

3. *Convergence*

   Technique: The patient is asked to focus on an object as it is brought closer to his nose.

   Positive: Poor focusing, lag in one eye, or pupillary abnormality.

V. *Laterality*

1. *Right-left identification*

   Technique: The child is asked to raise right or left arm, or legs. Then the child is asked to point to examiner's right/left arm and leg. Finally, he/she identifies examiner's crossed arms/legs.

   Positive: This depends on age; school-age children should make no mistake in orientation.

2. *Punching a bag*
   Technique: The child punches an imaginary bag. The arm first used is noted as probably indicating handedness.

3. *Kicking an (imaginary) football or pretending starting to march*
   Technique: As the title implies, the child then reveals his basic laterality by the leg he/she used first.

4. *Eye dominance*
   Technique: The child is asked to look through a toy telescope or tube of paper, or to "make a telescope" with his/her hands.

VI. *Sensory integration*

1. *Double simultaneous stimulation* or *face-hand test*
   Technique: The child is seated, eyes closed, and, after appropriate explanation, is touched lightly on the cheek of one side and on the hand of the other side. The child then points to the parts touched.
   Positive: Error on both the first and second trial.

2. *Stereognosis*
   Technique: Placing familiar objects into the child's hand after first presenting them for visual identification.
   Positive: More than one mistake when using three objects in different sequence.

Summary and commentary

Each clinician tends to evolve his or her "pet" tests. Among the nonfocal signs just enumerated, the presence of choreathetoid movements, poor finger-opposition, rough visual tracking, the presence of synkinesis, and a positive Denckla test are, in these authors' experience, consistently reliable signs of developmental lag, sometimes called "dysmaturation." They should not be overrated, but used as a porthole to get a closer view of the child's neurological development.

Whether a sign is judged to be "positive" or pathognomonic depends on the child's age. The reader is not expected to memorize tables of correlations of nonfocal signs to developmental stage, however. Suffice it to say, the beginning of school (i.e., age 6 years) is a reasonable demarcation line between considering most of these signs as being pathognomonic (in the school-aged child) versus having uncertain significance (the preschooler).

Other specific areas of observation will be discussed under the subsequent headings. A considerable portion of the *mental status* can be inferred from our clinical *observations*. However, later on, we will summarize separately the evaluation of the mental status.

VERBAL INFORMATION

It is a misconception that a child's play forms the main basis for the diagnostic workup of the child. Play is but *one* of the components. The child's verbal productions are another. Their relative values depend on the particular case; however, verbal communication reveals more in a shorter time.

The components of this section of the examination again can be presented in a checklist format:

- *Speech*—The "mechanical" part of articulation. Important clues can be obtained here regarding the child's level of maturity.
- *Voice*—Type and amount of inflection, in addition to "organic" markers, such as low voiced, hoarseness, and the like. Lack of normal voice inflection may be a sign of childhood psychosis.
- *Vocabulary*—This should be matched to the child's age. Not only "baby talk," but also generally immature vocabulary should be noted; on the other hand, excessively adult, affected, or stilted words or phrases may reflect a variety of influences in the child's environment (excessive parental or other pressures for sophistication, lack of peer contacts, or, indeed, too much association with adults, etc.).
- *Message content*—This, of course, is the crux of all verbal communications. Communications are evaluated as to age-appropriateness and gender-appropriateness, apart from the specifics of the substance of messages. The examiner should be prepared for a wide range of possibilities, from monosyllabic answers to direct questions to incessant voluntary productions, from seemingly candid statements to "pseudologia phantastica." Everything, or practically everything, goes and should be listened to with indulgence and caution, the basic question being: What is the overall message here? In addition, details may be significant: trauma or abuse may be reported; the child may boast excessively; or "woe is me" may be repeated over and over by a depressed child or an insightful neurotic one.

A few technical suggestions are in order: the examiner should not descend to the same level of immaturity as the child in his/her speech; however, the examiner must be careful to keep his/her speech simple enough to be clearly understood. Statements such as, "Wasn't this anxiety-provoking?" are either unintelligible to the child, or, if the child is older, he/she may require time to reflect on and "translate" the word "anxiety-provoking" into "child language." "Did that scare you?" may be better. Hypothetical situations have to be advanced with extreme caution and linked to concrete examples from the child's life, since the child's abstract reasoning is limited by the stage of cognitive development. Even some straightforward questions are difficult for the child to answer: "What makes you angry?" may lead to informative statements by a 12-year-old, but when the child is below 10 years of age, the way to ask this is to say something like: "You got mad when Mom did not let you go with Kevin. Do you get mad when she doesn't let you go out? Tell me what she doesn't let you do." A sure-fire rich subject is anger at younger siblings. The younger the child, the more concrete the examiner's inquiries should be.

One way to stay with this principle of concreteness is to have a good supply of examples of the patient's behavioral difficulties in the presenting complaints.

Thus armed, the clinician can make specific inquiries and compare the child's answers to the parents' and school teachers' reports.

The beginning clinician will probably feel most comfortable with a more structured approach (warning: excessive structure bordering on rigidity is counterproductive). A child can be made to feel at ease by being asked about his/her age, address, name of school, siblings, and from there: What do you like to do best? worst? After that, the clinician can proceed to interpersonal relationships: How do you get along with your teacher, peers, siblings, mother and father? Of course, most children will say "Fine!" to the last item, and the inquiry has to be pursued with specifics: What does your mother like you to do? What does she hate? What gets you in trouble with her? and so on.

The beginning clinician, especially the clinician who is used to working with adults, should remember that rephrasing a question is a very necessary part of interviewing technique with children. "How did that happen?" "What did you do?" and the like must at times be said over and over in different wording. "*Why* did you do it?" has been frowned upon by some as implying criticism and may have to be avoided more often because children simply cannot answer questions about their motives.

PLAY

The examiner should remember that the purpose of play is to communicate, i.e., to express what the child will not, or cannot, express verbally. There is no "magic" in children's play; it is not the royal road to the unconscious, and it takes more time than verbal communication and gives messages that are less precise, less easily validated.

On the other hand, play approximates the adult's free associations, yet it is more condensed; therefore, although less economical than the diagnostic verbal interview, play is more economical than free associations, which children often find difficult.

Finally, play is *not* an indispensable ingredient of every diagnostic session. Verbal facility, pressure of events (e.g., recent trauma), the child's own preference, or pressure of time (hopefully not a routine event in the clinician's life) are all factors that allow for omission of play.

Play requires play materials. A common mistake for the novice is to provide too many toys. This is distracting. A basic supply of puppets, including some animals, a vehicle or two, perhaps a house, and paper and pencil (or crayons) is often all that is needed. A few board games help with older children.

A basic principle of diagnostic play is that the purpose is *not* to *play with* the child, but to *observe* the play and usually the interaction with the examiner during the play. At the conclusion of the play session, the examiner should have learned something about the child's style of relating to the impulses within the child and to the world around him/her, and what concerns the child most. The examiner need not stand by (or sit) in reverent silence, either. Although the child should not be excessively distracted by incessant questioning, some questions and comments may be addressed to the child, or to the child's play. Most children will not mind explaining or accounting for what is going on.

Here, as in the child's drawings to be discussed below, the technique of discussing events in the third person, rather than in the child's first person, is useful. That is, the examiner allows and helps the child to give "a story" about what happens in play, rather than relating the events to himself/herself, which is, initially, more threatening.

THE CHILD'S DRAWINGS

This form of expression can be placed somewhere between talk and play. Drawings incorporate advantages of both, with the additional benefit of giving special clues about the child's neuropsychological-developmental level. Moreover, drawings leave the examiner with a permanent record. The same reasoning applies here as it does with play: drawings are not indispensable, and depend, even more than play, on the child's inclination and the availability of the other avenues of communication.

As with play materials, drawing materials should be simple. Watercolors are popular but potentially messy and, more important, potentially distracting and time-consuming. Paper and pencil (or crayons) are quite adequate.

Depending on the examiner's and the child's styles, the invitation to draw may be open-ended, or the examiner may ask for specific scenes, especially if too little is forthcoming with the open-ended approach. Specific techniques are the Goodenough-Harris Draw-a-Person (Harris, 1963) or House-Tree-Person test (Buck, 1948), the Kinetic Family Drawing (the child draws members of the family "doing something together") (Burns & Kaufman, 1970), or the game of Squiggles (devised by Winnicott [1971], in which either the child or the examiner completes a "squiggle"). At its very simplest, the examiner can draw a set of geometrical figures and ask the child to copy them, as a preliminary neuropsychological screening test (Bender Gestalt). Another simple test is to ask the child to draw a picture of himself/herself, or, if that is resisted, of a friend.

The pictures produced by children may or may not be revealing by themselves in terms of content; the examiner should use them as a springboard for discussion. The child may wish to complete the picture first or may readily participate in a running discussion about it. Many areas can be explored in that manner, and the examiner should not try rigidly to stay with the one topic that the picture portrays. Again, the purpose is *not* to produce a picture, still less a work of art. The purpose is to communicate about what hurts, upsets, scares, angers, or saddens the child, and how (s)he deals with it. The "third person narrative" (a story) can again be employed to great advantage. It is very easy to do this as the child sketches a house, tree, or person and tells "an exciting story" about what (s)he has drawn—how the house feels in different parts of the story and how it all turned out for the house (or tree or person).

GAMES

Age-appropriate puzzles may be used with the preschool child, but board games are the mainstay of many offices or playrooms catering to the grade-schooler. Many authors consider games an essential tool for play therapy, but they may be less important for the diagnostic interview.

If the examiner chooses to use board games, a caveat parallel to that in play applies: this is *not* a *game*, or contest, between the child and the examiner. It is a way of "making the unconscious visible" and an opportunity to see a gamut of the child's techniques for tackling problems and handling the excitement of success or the frustration of defeat. The examiner must, therefore, resist the temptation to engage in real play; playing a game with a child is done for professional work reasons.

Not all diagnostic examinations need include board games, since these are more time-consuming and give a lower yield than verbal interchange alone or graphic productions (drawings).

THE MUTUAL STORY-TELLING TECHNIQUE

This is a therapeutic technique pioneered by Gardner (1971) which can occasionally come in handy as a diagnostic approach to encourage and structure verbalization. The examiner asks the child to make up and tell a story from which the examiner picks out the relevant psychodynamics and then tells a story of his/her own, which highlights and further explores the child's defenses. When used diagnostically, this technique gives insights into the psychodynamic background of the problem as well as into the child's adaptability and ability to use alternative solutions in fantasy—a "window" on the child's cognitive abilities and maturity.

THE MENTAL STATUS EXAMINATION

In child psychiatry the formal assessment of mental status is of less crucial or immediate importance than its counterpart in adult psychiatry. The chief reason is the much smaller "yield" of grossly abnormal findings on children's mental status examinations. Simply stated, most children's mental status will be within normal limits *if* formal criteria of general (i.e., adolescent and adult) psychiatry are applied. The number of children showing signs of psychosis is smaller than that of adolescents or adults, i.e., fewer children are "crazy." However, it takes different criteria and an adolescent/adult developmental level to develop the attributes by which a cognitively fully developed individual can be defined as functionally psychotic. Also, the mental status examination is not performed only to determine presence of psychosis or organic impairment, although this is one of its main benefits, but is done to organize the examiner's general observations so that all observations and results of interactions can be presented in a clear, succinct, and systematic format that can be understood with precision by other professionals.

Children's cognitive and affective development does not yet allow for the crystallization and compartmentalization (and thus specific and clear expression) that enable us to formalize the adult's mental status exam so neatly (and often rigidly). Therefore, the child's mental status is arrived at more indirectly, by general, open-ended observation, and much less by questions and answers. It will include the points covered under all the previous sections, especially. Observation of nonverbal behavior in many, if not most, instances represents only another, more formal way to record the findings.

Table 1–2 gives a brief outline of what should be covered and recorded in the child's mental status evaluation. An example of the application of the mental status examination is provided in Chapter 5.

TESTS AND CONSULTATIONS

Having made *observations* of the child, the parents, and the child in interaction with parents and sibs, including observations about *the reported history* and the *child's mental state*, we are now ready to complete the diagnostic workup by requesting any *special tests or consultations* that are indicated by what has been disclosed.

The child will need a current physical examination, by the clinician or the referring doctor, or the psychiatrist may request a pediatric consultation. Other consultations frequently requested include those of our clinical psychology colleagues and colleagues in neurology, genetics, and communication disorders. The diagnostic questions on which we need consultation should be asked directly but not in a way to specify the exact tests or evaluation procedures that our consultant will employ; that selection is left to the consultant's discretion.

Table 1-2
Child Mental Status Examination

1.   Overall demeanor, attitude, and orientation
2.   Motor activity and coordination
3.   Cognition
         Alertness
         Attention span
         Intelligence
         Ability to communicate (see also "Language")
4.   Emotions
         Mood
         Anxiety
         Anger
         Other feelings
5.   Language
         Speech
         Formal characteristics: vocabulary, grammar, usage
         Content
6.   Thoughts
         Associations
         Preoccupations
         Dreams, fantasies
         Wishes
         Richness/poverty of ideation; talent
         Hallucinations
         Delusions
7.   Social interaction
         Eye contact
         Openness
         Shyness
         Cooperation
         Aggression
8.   A brief statement of the reactions of the examiner to the child
9.   Summary and diagnostic impression

PSYCHOLOGICAL TESTS

Among the valued consultants to be invoked in a diagnostic workup for a child is
the child clinical psychologist. Psychological tests are sometimes viewed as the
counterpart of the "laboratory workup" or "lab tests" of the clinician in other
fields of medicine. This, of course, is a very rough approximation and will raise
justified objections from psychologists, mainly on the grounds that the testing
process relies on interpersonal observations as well as the test instrument or
protocol itself. The psychologist administering the test is a health team member
who, when consulted by a physician, observes the child's behavior, attention
span, motivation, and other reactions during the test-taking procedure. The

clinical skills demanded by such observation are viewed as part of the testing and part of the consulting procedure.

We present here the most commonly used psychological tests along with brief commentaries on their clinical applications. The clinician ought not expect to, or need to, attain expertise in administering most of these tests unless (s)he is a fully trained psychologist. Testing is best done by an expert, and the clinician makes use of that expert's report.

Psychological tests often used can be grouped, according to their purpose and function, into cognitive, developmental, academic, perceptual-motor, and personality measures. Our suggestion is for the interested reader to learn more by consulting with an excellent child clinical psychologist. A standard reference is Anastasi (1982); it gives complete citations for each test mentioned in the following discussion.

1. Intelligence (or cognitive) tests

These tests are used to assess the child's intelligence on the basis of the formula: $IQ = MA/CA \times 100$. The intelligence quotient is the ratio of mental age to chronological age, multiplied by 100. A normal IQ is 100 or any score between 90 and 110.

The best and most widely used intelligence tests are the Wechsler Intelligence Scales for two age groups of children.

(a) Wechsler Intelligence Scale for Children—Revised Version (WISC-R). This test is used for children aged 6 to 15 years. The full-scale intelligence quotient is derived from the two subscales, verbal and performance. This gives us additional information about a child's cognitive functioning, since some children with perceptual or perceptual-motor dysfunctions will show combinations of deficiencies on one or both subscales, and children with developmental language or reading disorders may similarly be screened in a preliminary way. This kind of interpretation of the subscales requires a great deal of knowledge, experience, and caution on the part of the psychologist, because there are no hard and fast rules. The simple relationship of performance IQ to verbal IQ, previously thought to be indicative of brain damage or language disorders, is not very reliable. While many brain-damaged or attention-deficit-disordered children perform poorly on the performance scale as compared to the verbal scale, the reverse may be found, too. The classic finding is of a performance IQ 15 points above (Conduct Disorder) or below (Attention–Deficit Hyperactivity Disorder) the verbal IQ.

(b) Wechsler Pre-School and Primary School Intelligence Scale (WPPSI). This is a modification of the WISC-R to allow for testing of younger children (age 4–6 years).

(c) Stanford-Binet Intelligence Scale (Form L-M). The original intelligence test by Binet has been revised several times, and the L-M form has been used for children from age 2 years up. The fourth revision is now available. Although it is "spread out" over perceptual and motor tasks, too, the Stanford-Binet test relies more on verbal skills than the Wechsler Scales. Although less frequently used nowadays than the WISC, it is a reliable test except for socioculturally different or deprived children.

(d) The Colored Progressive Matrices (Raven). As the name implies, the test consists of designs or "matrices" which the child has to complete. The test is "nonverbal" and therefore suitable for deaf children or children with other verbal handicaps. Its scope is obviously limited compared to the WISC-R or Stanford-Binet, and although its results are also expressed as an intelligence quotient (IQ), it should be used as a screening device or preliminary estimate only.

(e) The Peabody Picture Vocabulary Test (Revised) and the *Slosson Intelligence Test* are used for quick assessment of intelligence. The Peabody Test is also suitable for evaluation of receptive language abilities and therefore often used by speech pathologists with children who are nonverbal.

Merits and demerits of intelligence tests. The chief advantage of intelligence tests lies in their general reliability (in the hands of a competent psychologist), their validity, and their good correlation with school performance. Overestimates of IQ are so rare that they are practically nonexistent; underestimates usually will be detected by an experienced examiner when confronted with a culturally different or mentally disordered child. The main reasons for underestimates are social or cultural, i.e., some ethnic and economic subcultures and practically all deprived environments provide insufficient verbal interaction, not permitting the child to learn enough words in order to use them in coping and adapting. Again, the alert psychologist will note the child's background and give a reasonable guess of the child's "potential."

2. Assessment of young children—the developmental scales

For very young children, a number of instruments have been devised which give a developmental quotient (DQ) according to the formula:

$$DQ = \text{Developmental Age (as tested)/Chronologic Age} \times 100.$$

The best known of these scales is the *Gesell Developmental Schedule*, which is used for children from 4 months to 4 years. Other similar instruments are: the

Cattell Scale, the *Merrill-Palmer Scales*, and the *Bayley Scale of Mental and Motor Development*.

3. Tests of academic achievement

We use such tests to get a relatively objective measure of what the child actually knows in terms of formal school subjects. These scores are useful for assessing a child's school achievement without the subjective bias of the teacher, but they are even more helpful when their results are combined with teachers' and other school reports, intelligence and other psychological tests. In that expanded context, the achievement tests help to pinpoint specific academic problems and possibly Specific Developmental (learning) Disorders.

One of the best known achievement tests is the *Wide Range Achievement Test* (WRAT). It assesses the child's ability in reading, spelling, and arithmetic. It is relatively superficial, but easy and quick to administer, and is a very handy screening test.

The Peabody Individual Achievement Test (PIAT) also assesses the child's achievement in the three "R's" and in general information. *The Woodcock-Johnson Psychoeducational Battery* is less commonly used, but more detailed. An achievement test that measures reading only is the *Gray Oral Reading Paragraphs Test*, whereas the *Key Math Diagnostic Arithmetic Test* measures solely mathematical ability.

4. Tests of perceptual-motor abilities

A child's ability to organize and integrate incoming sensory stimuli and process them towards appropriate motor responses can be measured by specialized tests. These tests are useful for detecting and quantifying central nervous system dysfunction, including Organic Brain Syndromes and Developmental Disorders.

The best known in this category is the *Bender Visual-Motor Gestalt Test,* scored on the basis of number of errors made by a child when copying a series of nine designs. Moreover, the examiner's observations on how the child tackles and executes the test are part of the assessed performance.

The *Test of Visual-Motor Integration (Beery-Buktenica)* or *VMI Test* is similar to the Bender Gestalt Test in that it also requires the copying of geometrical designs. The test is scored according to age-level norms and is well suited to young children.

There are tests for only one or the other of the components of perceptual-motor functions. For the visual component only, the *Frostig Test of Visual Perception* can be used. For the motor ability, the *Lincoln-Oseretsky Motor Discrimination Test* even gives a "motor development quotient."

Certain parts of the WISC-R can also be used for assessing the child's perceptual-motor functions, and the WISC-R may thus be used as a "screening test" for perceptual-motor dysfunction, to be followed by more specific testing should certain items suggest perceptual-motor deficits. A 15-point discrepancy between the verbal and performance parts of the WISC-R used to be considered pathognomonic of perceptual-motor problems or "brain dysfunction." Also, poor performance on certain subscales—Arithmetic, Coding, Information, and Digit span (hence the acronym ACID)—was taken to bespeak perceptual–motor disorder. However, many psychologists have become disenchanted with both of these facile summations.

5. Personality tests

These tests give structured data on a child's conflicting motives or impulses and the psychological defenses against them, i.e., they give a "window" on drive-defense constellation and enable us to judge inner conflicts on a number of parameters.

All personality or projective tests work on the same principle: the child is presented with an ambiguous stimulus (usually a picture, but it can be an incomplete sentence) and asked to respond to it. The expectation is that the response will reflect the child's personality projected onto that situation. The child's response will give clues to the child's psychological needs, impulses, affects, reality testing, self-image and self-esteem, and relationship to parents, to defense mechanisms, and to coping devices.

Indications for the use of projective tests are complex psychological situations, suspected psychosis, or occasionally, additional evaluation of suicidal risk or other risk of loss of control, e.g., when a child is very shy, inhibited, and communicates poorly. A modicum of cooperation is required, i.e., totally negativistic, noncommunicative, and uncooperative children are not suitable.

The validity and reliability of the results depend primarily on the expertise of the psychologist who administers and interprets the tests. Secondarily, for a child's benefit, a lot depends on the acumen of the clinician who integrates the test results into the overall clinical picture.

The following is a listing of projective tests commonly used:

(a) Thematic-Apperception Test (TAT) for ages 8 years and older and Children's Apperception Test (CAT) for ages 3 years to 7 years. Both tests' unstructured materials consist of cards that show children and adults in a variety of interpersonal situations, always ambiguous, so that the same card can be interpreted in a variety of ways by a variety of persons.

(b) The Rorschach Test. This is the famous inkblot test and is the least structured and most ambiguous of all projective tests. A Rorschach can be used in children 5 years or older and, again, requires a skilled clinical psychologist to administer, evaluate, and report it. The Rorschach Test gives information especially about reality testing, imagination, handling of affects, and interpersonal relationships.

(c) Incomplete Sentence Tests. As the name implies, the child is asked to complete the part of the sentence that has been left out, and his/her response may be indicative of fairly immediate stresses, worries, and the coping devices and defense mechanisms used to deal with them.

(d) Personality Inventories. These are included here because they measure certain personality traits and compare them to a normative sample. However, they are not projective tests, there being no ambiguous stimulus or situation presented to the child. Instead, the parent responds to true/false questions.

The prototype of these tests, the *Minnesota Multiphasic Personality Inventory* (MMPI), is not used for children; its derivative, the *Personality Inventory for Children* (PIC) consists of 600 true/false questions, dealing with affect, conscience, somatic complaints, peer relations, self-concept, and anxiety.

6. Tests of adaptive behavior and social adjustment

The chief example of these is the *Vineland Social Maturity Scale* (VSMS). It is based on information gathered from the parents in an interview. The examiner must be skilled in interviewing techniques as well as in evaluating the material obtained, as (s)he has to organize and rate it. The information obtained is organized into eight clusters, such as several types of self-help, locomotion, communication, and socialization. A "social quotient" (SQ) can be obtained similar to the intelligence quotient.

Other newer scales of social competence exist, but are less widely used. The Vineland score can be used to document the clinician's rating on Axis V (adaptive functioning) of the DSM-III-R; the *Children's Global Assessment Scale* (GGAS) likewise gives an adaptational rating.

7. Rating scales

Rating scales are not the exclusive domain of the psychologist. They are used across professional boundaries, and there are so many of them and so many new ones being devised for research purposes that there are few nationally accepted, standard rating scales. The reason for this bewildering number of rating scales is that they are all specialized for a certain diagnostic or behavioral category. Thus, there are a number of scales measuring activity level, attention span, and related behavior in hyperactive children (Attention–Deficit Hyperactivity Disorder). The best known are those devised by Conners, namely, the *Conners Parent Symptom Questionnaire* (PSQ) and the *Conners Teacher Rating Scale* (TRS).

The PSQ (in its recent factor-analyzed version) is a 48-item scale with groupings of conduct, inattention, psychosomatic problems, hyperactivity, impulsivity, and anxiety. The TRS has 39 items, covering behavior and activity in the classroom, impulsivity, and relationship with peers and teachers.

There are several depression rating scales, e.g., the *Childhood Depression Inventory,* by Kovacs and Beck, and the *Children's Depression Rating Scale,* by Poznanski et al.

8. Neuropsychological tests

This type of testing is more extensive and more specialized than standard psychological tests and requires special training on the part of the psychologist-examiner. It is used to determine the existence, the extent, and, to a significant degree, the localization of brain damage in children, as well as the functional sequelae of brain damage. Its practical applications therefore comprise both the diagnosis of various types of brain damage and the assessment of the potential for rehabilitation.

Two such tests are in current use—the first is the *Halstead-Reitan* and the second the *Luria–Nebraska Neuropsychological Battery.* The first is probably the most sensitive and accurate psychological test of brain function, because it distinguishes between normal and brain-damaged children with a high degree of reliability.

As the name implies, this is a *battery* of tests: these include such standard instruments as the WISC-R and one of the academic achievement tests; in addition, there are eight other tests, several of them essentially physical (neurological) examinations of motor coordination and visual-motor integration. The test battery is suitable for children from 5–14 years of age.

The *Luria–Nebraska Neuropsychological Battery (Children's Revision)* consists of 11 summary scales, which (as in the Halstead-Reitan Battery) combine observed motor and coordination performance by the child with tests of verbal, academic, and general intellectual abilities. The Luria–Nebraska has a narrower age range of applicability (8–12 years of age).

Questions to ask of a consulting psychologist. It is not decorous to request a specific test of a clinical psychologist. The latter is a professional colleague, not a laboratory technician. Still, asking about *learning capacity* will bring about a report of IQ scores and achievement scores; asking if there are any *signs of a thinking disorder* will obtain for us the psychologist's intelligence and projective test scores on the given child. Similarly, if we request the psychologist's opinion about a child's *basic conflicts, coping (or defense) strategies, views of self in the family, or ways of interpersonal relatedness,* we usually elicit Rorschach, TAT, Sentence Completion, or similar projective test results. The consultant is not constrained to use specific instruments as (s)he responds to our consultation request, but only to help us to further our understanding of the child. And it is illuminating to have a child tested, interviewed, and evaluated by a competent professional colleague, whether the colleague is a psychologist or a neurologist.

Laboratory tests and procedures are costly and for that reason should not be requested too hastily. Obviously, screening tests for kidney, lung, liver, and hematopoietic functions should be done if there are any indications that they are required. Beyond those, in child psychiatry the EEG is a vital procedure and the CT scan and NMR are no longer prohibited by great costliness if needed for diagnostic reasons. Clinical toxicology laboratories play an important function when we need to determine therapeutic blood levels of psychotropic drugs. Truly, today's diagnostic procedures are elaborate.

DIFFERENTIAL DIAGNOSIS

Once the clinician has narrowed down his/her impressions of what the disorder is and has invoked the laboratories and consultants to aid further diagnostic honing, the next move is to the purely "mind game" of medicine, the differential diagnosis. In carrying out the mental activity, the reasoning is as in the following example:

> Many signs point to the diagnosis on Axis I of Conduct Disorder (although the full criteria are not met) and on Axis II of a Developmental Reading Disorder, but I must rule out Depression, Organic Personality Syndrome and Oppositional Defiant Disorder on Axis I. Depression, however, is unlikely for reasons a, b, and c. Also, Organic Personality Syndrome must be ruled out by further diagnostic workup but seems unlikely at this point for reasons c, d, and e. Oppositional Defiant Disorder is unlikely for reasons c, f, and g, and the child's clinical picture fits more nearly the descriptive criteria of DSM-III-R's Conduct Disorder.

In other words, the differential diagnosis is a bit of detective work, of reasoning to make certain that the clinician has not missed recognizing the "correct" disorder. So the examiner goes through a process of asking, "Could it possibly be something else?" To do a sensible differential diagnosis the clinician must know a broad range of diagnostic categories and clinical pictures and, furthermore, know a lot about how psychopathology changes with a child's developmental stage. (S)he must have a firm grasp on child development generally.

TREATMENT PLANNING

The treatment is solving the problem. Sometimes the treatment can be preventive work, forestalling a more serious disorder by helping the child (and others) to make changes that will promote health and protect against disease and disorder. All treatment aims to work on one or more of these fronts: 1) relief of symptoms; 2) preventing recurrence of the disorder; 3) reorienting the behavior, feelings, and thinking of the child towards healthier functioning; 4) restoring or building a more wholesome interpersonal network to support the child's welfare as a dependent and immature person.

In more practical terms, we attempt the following:

1. We try to make the child feel better—happier—because anything that does that *is* therapeutic.
2. We try to institute adequate treatments that will really reduce the child's risk in the future—an immunizing operation, so to speak.
3. We want to go beyond the surface symptoms and see the child change towards being more competent (in doing, feeling, and thinking) and to become a different child, one who will have learned and been changed by the experience of having a mental disorder, i.e., the child will have some understanding of how to live life better.
4. We want the child to be more loving, surrounded by adults who love him/her, and to learn how to give and take, live interdependently, and find dependability in those around him/her.

Or more simply stated, treatment aspires to the following aims:

1. Relieve suffering in the present.
2. By helping the child, and the child's family, to solve the presenting problems, ensure continuation of normal development.
3. By a constructive approach to the problems at hand, enable the child and his or her family to take constructive approaches to future problems (the "immunizing value").
4. Encourage the child's talents to emerge, thereby contributing to a generally happier and emotionally richer personality.

Consequently, the plan of remediation or treatment can span things to be done with the child, things with the parents, things with the entire family group, and usually, also, things with the child's academic career, peers, and community resources to help children—all of which are the subject of Chapter 2.

PUTTING IT ALL TOGETHER

Out of the plethora of data, the clinician has to put together an intelligible body of information and then act. This may consist of the following schema:

1. History (and clear delination) of the *problem*.
2. Examination with special emphasis on *observation*.

3. Diagnostic workup.

4. Differential diagnosis—the composite of all the information that has been gathered and processed, along with the clinician's knowledge of normal child development and of psychopathology (of related disorders, similar disorders), so that cogent distinctions and differentiations can be made.

5. Treatment plan—a set of achievable goals and how to attain them.

Questions for Study and Action

1. Some research projects distinguish between a "clinical population" of children and a "nonclinical sample." Does the distinction mean that undetected cases do not exist in the nonclinical group? What mental disorders, untreated and undetected, might have a fairly high incidence (up to 10–15%) in a *nonclinical* group of school children? Try to reason it out, even if you do some guessing; you can check it out later.

2. Devise, in outline form, a clinical skills examination for certifying the basic clinical competence of third-year medical students. Show how you would arrange to evaluate their interviewing, physical exam, history taking, diagnostic steps, treatment planning, and ability to "put it all together."

3. Can you think of any ways to avoid being so *problem-oriented* as you do clinical work with and for a child patient? List three or more concrete ways to interact with a child that would focus on strengths as well as pathology and still not deviate too much from the professional relationship.

4. What did Leo Kanner, the first author of an American textbook in child psychiatry, mean when he referred to the parents' complaints for the child as their "admission ticket?" Once they are "in," what latent problems might you expect to surface? Would you expect problems of the parents themselves to emerge? Explain.

5. Ask four parents in a child psychiatry or pediatric clinic to describe, in 5–10 minutes each, what they did—what their life situation was—when they were at the current age of their child, the identified patient. Do you see any empathy for the child in their responses? Do they identify positively with the child? Try to explain your findings from this quick survey of parents.

6. If you are evaluating a nine-year-old boy who reads at second-grade level, list all laboratory procedures and consultations that you would request in aid of your *diagnosis* (i.e., thorough understanding).

7. Assuming that you settle on a psychogenic or motivational learning block—under-achievement—as the most likely diagnosis for the boy in Question #6, name three other possible diagnoses and show how you would differentiate each from underachievement.

8. Did you consult with any schoolteacher as part of your answer to #6? Should you? Would you want to collaborate with the boy's school in getting a treatment program into operation? Explain.

9. Ask three children whom you see in a clinic or on an inpatient service to draw a house quickly and make up an interesting story about the house. Give emphasis to the story, not the drawing, and let the story be "exciting," asking how the house feels at each turn in the plot. Read back the story as you have written it down, asking the child if anything was left out. Then, later, view the house's story *as if* it were *the child's autobiography*, a story of her or his own world. What do you make of it?

10. What other techniques for eliciting a child's fantasy do you know about? Name six, including the "how-to" part.

For Further Reading

Anastasi, A. *Psychological Testing* (5th edition). New York: Macmillan, 1982.

Buck, J.N. The H-T-P technique: A qualitative scoring manual. *J. Clin. Psychol.*, 4:317–396, 1948.

Burns, R.C., & Kaufman, S.H. *Kinetic Family Drawings*. New York: Brunner/Mazel, 1970.

Doll, E.A. *Measurement of Social Competence*. Educational Test Bureau, 1953.

Gardner, R.A. *Therapeutic Communication with Children: The Mutual Storytelling Technique*. New York: Jason Aronson, 1971.

Goyette, C.H., Conners, C.K., & Ulrich, R.F. Normative data on revised Conners parent and teacher rating scales. *J. Abnormal Child Psychol.*, 6:221–236, 1978.

Harris, D.B. *Children's Drawings as Measures of Intellectual Maturity: A Revision and Extension of the Goodenough Draw-a-Man Test*. New York: Harcourt Brace and World, 1963.

Hertzig, M.E. Stability and change in nonfocal neurologic signs. *J. Amer. Acad. of Child Psychiatry*, 21:231–236, 1982.

Kanner, L. *Child Psychiatry* (3rd Ed.). Springfield, IL: Charles C Thomas, 1957.

Kovacs, M., & Beck, A.T. An empirical clinical approach toward a definition of childhood depression. In J.J. Shultzbrand & A. Roskin (Eds.), *Depression in Childhood. Diagnosis, Treatment and Conceptual Models*. New York: Raven Press, 1977.

Lewis, M. *Clinical Aspects of Child Development* (2nd Ed.). Philadelphia: Lea and Febiger, 1982.

Poznanski, E.O., Cook, S.C., & Carroll, B.J. A depression rating scale for children. *Paediatrics,* 64:441–450, 1979.

Reitan, R.M., & Davison, L.A. (Eds.). *Clinical Neuropsychology: Current Status and Applications.* Washington, DC: V.H. Winston & Sons, 1974.

Robson, K.S. (Ed.). *Manual of Clinical Child Psychiatry.* Washington, DC: American Psychiatric Press, 1986.

Simmons, J.E. *Psychiatric Examination of Children* (3rd Ed.). Philadelphia: Lea and Febiger, 1981.

Salvia, J., & Ysseldyke, J.E. *Assessment in Special and Remedial Education.* Boston: Houghton Mifflin, 1978.

Sattler, J.M. *Assessment of Children's Intelligence and Special Abilities.* Boston: Allyn and Bacon, 1982.

Thomas, A., Chess, S., & Birch, H.G. *Temperament and Behavior Disorders in Children.* New York & London: New York University Press, 1968.

Winnicott, D.W. *Therapeutic Consultation in Child Psychiatry.* London: Hogarth Press, 1971.

Special References

The following textbooks stand as standard references throughout this book. They are listed here and will not be repeated at the end of each chapter. The reader is reminded that (s)he can use these references for further reading with most of the chapters that follow.

American Psychiatric Association. *Diagnostic and Statistical Manual of Mental Disorders* (3rd Ed., revised). Washington, DC: American Psychiatric Association, 1987.

Connell, H.M. *Essentials of Child Psychiatry* (2nd Edition). Melbourne, Australia: Blackwell Scientific Publications, 1985.

Josephson, M.M., & Porter, R.T. (Eds.). *Clinician's Handbook of Childhood Psychopathology.* New York: Jason Aronson, 1979.

Kaplan, H.I., & Sadock, B.J. (Eds.). *Comprehensive Textbook of Psychiatry* (4th Ed.). Baltimore: Williams & Wilkins, 1985.

Noshpitz, J.D., Call, J.D., Cohen, R.L., & Berlin, I.N. (Eds.). *Basic Handbook of Child Psychiatry, Vols. I–IV.* New York: Basic Books, 1979.

Rutter, M., & Hersov, L. (Eds.). *Child and Adolescent Psychiatry: Modern Approaches.* Oxford, England: Blackwell Scientific Publications, 1985.

2

Treatment in Child Psychiatry

The acid test of our clinical skills comes *after* we have done a physical examination, taken a detailed and complete history, interviewed parents and child, done a mental examination with the child, ordered laboratory studies to be done, called in the pertinent consultant colleagues, completed our diagnostic workup and differential, and turned our scientific and practical skills to formulation of a treatment program, or treatment plan. The treatment plan in child psychiatry incorporates all the supportive, healing, comforting, educating, and advocacy measures that need to be undertaken to save the child and advance the child's healthy progression in her or his life cycle. That is to say, we need to work out a plan for treatment that includes the child as a young scholar; as an individual person with deficits, conflicts, and strengths; as a young animal for whom biological treatments may be highly appropriate; as a member of a family; as a young person in need of good peer relationships; as a being whose behavior—and feelings and cognition—are shaped and reinforced by environmental influences.

In this chapter we consider the major types of treatments that are available in child psychiatry. As a result, we have divided the discussion in Chapter 2 into the following: *pharmacotherapeutic* modalities; followed by *psychotherapies,* including *individual* modalities of the behavioral, cognitive, emotive/expressive varieties; *peer group, family group,* and *heterogeneous group;* and *socioenvironmental* therapies.

PHARMACOLOGICAL TREATMENT OF PSYCHIATRIC DISORDERS IN CHILDHOOD

There is no absolute indication for the use of psychotropic medication in childhood, since there is hardly any disorder for which pharmacological treatment alone is lifesaving or even specifically indicated. Put differently, there is no psychiatric disorder of childhood which cannot be treated by alternative nonpharmacological measures. Then, why drugs in child psychiatry?

The statements just made, while true, leave out several important considerations:

1. The magnitude of environmental leverage necessary to produce the same effect alone compared to being combined with pharmacological treatment. In many cases, the number of trained staff required is either simply not available or propels the cost to practically unattainable heights.
2. The considerable length of time necessitated by alternative, nonpharmacological treatments, thereby prolonging the patient's suffering.

At the present state of the art, pharmacotherapy is not yet curative but is an important adjuvant modality, often producing changes in mood or feelings, behavior and thinking. There are four main groups of psychotropic medications used in the treatment of children: stimulants, antidepressants, neuroleptics, and antianxiety agents. The clinical use of stimulants and antidepressants is described now, then again later in chapters on Attention–Deficit Hyperactivity Disorder (ADHD) (Chapter 21) and Mood Disorders (Chapter 15). In that context, some pharmacotherapeutics will make more sense, we hope. (*Note:* We use the standard DSM-III-R nomenclature for disorders we refer to throughout this book.)

The indications are clearest for using *the stimulants,* since the diagnostic criteria for ADHD are well established; those for the antidepressants are somewhat less clear only because of the relatively recent emergence of generally accepted diagnostic criteria for childhood depression and the broadened use of antidepressants in ADHD also. Nevertheless, the clinician knows that tricyclic *antidepressants* (TCAs) are nearly always used for three clear-cut indications: depression, separation anxiety and enuresis with certain features.

When we come to the next two categories, *the neuroleptics* and *antianxiety agents,* the indications for use with children are often less definite and more dependent on alternative treatment approaches.

The stimulants and antidepressants will be summarized first; their detailed clinical use can be reviewed under Attention–Deficit Hyperactivity Disorder, Mood Disorders (Childhood Depression), and Functional Enuresis. Next, we shall consider neuroleptics and anxiolytics.

THE STIMULANTS

Description and mechanism of action

Three chemically different, but pharmacologically similar, substances are most frequently used. All three act by potentiating the catecholamine neurotransmitters (norephinephrine and dopamine) in the central nervous system, both by stimulating their production, and by preventing their reuptake at the synaptic cleft, thus inhibiting their metabolism and breakdown. The net result is higher levels of active catecholamine neurotransmitter substance. Whether the same is true for the other major category of neurotransmitters, the indoleamines, is an unresolved issue. The stimulation of production of neurotransmitters is the mechanism that distinguishes the stimulants from the tricyclic antidepressants; the latter act mainly by preventing the reuptake of the neurotransmitters.

1. *Methylphenidate (trade name: Ritalin)*—This is the most commonly used, but strictly controlled, substance. Dose range is 0.3–0.8 mg/kg/dose with a duration of pharmacological action of about four hours. A good practical system is that of slow "escalation": below ages 6–7, the operational unit is the 5 mg tablet, of which one is given in the morning and increased by 2.5 mg increments (½ tablet) every few days until an effective dose is reached. The afternoon dose, if necessary, is titrated in the same manner. Maximum daily dosage rarely must exceed 10–15 mg in this age group. *Note:* Before kindergarten age, the results are confusing and equivocal; therefore, stimulants should seldom be used in preschool-age children. Above ages 6–7, the operational unit is the 10 mg tablet, with increments at 5 mg (½ tablet) at 3–5 day intervals. Maximum daily dose is dependent on age, but dosage that exceeds 60 mg is no more effective and the apparent need for higher dosage is more likely due to environmental factors or to the fact that the child is about to outgrow the usefulness of stimulants.

2. *The amphetamines*—Although both levoamphetamine and dextroamphetamine may be used, the former is rarely selected. The dosage range of dextroamphetamine (trade name: Dexedrine) is 0.5–1.5 mg/kg/day, not to exceed a total dose of 60 mg per day, and the titration regimen is the same as described with methylphenidate, although duration of action may be 1–2 hours longer. Nowadays it is less commonly used, although there is no sound pharmacological reason for avoiding dextroamphetamine. It is a controlled substance.

3. *Pemoline (trade name: Cylert)*—This is the most recent, least potent, but longest-acting drug in this category. Its prescription is not as highly controlled as amphetamine or methylphenidate. Duration of action is at least 12 hours and, unlike the previous two substances, pemoline requires a "build-up" period of regular administration of up to a month. Dosage range is 18.75 to 150/mg/day (no available standard data on per kg dosage). The available tablet strength is 18.75 mg, 37.5 mg, and 75 mg, and increments are best made in 18.75-mg-per-day units every 3–7 days.

Side effects

1. Paradoxical alteration of mood, usually in the form of whining, easy crying with commensurate provocation, occasionally paradoxical depression. These are usually related to relatively higher doses, sometimes excessive response even to lower doses, and are reversible with dose reduction or discontinuation of the medicine. Pemoline is least likely to show this reaction and can sometimes be used in cases where the other stimulant drugs have produced it.

2. Excessive response—overcontrol, slightly zombielike appearance. These side effects are reversible and again least likely with pemoline, since pemoline is the least potent of the stimulant drugs.

3. Decrease in growth rate was at one time a source of concern, but careful reassessment strongly indicates that even the small growth retardation previously claimed was not sufficiently substantiated and is refuted by long-term follow-up.

4. Anorexia and weight loss are rarely marked in children and often abate after 3–4 weeks. If persistent and a source of worry, reduction of dose or temporary discontinuation of the stimulant may be helpful.

5. Occasional paradoxical irritability and restlessness are reported in children whose attention span is well controlled with stimulant medication. This usually happens early in treatment and may be a spurious finding, i.e., it represents parental anxiety and ambivalence, although it may occur as a "genuine," though transient, side effect.

6. Insomnia is an unpredictable effect. Some children whose hyperactivity is such that they get very little sleep usually sleep better with a late afternoon dose of stimulant medication. Others may have difficulties getting to sleep and the second dose of stimulant medicine has to be given early (around noontime). Rarely is insomnia a significant problem, unless the physician has a personal need to control the attention deficit disorder and hyperactivity completely at all times, which is clinically impossible.

7. As we shall show in the chapter devoted to Tic and Habit Disorders (Chapter 13), the stimulants can worsen a preexistent Tic Disorder or unroof a latent one and can make picking at the skin, a Stereotypy/Habit Disorder, dramatically worse in some children.

THE ANTIDEPRESSANTS

Description and mechanism of action

For all practical purposes, only the tricyclic antidepressants (TCAs) are used in child psychiatry. Some of the other, newer categories of antidepressants, such as trazodone (trade name: Desyrel) are showing great promise, but their safety and effectiveness in children still have not been shown conclusively enough.

The mechanism of the antidepressant action of the TCAs is not completely understood, but what is known points to the prevention or blocking of the reuptake of catecholamines or indoleamines at the synaptic cleft, as the main antidepressant mechanism. They differ from the stimulants, with which they share this mechanism, in that they do not stimulate the production of these neurotransmitters and do not potentiate them by any other known means except to prevent their reuptake and deactivation. Other mechanisms, especially anticholinergic activity both centrally and peripherally, account for other effects and especially side effects.

The following preparations are used in pediatric practice:

1. Tertiary Amines
   (a) *Imipramine (trade name: Tofranil)*—Dose range is 1.5 to 5 mg/kg/day or 10–150 mg total per day.
   (b) *Amitriptyline (trade name: Elavil, Endep)*—Dose range is similar to imipramine.
   (c) *Doxepin (trade name: Sinequan, Adapin)*—Dose range is similar to imipramine. Is available in liquid form.

2. Secondary Amines
   (a) *Nortriptyline (trade name: Aventyl, Pamelor)*—Dose range is similar to imipramine with the caveat that it has been shown to have a "therapeutic window" at between 50–150 ng (nanograms) per ml; i.e., doses above and below this blood level are not likely to be effective (Geller, et al., 1983). It is available in liquid form.
   (b) *Protriptyline (trade name: Vivactil)*—Dose range in *older* children (around 12 years of age) is usually 5–10 mg total daily dosage. In the authors' experience, it is least likely to produce excessive sedation as a side effect, but is used mainly in treatment of adolescents and adults.
   (c) *Desipramine (trade name: Norpramin, Pertofrane)*—The dosage range of desipramine is the same as that of imipramine, i.e., 10–150 mg total per day. Desipramine has the added advantage of easy laboratory determinations of blood levels, which are, after all, the decisive metric for assessing the dosage needed. Moreover, desipramine has a low incidence of drowsiness and is generally well tolerated by children.

Note: The clinician is well advised to use the lowest effective dose.

All three secondary amines may have a faster onset of action (1–2 weeks) instead of the 1–4 weeks required for the tertiary amines.

The therapeutic effects of antidepressants are simply the relief of depression. Being "pepped up" or euphoric is not a pharmacological effect of antidepressants. The effect in enuresis is due either to the decrease of stage 4 or REM sleep, or to a direct effect on bladder musculature (Rapaport et al., 1980). The beneficial results of use of tricyclic antidepressants in school phobia may be due to their antidepressant effect or else to an effect akin to that seen in adult panic states.

Recently, there has been a revival of interest in the use of tricyclic antidepressants as an alternative to the stimulants in the pharmacological treatment of ADHD. TCAs may be considered for children with ADHD who are unresponsive to the stimulants or when the stimulants have an excessively short duration of action (Pliszka, 1987).

It should be noted that only imipramine is recommended officially for children ages 6–12 years; the other antidepressants do not have the manufacturer's recommendation for use below age 12. However, they are used in school-age children and are no more dangerous than imipramine. The side effects, and especially the caveats listed under cardiovascular side effects, apply to all of them.

Side effects (untoward effects)

1. Cardiovascular:
   (a) Increase in cardiac conduction time and a lengthened QRS complex may result in arrhythmia and, rarely, even cardiac arrest. This is the basis for the lethality of neuroleptics in overdoses. Even in therapeutic doses, the child's pulse should be regularly monitored and any arrhythmias promptly noted, checked by EKG, and the medicine discontinued until the nature of the EKG abnormality is determined. From then on, it becomes a matter of weighing the risks versus the benefits of continued pharmacotherapy with this particular or related tricyclic compounds, even at reduced doses.
   (b) Increased or sometimes decreased blood pressure usually presents few problems, if any, with therapeutic doses. The same is true of reported decreased cardiac output.
2. Drowsiness, sleepiness, or dizziness are frequent side effects, the importance of which lies in interference with schoolwork. Parents and children react negatively because these side effects are so visible and remind them that the child is "drugged," but they are not dangerous.
3. Anticholinergic side effects: dry mouth is the most common, followed by blurred vision. Constipation is rarely encountered. Dry oral mucosae may interfere with the natural lubrication of the throat and predispose to infection, and discontinuation of the medicine may then be necessary. Mild hyperthermia may be seen in children medicated with TCAs when they engage in strenuous (usually competitive) exercise in hot, humid, weather.

Agranulocytosis is a rare, but important side effect. (For management, see under Neuroleptics.)

THE NEUROLEPTICS

Description and mechanism of action

Neuroleptics (synonyms: antipsychotics, "major tranquilizers") comprise a chemically dissimilar and heterogeneous group of substances, all of which have the same pharmacological effect—dopamine blockade at the postsynaptic receptor. The effects of this are most prominent in the subcortical structures of the central nervous system—the limbic system and surrounding structures, thereby producing a calming and "regulating" effect on emotions and the processing of stimuli. These drugs are antipsychotic, counteracting delusional thinking and hallucinations.

Since childhood psychoses do not show the clear manifestations so prominent in adult psychoses (delusions, hallucinations, peculiarities of thought and affect), these agents are commensurately less effective in children. Their main use is in calming the agitation, hyperactivity, and aggressiveness of the psychoses of childhood.

The following compounds are used in children:

1. Phenothiazines
    (a) *Aliphatic—chlorpromazine (trade name: Thorazine)*—This is the oldest neuroleptic. The basic dose is 2.5 mg/kg/day, usually amounting to 10–100 mg or more per day.
    (b) *Piperidine side chain—thioridazine (trade name: Mellaril)*—Dose range is the same as that of chlorpromazine. (There is a caveat of never exceeding the dose of 800 mg per day. Although this pertains to adults it is worth keeping in mind, since doses above 800 mg per day cause serious ophthalmic side effects: pigmentary retinopathy and opacities of the lens.)
    (c) *Piperazine side chain—trifluoperazine (trade name: Stelazine)*—This is an example of a high-potency-per-milligram phenothiazine. Dose range is 0.25 mg/kg/day or less (range from 2 to over 10 mg per day, with appropriate caution, see section on Side Effects).
2. Butyrophenones
    The only representative so far approved in the USA is haloperidol *(trade name: Haldol)*. Its use has steadily increased. It is the most potent (per milligram dosage) neuroleptic in use today and is the treatment of choice in Tourette's Disorder.

Side effects

Although the neuroleptics have a much broader therapeutic range than the antidepressants and lethality is practically unknown, this is the class of psychotropic medications that has the longest list of side effects.

They will be discussed in order of frequency.

General CNS side effects.

1. *Sedation*—This is the most common side effect of all the neuroleptics used with children. There is no doubt that the low-potency-per-milligram (high-dose, low-potency) neuroleptics produce sedation with drowsiness and sleepiness (the sedative-hypnotic effect) more predictably than the high-potency-per milligram (low dose, high potency) ones. The former have therefore also become known as "sedating phenothiazines." The prime examples are chlorpromazine and thioridazine. However, the clinician dealing with children must realize that the claims made for "nonsedating" or even "energizing"

properties in the high-potency-per-milligram neuroleptics apply chiefly to adults, and that in children all of these bets are off. Sedation may occur in the most "nonsedating" neuroleptic.

2. *Lowering of seizure threshold*—This side effect is most likely to occur with chlorpromazine and least likely with haloperidol (and probably thioridazine as well).

3. *Weight gain*—This is probably due to hypothalamic stimulation and is fairly common. It appears to occur more frequently and with greater increases in weight with high dose, low potency preparations.

Extrapyramidal side effects. Dopamine blockade is not limited to those subcortical structures dealing with emotions but affects other parts as well. Therefore, this effect will take place in the basal ganglia and produce extrapyramidal effects which, since we are not looking for them, are considered side effects. The higher the potency-per-milligram, the more pronounced the extrapyramidal effects are. Thus, the low-potency-per-milligram neuroleptics such as chlorpromazine and thioridazine are much less likely to cause these effects than such high-potency-per-milligram ones as haloperidol, thiothixene, and trifluoperazine.

Thioridazine is in a class by itself in that it also has the most pronounced anticholinergic effects; in this way, it carries "double protection" against extrapyramidal reactions.

The specific extrapyramidal syndromes resulting from neuroleptics are listed below:

1. Acute dystonic reactions are the most obvious and frightening side effects, although they look more dangerous than they are. Theoretically, any group of striated muscles may be affected, but in reality, spasms of the muscles of the neck, trunk, and buccal-masticatory-deglutition area are the most frequent, often combined with spasms of external ocular muscles referred to as oculogyric crisis. The patient first complains of pain in the nuchal or dorsal region, followed by spasm of those muscles. If the spasm involves the sternocleido-mastoid muscle on one side more than the other, the head is turned to one side; torticollis spasms in the facial muscles produce grimacing. Difficulty in articulation and swallowing is common, especially in young children who become frightened and restless (often combined with simultaneous akathisia, see below) and cannot tell what is hurting them. The eyes are often turned upward in oculogyric crises. Saliva drools from the mouth as the tongue protrudes and food cannot be swallowed properly. These reactions last several hours if untreated and gradually subside as the blood level of the neuroleptic decreases.

2. Parkinsonism is manifested by tremor, masklike facies, and bradykinesia (slowed movements).

3. Akathisia is a feeling of restlessness without the feeling of anxiety. Instead of being calmed by the neuroleptic, the child is unable to sit (or lie) still and moves about all the time.

4. Dyskinetic movements, usually in the extremities, look like mild choreiform or hemiballistic movements. They reflect the inability to correctly "dose" the balance of agonist and antagonist muscles.

    The diagnosis of all these extrapyramidal side effects is made on the basis of history and physical examination. The latter includes checking for "cogwheeling," i.e., moving the patient's relaxed forearms (flexion and extension of elbows) and getting the feeling as if moving over a rough, "pebbly" surface. The treatment is discontinuation of the neuroleptic and usually the use of an anticholinergic (antiparkinsonian) medication.

    When the extrapyramidal syndrome is acute and severe, intramuscular antiparkinsonian agents or diphenhydramine provide rapid relief.

5. Tardive dyskinesia is rare in children but, because of its medicolegal significance, must be listed as one of the warnings given to parents. Typically, it consists of circumoral and lingual abnormal movements, but can start elsewhere as well. Unlike the other extrapyramidal effects, tardive dyskinesia develops late in treatment, usually after a long course, and often "surfaces" on discontinuation of the neuroleptic. (This observation lends support to the denervation-hypersensitivity hypothesis of its mechanism, i.e., prolonged dopamine blockade produces denervation and subsequent hypersensitivity of the dopamine receptors.) The common extrapyramidal symptoms, on the other hand, typically occur early in treatment and disappear completely upon discontinuation of the neuroleptic. The anticholinergic agents, which are effective in the other extrapyramidal syndromes, are ineffective in tardive dyskinesia.

    Tardive dyskinesia is reversible in its early stages. Therefore, clinical vigilance is the best method of prevention. Examination of the tongue for fasciculations is an easy and most effective diagnostic tool (the tongue should not be outstretched, but should be inspected, while resting in the mouth, with adequate lighting).

6. "Withdrawal Emergent Syndrome" or withdrawal dyskinesia (McAndrew et al., 1972; Polizos, Englehardt, & Hoffman, 1973) is a rare complication of neuroleptic therapy. It consists of various combinations of previously described dystonias *plus* nausea, vomiting and diaphoresis (sweating). It follows sudden (planned or incidental) withdrawal of the medication, appearing within a few days to two weeks. It usually remits in the following (up to 12) weeks. A few patients, however, need resumption of medication for remission to occur. The relationship of this syndrome to tardive dyskinesia is not clear, but they certainly show some similarities.

7. The neuroleptic malignant syndrome (Delay, Pichot, and Lemperière, 1960) is an extremely rare side effect in children. It is characterized by muscular rigidity, fever, autonomic dysfunction, and altered consciousness. We mention it because it is potentially fatal; as soon as it is suspected, all neuroleptics should be immediately stopped, and the child hospitalized for intensive supportive measures (Levenson, 1985).

Systemic side effects.

1. *Anticholinergic*—These are similar to the ones described for antidepressants, but of lesser intensity. Only thioridazine is likely to produce clinically significant dry mouth or mydriasis, and only when used in higher doses.

2. *Dermatological*—There are usually allergic skin rashes. Photosensitivity is of practical significance with chlorpromazine in summer months (or in areas of intense sunshine). It very rarely occurs with any of the other phenothiazines.

3. *Hematological and hepatotoxic*—These are rare nowadays. Agranulocytosis or neutropenia is probably the one encountered by the practitioner. While rare, it is a serious side effect.

   There are two schools of thought concerning the clinical approach to these hematological/hepatotoxic side effects. On one hand is the philosophy of regular laboratory follow-ups (CBC [complete blood count] or at least WBC [white blood count] and liver enzymes). On the other are the proponents of clinical follow-up with a high index of suspicion whenever any upper respiratory tract or urinary tract infection appears. This school of thought cautions that rarely will a patient oblige by having an abnormal laboratory test just when the test is scheduled. The majority of clinicians now favor the second ("clinical") approach.

4. *Cardiovascular*—Cardiac side effects are rare and are based on the anticholinergic properties. Effect on heart rate is negligible.

   Hypotension is thought to be due to alpha-adrenergic blockade, but is not nearly as significant as in adults. Vascular collapse (shock) from phenothiazine overdose should never be treated with epinephrine since that could be fatally cardiotoxic, but with norepinephrine only.

THE ANTIANXIETY ("ANXIOLYTIC") MEDICATIONS

Description and mechanism of action

These medications include two chemically different groups of drugs, the benzodiazepines and the antihistamines.

1. *The benzodiazepines*—These compounds inhibit or "dampen" CNS excitation, especially in the limbic system, by acting on benzodiazepine receptors. These are of two types, antianxiety and sedative. There is a close relationship between the benzodiazepines, their receptors, and GABA, an inhibitory CNS transmitter substance. Although there are now many benzodiazepines on the market, only a few are used in child psychiatry and these are used rarely.

   The favorite seems to be lorazepam (trade name: Ativan), a short half-life benzodiazepine. Oxazepam (trade name: Serax) is another short half-life representative of this group with occasional use in older children. Diazepam (trade name: Valium) is a long half-life benzodiazepine whose only drawback is its notoriety as a popular substance of abuse. Alprazolam (trade name: Xanax) is effective but not to be used longer than 6–8 weeks.

   These medications are given in appropriate pediatric doses as adjuvant therapy to psychotherapeutic management of an anxiety disorder, especially school phobia (Separation Anxiety Disorder). They should be used very selectively.

2. *The antihistamines*—These are frequently used by the pediatrician for their general calming effect. This is an exploited side effect of diphenhydramine (trade name: Benadryl). The favorite in this category, however, is hydroxyzine

(trade names: Atarax, Vistaril), which has definite, but mild, tranquilizing properties.

Note: Buspirone, a new anxiolytic drug that is not a benzodiazepine, can be used in treatment of children but with caution until its safety has been assured.

Side effects

This group of medications is characterized by a relatively benign profile of side effects:

1. Drowsiness and fatigue are the most common side effects for both the benzodiazepines and the antihistaminics.
2. Mild depression may occur with benzodiazepines, and possibly with antihistaminics as well.
3. Anticholinergic side effects occur with antihistaminics, and, apart from causing the characteristically dry mouth, may occasionally lead to hyperactivity, especially in children with Conduct Disorder.
4. Rage reactions because of cortical disinhibition could theoretically occur, especially with the benzodiazepines, but to date have not been described in children.
5. The one potentially serious side effect occurs with benzodiazepines: abrupt cessation after prolonged use (more than six months) may produce convulsions, especially when short-acting benzodiazepines are used. Tapering the medication is therefore always necessary when it is discontinued.
6. Dependency can theoretically occur, but we have never seen it in children. What we do witness occasionally is a rebound of anxiety when the anxiolytic medication is discontinued. This can easily be handled by tapering the medication upon discontinuation.

SUMMATION OF THE MAIN GUIDELINES OF PHARMACOLOGICAL TREATMENT

1. Proper diagnosis is essential.
2. The indications are clearest for the use of the stimulants in Attention–Deficit Hyperactivity Disorder, followed by their use in certain Conduct Disorder cases. Antidepressants are appropriate and effective in strictly diagnosed Childhood Depression and in severe Obsessive-Compulsive and Phobia Disorders. They are also effective in some forms of Enuresis.
3. The indications for the neuroleptics are more difficult to establish for the nonspecialist. The use of the antianxiety–antihistamine, hydroxyzine, is appropriate for the primary care physician as an adjuvant to other measures.
4. The acute side effects are most dangerous in the antidepressants, where strict preventive measures against overdose are imperative. The overall and long-term side effects are most numerous in the neuroleptics.

PSYCHOTHERAPIES

Whenever one person—a trained therapist ideally—aids another person (or a small group of persons) with a mental disorder to change in behavior, feeling, or thinking, that is psychotherapy: people helping people to change, even sometimes to change their whole lives and outlooks on self and world.

Although overlapping modalities are often employed at the same time, it makes sense to conceptualize the psychotherapies as either 1) individual or 2) group. The individual psychotherapies are (a) behavioral, (b) cognitive, (c) emotive, or (d) a combination of those three. Group psychotherapies can be subdivided into (a) family, (b) peer group (all children of roughly similar age), and (c) heterogeneous group (diverse ages). Each of these modalities will be characterized briefly since our intent is to survey the treatments used in child psychiatry and not to supplant therapy textbooks.

INDIVIDUAL PSYCHOTHERAPIES

1. Behavioral

Behavioral therapies used in child psychiatry include reciprocal inhibition or systematic desensitization, response prevention, flooding or implosion, modeling or imitating, operant conditioning, sensitization or aversive control, self-monitoring and self-reinforcement, assertiveness training, social skills training, biofeedback, and others. Although behavior modification or change is the focus of the behavioral therapies, they are in general congenial to a multimodal therapy plan that incorporates drug, cognitive, and emotive individual therapies, as well as group and environmental therapies. Some behavioral therapies rely on cognition-oriented and affect-oriented therapy as integral to the behavioral focus.

Systematic desensitization is a behavioral therapy originated by the psychiatrist Joseph Wolpe, based on the assumption that a relaxed child will not be tense or anxious at the same time. Hence, the first step is to induce relaxation (sodium pentothal, hypnosis, guided imagery, progressive relaxation), then to have the child encounter (usually through imagination) several increasingly dreaded or upsetting scenes, until finally—staying relaxed—the original scene be confronted without terror: for example, the change of burn dressings, or the phobically dreaded dog.

Response prevention is a behavioral therapy that may appear old and plain, but it needed contemporary academic psychologists to revive it as a therapeutic approach in individual behavior therapy. If, as an example, a child fears elevators, a benign adult may hold the child for one flight down, one flight up, with the child's eyes closed, and then with eyes open for further flights until the child's fears are no longer activated by elevator rides. The fear response is prevented by reassurance, distraction and praise until it is no longer a problem.

Flooding or implosion, often used together with response prevention, consists of real exposure to an object or situation that provokes a strong reaction but does not allow the child to leave the scene. The full extent of panic that occurs is not overwhelming to the child, so becoming flooded with fear is seen, henceforth, as something that can be weathered, survived. The flooding with negative feelings soon lessens so that the behavior has been altered, the problem solved. For example, the dentist can work with a cooperative child afterwards.

Modeling or imitating, given close attention by the psychologist Albert Bandura, is another behavior therapy that is consistent with ancient traditions: one child shows another how to act and an adult praises the new behavior. Coaching, rehearsing, taking trial runs, while encouraged and reinforced for every correct imitation, clinch the learning of new ways of behavior.

Operant conditioning of behavior, thanks to Burrhus F. Skinner the most popu-larized form of behavior modification, is also known as *instrumental conditioning* or *response-contingent reward and punishment.* It is a form of "applied behavioral analysis," both a research and treatment device. Whereas classical conditioning (as by Pavlov) worked by manipulating concurrent stimuli, operant conditioning manipulates the effects of responses. Even a self-mutilating psychotic child is not continuously mutilating herself or himself, so rewards can be used to strengthen or reinforce nonmutilative behavior. The therapist is called on to find superb reinforcers, not effective stimuli. Candies, praise, pleasure outings, and tokens to be cashed in for later rewards can all be used effectively with retarded, autistic, psychotic, delinquent, poorly learning, aggressive, enuretic, and other troubled children. Times out from reinforcement and random rein-forcement only augment the yield. The child's insight, verbal feedback, and "cooperation" are not necessary during operant conditioning. No "black box" has to be reckoned with until contingency contracting is introduced.

Sensitization or *aversive control* can be used in either operant or Pavlovian conditioning, depending on whether the punishing shock or reproach accompanies the stimulus or is response-contingent—whether the cookie jar itself gives off a sensitizing shock *or* the cookies in it are plastic and inedible when taken by the young cookie thief! Aversive techniques are controversial, to be sure, even with low-functioning autistic children, and in general they are less efficient than positive reinforcement strategies with all young children.

Self-monitoring and *self-reinforcement* are behavior-therapy techniques useful with children, as parents know when they devise checklists for their children's toothbrushing, bathing and doing household chores. The child monitors and records parentally approved behavior and may even be awarded gold stars that can be turned in for toy or treat money each week.

Assertiveness training is a particular behavioral therapy for shy, overly passive, or isolating children. The problem with many American children today is hardly their lack of self-assertion, unfortunately. Role playing is coached and encouraged so that the passively withdrawing child learns to speak "loud and clear," practice eye contact, and suggest other ways than what the adult has offered. Behavioral rehearsal is carried out, and positive reinforcers administered by the therapist strengthen the newer, assertive behavior as a part of the child's everyday repertoire. Obviously, modeling, operant conditioning, and other techniques are interwoven into assertion training.

Social skills training may go beyond assertion training in implanting the skills of more graceful social interaction into the child's behavior repertory. "Activities of daily living," as coached and rewarded by occupational therapists, are fundamental social skills needed by children. Tying one's shoelaces cannot be expected today in six-year-olds who have known only velcro fasteners, hence expected social skills vary from time to time but can be taught when learning environments are conducive to learning. Saying hello, introducing two strangers, getting acquainted, paying attention to what others say and do, eliciting and making suggestions, negotiating differences and conflicts—all these are important social skills needed by a child who is to feel competent in interpersonal relations.

Biofeedback entails autonomic or vegetative conditioning; it may rely on operant conditioning and other modes, too. Overt behavior is altered by monitoring and altering its autonomic concomitants. A child can learn to control fear or anger by receiving on-line information about blood pressure, heart rate, gut motility, sweating, and galvanic skin response when anger mounts. Even the EEG can be controlled through relaxation and meditation, teaching the child valuable prosocial techniques. Biofeedback may prove to be an increasingly useful behavior therapy stratagem for children with asthma, peptic ulcer, and other disorders in which faulty habits lead to physiological dysfunction or physical ills have psychic contributions made to them.

There are other behavior therapy possibilities, but since they rely on changing affect or cognition more than behavior they will be considered in later sections.

2. Cognitive

It is of historical interest, at least, that some radical behaviorists who formerly shunned thinking and "intrapsychic" processes have recently come to incorporate cognitive therapy and affect-oriented therapy into their more eclectic therapy program. Although some purists may object, today, more than ever before, various modalities are used to help children without cultist limitations being imposed by the therapist. There is, as a result, much less one-treatment dogmatism when therapies are selected to fit the child's needs and not the therapist's prejudices. The cognitive therapies that we present in brief overview include didactic instruction, giving the treatment's rationale, thought stopping, self-instruction, satiation training, hypnosis, guided imagery, sensory awareness training, and repetition extinction.

Didactic instruction consists of verbal explications, checking out the child's reasoning and understanding, advising and coaching, praising and encouraging. It might be said that it is the "therapy" to which parents and schoolteachers find themselves naturally drawn. It would be of obvious importance in working with a child who needs to give herself insulin injections, who has a learning block, who is misinformed, who is unaccustomed to remembering dreams, or who asks direct questions of an adult or another child. Researchers continue to reveal that not only individual tutelage but also group sessions are more effective when group leaders do this kind of self-conscious teaching and explaining to the child(ren) and do not rely entirely on behavioral or emotive techniques. Hence, cognitive therapies are enriched and informed by learning theory principles; for example, the rate of learning many things is quickened if the child's fantasies, longings, interests, and attitudes are brought to bear in the learning sessions. If a child's insight is to be enhanced, instructional measures are highly appropriate even if offered tentatively by the instructor.

Rationale giving by both therapist and child is a cognitive therapy that is often employed, since it facilitates consensual validation of perceptions, attitudes, and beliefs and encourages the child's search for meaning (of symptoms, perplexities, uncontrolled affects, and so on). The tentative provision of the rationale of treatment modalities prepares the ground for later interpretations and cognitive masteries. A common instance of rationale giving used by the authors is to describe the importance of a child's remembering dreams and working with them while with the therapist: the dream is intensely personal, relatively unaffected by anyone else; the dream tells us in symbolic form something that we know already but do not know that we know; the dream is like an unopened message from our "unconscious"; the dream is a biological necessity for the human being; we all dream every night after several minutes of deep sleep, and on and on. Children will change gladly if a trustworthy adult therapist guides them and helps them to integrate their learning to change in empathetic, true encounter.

Thought stopping is a cognitive therapy rather similar to the behavioral therapy of response prevention, but in thought stopping the emphasis is cognition-oriented. An example would be the interruption of a depressed child's ruminations about helplessness and hoplessness by valid counterarguments or by encouraging the child to demonstrate power skills by lifting weights or calisthenics or a quiet walk with the therapist or an active game with another child. At times, the therapy is as simple as saying, "Oh, stop that!" The obsessive child provides a good illustration of unproductive thinking that parents learn, through trial and error, that there are a variety of ways to bring to a halt. The child benefits, sometimes, even when it is pointed out that his/her tugging at mental windmills seems to be an unreasonable claim to moral glory and superiority. A child who is "a nut about robots" can stop the preoccupation when lovingly diverted into other, sexier topics by agemates.

Self-instruction is an elaborate cognitive therapy of self-control or self-guidance, wherein the child provides her/his own direction giving. At first, the child may say aloud the autosuggestive admonitions and later repeat them subvocally. For instance, an impulsive child may count to 10, then say aloud, "Don't hit. Slow down. You'll feel better if you just say you are angry but don't lash out," later giving himself (or herself) the same silent admonitions about hair-triggerlike reactions. Here is another example: A foster child who can think, *My new foster mother is not my real mother; she is neither my ideal nor the worst person on earth,* is on the way to a realistic modulation and control of thinking (also of doing and feeling).

Satiation training is a technique of stimulus satiation—like letting (or forcing) the firesetter to strike a couple of large boxes of kitchen matches until he "gets sick of it" and concludes he has had enough of firesetting. The psychologist Knight Dunlap first reported stimulus satiation in 1930. Because of its heavy load of affect, we discuss this later under "Emotive/Expressive Therapies: Negative Practice" (p. 50). It is a form of conditioned inhibition.

Hypnosis is a cognitive therapy adjunct that is increasingly used in child psychiatry. When it becomes *hypnotherapy,* it is not merely an adjunct but a mode of therapy. Under hypnosis, the child *dissociates* his thought processes in order to enter a trancelike state in which the peripheral environmental cues are shut out and an intense concentration on the therapist is produced, with a vibrant awareness of the relation between hypnotist and subject. Within the framework of being only aware of relatedness, the child, already close to sensorimotor experiencing, dissociates from the global awareness that typifies wakefulness and "regresses in the service of the ego" to a highly sensitive interpersonal relatedness, enabling the child to attain new insights, changed attitudes, and comprehensions. All of those cognitive changes are confirmed in posthypnotic suggestion. Some hypnotherapists believe that the very experience of recapturing the earlier sensorimotor mode of cognition can be therapeutic because it means derepression and a new integration with later, current cognitive techniques and styles.

Guided imagery is a cognitive therapy technique that can easily be interspersed with behavioral and emotive (dynamic, expressive) individual psychotherapies. For example, a boy who fears riding in an elevator may be asked what it would take to overcome the avoidance of elevators and he may reply that it would take Superman. Thereupon, the therapist may ask the child to close his eyes and imagine Superman getting on an elevator and going up 20 floors. The child describes the details of his imagery to the therapist, then opens his eyes and is told to close his eyes and now imagine accompanying Superman to the elevator door, then after describing that in detail, to open his eyes, then to imagine getting on the elevator with his hero and riding up as many flights as he can, and so on. Ultimately, through such guided fantasy or imagery, the child (at least intellectually) can master an elevator ride. Many of the exercises of Gestalt therapy employ guided imagery, as shown in the children's book, *Put Your Mother on the Ceiling* (de Mille, 1973).

Sensory awareness training, also frequently used in Gestalt therapy, is related to guided imagery in that it encourages fuller awareness of sensations and alternatives to conventional thought processes and contents. Like the drama student of Stanislavski, the child is encouraged to be aware of her own senses or sensations, to attend to exteroceptors, interoceptors and proprioceptors, to use one's body in sensory awareness training. The aliveness that is produced when a child knows her own sensations is the goal of such therapy. As in meditation, the child hears natural and mechanical sounds of which the child was earlier unaware, sees sights unimagined previously, smells new odors, knows what hunger and thirst are, and feels herself (proprioception = self-feeling) as never before. The child who has had fuller sensory awareness is not going to be easily faked out or brainwashed. *Born to Win* (James & Jongeward, 1973) was a book that emphasized sensory awareness as a pathway to authenticity for children. Cognitive awareness of one's bodily sensations is the therapeutic goal of this training. It is a system better developed in the Orient than in western cultures.

Sensory extinction is a technique used to extinguish operant behavior that produces sensory consequences. Extinction of naturally occurring behavior is done typically through *removal* of consequences such as praise or fantasy or attention to the child. The psychologist Arnold Rincover and his associates (1979) noted that some compulsive acts (turning a clicking light switch off and on repetitively) do not seem to be ways to reduce anxiety. That is, they suspected that anxiety reduction was not the negative reinforcer in compulsive acts, but instead the light produced by switch flicking was what the child liked. Proving again how important a meticulous behavioral analysis can be, they found that one child was reinforced by the changing light (a visual experience) but one was influenced by the clicking sound (auditory).

It is very likely that anxiety has been overdrawn generally in child psychiatry, and certainly it is not enough to account for such compulsive behavior of children. The sensations may be what matter.

3. Emotive/expressive

There is a plenitude of affect-oriented therapies for individual children, therapies that range from affective education and giving comforting support and reassurance on a crisis basis, through abreaction and catharsis, negative practice, and paradoxical intention to art therapy and on to long-term dynamic-verbal psychotherapy, including psychoanalysis. Most of these expressive therapies incorporate cognitive and behavioral techniques; thus, some might claim that psychoanalysis (for example) is largely a cognitive therapy, but we somewhat arbitrarily emphasize its expressive, emotional component in our review that follows.

Affective education consists of training a child to acknowledge and monitor emotions, the affects of both the child and others. This therapy technique appears in nearly all the expressive therapies to follow and again as a vital part of an environmental therapy, *psychoeducation.* It is reminiscent of Adolf Meyer's "mental hygiene teaching" on a one-to-one basis.

Children need to know their feelings and how to recognize and moderate them. They also need to be cognizant of others' feelings. This emotional training relies on cognitive therapy to help moderate affects, a certain benefit to uncontrolled and impulsive children.

Using the illustrations in Charles Darwin's book, *The Expression of the Emotions in Man and Animals,* has been helpful to show children how bodily positions and facial expressions change during emotions, asking the children to imitate the varied emotions. This technique has proved especially effective with poker-faced children suffering from psychophysiological disorders ("Psychological Factors Affecting Physical Condition" in DSM-III-R classification) such as asthma, ulcerative colitis, headache, and vomiting.

Crisis ventilation and support is brief emotional therapy that can be quite helpful to a child under acute emotional stress. Examples of trauma and crises are kid-napping, abuse, witnessing the death of a parent, being in a tornado or hurricane, and being abandoned by parents. Given an opportunity to cry, to revitalize the horrors of the upsetting event or situation, the child derives both comfort and a new perspective on the trauma. Since a child's crisis reaction lasts, usually, no more than six-to-eight weeks, the child may need to be seen only once or twice weekly for about six weeks in order to regroup, reequilibrate, and return to a more normal status emotionally. If the crisis care, centered on feelings but coupled with cognitive and behavioral approaches, is also supplemented by environmental changes that restore the child to good relationships with depend-able adults, the child goes from feeling insecure to feeling secure.

Abreaction and catharsis are closely akin to emotional flooding, the abreaction being an intense emotional expression and catharsis being the healing integra-tion that occurs when symptoms are relieved following abreaction. Emotional release, especially of old experiences long buried or repressed, can be highly beneficial for a child, provided the child is helped to put feelings into words. Nonverbal abreactions can produce brief benefits and lead to a subsequent state of relaxed exhaustion, but verbally defined and experienced abreactions last longer and seem to produce a greater desensitizing of the child.

Both abreaction and catharsis originally came from the theater (German and Greek, respectively), where speaking and verbalizing are of utmost weight. Psychodrama, role playing and imagery are all good theatrical settings for the release and relief that come from abreaction and catharsis. So is hypnosis, an early way of attaining catharsis.

Negative practice is also called massed practice or overpractice and involves having a child with a simple motor tic, for example, or compulsive hand washing, as another example, overdo the symptomatic behavior. The tic or hand-washing symptoms may actually diminish unpleasant emotion, so encouraging overpractice of the symptom brings negative emotion to the forefront and, once exhausted by overdoing both the symptom and the unpleasant negative affect, the child rests, feeling relief at having neither symptom nor affect. The symptom, then, is said to have undergone a *conditioned inhibition*. It must be apparent to the reader that the child would also be talked to, and also do some talking, while engaged in negative practice. Luckily, the child usually talks of getting tired, having enough of all this, and gets the point of the ordeal to which he or she is subjected.

Paradoxical intention therapy is akin to negative practice in that the therapeutic goal is the opposite of what is *being done*. However, in paradoxical intention therapy overpractice is not an element nor does inhibition conditioning usually occur. George Fox, the early Quaker, employed paradoxical intention in the following interaction with William Penn. Penn, from a class of men who wore swords, asked Fox what he could do about the sword, without which he felt undressed but with which he did not feel like a consistent pacifist. Fox told Penn, "I would advise you to go on carrying your sword as long as you can." Thereupon, Penn discarded his sword.

Even a child can comprehend the subtlety of paradoxical intention. For example, a boy with daytime enuresis is told to let the therapist know whenever, during a therapy session, the child is ready to wet his pants. Or a compulsive toothbrusher is given a new toothbrush and asked to demonstrate "what this brushing is all about." Or a young thief is asked if (s)he has seen anything in the consulting room that (s)he'd like to steal while the therapist leaves the room. Such tactics are not without some risk of backfiring, but they do convey to a child that feelings, unvarnished and undefended, are to be talked about during psychotherapy. Although socially when in the house of the hanged we do not mention rope, professionally we do sometimes speak of unmentionable matters and mobilize strong affects when we do.

Art-expressive therapy employs sculpting, drawing, painting, and storytelling to enhance strong emotional expression and verbalization of conflicted feelings.

The child psychiatrist Richard Gardner (cited in Chapter 1) has developed extensively the mutual storytelling technique; art therapists also encourage emotional expression with the media of clay or plasticene, paints, and drawing materials. Although it is called art therapy or simply expressive therapy, the artistic or aesthetic dimension is not the focus of such psychotherapy; instead, it is centered on the expression of the child's affects and uses the media of genuine art but only for facilitating emotional release.

Dynamic-verbal psychotherapy has many similarities to psychoanalysis and shares the psychoanalytic heritage of theory and techniques to an extent. Also called *uncovering therapy, relationship therapy, insight-oriented therapy,* and *brief dynamic therapy,* the dynamic-verbal psychotherapy that we refer to is a highly emotionally centered form of individual "talking psychotherapy." One of us (PLA) has published a basic text about this form of individual work, *A Primer of Child Psychotherapy* (1982), so we shall not undertake to summarize that here.

The principal features of dynamic-verbal psychotherapy are that it is affect-oriented, problem-centered, curious about motives and longings, and entails some comforting, educating, and advocacy in the professional therapeutic relationship; the interactions are respectful of the child, bound by medical ethics, and equip child and parents to live together more productively. The relationship is one that ends; it does not last forever, but restores the child whose conflicts have been resolved and symptoms relieved to the real relationships of love–hate with family and friends. Both therapist and child monitor the professional relationship for signs of distortions by transferences, countertransferences, and other strayings from their professional tasks, giving the child an object lesson in wholesome interactions that (s)he can use in other relationships. In the process, the child's fantasies, dreams, perceptions, and imaginative productions are given importance, as are the child's attitudes, opinions, notions, longings, and cravings. Many specialized techniques may be drawn on—role playing, dream analysis by the child, play, squiggles, drawings, storytelling, relaxation, identifying episodes of strongest feelings between sessions, problem solving in vitro and in vivo, asking and answering questions, and so on.

Again, there are cognitive and behavior therapy adjuncts to dynamic-verbal psychotherapy even if the emphasis is on emotions. Flexibility—valuing the child's true self—is stressed more than orthodoxy of style or technique. Parents and sibs are included in some sessions with the child, so group psychotherapy techniques and methods are brought into the work, too. Psychopharmacotherapeutic agents are employed if and whenever indicated. Hence, at issue is a veritably multimodal therapy that keeps focused on affect, differences, and relatedness.

Child psychoanalysis as it is actually practiced, not as it is conceptualized, is quite similar to the dynamic-verbal psychotherapy just depicted. Today's child analyst also practices a highly flexible, eclectic, or pluralistic approach, although on a more frequent and intensive basis of scheduling. The child analyst has always undergone a personal analysis with a training or supervising analyst and has conducted a small number of analyses under close control by a supervisor; the dynamic-verbal psychotherapist has not always done that. Hence, quality control would be expected to be stricter in the training of the child psychoanalyst.

Anna Freud is the originator of a child psychoanalysis that is more similar to dynamic-verbal psychotherapy than the school that owes its impetus to Melanie Klein. The latter group are also more like orthodox Freudian analysts who work solely with adults. Although the American Psychoanalytic Association ordinarily did not certify the London Institute graduates, a child analyst from the London Institute (and most others throughout the world) may not have had medical training and certification, thus being restricted by practical matters, as well as beliefs, from carrying out physical exams, prescribing pharmacotherapeutic agents, having hospital privileges, and so on, in this country.

Several standard works are available for learning about the theory and practice of child psychoanalysis. Some of these are listed in "For Further Reading" at the end of this chapter.

4. Multimodal

Since children are not obliged to fit into what the one-approach therapist can do, a multimodal therapist works best for a range of children. Multimodal individual psychotherapy provides a wide range of knowledge, skills, and possibilities for helping children: biological treatments in inpatient and outpatient settings; behavioral, cognitive, and emotive therapies; and diverse group therapies and environmental interventions, too.

GROUP OR PSYCHOSOCIAL THERAPIES

Because a child needs to belong and be a sociable person, however uniquely different from others, group socialization therapies are needed in child psychiatry. A therapist serves as group *leader* or convener and others are *members* of the group. Many group therapists working with children opt for a co-therapist of the other gender. Certainly, if the members of the group are male *and* female, a male and a female as co-therapists is preferable. In forming a group, our plan has been to have the co-therapists interview each child before entry to explain the group's *raison d'être* (talk about problems in a group with other children, etc.) and to inform the child of the group's rules (no violence, regular attendance, punctuality, and confidentiality). If the child subcribes to the rules, the child is accepted into the group.

Peer group

When children of a particular age are brought together into a group, the convention is to call this a peer group. Age is a very rough index of developmental level but it makes for some manifest similarities that may lend cohesion to the group initially. The peer therapy group is ordinarily a group of outpatients. They usually meet with the co-leaders once or twice weekly. At the group's first meeting, the children by turns introduce themselves, mentioning a problem with which they are grappling and for which they need help from others. Others are encouraged to join in, asking questions if they have any. After polling the group, the co-therapists may make some very general remarks and then review the rules of the group.

The peer group meeting in subsequent sessions is a time for verbal interchange about problems both in reality and fantasy, but can also be an activity group doing woodworking, cooking, or field trips. Cooperation, individuation, and self-expression are moved forward in a peer group. Transferences can be analyzed readily and this benefits the group members.

Family group therapy

Following the early pioneering work of Nathan W. Ackerman, a child psychiatrist, family group therapies have proliferated in the United States over the last three decades. Most employ *systems theory* in some form—viewing the family as an open system that changes over time and functions, under guiding rules and principles, in relation to a broader sociocultural system. (See Chapter 37 for discussion of Systems Theory.) Patterning and systematization of roles and relationships are stressed, although simple linear causal explanations are abandoned and replaced with postulates of equifinality (totally different outcomes of the same origin) and mutual dependence (any alteration is an interdependent cause *and* effect within the system). Communications are closely studied as the social matrix of relationship, and they change when the system shifts and changes. Moreover, most family group therapies reason and analogize according to the conservative paradigm of equilibrium theory or homeostasis, as if only rebalancing and not novel reorganization were needed when families are in crisis. The ensuing discussion follows mainly the formulations of Froma Walsh (1982).

Accepting the systems perspective, but with varied emphases, are these models of family therapy: structural, strategic, learned behavioral, psychodynamic, differentiation, and experiential. The *structural* model (Minuchin) focuses on hierarchical subsystems (parental, sibling, spouse, or conjugal) and roles, and the *boundaries* of the family as a whole and between its subsystems. The *strategic* model (Haley) looks also at hierarchies and patterns (coalitions, triangles) that appear as strategies for solving problems. The strategic model sees the problem-solving strategies as *the* family problem. The *learned behavioral* model (Robert L. Weiss), derived from social psychology, stresses the array of contingencies (rewards and punishments) that facilitate or inhibit learning of social behavior and social influence and control within families. The *psychodynamic* model of family therapy (Framo, Lidz, Ackerman) focuses on the unconscious dynamisms (carry-overs from families of origin) that influence interpersonal relations within the family; this model is sensitive to scapegoating and projections and gives a reminder that former generations have influences on the two generations present within a family. The psychodynamic model, like Minuchin's structural model, emphasizes structural–functional concepts such as the parenting coalition, boundaries between the generations, and sex roles within the family. The *differentiation* model of family therapy (Bowen) emphasizes the family as a collective, "undifferentiated ego mass," from which individuals hatch and within which, barring too great anxiety, they are able to differentiate and individuate. The *experiential* model of family group therapy (Satir, Whitaker) is shorter on theory than most models but does center down on the here and now of the family as a whole, helping the members of the total system to communicate their feelings more clearly and directly, be more flexible about rules and standards, and be both more open to the outside and more playful and experimental in their interpersonal relationships.

Some form of family group therapy is needed in child psychiatry. Ordinarily, the most-used would be a combination of the *psychodynamic* and of the *learned behavioral* models and the sessions would keep a focus on the child, thus retaining some flavor of child advocacy.

Heterogeneous therapy groups

When age ranges are not strictly observed and children (themselves of diverse ages) from several families are brought into a heterogeneous therapeutic group, both advantages and disadvantages accrue. For one thing, it may be a first-time opportunity for the child to be with adolescents and older adults who speak candidly while showing compassion for each other. But, on the side of risks, the child often tends to be demeaned and neglected in such a heterogeneous group.

Sometimes groups are composed of several parents and several children, usually to a total of eight-to-10 persons. These groups can take cognizance of both personal and family problems in their working agenda and that may be advantageous. Again, however, children need advocacy by the group leader if they are not to be shoved aside and ignored in such groups.

Heterogeneous therapy groups are not as widely used as peer groups and family groups in child psychiatry.

SOCIOENVIRONMENTAL THERAPIES

Child psychiatry, influenced by preventive medicine, includes among its available treatments a number of interventions into the child's daily social environment. These are mainly directed to changing the setting in which the child lives, sometimes removing the child from home and school in the community and making the child into one of approximately one million American children who live away from parents in special children's institutions. Sometimes, other environmental manipulations, probably superior to institutionalization as a rule, can be carried out in an outpatient or day care program, permitting the child to live at home. All of the different settings that we shall consider in this brief introduction have sprung up as much to "protect the community" from the wayward child as to protect and serve the child. Also, the efficacy of each institution depends on how well it serves children, or a particular child, with a mental disorder. That is to say that not all manipulated environments are efficacious in meeting the needs of growing children.

In this preliminary survey we have elected to consider:

1. hospitalization
2. residential treatment or milieu therapy
3. psychiatric day care and after-school care
4. psychoeducational programs
5. family support services
6. foster care
7. courts and correctional facilities
8. recreational and camping programs
9. boarding schools

Hospitalization

Hospitalization is indicated whenever a mentally disordered child's care becomes too much for the parents to manage; that is the final criterion in any decision to send a child to a mental hospital. Children who endanger themselves or others, who also have a serious mental disorder treatable in the mental hospital but not in any less restrictive setting, and who are under 14 years of age can be admitted involuntarily in most areas of the United States. Even so, court reviews and children's access to attorneys safeguard children's rights.

There is no mental disorder per se that requires hospitalization, since family coping abilities are the determinative condition, but, generally speaking, extremes of disruptive conduct or behavior, suicidal attempts, psychosis, developmental disorders, life-threatening psychophysiological or somatoform disorders, and organic mental disorders do warrant hospitalization. Furthermore, hospitals are good places to carry out complicated diagnostic workups and establish treatment programs for the future.

A rule of thumb in child psychiatry is that children belong at home with their families, hence hospitalizations, aside from costliness, should be kept as brief as possible. That rule holds true even for autistic children who have been found to reach maximum benefits from no more than four months of hospitalization. It is tragic to see children, who have learned the ropes during prolonged hospitalization, unable to cope when they finally are discharged. Most hospitals are overly structured and hierarchical to a fault, so they do not encourage a child's readiness for democratic living.

Milieu therapy (residential treatment)

When groups of children are in hospital or residential care, the entire staff (usually working with leadership from a clinical director) are the child group's milieu therapists. An individual therapist might engage the child in a therapeutic alliance. The staff as a group, however, plan the psychiatric care for the individual child and carry that out according to an organized plan that balances individual and group emphases. Hence, the whole environment is scrutinized and changed so that it will be therapeutic in an active manner and envelop the child in a unified setting. That may give equal importance, at times, to the work done by a child care worker, child psychiatrist, occupational therapist, teacher, pediatrician, social worker, psychologist, cook, psychoanalyst, gardener, recreation therapist, art or music therapist, nurse, and others. The child enters into a therapeutic alliance with the total milieu. The children may practice self-governance through their own council or assembly, and negotiate and bargain collectively and rationally with the adults, as part of the therapeutic milieu.

Milieu therapy in residential care works best when it is made available for long periods (one-to-five years) to children with severe disorders who are unable to function in a more noxious, unstructured environment of home and community school. Considering the severity of the disorder and the pathogenicity of previous living arrangements, it is no wonder that a therapeutic milieu is of prolonged duration.

Psychiatric day care

When a child and the child's family see that both day and night hospital care are not needed but the child is not ready to go home or to school, psychiatric day care or day treatment is an excellent option to have available. Further, some children who have been outpatients may need day treatment temporarily in lieu of hospitalization.

Psychiatric day care for children often provides both a school program and a full range of multidisciplinary psychiatric services. Day care programs often are able to accommodate children from the time they leave school until the end of the day, if the child can attend a regular school. Overall, day care is cost-effective and beneficial to children with mental disorders, being more effective for adjustive and stress-related disorders than for those of chronic, insidious onset. Also diminishing the benefits of day care is severe family pathology and, at times, removal of the child from mainstreaming in the school and neighborhood may not be optimal.

Psychoeducational programs

When the child moves from hospital to day care to community schooling, some school systems provide special schools, or special classes, for children with mental disorders. These programs, like day care and other specialized settings, incur the risks of becoming segregated islets or ghettos, so careful calculation of cost/benefit ratio must be made in each case. If benefits clearly outweigh the risks, a psychoeducational (sometimes called *affective education*) program can be used to help a child both cognitively and emotionally.

If a psychoeducational setting is fully effective, it will teach both academics and mental health to the children, interwoven as both are in ordinary life, fused with values of autonomy with responsibility.

Family support services

In America, where there is no national policy for families with children, and where services to families are low-budget and low-priority concerns, helping families to link up with community services is an ordeal—like being a broker when there is precious little to buy, steal, sell, or barter. Families are needful, however.

Families may need better jobs for the adults and income supplementation if they are to survive; medical care if they are not to become disabled or die; housing and shelter; homemaking services; vocational guidance; help in relating to the schools their children attend; adequate food to prevent malnutrition (food stamps, Aid to Families With Dependent Children); counseling services for sexual problems, alcoholism, and drug abuse; and so on. Ordinary families need many things that they lack when they are functioning moderately well and need much more when they face problems, crises, and stresses.

Social workers have ordinarily helped the child psychiatry patient's family to establish supportive networks in linkage to community resources. Social workers still do this, but the child psychiatrist herself (or himself) has to stand ready to be a patient advocate and add emphasis to the needs of families when contacting support services in the community.

Foster care

In family emergencies that attend disablement of the parents, the child may need fostering. Foster care ranges from short-term boarding arrangements to longer placements lasting 10 years or more. Some foster care becomes coterminous with childhood itself, at age 18 years, especially if the child cannot be adopted. Foster care occurs in two settings, one the rather impersonal children's institution and the other a replica of nuclear family life.

Children may go into foster care if one or both parents die, go to a cancer or mental hospital or nursing home, abandon them, neglect or abuse them. Still the child feels a strong bond to those parents and may need to retain contacts with the biological parents who failed the child. But it is sometimes difficult for foster parents to promote or even allow such contacts, especially if the foster parents regard the original parents as unworthy or malevolent.

Foster care is poorly subsidized out of welfare department budgets. Foster parents are often working-class people who give fostering to relatives and acquaintances, fortunately, without claiming *any* remuneration. Oddly, middle-class Americans seldom do that for homeless children, although they could afford it more readily. Subsidized foster care—or we should say: meagerly subsidized foster care—places the fostered child at risk of neglect, a cold reception, undernutrition, and even sexual and physical abuse when in the foster home. Paul Fine, a child psychiatrist in Omaha, has reported an unusually positive and successful program of *primary prevention* through a child psychiatrist's supportive services to foster parents—compassionate help in individual and group consultation, aiding the foster parents to form child advocacy networks, to upgrade the licensure and competency (and pay) of foster parents, and to form a network of community support among themselves and between foster parents and others in Omaha. Such efforts are all too rare, so *group homes* for homeless children may be superior to the foster homes in many parts of our nation.

Courts and corrections

Hundreds of thousands of children in the United States have been adjudicated delinquent and sent to correctional facilities. White children are more likely to wind up in mental health clinics or hospitals, while black children are more likely to be sent into a "correctional facility," the contemporary equivalent of the old reform school. Although outcomes of the two placements may be hard to document, available studies show a superior outcome for those who are deflected into the psychiatric system.

Nevertheless, correctional programs are needed for delinquent children (those with Conduct Disorders) and the children often fare better under the structured overseeing by court and probation workers than in outpatient child psychiatry centers. A compromise, often working well, is to have the court mandate regular attendance for psychotherapy as a condition of the child's probation. Required psychotherapy is surprisingly efficacious.

Recreational and camping programs

Summer camps for children with mental disorders have a noble history, but only during the 20th century. Children can take respectable leaves from parents and sibs; they learn new skills; they benefit from peer interactions and relationships with older counselors who serve as ego ideals. Many children with mental disorders return from a camping experience with evident ego-strengthening and ego-expanding having occurred.

Recreational opportunities for children with mental disorders are important. In Norway, where services to all children are voluminous, recreational programs are given great emphasis. Children in crowded cities all over the world benefit from recreation and it is a splendid adjunct to other psychiatric therapies. In the United States, organized charities (United Way, Police Athletic League) and private agencies (churches, Boys Club, Scouts) provide most of the available funding for needed recreational programs.

Boarding schools

"When the chemistry is bad" between parent(s) and child, a boarding school, expensive as it usually is, may provide respite care during an acceptable separation of child from parents. That arrangement for middle-class Britons has become practically institutionalized, expected. American or British children may find boarding school better than unrewarding and unrelenting conflicts between a child and parents.

Some boarding schools wish to attract children with developmental or other mental disorders. Others will enable a child to get "extra," specialized help for mental disorders on an extracurricular timing. All the advantages and disadvantages of parentectomy inhere in any type of boarding school for young children.

RELATING CHILD PSYCHIATRIST, CHILD AND PARENTS, AND SCHOOL

The prevalent cliché holds that there should be close cooperation between the child psychiatrist and the school. Many child psychiatrists describe procedures for, with the parents' permission, communicating with the child's teacher(s) early in the diagnostic process and continuing to do so as treatment proceeds. This is often imperative in Attention–Deficit Hyperactivity Disorder. For their part, many educators are interested in cooperating closely with child psychiatrists.

Unfortunately, the relationship between child psychiatry and school does not always work out as smoothly as each party expects. The two main reasons are: the lack of realization that the two professions inhabit two different universes and the failure of both to engage the parents fully. In other words, child psychiatrists and teachers may be eager to talk to each other, but they often do so without drawing sufficiently clear lines of demarcation for who is going to do what, and without realizing the need to explain their respective goals to the parents and to obtain the parents' agreement and support.

The parents, for their part, will often make a stark distinction between the respective functions of the school and the clinician and request confidentiality vis-à-vis the school system. Another reason, of course, is the parents' pathological defense mechanism of projection or displacement of blame onto a teacher. Parents may feel that psychotherapy is between them/their child and the doctor, and is not the teacher's business. At that point, the clinician will do well not to be dogmatic, but to vary and individualize his/her approach, not only for each case, but for the same case in the course of treatment, as the parents' attitude may change.

Most parents, alas, may have a valid point when they claim that the child may be stigmatized among his/her peers and may be treated differently by the teacher who knows of a child's psychiatric involvement. In practice, it is often the child who "spills the beans" about seeing a psychiatrist to his/her peers; teachers rarely do. The parental anxiety may be about there being "a record" that will haunt the child in later life. There is little realism at the base of this fear because the future adult may genuinely forget childhood psychotherapy and can, therefore, answer "No" to questions about past mental disorder on employment questionnaires. What is realistic is that knowledge about psychiatric treatment will somehow leak out, via the school system, and that this is indeed more likely to happen if the teacher knows about it. How much harm it actually does is another matter. It depends on the attitudes in that particular community, the professionalism of the teachers and counselors, the adherence to confidentiality standards among the school clerical staff, and finally and most significantly, the child's psychopathology and the coping style of the family. In the worst case, the child is taunted by peers and made to feel inferior and different by the teacher. However, the parents may be given only this side of the story or choose to hear only of their child's plight. What they do not hear, or do not want to hear, is that since all interpersonal transactions are two-way events, the child may have brought much of this scenario on him/herself by being provocative, aggressive, or vengeful. It is this one-sided scenario that is presented to the child psychiatrist, and it is then the mental health professional's role to disentangle the web of secrecy and intrigue.

It has been our overall experience that most parents are protective enough of their children vis-à-vis the school system, so that there is rarely a need for the clinician to intervene to protect a child. It is tempting to become an activist, but that means abandoning the psychotherapeutic skills that are the reason for the parents' consulting the clinician in the first place. We, therefore, propose the following approach:

1. The clinician should be flexible and clinically circumspect—not all parents are alike, not all teachers are alike. Many, perhaps most, parents will reach a reasonable accommodation with the teacher(s). Whenever this is not the case, the clinician will find out why: Is it parental or family psychopathology, or the teacher's attitude, or the peculiar sociocultural "mix" of the particular school? The clinician may suspect and, in due course, diagnose psychopathology in the parent(s); (s)he should never do so regarding the teacher. The opportunity to interview/examine the teacher in a psychiatric sense is never given in this context, and the clinician must beware of "loose lips," i.e., making even a suggestive statement implying a psychiatric diagnosis of a consulting or consulted teacher. Expressions such as "the teacher sounds like an angry, or rigid, paranoid, person" have no place in the mental health worker's discussion with the parents. Although this seems at first unfair (after all, teachers are not immune to mental illness either), anything but strict adherence to professionalism on the part of the clinician opens up the teacher to stigmatization.

2. Unless (s)he is working as the school's consultant, the clinician has been consulted by the child (i.e., the child's parents) and therefore owes confidentiality and service to the child. In very practical terms, this means that the clinician works for the child's best interests. Optimally (and actually this is frequently done) this includes communication with the teacher; if this is precluded, the clinician can expect to achieve a surprising amount of success through work with the child and family alone. As a matter of fact, even under circumstances of parental support for communicating with the teacher, direct communication is not always necessary; making the parent(s) assume the active role of intermediary with the school may serve several positive functions: enhancing their parenting and advocacy skills and improving parental self-esteem by entrusting them with an important role, providing an opportunity for corrective emotional experiences between parents and educators, and freeing valuable clinical psychotherapeutic time. Some teachers—even entire school systems—are very interested in learning how to take care of emotional problems in children; the teacher's education in that respect should not be funded by the patient's family or by the psychiatrist. Teachers can arrange in-service training sessions to upgrade mental health skills and knowledge.

Our conclusion is that when the clinician asks but is refused child or parent consent to give information to the school, (s)he has no choice but to abide by this, except in cases of emergency—which rarely, if ever, call for an urgent communication with the school. One of the pitfalls of confidentiality is a school system's inquiring as to whether an appointment has indeed been made for a particular child, as the school was most anxious to have the child seen by the mental health professional. Despite the mental health profession's interest in good relations with the school system, such an inquiry must be refused, since it is confidential information which needs a signed release to be divulged.

3. The best way to bridge the natural gap between the educational and mental health systems is by formal consultation. It is usually contracted and paid for by the school system, and in its simplest and most effective form is "consultee-oriented," the consultee being the school system (i.e., various individual teachers or counselors). This obviates the need for obtaining parental consent for contact with the child, as the "patient," or rather consultee, is the teacher, the child's identity being unknown to the consultant.

A more complex form of school consultation consists of an actual examination of the child, or at the least classroom observation, by the clinician personally, in addition to the conferences with the teacher previously outlined. Parental permission needs to be secured, and the parents themselves are usually present, involved in the process. The focus may shift from strict consultee-oriented consultation to varying degrees of traditional patient-doctor relationship in the context of the school. This is a difficult role, calling for considerable experience on the part of the clinician, and is not recommended for the beginner. The model just described lends itself best to a school with a specialized function and circumscribed population with relative uniformity of pathology, e.g., schools for children with sensory handicaps (schools for the blind, the deaf), or with severe learning disabilities or mental retardation. The clinician works in an environment structured by the school, with a great deal of support from the school, which ensures the success of the clinical work. Unless such support is forthcoming, the clinician had better not undertake the job but work on setting up the support system first.

If there is one statement of summary advice we would give, it is for the clinician to base him/herself on a good rapport with the parents: they are ultimately responsible for and in charge of the child, and they can be accessed for treatment. The educator can be a most valuable ally, but the clinician ultimately has much less leverage with educators than with the child and the parents.

Questions for Study and Action

1. Psychiatry has been defined as "a branch of medicine dealing with disorders of thinking, feeling, and doing." Name two therapeutic modalities for each of the categories of *thinking*, *feeling*, and *doing*.

2. Are psychoactive drugs available to ameliorate problems of doing, feeling, and thinking? Name *one drug for each* type of disorder: a thought disorder such as Schizophrenia, a mood disorder such as Mania, a behavior disorder such as Attention–Deficit Hyperactivity Disorder.

3. Sometimes parents and children are noncompliant with treatment programs. Name five ways in which a child would show noncompliance or resistance.

4. Name five ways in which parents would show noncompliance or resistance to a treatment program outlined by their doctor.

5. Name five ways in which a compassionate physician would deal with noncompliance. Is it merely accidental that a *doctor* (Latin, *docere*) has always been seen as a *teacher?* Explain your answer.

6. Why is most practical, commonsense individual psychotherapy of a kind that uses behavioral, emotive, and cognitive approaches? Use mild mental retardation as an example.

7. How would you account for the proven efficacy of individual psychotherapy for fearful, inhibited children and of group/socioenvironmental therapies for delinquent, Conduct Disorders children?

8. In recent years, specialists in branches of medicine such as family practice, pediatrics, and internal medicine have emphasized that they have "cognitive skills" as well as "technological skills." Name five cognitive skills, each of which may take more of the doctor's time, that you'd want to find in your personal physician.

9. Leading psychopharmacologists insist that drug therapy in any field of psychiatry is always secondary or auxiliary to an overall program of psychosocial therapies. Why? Why couldn't a child psychiatrist prescribe a psychostimulant drug for ADHD and let the rest go?

10. What differences do you see between "intellectual insight" and "emotional insight or working through?" Explain.

For Further Reading

Adams, P.L. *A Primer of Child Psychotherapy* (2nd ed.). Boston: Little, Brown, 1982.

Biederman, J., Gastfriend, D.R., & Jellinek, M.S. Desipramine in the treatment of children with attention deficit disorder. *J. Clin. Psychopharmacol.*, 6:359–362, 1986.

Campbell, M., Cohen, I., & Small, A. Drugs in aggressive behavior. *J. Amer. Acad. of Child Psychiat.*, 21:107–117, 1982.

Cantwell, D., & Carlson, G. Stimulants. In J. Werry (Ed.), *Pediatric Psychopharmacology.* New York: Brunner/Mazel, 1978, pp. 171–207.

Darwin, C. *The Expression of the Emotions in Man and Animals.* Chicago & London: The University of Chicago Press, 1965.

Delay, J., Pichot, P., & Lemp.erière, T. Un neuroleptique majeur non phenothiazine et non reserpinique, l'haloperidol, dans le traitement des psychoses. *Ann. Med. Psychol.,* 118:145–152, 1960.

de Mille, R. *Put Your Mother on the Ceiling: Children's Imagination Games.* New York: Viking, 1973.

Donnelly, M., Zametkin, A.J., Rapoport, J.L., et al. Treatment of childhood hyperactivity with desipramine: Plasma drug concentration, cardiovascular effects, plasma and urinary catecholamine levels, and clinical response. *Clin. Pharmacol. Ther.,* 39:72–81, 1986.

Geller, B., Perel, J.M., Kuitter, E.F., et al. Nortriptyline in major depressive disorder in children: Response, steady-state plasma levels, predictive kinetics and pharmacokinetics. *Psychopharmacol. Bull.,* 19:62–65, 1983.

Graziano, A.M. (Ed.). *Behavior Therapy with Children.* Chicago: Aldine, Vol. I (1971) and Vol. II (1975).

Gualtieri, C.T., Quade, D., Hicks, R., et al. Tardive dyskinesia and other clinical consequences of neuroleptic treatment in children and adolescents. *Am. J. Psychiatry,* 141:20–23, 1984.

James, M., & Jongeward, D. *Born to Win: Transactional Analysis with Gestalt Experiments.* Menlo Park, CA: Addison-Wesley, 1973.

Kendall, P.C., & Braswell, L. *Cognitive-Behavioral Therapy for Impulsive Children.* New York: Guilford, 1985.

Levenson, J.L. Neuroleptic malignant syndrome. *Am. J. Psychiatry,* 142:1137–1145, 1985.

Noshpitz, J.D. (Ed.-in-Chief). *Basic Handbook of Child Psychiatry, Vol. III: Therapeutic Interventions* (Harrison, S.I., Ed.). New York: Basic Books, 1979.

McAndrew, J., Case, Q., & Treffert, D. Effects of prolonged phenothiazine intake on psychotic and other hospitalized children. *J. Autism Child Schizophrenia,* 2:75–91, 1972.

Pliszka, S.R. Tricyclic antidepressants in the treatment of children with attention deficit disorder. *J. Amer. Acad. of Child Adol. Psychiatry,* 26:127–132, 1987.

Polizos, P., Englehardt, P., & Hoffman, S.P. Neurological consequences of psychotropic drug withdrawal in schizophrenic children. *J. Autism Child Schizophrenia,* 3:247–253, 1973.

Rapaport, J.L., Mikkelsen, E.J., Zavadil, A., et al. Childhood enuresis II. Psychopathology, tricyclic concentration in plasma, and antienuretic effect. *Arch. Gen. Psychiatry,* 37:1146–1152, 1980.

Rincover, A., Newsom, C., & Carr, E. Using sensory extinction procedures in the treatment of compulsivelike behavior of developmentally disabled children. *J. Consult. Clin. Psychol.,* 47:695–701, 1979.

Walsh, F. *Normal Family Processes.* New York: Guilford, 1982.

Weiss, R.L. The conceptualization of marriage from a behavioral perspective. In T.J. Paolino & B.S. McCrady (Eds.), *Marriage and Marital Therapy: Psychoanalytic, Behavioral and Systems Perspectives.* New York: Brunner/Mazel, 1978.

Werry, J.S. (Ed.). *Pediatric Psychopharmacology: The Use of Behavior Modifying Drugs in Children.* New York: Brunner/Mazel, 1978.

II

DISORDERS OF CHILDHOOD: DOING, FEELING, THINKING, AND BEING VICTIMIZED

In the second part of this book, we shall consider the major categories into which clinicians have allocated children's mental disorders. Each disorder is described, and information, when available, is provided concerning its epidemiology, clinical course or prognosis with and without treatments. We have given particular attention to furnishing the reader with over 120 case vignettes that illustrate the disorders in question. We call attention here to the Questions for Study and Action that are appended to each major subdivision of the text, since our field testing has demonstrated that the reader's review and grasp of the clinical materials given in the text will be both imprinted and extended by a thoughtful attempt to respond at some length to each of the questions posed. Some of the questions are straightforward encouragements to review and apply the content of the text itself, while others may entice the reader to go further in some clinical action research which is a very good way to have learning experiences.

Child psychiatry is defined by most dictionaries as the scientific study and practices devoted to children's disorders of thinking, feeling, and behavior. We have found that very traditional conceptualization to be useful. Therefore, we devote the first three sections of Part II to Doing or Behavior Disorders *(Section A),* Feeling and Mood Disorders *(Section B), and* Thinking and Central Processing Disorders *(Section C). Having made that decision, we realized that some very damaging things occur for many children, things that were left out by the traditional classification system, so we have added a fourth Section D,* Being Victimized. *Becoming a victim is very much a part of the child's existential situation in our current era, and victimization is disordering and maddening in a variety of ways. At the end of Section D, we have included a brief chapter for the clinician who may have to appear in court on a child's behalf; this is a survey, for beginners, of forensic child psychiatry.*

SECTION A

DOING OR
BEHAVIOR DISORDERS

DSM-III-R sensibly lumps together Oppositional Defiant Disorder, Conduct Disorder and Attention–Deficit Hyperactivity Disorder as "Disruptive Behavior Disorders." We have arbitrarily chosen to save the Attention–Deficit Hyperactivity Disorder (ADHD) for Section C on Thinking and Central Processing Disorders; we took that option because we feel that ADHD is more pervasive and sets up a style of living for the child that direly influences cognition and feeling, as well as behavior. We have concluded that ADHD is a disorder that belongs with other disorders of cortical learning and functioning. Nonetheless, we acknowledge that ADHD is a *disruptive behavior disorder* too.

Since the human organism and person are of one piece, individual in the strict sense of indivisible, it is only to be expected that all of the behavior disorders in childhood will have heavy components of cognitive and emotional or affective derangement as well. That expectation holds for Conduct Disorder, Oppositional Defiant Disorder, Episodic and Organic Disorders, Factitious Disorder, Firesetting, Functional Enuresis, Functional Encopresis, Eating Disorders, Sleep Disorders, Gender and Sexual Disorders, and Tic and Habit Disorders—all being the subjects of Chapters 3 through 13. Since these disorders show behavior as somehow remarkable, we assign all of them to this Section A.

Note: Many of our discussions follow DSM-III-R, but we have decided not to slavishly conform to DSM-III-R when clinical judgment may dictate nonconformity.

3

Conduct Disorders

S ince "behavior disorders" were poorly defined, the category of Conduct Disorders, formerly a stepchild of child psychiatry, was resorted to as a "wastebasket diagnosis." It was something to call those children with troublesome behavior. Today, however, combining clinical experience, reexamining previous data, and using new empirically based diagnostic criteria, we see Conduct Disorders have emerged as an important and clinically viable category. The clinician can expect to see Conduct Disorders fairly frequently, especially those that overlap with the syndromes of Attention–Deficit Hyperactivity Disorder, Neuroses, or Anxiety Disorders and Mood Disorders. A large number of patients with Conduct Disorders can be expected to be encountered, an expectation borne out by repeated clinical experience. Conduct Disorders are the most frequently diagnosed cases in a child psychiatric clinic setting, although not necessarily in the physician's office.

DEFINITION

The Conduct Disorders in DSM-III included four diagnostic subcategories, following their particular combining of the factors of aggression and socialization. They all share the following two characteristics:

1.   There is a deficit in empathy, the ability to feel for others. While this differs in

69

degree between the socialized and undersocialized subtypes, all Conduct Disorders contain this defect.

2. Either actively or passively (depending on the subtype), these children do not fit in with the rest of society and its demands for inner values and outward conduct.

These are the children who, with unchanged behavior, will grow up to be Antisocial Personality Disorders. Children with Conduct Disorders have difficulties at home, at school, on the playground—everywhere that rules apply and loyalty or affection or fair play may be enforced and expected.

The DSM-III-R Work Group announced late in August 1986 that four items, from a list of 17 antisocial acts (and appearing during more than six months), would be needed to diagnose a case of Conduct Disorder. Also, DSM-III-R revived an old question of whether the neatly delineated four subtypes were valid clinically or conceptually. Ultimately, it appeared that DSM-III-R and DSM-IV might contain but a single category of Conduct Disorder, 312.90; yet DSM-III-R in 1987 contained three subtypes: 312.00, solitary aggressive type; 312.20, group type; and 312.90, undifferentiated type.

For purposes of exposition, we will describe the four subtypes that were listed in DSM-III, while recognizing that their didactic and clinical utility is limited.

ETIOLOGY

Considerable controversy regarding etiology revolves around nature versus nurture, thereby providing one more example of the fallacy of this dichotomy. Very likely, the Conduct Disorders arise as a result of a combining of inborn constitutional–temperamental characteristics of the child with the attitudes about and responses to those characteristics by the caregivers (parents).

Commonly seen is a "poor fit" between either excessively aggressive or excessively passive (withdrawn) reactions in the child, and the inability of the parent or parents to respond to those reactions in a way that will "smooth them out" eventually. A large area of overlap between Attention–Deficit Hyperactivity Disorder and Conduct Disorders connotes added weight for constitutional factors. Medical histories, psychological tests, some physiological tests (e.g., galvanic skin resistance), and careful neurological evaluations have all pointed towards developmental delays and neurologic deficits, as well as perceptual and learning difficulties, in conduct-disordered children. Yet Conduct Disorders are more frequent in children of antisocial and alcoholic parents, and this stresses the contribution of parental attitudes and defective, sometimes abusive, child rearing, as well as possible genetic contributions. Daily clinical experience confirms the fact that Conduct Disorders predominate in poorly structured families who lack sufficient practices of good conduct or appropriate discipline, or who engage in profound conflict over basic values while putting children "in the middle." Obviously, again, genetic and environmental factors are interwoven.

It follows that we can find certain predisposing factors in both the organic and interactional spheres. Attention–Deficit Hyperactivity Disorder, learning disabilities, and being adopted are found in a high proportion of these children. Some environmental predisposing factors are: parental rejection and/or severe neglect, changes in caretakers (e.g., from parents to multiple foster parents), impersonal and emotionally depriving institutional living, and single-parent (maternal) upbringing when that single parent is significantly handicapped or deficient in child-rearing capabilities. Interestingly, large family size has also been found to be correlated with Conduct Disorder. Finally, boys are more predisposed to Conduct Disorder than girls (4:1 to as high as 12:1) (Richman, Stevenson, & Graham, 1982; Rutter, Tizard, & Whitmore, 1970; Wolff, 1985).

Conduct Disorder, Undersocialized, Aggressive (312.00)*

CASE 3-1   Eleven-year-old Sean was referred to a mental health clinic by the probation office because of *incorrigible behavior* both in school and in the community generally. He was repeatedly expelled from school because he would *fight and injure* other children, at times *severely*. At home, he would threaten his younger siblings, and he had set several fires. He had practically *no friends*.

Sean came from a single-parent family. His father had deserted the family when Sean was three years old and was subsequently sent to a state penitentiary. Mother divorced and remarried, but that husband, in turn, left soon afterwards. A succession of Mother's boyfriends provided *no stability;* instead, it produced severe physical *abuse* at the hands of two of those boyfriends.

All attempts that Mother made to *discipline* Sean were unsuccessful. Likewise, he showed *no response* to the measures the school instituted either to inspire him or to punish him. In addition to violent and uncontrollable behavior, he was *unable to sit still*. He made few friends, and invariably lost them, partly because he would turn against them on the slightest or even a nonexistent provocation, and partly because he showed *no loyalty* to them. Moreover, he would indiscriminately *steal* from them and attempt to *blame them,* or anybody else, in order to extricate himself from any difficulties.

He showed *no fear or revulsion* about his cruel acts. On television, he watched horror movies with great delight, subsequently reveling in descriptions of how

*DSM-III code.

"bugs were crawling out of the dead man's eye sockets," or "he crushed the man's skull and the brain oozed out." He gave the impression of "stimulus hunger" for cruelty.

Comment. This case history illustrates how a Conduct Disorder of aggressive, undersocialized type can be defined by a simplified triad:

1. A pattern of antisocial and aggressive behavior.
2. Lack of bonding with other people and disregard for the feelings of others.
3. Persistent behavior difficulties, especially at school, generally resistant to discipline.

CASE 3-2   Ten-year-old Chuck was seen by the child psychiatrist at the behest of the school and the Department of Social Services because of their concerns over Chuck's precocious and aggressive sexual interest in girls, as well as their suspicions of *repeated* marijuana use. In addition, he was *ostracized* by his peers because he would *tattle* on them and *tease* and often torture them physically. In the process, he would *extort* their lunch money from them.

Past history of Chuck showed his having always been a stubborn, *willful* child who was given to *frequent aggressive outbursts* when his wishes were not immediately satisfied. He seemed *unable* to learn from experience.

During the psychiatric interview, Chuck was *sullen, hostile, and generally uncooperative.* He *blamed* others for all his difficulties and appeared to *lack* feelings of affection or tenderness. He repeatedly emphasized his *boredom* except in circumstances of *high excitement* which almost invariably boiled down to *aggressing* against somebody else and seeing that person *squirm or suffer.* He acknowledged his interest in girls—with the implication that he *derived pleasure* from their fears, embarrassment, and *his power* (even temporarily) over them. None of the girls he pursued had ever liked him.

He had started stealing Mother's cigarettes and smoking them at about age five, and by the time he was in third grade, Chuck was *smoking marijuana regularly.* He experimented with amphetamines, barbiturates, and occasionally LSD, obtaining the money for procuring them *by theft and bullying* of peers. He had *no remorse or guilt* about his actions, *nor* did he develop any close ties to any of his peers.

Comment. Case 3-2 shows two special features of this type of Conduct Disorder: precocious sexuality and drug abuse, in addition to the "core" characteristics.

The diagnosis is made on the basis of the persistent pattern of callous aggressiveness or criminality ("thefts outside the home involving confrontation with the victim," according to the DSM-III, 1980, definition, p. 48), severe and persistent defects in relatedness to others, including lack of consideration, remorse, or guilt, and severe and persistent behavior problems at home and at school.

DIFFERENTIAL DIAGNOSIS

This includes, first of all, *isolated* antisocial acts or behaviors, but without their persistent, long-term, practically lifelong duration. Adjustment Disorders can be distinguished by the emotional relatedness to people and by the context in which they occur, as well as precipitating stressful factors. Oppositional Defiant Disorder is similarly characterized by basic respect for the rights and feelings of others in spite of intolerance of authority. Finally, Attention–Deficit Hyperactivity Disorder is often *part* of the Conduct Disorder, so the two diagnoses may need recording on Axis I.

TREATMENT

Always difficult, treatment of youngsters with this undersocialized and aggressive disorder should, ideally, be undertaken in long-term, high-quality residential treatment centers because of the accompanying profound affective and cognitive deficiencies inherent in this disorder of behavior. Residential care is impossible for all, given their large numbers, their derivation from socioeconomic strata that are often dependent on community support for their very existence, let alone paying for such treatment, and the fact that so many are funneled into corrections, not mental health. Therefore, only those who cause the greatest trouble in the community are referred to residential facilities, which are often correctional institutions. The treatment outcomes are mixed at best.

If ambulatory treatment is undertaken, it must include the parent or parents, since the goal is to help parents manage the child more effectively by a combination of acceptance of the child as a person and consistent, firm guidance and discipline. The latter should be of the "preventive" kind, i.e., trouble should be anticipated and prevented; this is more effective and easier on the parents than punishment after the transgression. Although few parents of these children, burdened as they are with significant pathology of their own, can do this fully, even partial success at management is potentially helpful and, as a matter of fact, indispensable.

Individual treatment of children may be attempted in connection with parental counseling and consists of building up a relationship with the view towards identification of the child's healthier "ego" with the therapist. A cautionary remark is in order here: psychotherapy of the traditional uncovering or analyzing type is *not* indicated, since it may worsen the disorder if done before establishing a therapeutic alliance.

Pharmacotherapy is probably the best individual therapeutic modality we have at our disposal, whenever there is sufficient overlap of the Conduct Disorder, undersocialized aggressive type, with Attention–Deficit Hyperactivity Disorder. In such a case, the usual pharmacologic agents—viz., stimulants (methylphenidate and others) are effective both for the usual symptoms of Attention–Deficit Hyperactivity Disorder and the impulsivity characteristic of both disorders. Aggression is thereby held in check to a considerable extent, which, in turn, prepares the ground for other measures—usually guidance and "preventive discipline." Thus, pharmacotherapy, as is always the case in child psychiatry, cannot succeed by itself and must be used in combination with other measures.

When there is little or no overlap with Attention–Deficit Hyperactivity Disorder, pharmacotherapy is much less effective. Stimulants seldom work, and the "second line" agents are sometimes tried—neuroleptics and tricyclic antidepressants— often with no effect, even though neuroleptics should decrease aggression. However, this does not always happen with Conduct Disorders; aggression contin- ues to be present even when side effects (most commonly, sedation) have set in. The tricyclic antidepressants have been found to be more effective than origi- nally thought. They have been found to decrease impulsivity even when no depression is diagnosed. Of course, there is a moderately greater probability of successful treatment of depression than of Conduct Disorder generally. Never- theless, even though there is no good predictability of success by the antidepres- sants, they are worth trying as part of any treatment program. Lithium carbonate has been found to be occasionally effective in reducing violent behavior, and may be tried in appropriate cases. The need for strict clinical and laboratory supervision (serum Lithium levels) makes this a more complicated procedure, especially considering the fact that so many of these families are unreliable and do not follow through with medical advice.

In summary, the general physician should be cognizant of the difficulties in treating *any* Conduct Disorder and refer the child to a specialist.

COURSE AND PROGNOSIS

The undersocialized, aggressive type of Conduct Disorder has the worst progno- sis of all the Conduct Disorders. Nevertheless, the course and prognosis vary with the severity. Severe cases develop into Antisocial Personality Disorders, often in spite of treatment. Milder cases, especially if adequately treated, develop sufficient controls in the course of maturation to achieve stability by the time the individuals are in their twenties. Unfortunately, all these patients are prime recruits for the ranks of delinquents and criminals.

Conduct Disorder, Undersocialized, Nonaggressive (312.10)*

The distinguishing feature of this type is the nonaggressive nature of the antisocial behavior; its essence can best be captured by the definition "sneaky" or

---

*DSM-III code.

"devious," all other characteristics being roughly the same as for the aggressive type.

In psychoanalytic terms, we would refer to these children as "passive-aggressive." Some are shy and may be exploited by others; others are exploitative themselves. It is possible that they resort to these mechanisms because, as a group, they are physically less robust; they feel weak and handle their anger by devious revenge.

CASE 3-3   Jeffrey, age nine, was seen after he had *run away* from home follow-ing an altercation with his parents. He had hidden for over a day in a wooded area bordering the river near his home, and, when found, seemed to *enjoy* the concern everybody had felt because of the possibility that he may have drowned. This was not the first runaway episode, but it was the longest. His history was replete with *failures*—poor schoolwork, no lasting friendships, and a reputation among peers and neighbors of being a *thief and a liar.* Neighbors did not allow him to play with their children as they feared that he was *a bad influence* and, at any rate, seemed only to *use* them, since he seemed to cultivate all other interpersonal relationships purely for *his own gain.* The teachers described him as an *ingratiating and superficially friendly* lad who could, however, *never* be trusted. He was often *truant* from school. He was *dominated* by his peers, with only one of whom he seemed to have developed a more than casual relationship. Actually, this was an older boy who eventually was caught *sexually molesting* Jeffrey.

Jeffrey's *parents* had almost *given up* on him. They *had never* shown a great deal of affection for him, although he was their only child. Instead, they were preoccupied with getting ahead socially, although the father's business dealings were sometimes considered *"shaky."* Jeffrey admitted that the runaway episode was more for *revenge* against his parents than anything else.

Comment. The preceding case highlights the passive-aggressive aspects of this type of Conduct Disorder, as well as the fact that these children are at prime risk for sexual exploitation. The cases show undersocialization but a less overt aggression.

TREATMENT

This is no less difficult than for the aggressive type because of the lack of significant overlap with Attention–Deficit Hyperactivity Disorder, thus eliminat-ing effective trials of pharmacotherapy. On the other hand, this barrier to a feasible treatment is partially offset by the somewhat greater availability of these youngsters for traditional educational and eventual psychotherapeutic approaches.

Behavior modification techniques have been used with some success in this disorder, in combination with the other individual treatment modalities. Again, involvement of the parents is imperative and, of course, the treatment should be left to a specialist, and an imaginative and patient one at that.

Course and prognosis are probably slightly more favorable than in the aggressive type, although development of severe character disorders is the rule rather than the exception.

Conduct Disorder, Socialized, Aggressive (312.23)*

The characteristic features are persistent *aggressiveness*—physical violence against people or property or aggressive thefts (e.g., extortions, burglaries)—combined with *group* loyalty and capacity for empathy and guilt confined mainly to one's group of peers.

CASE 3-4   Johnny was almost 11 years old when he was seen for the third time by the child psychiatrist. He had been known to the police for several years, having been a junior member of a notorious inner-city *street gang*. As such, he had been an active participant in several *burglaries and purse snatchings,* and had even been *an accomplice* in an armed holdup. The gang was known as "The Young Warriors" and its members had taken a "blood oath" of *loyalty.* Johnny indeed observed that loyalty. In other situations, however, he was *crafty and devious.* Moreover, he was *generally a "loser":* poor school record, not particularly popular, and generally not possessing any particular skills.

Comment. The patient described in this case vignette represents the prototypical Conduct Disorder—socialized, aggressive type—the member of a gang, loyalty to which is a source of identity, strength, and self-esteem and, at the same time, a source of morality—a morality at variance with the norm of society, however.

The nonspecialist physician should be aware of sociological views on this particular type of Conduct Disorder which consider it as an adaptive response to family and urban ghetto inadequacies and declaim against our medicalizing the condition. Often arising in the context of a large family with some, but not abject, economic hardship, socialized aggressive Conduct Disorder may be a way of life for many poor children. Discipline is inconsistent but intrafamily relation-ships are never as rejecting or abusive as in the undersocialized Conduct Disorders.

The aforementioned findings are helpful in the *differential diagnosis* of delin-quency: they differentiate the socialized from the undersocialized Conduct Disorders, since both types result in delinquency.

We will discuss the course, prognosis, and treatment of aggressive socialized Conduct Disorder together with the nonaggressive type of socialized Conduct

---

*DSM-III code.

Disorder, since it is the social awareness of these children that makes them more amenable to treatment and allows for a better outlook.

Conduct Disorder, Socialized, Nonaggressive (312.21)*

CASE 3-5   Janet was 12 years old and *habitually* in trouble. Shy and self-effacing, she had nevertheless acquired a reputation of usually *winding up* with somebody in trouble or the companion of delinquents. She was a *follower* and could easily be talked into joining an individual or group for almost anything, as long as it involved *getting something or getting away* with something. This usually meant *petty thefts, smoking marijuana, or "playing hookey" from school*. She was usually friendly but could not be relied upon to tell the truth. Even when it was evident that her friends had led her into trouble and *used* her, she *would not* tell on them and continued to befriend them. For several years, the school's guidance counselor and social worker had tried to help her out of this *losing* pattern, but to no avail. Although the patient indicated *no guilt or remorse*, she was reported to have been *depressed* on several occasions.

Comment. Group loyalty and relatedness to others characterize this case as Conduct Disorder of the socialized type; the lack of confrontation with the children from whom she stole, together with the fact that Janet was passively involved in trouble, confirm the nonaggressive nature of her Conduct Disorder, according to DSM-III.

TREATMENT

As a group, these youngsters are still difficult to treat, but less so than the undersocialized group. The clinician is advised to heed the same warning regarding uncovering "dynamic" psychotherapy as was emphasized in the undersocialized Conduct Disorders: Don't use this therapeutic approach! It can make the patient worse.

Various other treatment approaches can be considered in individual cases, such as "reality therapy," behavior modification, and residential treatment with structure, support, and identification. This is a specialized set of tasks not to be attempted by the nonspecialist. Innovative programs, such as special camps, have shown promise. Poorly staffed residential treatment facilities or badly run

---

*DSM-III code.

correctional institutions have been counterproductive, but when well managed and well staffed, those facilities can be of great help by reorienting these children to different relationships through a prolonged exposure to fairness and predictability. Again, it is the child's basic relatedness to other people that helps to brighten the prognosis with treatment.

COURSE AND PROGNOSIS

Many, perhaps most, of these more socially aware youngsters have a better prognosis than the undersocialized group. They are less self-centered, and their capacity to relate to people make rehabilitation possible. A considerable number seem to "outgrow" their antisocial relationships late in adolescence. They are helped in this by new relationships, especially heterosexual relationships, relationships at school and work, and identification with employers, supervisors, or other stable adults.

CONCLUDING REMARKS ON THE CONDUCT DISORDERS

Conduct Disorders are a difficult category of child psychiatric disorders—not so much in diagnostic terms but rather in terms of therapeutic frustrations to the health professions. Physicians, by nature and by training, want to help. When it comes to Conduct Disorders, the nonspecialist physician, and very often the specialist as well, is left without being able directly to help them and with the frustrating role of incorporating parents' and teachers' fears that these children will continue their long-established patterns of poor functioning.

This, however, is an overly superficial picture. By correctly diagnosing the type of Conduct Disorder, the physician can steer the family, school, and agencies towards potentially helpful resources and thereby at least help diminish the overall suffering of all involved. For more socialized children, the physician can do more than comfort: s/he can be a peripheral, but important, model for positive identification. But the nonspecialist should not be misled into taking that child into a casual form of "treatment." "The road to hell may be paved with good intentions," and ill-advised, though well-meant, maneuvers will result in damage to both parties and spoil the clinician's usefulness for future patients.

Questions for Study and Action

1. How could a child clinical psychologist's testing aid in diagnosis and treatment of a child who has the reputation of stealing, fighting, lying, showing cruelty to

animals, firesetting, and absence of remorse? Write out four other *specific* questions you would ask of the psychologist.

2. How could an educator's evaluation of a conduct-disordered child assist the coordinating physician's diagnosis and treatment? List four *specific* questions you would put to the psychoeducational tester.

3. Other than psychiatric interviewing of child and parents (for mental status, developmental and family history) and psychological and educational testing, write out—in order to get into the practice of doing a proper diagnostic study—six other diagnostic tests or studies or consultations you would wish to have done (i.e., the physician should "order" to be done) for a child such as that described in Question #1.

4. In a subculture with rigid sex-role stereotyping, would deprivation of maternal care, with failure of attachment to her, be more or less influential than deprivation of paternal care? Explain your answer.

5. Child psychiatrists, focusing on the child's perspective, evaluate a child's lacks and intakes of total parenting—not mothering or fathering *per se*—in taking a conduct-disordered child's personal history. Why? Does this run counter to either patricentric or matricentric ideologies of child development? Explain.

6. In the juvenile law there are two classes of children with Conduct Disorders: status offenders and delinquents. Explain the differences between these two types of offenders. Are there any reasons for a physician to know this distinction? Does the legal distinction affect our diagnostic workup, differential diagnosis, treatment, or prognosis? How so?

7. On logical, plausible grounds, show how each of the following childhood traumata could influence a child to have an undersocialized, aggressive Conduct Disorder:
   (a) an eight-year-old girl's sexual abuse by her stepfather;
   (b) an 11-year-old boy's physical abuse by an alcoholic father;
   (c) a 12-year-old girl whose parents divorced after years of violent conflict with one another;
   (d) a 10-year-old boy whose mother is a liberal Catholic and whose father, following a career as a petty criminal, became "born again," converted to a pentecostal sect, and demanded the entire family accompany him to his church's services four times each week.

8. Why are parents' "superego lacunae" of concern to a family therapist when a 10-year-old son is a violent, undersocialized delinquent? What do these parental blindspots-in-conscience have to do with their son's acting out? with their parental empathy? with the child's identification with his parents? Explain, giving examples of parents' conscience deficits.

9. Why is any nine-year-old girl's lack of a close chum to whom she is loyal of psychiatric importance? List five possible disadvantages for a child of this age when there is no close bond to a friend who is not a relative.

10. Why are more black children, in contrast to white ones, at risk of being sent promptly into the justice and correctional system (not the psychiatric system) when they show the same serious misconduct? List four correlates of being black in America that add to that risk.

For Further Reading

Aichhorn, A. *Wayward Youth.* New York: Viking, 1974 (original in German, 1925).

Hersov, L.A., Berger, M., & Shaffer, D. (Eds.). *Aggression and Antisocial Behaviors in Childhood and Adolescence.* Oxford, England: Pergamon, 1978.

Lamb, M.E. Paternal influences on early socioemotional development. *J. Child Psychol. & Psychiatry,* 23:185–190, 1982.

Lewis, D.O. (Ed.). *Vulnerabilities to Delinquency.* New York: Spectrum, 1981.

Marriage, K., Fine, S., Moretti, M., & Haley, G. Relationship between depression and conduct disorder in children and adolescents. *J. Amer. Acad. Child Psychiatry,* 25:687–691, 1986.

Mednick, S.A., & Christiansen, K.O. (Eds.). *Biosocial Bases of Criminal Behavior.* New York: Gardner Press, 1977.

Mitchell, S., & Rosa, P. Boyhood behavior problems as precursors of criminality: A 15-year follow-up study. *J. Child Psychol. & Psychiatry,* 22:19–33, 1981.

Richman, N., Stevenson, J., & Graham, P. *Preschool To School: A Behavioural Study.* London: Academic Press, 1982.

Rutter, M., Tizard, J., & Whitmore, K. (Eds.). *Education, Health and Behaviour.* London: Longman, 1970.

West, D.J. *Delinquency: Its Roots, Careers and Prospects.* Cambridge, MA: Harvard University Press, 1982.

Wolff, S. Non-delinquent disturbances of conduct. In Rutter, M. & Hersov, L. (Eds.). *Child and Adolescent Psychiatry. Modern Approaches,* 2nd edition. Oxford: Blackwell Scientific Publications, 1985.

4

Oppositional Defiant Disorder

DEFINITION

Oppositional Defiant Disorder is a nondelinquent "conduct" disorder shown by children who are disobedient, defiant, negativistic, angry, and aggressive in their opposition to adults. DSM-III-R calls this Oppositional Defiant Disorder (313.81) and groups it with Attention-Deficit Hyperactivity Disorder and Conduct Disorders under "Disruptive Behavior Disorders." For at least six months the child has shown at least five of the following nine indicators:

1. frequent loss of temper
2. arguing with adults
3. frequent active defiance or refusal of adult requests or rules, e.g., refusing to do home chores
4. frequent deliberately annoying behavior, e.g., grabbing other children's hats
5. frequent blaming of others for one's own mistakes
6. frequent touchiness or easy annoyance by others
7. frequent anger and resentment
8. frequent spiteful and vindictive behavior
9. frequent swearing or obscenity in speech

81

The indicators must occur at times other than during the course of Conduct Disorder, Dysthymic Disorder, or an episode of hypomania, Mania or Major Depression, or an episode of Schizophrenia or Pervasive Developmental Disorder, if the diagnosis is to be Oppositional Defiant Disorder.

The "oppositional personality disorder of childhood" was described by the Group for the Advancement of Psychiatry (GAP) Committee on Child Psychiatry in 1966; for them the term was for a class of children who show prominent trends along the spectrum from passive to aggressive (passive-aggressive) or from obedient to defiant. It is very much like a prodrome of the Passive Aggressive Personality Disorder of adults (Axis II of DSM-III-R).

For some, it would not be conceivable that a child could be "oppositional" were the child and parents not living under the sway of the fourth commandment: *"Honor thy father and mother that thy days may be long on the earth"* (i.e., so they will not make you a victim of infanticide!). For others, some rules must be promulgated but they should summarize and enshrine happy, successful ways in which children have behaved already and not be rules imposed anew from out of the blue. "Discipline" means self-control more than punishment, some others assert. Discipline has more than a punitive referent; discipline is a kind of voluntary discipleship, for example, and has to do with one's own willing, sometimes eager, learning from a generous teacher.

Only against the context of adult authority (of both rational and irrational types) do the descriptors of Oppositional Defiant Disorder (ODD) make sense: disobedient, negativistic, confronting, resistive, provocative, dawdling, foot-dragging, defiant, argumentative, obnoxious. Those, being terms that critical parents would use, make ODD a disorder still to be documented as a true mental disorder of children. In community surveys, cases of oppositionalism are of too great incidence to be a mental disorder.

ETIOLOGY AND PATHOGENESIS

School and family difficulties rise to prominence in cases of oppositional disorder, hence the authority imposed by home and school may help to set the tone for the genesis of this disorder. The first signs of something like Oppositional Defiant Disorder emerge between 18 and 36 months of age as a normal developmental phase but the true disorder emerges only when the signs persist for at least six months, after 36 months and before 18 years of age. We have little information about predisposing and precipitating conditions but it seems logical to suppose that parents and teachers who impose arbitrary, irrational authority on children will exacerbate any temperamentally derived influences residing within the child. Again, a temperamentally "difficult" infant may grow into having a case of Oppositional Defiant Disorder. The "difficult" infant is characterized by irregular biorhythms, frequent and intense negative affect, withdrawal from novelty, and slow adaptation to change, but is still adjudged to be *difficult* by the caregiver.

The characterization of authority types by Erich Fromm (1944) remains apt. Irrational authority in Fromm's view is not based on love or reason but merely on brute force and hierarchy. It says, Tarzan-like, "Me adult, you child. As a stronger person with greater entitlements than you, I say *you must,* so you must. I do not have to give reasons but you must obey because I say so. I can make you do as I say." The more rational authority of adults has been well described by Summerhill's Alexander S. Neill, Paul L. Adams, and others (1971); rational authority is based on empathic love and fairness, and reasonableness.

CLINICAL DESCRIPTION

The diagnostic criteria given depict the condition as it appears clinically. The next case vignette exemplifies more of what a clinician observes in ODD.

CASE 4-1   David was 11 years old when his parents, moving to a new city, sought out the child psychiatrist to whom they had been referred. When the parents were seen initially, the father did most of the talking with the mother deferring to him but shaking her head in quiet disagreement with some of the father's pronouncements. David's problems dated back to kindergarten, the parents said.

The father declared, "David's problems are *lying, refusing to cooperate, threatening to run away,* and *getting upset* when we impose *strict discipline.* But he *eggs us on.* He shows *no respect or obedience.* He *argues* with us about everything and constantly *accuses grownups of being unfair.* He *bullies* his little sister and anyone else he can." The mother stated, "But my husband, not just David, is also the villain of the piece," for she felt her husband baited the boy and gave him arbitrary orders that were insulting and uncalled for.

David, seen alone, stated that his father and his little sister were "the problem" and encouraged the child psychiatrist to "psychoanalyze" his little sister. His whole tone was one of *"edginess"* and his talk was *sarcastic, demeaning of others, complaining.* He made the child psychiatrist feel that David was being a *first-strike "badmouther"* who seemed to feel deeply hurt and put upon.

David grumbled peevishly that his father, himself "a lazy oaf," made David work too hard; indeed, the lawn that the lad was required to mow each week was just under 2½ acres. The father was heard to scream at David in the waiting room, "You are *not* an adult. I can break you and I will. I am stronger than you are. You don't tell *me* what to do!"

Comment. Later, the parents recounted that David had been verbal and outspoken, indeed since kindergarten, but that his obstreperousness had begun only when he was eight years old when his father, losing his traveling job, had returned home to live for one year. The father had been depressed and irritable; the boy had become the father's scapegoat.

DIFFERENTIAL DIAGNOSIS

The Axis I diagnosis of Oppositional Defiant Disorder (ODD) is differentiated from other disorders in the following ways:

1. *Conduct Disorder*—by ODDs not violating others' basic rights, not violating major societal norms and rules.
2. *Oppositional behavior between 18 and 36 months of age*—by ODDs' age being 3-18 years.
3. *Parent-Child problem*—by the ODDs being more severe and not restricted to parents because peers, teachers, and other adults are involved.
4. *Schizophrenia or Pervasive Developmental Disorder*—if either of these is present, because they are more severe, the diagnosis should not be recorded as Oppositional Defiant Disorder. The same applies to Conduct Disorder and Obsessive Compulsive Disorder, both of which have more serious signs and symptoms than ODD. However, concurrent diagnoses of Oppositional Defiant Disorder and Attention–Deficit Hyperactive Disorder, Mental Retardation and chronic Organic Mental Disorder can be recorded.

TREATMENT AND PROGNOSIS

Untreated, the ODD may become a Conduct Disorder (Axis I) of childhood, a Passive Aggressive Personality Disorder (Axis II) of later life, or an Antisocial Personality Disorder (Axis II). The course is chronic and attended by much interpersonal pain, with school and family problems often waxing to the point of utter failure in both spheres and peer relations that are not truly rewarding and happy.

The treatment modalities for ODD are of three categories: *behavioral* (by working directly with the child or by training the parents in reinforcement strategies), *emotional and cognitive*, and *family group*. The family group approach may be used in addition to either of the first two treatment programs. Family group therapy centers on the interactions, then and there, of parents and child(ren). When behavior therapy is applied to children's aggression, it is to be remembered that ignoring misbehavior is more effective than responding to it, and best of all is the positive reinforcement of acceptable behavior. When emotive-cognitive therapy is used the therapist must remember to foster parenting, comforting, and attachment, as well as to use teaching and advocacy techniques.

Questions for Study and Action

1. Define each of the following terms clearly: passive noncompliance, active resistance; resistive behavior, negativistic behavior; rational authority, irrational authority; a child with initiative and spunk, an aggressive child, a difficult child (Thomas & Chess, 1977).

2. Propose a convincing and psychiatrically sound counterargument to the following:

    When he was principal of a Harlem school, Elliot Shapiro tried out a curriculum consisting mostly of expressing hostility—the children gave talks, wrote compositions, and acted out why they hated their parents, their siblings, the police, the school's principal. The procedure raised their IQs, for stupidity is a character defense of turned-in hostility.

3. An angry mother returned with her oppositional child for a second interview, demanding to be seen before the child psychiatrist saw the child. Write out an intelligent and workable response to the following message she had for the doctor:

    I do not intend to bring Rambo for a third appointment because it is obvious to my husband and me that you have no understanding of our lifestyle. You asked us if we gave the kid an allowance, a thing we definitely do not believe in; our idea is that children work for any money we give out. We are strict about that and have no wish to coddle Rambo or his brother and sister. And you also asked if there was any meal that we all sat down for; we are so busy running around doing all the chores that need doing that we do not even have regular meals individually. Each person eats at different times and it is usually some fast food snack picked up and brought home for the children.

    Be kind!

4. Since the diagnosis of Oppositional Defiant Disorder is more one of social or political polemics than of biomedical indexing and categorizing, make a case for its being placed on Axis II in a future version of the *Diagnostic and Statistical Manual of Mental Disorders*. What weight would you give in your argument to each of the following circumstances? The Group for the Advancement of Psychiatry in 1966 proposed it as a personality disorder, not as a well-crystallized syndrome or neurosis; the affected children are lacking age-appropriate ego strengths; the appraisal of the child depends so heavily on the moral valuations of parents and teachers; the ultimate outcome, when untreated, is both uncertain and consists mainly of legal problems; it is a congeries of symptoms that may underlie Depression, Schizophrenia, Sociopathic or Antisocial Personality Disorder, ADHD, Parent-Child Problem, Pervasive Developmental Disorder, Obsessive Compulsive Disorder, and so on.

5. Make an argument for David's case, in this chapter, as a parent-child problem and not a true mental disorder. Explain fully.

6. Successful parenting is often portrayed as a triumph of helping empathy over such distortions as projective identification, narcissistic identification, splitting, role reversal, and identification with the aggressor. These will be explained more fully in the section of this book entitled "Being a Victim." For now, write down *six actual behaviors* that David's father could have shown towards the boy to display an attitude of helping empathy. Explain how empathy is embodied in each behavior by the father.

7. The Bible, frequently cited by Jews, Christians, and Muslims alike, exhorts children to keep the fourth commandment, "Honor thy father and mother that thy days may be long on the earth." Believers have sustained an air of tension about the correct kind of relations between parents and children, because they also believe that parents should not "provoke children to wrath." Assort the following under two columns entitled *Honor parents or be killed* and *Don't provoke your children to wrath:* child battering occurred without any law against it until late in the 19th century; a high rate of infanticide in 19th century Paris; opposition to laws against child labor until it was finally outlawed in 1946 in the USA; child's keeping the secret that a father has incestuous relations with his young daughter; the popularity of Dr. Spock's *Book of Baby & Child Care;* the popularity of "free schools" (like Summerhill or Satori) among urban upper-middle-class parents; the greater prevalence of intersibling violence over child-against-parent violence in the USA.

8. In view of the complicated differential diagnosis for cases of ODD, map out the necessary diagnostic studies and consultants you would need for diagnosing accurately a child such as David. Explain each diagnostic endeavor.

9. Why would work with parents and school be essential with cases of ODD? How would you go about this work?

10. Outline an initial family group session with David, his sister, his mother, and his father, i.e., make an agenda for the first family group meeting. Explain each item on the agenda.

For Further Reading

Adams, P.L., Berg, L., Berger, N., Duane, M., Neill, A.S., & Ollendorff, R.H.V. *Children's Rights: Toward the Liberation of the Child.* New York: Praeger, 1971.

Fromm, E. Individual and social origins of neurosis. *Am. J. Sociology,* 9:3, 1944.

Group for the Advancement of Psychiatry, Committee on Child Psychiatry. *Psychopathological Disorders in Childhood: Theoretical Considerations and a Proposed Classification.* New York: Group for the Advancement of Psychiatry, 1966.

Thomas, A., & Chess, S. *Temperament and Development.* New York: Brunner/Mazel, 1977.

Thomas, A., Chess, S., & Birch, H.G. *Temperament and Behavior Disorders in Children.* New York: New York University Press, 1968.

5

Episodic and Organic Disorders of Behavior

A full listing of episodic and organic disorders would require an encyclopedic text and would include many disorders that are very rare in childhood. Hence, we include only a sampling of episodic-organic problems in this chapter.

Somewhat arbitrarily, we defer a discussion of the major Organic Mental Disorders to Chapter 24; because we want to emphasize the impedance of higher cortical functions in those disorders, we group them among Thinking and Central Processing Disorders. A quick inspection of Chapter 24 at this point shows their relation to central processing disturbances.

For this chapter, we consider "organic" disorders which have mainly *behavioral* oddities, outbursts, and cardinal signs: Organic Personality Disorder (310.10), which we take to include Intermittent Explosive Disorder (312.34) in children, and only these five Psychoactive Substance-Induced Organic Mental Disorders: Alcohol Intoxication (303.00), Alcohol Idiosyncratic Intoxication (291.40), Amphetamine Intoxication (305.70), Cocaine Intoxication (305.60), and Phencyclidine Intoxication (305.90). Although children may show aberrant behavior after ingesting many other substances, we believe the basics can be learned from our discussion of an abbreviated list.

DEFINITION

This chapter discusses children with outbursts of aggressive, disordered behavior occurring mainly in the context of a brain disorder. Child psychiatry keeps grappling with angry, assaultive, impulsively aggressive children, having to use a classification scheme that is modeled on the patterns of adults not of children.

Young persons regularly may be docile, passive, and peaceful but they intermittently burst out into flurries of aggressive behavior. We saw some of that unpredictability in the preceding chapters on Conduct and Oppositional Defiant Disorders—those who endanger others, set fires, and assault. The Disruptive Behavior Disorders in DSM-III-R include Attention-Deficit Hyperactivity Disorder (ADHD) (314.01), Oppositional Defiant Disorder (313.81), and Conduct Disorder (312.20, 312.00, 312.90); all may have some episodic flare-ups but they are not as dramatic as those we consider now.

The episodic nature of their children's strange behavior baffles the untutored parent or teacher, even while it gives strong hints of an organic mental disorder (or organic brain syndrome) to the physician. Any child showing off-then-on assaultiveness needs to have a central nervous system and mental state evaluation, a careful drug history, and perhaps a neuropsychologic test battery. We return to this under the subsections on Diagnostic Workup and Differential Diagnosis. In this brief presentation we cannot give a complete discussion of the multitude of considerations that are called for but we shall give a beginning consideration.

Episodic disorders of behavior are of multiple etiology and myriad form. All those listed under the title of this chapter are surely included but, in truth, some of the Mood Disorders and Anxiety Disorders may also be episodic in their day-by-day occurrence, just as all of the impulse control disorders may be (see especially the chapters on Firesetting, Conduct Disorders, and Oppositional Defiant Disorder). Indeed, aggression is a frequent finding among any "acting-out" children whose relations to others may be impaired. But it is the merging of acting out with organicity that engages our attention now.

ETIOLOGY

The major consequences of histogenic, genogenic, or chemogenic disorder, such as head injury, epilepsy, and PCP or amphetamine intoxication in children, may reside in the disturbances of their relations with others that their brain disorder triggers. Whatever the specific lesions of the brain, it is how they disorder the child's behavior in the interpersonal sphere that matters a great deal. What we desire to convey here is our conviction that, because of the nature of frontally corticated humankind with a highly elaborated prosencephalon, human biology cannot exclude the psychic and social from its comprehensive perspective. We regard the biopsychosocial model as the most useful one for conceptualizing etiology and pathophysiology, even with proven brain disorders. The forebrain's highest achievement may be that it enables us to use symbols that link us to one another; in short, our cerebral advantage is that we *can* live in fuller communication with our fellows. Hence, the interpersonal ramifications of a brain disorder may be very crippling.

EXPLOSIVE DISORDERS (OR DISORDERS OF IMPULSE CONTROL)

CLINICAL DESCRIPTION

Today, the human failure to curb and moderate our aggressive impulses is evident in conventional living as well as in deviant lifestyles (or chaotic lack of lifestyle). Aggressive outbursts are seen everywhere. According to DSM-III, now superseded, explosive disorders could be repetitive *or* unitary and isolated in frequency of occurrence. An Intermittent Explosive Disorder's diagnostic criteria would be these four:

1. Numerous episodes of aggressive outbursts that have led the child to assault others or to destroy property.
2. Aggressive episodes show a dyscontrol of assaultiveness or destruction that goes far beyond what may be warranted by any precipitating conditions.
3. Behavior other than during the episodes is not generally impulsive or aggressive.
4. The "berserk" behavior is not due to Schizophrenia or other psychosis, Conduct Disorder, Mania, or Intoxication by psychoactive drugs. (See DSM-III Quick Reference, p. 165.)

Since the symptom-free intervals of criterion 3 occur rarely *and* since most cases that do approximate the other criteria have proven to be due to central nervous system damage, these rather shaky diagnostic categories might have been subsumed, in DSM-III-R, under Organic Personality Disorder (explosive type) (310.10). Certainly, for child psychiatry we shall deal with the Organic Personality Disorder now instead of in its DSM-III-R listed sequence under the Organic Mental Disorders because that is, in our experience, what most "intermittent explosions" of children truly are.

Organic Personality Disorder (Explosive Type) (310.10)
(Includes Intermittent Explosive Disorder [312.34])

DEFINITION

The Organic Personality Disorder cannot be diagnosed in a child who meets only the criteria for Attention-Deficit Hyperactivity Disorder (ADHD), i.e., who is merely hyperactive, inattentive, and impulsive but without additional evidence of a specific brain disorder. But if the child meets all criteria for ADHD and shows the following characteristics, in addition to those of ADHD, the diagnosis can be made. These are the criteria (DSM-III-R) of the explosive Organic Personality Disorder:

1. Marked deviation in personality or behavior involving *at least one* of the following:
   (a) emotional lability—quick shifts from smiling to crying
   (b) sudden explosive outbursts of temper
   (c) impaired impulse control—deficient social judgment, sexual indiscretions, recklessness, stealing
   (d) marked apathy, indifference, or disinterest in former games or hobbies, "amotivational syndrome"
   (e) suspiciousness or paranoid ideation with no evident basis in reality
2. No clouding of consciousness—i.e., not Delirium; no prominent loss of intellectual abilities—i.e., not Dementia; no predominant disturbance of mood—i.e., not Organic Affective Disorder; no predominant delusions or hallucinations—i.e., not Organic Delusional Disorder or Organic Hallucinosis.
3. Evidence (from history, physical exam or lab tests) of a specific organic factor that can be tied etiologically to the disturbance.
4. Not entirely accountable to Attention–Deficit Hyperactivity Disorder.

CLINICAL DESCRIPTION

As we stated earlier, the child with the explosive type of Organic Personality Disorder (310.10) shows more "organicity" than the classic case of Attention-Deficit Hyperactivity Disorder and "harder" signs of neural impairment than the "soft" ones of ADHD. Organicity (or "organically impaired") is not a precise term but it has some sensible referents. The cardinal signs of organicity are: 1) impaired memory; 2) impaired judgment; 3) impaired speech and praxis; 4) impaired handwriting and figure drawing; and, sometimes, 5) a disturbance of orientation to time, place or person. To these five can be added for certain cases of organicity: 6) labile and shallow affect; 7) decreased attention or attentiveness;

8) impulsiveness; 9) hyperkinesis and agitation; and 10) concrete thinking with inability to deal with abstractions. All of these indicate that something may be awry in the cerebral functioning of the child. They indicate impairment of higher cortical functions—intellection, cognition, attention, memory, judgment, speech, and handwriting.

In the clinical interview with a child, especially in a formal mental state exam, memory can be tested readily and will show deficient recent, intermediate-term, and remote recall. A child who knows that (s)he has an impaired memory may respond, "I used to know (remember) that but sometimes I don't now." Or the child will fumble and say, "I tried to remember it but I couldn't." Or wild guesses will be made with or without apologetic concern, guesses that are oddly off the point. Occasionally, secondarily, such a child will confabulate to gloss over the memory impairment. Confabulation is not the same as lying when pressured, or imaginative fabrication of events, or *pseudologia phantastica;* confabulation is more like "jive talk," for it often substitutes a pleasant verbiage in place of directly answering a question that tests the child's errant memory and, if an answer were to be given, it would reveal the child's faulty remembering.

Impaired judgment may be displayed if the child shows, during interview, a lack of stranger-reticence: to ask the doctor, for example, "You like me, don't you? I like you," and to hug or kiss the doctor whom (s)he has just met. The child "behaves inappropriately," we say. Or a child may be reckless and dangerous in what (s)he does on the playground or in the heavily trafficked street. Or a lack of tact—disinhibition—may be manifest. Another term for tact is *social intelligence:* knowing not to assault an adult without provocation, not commenting on another person's missing finger or withered limb as soon as it is observed, not scarfing up the last five cookies, not urinating in the corner of a doctor's office, and so on.

Impaired speech and praxis are discernible whenever, for example, slurring occurs and is noted by the examiner, or when a child's speech is indistinct and overuses elision, sounding like the overdrawn TV inebriate's mispronunciation. If a clumsy dyspraxia, as shown by an inability to arrange match sticks in a simple pattern, and an unsteady gait accompany the impaired speech, the diagnosis would more likely be that of an Intoxication. In Organic Personality Disorder the dyslalia and dyspraxia are characteristically more subtle than would appear in acute Intoxication.

But the test phrases of earlier days in neuropsychiatry may still produce telling results. One asks the child, "Will you say *Methodist Episcopal?* Please say, '*Around the rugged rock the ragged rascal ran.*' Faster, please." If those phrases are repeated accurately and at quickened pace, there is likely no speech disorder denoting organicity.

Overenunciation and oversyllabization of speech are characteristic of multiple sclerosis' scanning speech, when the jerky enunciation of each syllable reminds the hearer of a poem being scanned.

Oh, MAry HAD a LITtle LAMB
Its FLEECE was WHITE as SNOW. . . .

Impaired handwriting and figure drawing can be elicited by giving the Bender Gestalt or Draw-a-Figure test. One of us likes to ask the child to write his signature, then on a separate paper to write down his favorite foods or an ideal menu. The signature is preserved intact in most cases but the constructed list will show unevenness, variations in letter size, tremors, and other signs of organicity borne in the handwriting alterations.

Disturbed orientation to time and place is almost as "cardinal" a sign of organic brain damage as are impaired memory, judgment, speech, and handwriting, and, if present, disorientation will be very influential for the diagnostician. Disorientation is tested in the three spheres of temporal, spatial, and interpersonal. The patient with organicity may have disordered bearings.

1. Time—does not know today's date, month, or year or whether it is morning, afternoon, or night;
2. Space—does not recognize in which state and city (s)he is being interviewed, in what clinic or hospital, etc.;
3. Person—lacks his/her bearings about the interpersonal significance of persons in his/her milieu. For example, he/she does not fathom that the interviewer is a physician, that the team member is a nurse or social worker, or that these are all professionals set up to help a child. Many beginners in child psychiatry misunderstand "orientation to person," believing that it includes only a knowledge of one's own name, but it also covers correct sizing up of the others around one and a grasp of what they are there for.

Labile and shallow affect is nearly always a cardinal sign of organicity and is a part of the behavioral mosaic resulting from fronto-parieto-temporal dysfunctions. It is a diagnostic criterion for Organic Personality Syndrome. Few children with organicity, in our experience, show as conspicuous an emotional lability as is frequently seen in demented, aged persons. Lability, like the explosive outbursts, may be unroofed surprisingly, however, with the barest frustrations that arise during an interview.

Inattention shows itself most readily when digit span is tested. A resident once said that such a child "repeats digits by jumbling them up like a dyslexic reading a word."

Impulsiveness will be characterized in Chapter 21 on Attention–Deficit Hyperactivity Disorder (ADHD) (q.v.). It is not wholly dissimilar from lability and explosiveness.

Hyperkinesis is defined under ADHD.

Impaired abstracting can be tested by asking the child, "What's funny about . . . ?" and relating a simple joke. Also, one can ask the child to interpret proverbs like "A stitch in time saves nine," or "You can drive a horse to water but you can't make him drink," or the old favorite, "People who live in glass houses should not throw stones." Computing serial sevens or threes, three times five, four times 19 are calculations ordinarily done correctly by a sixth-grader, but will be impaired in some cases with organicity.

CASE 5-1   Miguel was 10½ years old when he was riding in the front seat of his family's automobile, not wearing a seat belt. Although his mother was driving slowly and carefully on an expressway, locally called The Mixmaster, with numerous levels of curving lanes of highway crisscrossing, there suddenly appeared a truck—falling from two tiers above them onto their car. Miguel's *mother died instantly* and Miguel spent the next 17 days in *a comatose state* in neurosurgical intensive care. On the 17th day, having had his certain death foretold by the doctors, Miguel sat erect on his bed and asked if there was anyone with whom he could play "Dungeons and Dragons." There was much talk of *the miracle* of his survival and many comparisons of his recovery of consciousness to a *resurrection from death.* His father said that *only divine intervention* could have saved Miguel, and the father made promises to live in celibacy and to make novenas of gratitude and joy for his son and retreats and pilgrimages of respectful sorrow for his departed spouse.

Miguel had been promoted to the eighth grade before the accident occurred, for he was *a superior student* who had been allowed to skip past both third and sixth grades. He was the only Latino in his class who had been placed in a special program for *talented and gifted* students. At school he was eager, teachable, and docile. He was *an only child,* much *pampered* and beloved by both of his parents, and he had been *treated as special* because he was just that—before his head injury.

After the accident, Miguel took *little interest in school work* and could not stay in the gifted child program, but during the eighth grade his teachers remained lenient, reassured by the fact that, although he did no homework and spent his class periods *fidgeting* and *distracted,* Miguel's standardized achievement testing was still *above his grade level* and his reading *scored at the 11th grade level.* At home, Miguel's father noted that the 11-year-old had had a decided *change of personality.* Miguel became *unkempt* and *disheveled;* just getting him to bathe even once a week was an ordeal; he became *chronically tardy.* He claimed he *hated school,* his teachers, and his classmates. He would *flare up in belligerency* against his father even though his father compulsively spoke quietly to Miguel and attempted never to rattle or upset him. Miguel ceased being as enspirited and enthusiastic about life as he had seemed before the death of his mother.

For a month or more, Miguel cried some about his mother's death but far more of his later tears were angry, frustrated tears of *exasperation outbursts* both at home and at school. He was called "very *explosive,* very *changeable* and changes moods very suddenly" by the school counselor. His homeroom teacher saw him as "having one *microtantrum* after another." He quickly lost both his best chum and some of his more casual playmates; thus, by the end of the eighth grade he was *friendless and lonely.* At home, in rages, he broke up dishware and radios. He often *looked perplexed* and made some comments to his father which sounded bizarre: "I am immortal. I am impervious to harm. I rose from the dead." Hence, in the summer before Miguel entered ninth grade, when he was still 11 years old, his father sought a psychiatric evaluation for Miguel.

Miguel was a handsome, small lad who looked more *indio* than *castellano* (more American Indian than Spaniard) and was at the eighth percentile for height and weight, so he looked a bit like an addlepated little Hispanic professor to the examining psychiatrist. His speech was appropriate as far as his vocabulary was concerned, but occasionally he made *comments that seemed off-the-point* and he would not explain or rephrase what he had said. At times, he seemed to be *searching for the correct word* and, not finding it, would change the subject. His speech seemed both *overly deliberate* and slightly *slurred* and dysarthric. Digit-span testing revealed *inattention* and *impatience.* "Stop that shit," he would yell out, *menacing* his clenched fists to the examiner. He was *well-oriented* for time, place, and person, but his *handwriting was crude, irregular, and clumsy* for a boy so bright and verbal. He *wrote his name clearly* and without any abnormality. IQ testing showed *deficits in performance IQ,* notably in *block design, coding,* and *object assembly,* but a *verbal IQ of 130* with some evidences of having been higher in the past, according to the clinical psychologist. His Bender Gestalt test was abnormal. EEG, CAT scan, and skull roentgenograms were *not diagnostic of any cranial abnormality.* The father concurred when the child psychiatrist met with him to interpret the findings and to offer a diagnosis of Organic Personality Disorder following a closed head injury.

During the sixth month of once-weekly visits designed to help Miguel obtain a better view of himself and his milieu despite his organicity, the boy became starkly paranoid, believing that his father had engineered the truck falling onto his mother's car. Himself suspecting some interpersonal, father-son storm, the psychiatrist asked the father to join Miguel and him for a few sessions. It was revealed that father had "toughened up his act with Miguel," having become less attentive and solicitous when Miguel had an angry, explosive outburst. Father's *walking away and "ignoring the tornado"* had reduced the frequency of the firestorms.

Miguel, on hearing this, apologized to his father but claimed that *some of his rage attacks could not be prevented,* that he felt *powerless to control them.* The father had also "reentered the sex market," he said, but he felt guilty that he had been patronizing "bad women" and wondered if Miguel would "permit me to date nice women," whereupon Miguel "pitched a fit," wept, and whined, and accused the father of wanting to "betray mama." Within six more months, Miguel was much better organized, happier, and had a positive attitude towards his new stepmother.

Comment. Miguel had several of the signs of organicity to warrant his case being diagnosed as one of Organic Personality Disorder. He misperceived, was both suspicious and grandiose, but was not psychotic. He met the diagnostic criteria for ADHD but went beyond that less ominous diagnosis. Although he was able to think abstractly and stay well oriented, to give apt interpretations of proverbs, to subtract serial sevens and do calculations, he showed:

impaired memory
impaired judgment
impaired speech and praxis
impaired handwriting and Bender Gestalt drawings
labile affect
deficient attention
impulsiveness
explosive rage outbursts
hyperkinesis

Organicity, it must be conceded, is a diffuse concept for organic brain dysfunction, but for a case like that of Miguel it has some utility. Miguel had no hard and stark signs of intracranial pathology but his history of prolonged coma can be taken to denote a closed head injury, the organic etiology of his organic personality disorder. It must be obvious that his interactions with his father, stepmother, teachers, peers, and child psychiatrist were also telling circumstances, along with his head injury.

DIAGNOSTIC WORKUP FOR ORGANICITY
(ESPECIALLY FOR ORGANIC PERSONALITY DISORDER)

Having taken a detailed history of both the child's premorbid functioning and the child's present dysfunctions, the diagnostician observes the child and notes carefully any indices of organicity as they have been discussed in the foregoing subsections. The mental state examination is extremely important as a way of systematizing and codifying one's efforts to understand more about the child's mental disorder. The physical and neurological examinations may give further knowledge. Next, after observation (looking, listening, palpating, percussing) has been done well, two other options arise for the doctor's progression towards more effective understanding: 1) laboratory studies and 2) consultations with others on the health team.

Laboratory studies that may be ordered in a case such as Miguel's would be: radiologic studies of the skull and other bones (for fractures of the skull and for bone age determination); electroencephalogram (preferably after sleep-deprivation); computerized axial tomography (CAT); or other radio-imaging devices such as nuclear magnetic resonance. Spinal fluid tap (for chemical analysis and dynamics) did not seem to be indicated for Miguel. More familiar screens for ruling out anemia and for measuring thyroid or renal or hepatic functioning might also be requested, since they can be included in chemical laboratory assays that are not terribly expensive and provide some reassurance that the child is a healthy physical specimen. A similar cost-to-benefit ratio applies to a urinalysis and complete blood count.

Consultations with other health-team members may include a speech-and-language expert (called communication disorders specialists in some settings), a pediatric neurologist, a neurosurgeon, and a clinical psychologist.

Then, besides those in the hospital or medical center, there are certainly some school personnel whom the clinician will wish to consult. The school personnel can be engaged through mail correspondence or, preferably, during a school visit by the physician. At such a school-based conference, the doctor would hope to see assembled the homeroom teacher, the principal, the father (in Miguel's case), Miguel himself, and any school psychologist, social worker, or counselor who has had some true contact with the child both before and after his head injury.

Now, returning to those who are at the medical center, the reader may wonder why we would suggest calling in the communication disorders specialist, and neurological, neurosurgical, and clinical psychology experts. The professional work of each of these would be of value: the communication disorders person to do psycholinguistic testing and to identify the speech difficulty and any suggested treatment for it; the pediatric neurologist to assess current status and make prognostication and occasionally to aid in treatment planning (epilepsy, focal lesions); the neurosurgeon to comment on the history and previous treatments as well as to help assess his current functioning; and the clinical psychologist to help assess intellectual, emotional, and behavioral status. The clinical psychologist's testing of IQ joins with her/his testing of imaginative productions or projections and testing of scholastic skills to produce a highly worthwhile interchange between psychologist and child psychiatrist. The child benefits from the work of all the team. Unfortunately, all of the team's heads put together usually do not determine the location or extent of the child's brain pathology.

Although the specific etiology for Organic Personality Disorder can include degenerative, proliferative, infectious, and toxic conditions, all of which must be considered, it is the head injury—as in Miguel's case—following a traffic accident that most often provokes the chronic brain syndrome and, moreover, becomes a major killer of young persons.

DIFFERENTIAL DIAGNOSIS

We cannot be complete and exhaustive here but Organic Personality Disorder (OPD) can be differentiated from some other disorders in the following ways:

1. *Dementia*—OPD shows a lessened degree of intellectual decrement.
2. *Organic Affective Disorder*—In OPD there is lability but not a sustained mood disorder, manic, depressed, or mixed.
3. *Organic Delusional Disorder*—A case of OPD does not show prominent delusional thinking.
4. *Organic Hallucinosis*—The OPD case is not hallucinating.
5. *Delirium*—The OPD case shows no real clouding of consciousness and is not as "off-base" as the delirious child (e.g., with a high fever).
6. *Organic Anxiety Disorder*—The case of OPD lacks panic attacks or generalized anxiety.
7. *Amnestic Disorder*—OPD does not show severe memory loss as its main symptom.
8. *Intoxication*—This one is tougher but can be differentiated by urine and serum screens and a detailed drug history that are negative. Unfortunately, many of the antiepileptic drugs may prompt or exacerbate many signs of OPD.
9. *Epilepsy*—If seizures *are* present, they are coexistent with OPD and should be recorded on Axis III. Complex partial/psychomotor/temporal lobe epilepsy often shows in behavior disorders, automatisms, and rage outbursts, so these need to be ruled out in any episodic behavior disorder.

TREATMENT AND PROGNOSIS

The treatment encompasses the parent(s), the child's behavior problems, educational or learning problems, cognitive impairments, emotional outbursts, and difficulties in peer relationships. If a comprehensive treatment program is devised, it can alter the otherwise grave prognosis, but the prognosis even when a child's brain has been injured is not as gloomy as in an adult with a similar lesion. The plasticity of even neural tissue in children may account for the favorable adult outcome of brain-damaged children who had, in their childhood, profound psychiatric disorders, but a treatment program is urgently required.

The treatment modalities for helping parents are mainly counseling, or "talking therapy," to alleviate their perplexity in knowing how to relate to their changed child with a newly manifested Organic Personality Disorder. The parents are helped by ventilating their doubts about their own competency, fears for the future, and quandaries in the present. They require encouragement to talk with the child, to empathize with their handicapped child, not to abdicate their parenting role(s), and to assist in carrying out the treatment plan for the child. Eventually, they will see that, with their and the psychiatrist's help, the child is still mainly a child and that (s)he has kept intact some of his/her premorbid capabilities. The brain damage seldom is totally debilitating and, given help, the child will learn more adaptive coping and be able to participate in many facets of normal childhood.

The child's treatment may include the following: behavior therapy, for, after all, his/her episodic behavior disorder and social skills deficit are a major part of the presenting picture; dynamic–verbal, or "expressive," therapy for gaining better emotional and cognitive control; an individualized educational program to minimize the cognitive, perceptual memory and motor problems; and psycho-pharmacologic agents to reduce some of the symptomatic behavior.

The pharmacotherapeutic agents to be employed do have some potential disadvantages. The major tranquilizers—even thioridazine which is often favored—add to the sedation and withdrawal that a child may manifest between outbursts, even if he/she reduces the outbursts' incidence. Thioridazine, like the other neuroleptics, may interfere with the child's sexual feelings and capabilities, too. And, finally, the major tranquilizers have parkinsonian effects (euphemistically called "side effects") immediately, and there lurks the possibility of tardive dyskinesia.

If we turn to psychostimulants and antidepressants, we find that methylphenidate may enhance rote learning and memorizing as a result of increased concentration, just as it does with ADHD cases—a desirable goal at times, but it restricts the focalized learning by blocking out all peripheral cues that are so indispensable in making learning and discovery enjoyable for most children. Imipramine, the drug of choice for many young persons with a clinical picture like Miguel's, could worsen the epileptic seizures of those children who are by history seizure-prone and may induce the first seizures in others. Cost-to-benefit ratios have to be considered in each single case, therefore.

The antiepileptic drugs often exacerbate the brain-damaged behavior picture, but on the other hand, each uncontrolled or unprevented seizure may worsen even more the decrements seen. Notably, diphenylhydantoin may be toxic to a child who needs it to control her or his epilepsy. Therefore, choices are not easy.

The use of lithium salts to control explosive attacks in brain-injured children remains experimental—promising but of unproven value. A few may benefit from an old standby, diphenhydramine, at bedtime, or from one of the beta-adrenergic-blockers (e.g., propranolol) during the day, or from diphenylhydantoin even when there are not seizures, or from carbamazepine; but in the final analysis the trial of all these drugs is more empirical than rational in its inspiration.

PSYCHOACTIVE SUBSTANCE-INDUCED ORGANIC MENTAL DISORDERS

Out of the plethora of mind-altering toxins made available to children (by rarely apprehended criminals), we must select only alcohol, uppers, and PCP, neglecting many others (LSD, psilocybin, mescaline, cannabis, inhalants, etc.) that are less commonly causes of childhood mental disorders. These are all chemogenic brain noxae that may lead to brutally aggressive episodes that mimic the psychosis of brain tumor, head injuries, cerebrovascular accidents, subdural hematoma, infections, anticholinergic intoxication, or mania that shows a lot of anger and aggression.

Alcohol Intoxication (303.00)
Alcohol Idiosyncratic Intoxication (291.40)

DEFINITION AND DIAGNOSIS

Simple Alcohol Intoxication gives a history of recent ingestion of sufficient alcohol to yield a blood level of 0.11–0.20%, the range between being "drunk" and being "drunk and disorderly," as the police term this. By contrast, the blood alcohol level of a child with Alcohol Idiosyncratic Intoxication is well *below* the 0.11 figure, the point being that the smaller amount, recently consumed, triggers an episode of aggressive or assaultive behavior that is atypical for the child when not drinking. The small amount consumed would never induce simple Alcohol Intoxication and may not be enough to produce the odor of an alcoholic breath. The details of amount consumed, confirmed or not by blood levels below 0.11% alcohol to blood, will distinguish which disorder is present.

The importance of an accurate history, difficult to elicit from most intoxicated informants, must be emphasized. A history of drinking alcohol regularly and frequently will usually rule out Alcohol Idiosyncratic Intoxication and rule in simple Alcohol Intoxication and provide us, furthermore, with a diagnosis of Alcohol Dependence.

CLINICAL DESCRIPTION

That children may be dependent on alcohol does not astonish anyone who knows about fetal alcohol syndrome, the increasing incidence of alcohol consumption by ever-younger children, and the risk that 50% of the same-sex offspring of alcoholic parents will also become alcoholics. Alcohol is the toxin easiest for children to obtain—and on more occasions than family celebrations. Adults, then adolescents, and then children show alcoholism in decreasing frequency.

CASE 5-2   Reginald, a nine-year-old fourth-grader in a special class for slow readers, declined repeated offers by his two closest chums, classmates, to "sip some vodka" from a flask one or the other replenished daily from the home bar of his father. One morning, during a recess when some of the boys congregated in the toilet to smoke cigarettes and pot or to drink alcohol, Reginald decided to give the vodka a try. Initially, he made a face and then teasingly pretended to stagger and speak with slurring speech. Within five minutes, however, he *ran amok.* He *kicked* over trash cans, *cursed* the teacher and *hit* her, threw a chair through the classroom window, "*looking very wild,* like a maniac." The teacher, a veteran, thought he might have been smoking pot laced with PCP and called for the vice-principal of the inner city elementary school. Reginald *previously had not shown* this kind of *violent behavior.* He had a *history of a skull fracture* at age four years, possibly a sign of physical abuse by his alcoholic stepfather.

Comment. Reginald's special class for poor readers had a high incidence of children with Conduct Disorder but Reginald himself was not a "bad egg," although it was suspected that his parents had abused and neglected him. Reginald did not try drinking alcohol again until he was an adolescent; the wild rage attack recurred at that time. His diagnosis was Alcohol Idiosyncratic Intoxication and that of his two classmates was Alcohol Dependence *and* Conduct Disorder.

TREATMENT AND PROGNOSIS

For best results, the child with Alcohol Intoxication needs to be studied as an outpatient, determining the extent of his or her problems. If (s)he is alcohol-dependent which was brought to attention during only one of many episodes of intoxication, the child may need to be hospitalized for ease of studies of liver and psychologic test performance, and for studying his parents and getting their assistance in depriving the child of access to alcohol. Sometimes the hospitalization is warranted to control malnutrition, dehydration, and alcohol withdrawal delirium that may ensue.

If the diagnosis is Alcohol Idiosyncratic Intoxication, it is equally or more urgent to work with the parents to deprive the child of the toxin that sends him into a psychotic rage. Also, this child should be hospitalized for skull films, CT scan, and EEG to see if there is an old head injury. The occult head injury may have been producing other symptoms that had not been identified previously. Nocturnal major seizures or psychomotor seizures would be examples of conditions to be medicated, while dural scars or adhesions and a chronic subdural hematoma may be helped surgically.

The facts stand that alcohol-abusing children are at great risk of later pathology, including worsening Alcohol Dependence. They may need better nutrition with vitamin supplementation, help in improving wholesome peer relations, special help for school deficits, and surely counseling on how to stay out of trouble with illegal drugs.

Alcohol abuse runs in families; total abstinence also has a high familial incidence, but the offspring of teetotalers may become moderate social drinkers or alcoholics, too. A detailed family history of both parents and their first-degree relatives seems a useful document for psychotherapeutic work with the child and parents. No serious harm can be documented from children's drinking moderate amounts of wine at family celebrations of Christmas, Passover, weddings, and wakes, if not proscribed by family customs and values.

Amphetamine or Similarly Acting Sympathomimetic Intoxication (305.70)

DEFINITION

Amphetamine Intoxication can be diagnosed if four criteria are met, according to DSM-III-R. These could be paraphrased as follows (see DSM-III-R for the precise statement):

1. Recent use of an amphetamine or similar substance, by history.
2. Within an hour after use (I.V. or oral), *at least two* of these mental symptoms:
    psychomotor agitation
    elation or hyperalertness
    grandiosity, mental expansiveness
    loquaciousness
    hypervigilance or suspicion
3. With an hour after use, *at least two* of these physical symptoms:
    rapid pulse rate when at rest
    pupillary dilatation
    blood pressure elevation
    sweating or chills
    nausea, vomiting, or retching
4. Clinical picture is not attributable to any other physical or mental disorder.

CASE 5-3   The first example of severe amphetamine intoxication ever seen by one of us (PLA) was of Hector, a very *paranoid, restless, assaultive* six-year-old boy who had *"gotten into my diet pills,"* as his overweight mother told of the etiology of his combative behavior. She had mixed a bottle of dextroamphetamine capsules prescribed by a family doctor with some fenfluramine hydrochloride tablets prescribed by an internist and some methylphenidate tablets that a pediatrician had prescribed for her nephew. The latter's prescription was being abused by both the nephew's mother and aunt. The mother carried the three medications because she had discerned that no single one curbed her appetite for more than five to seven days at a time. She *could not give any estimate of how many* of each medication had been ingested by her son about an hour earlier. Hector himself *did not know* or *would not tell;* it was *uncertain that he understood* the emergency physician's questions. He appeared *unable to communicate rationally* as he *took a position of vigilance* in the corner of the examining room, looking *wild-eyed* with *dilated pupils, jumping nervously* at hearing the slightest noise, and *flailing an armboard* (for venipunctures) at anyone who came near him, *screaming "Don't kill me!"* A kindly male orderly, speaking softly, subdued and restrained the *sweaty and tachycardic* Hector so that the boy could be examined and made to undergo gastric lavage.

Comment. To clarify the diagnosis (beyond detecting the three drugs, in Hector's case, that were in the gastric washing), it is important to look closer at Hector in his family. Is he neglected? Is he accident-prone? Is the mother amphetamine-dependent? Do both parents need drug education? Is the mother self-medicating a dysthymic life? What is the story on the other children? Is theirs a multiproblem family? Would the mother try a weight reduction program in a group of her peers? Have they frequented the poison control center previously? What are the family's needs? How is it that a child of Hector's age ingests capsules and pills that he sneaked from his mother's purse? Are there other indices of a Conduct Disorder? Other pathology?

DIFFERENTIAL DIAGNOSIS

Amphetamine Intoxication can be distinguished from other conditions in ways that we indicate below:

1. From Cocaine Intoxication or other "uppers" intoxication by blood and urinary toxicological studies, the history, and by the fact that "crack" is usually smoked in pipe, not ingested by mouth.
2. From Phencyclidine Intoxication by amphetamines' lack of certain PCP symptoms (slowing of perceived time, numbness, synesthesias, for example), as well as by laboratory and drug history studies.
3. From Mania by amphetamines having been used and by clinical picture. The latter is not always easy since some manics may be more belligerent, assaultive, and angry than euphoric or suspicious. The *suspicious and angry* manics are difficult to differentiate clinically. Time and detailed observation will aid the

differentiation, best done in a hospital if Mania is suspected. It also helps to keep in mind that Mania is very rare in children.

The clinical picture and history of intoxication does not confuse the adept clinician into seriously considering Delirium, Organic Delusional, Mood, or Hallucinosis syndromes in the differential.

TREATMENT

The treatment for an almost accidental ingestion of a toxic dose of amphetamines was suggested under the "Diagnostic Workup for Organicity." The treatment does vary with the nature of the disorder.

However, if a child has developed an amphetamine dependency, hospitalization, with monitoring, milieu support, and family and individual psychotherapy, is indicated. The treatment program should include careful drug education, environmental manipulation, peer group therapy, and perhaps continued outpatient personal psychotherapy.

PROGNOSIS

Although psychiatrists no longer hold to an "addictive personality" to support gloomy prognostications, the high mass incidence of children abusing drugs has become a public health concern without a bright prognosis. Drug-dependent children do not have a wholesome childhood or adolescence; if they are untreated, they are at risk of antisocial problems, poor work opportunities, school failure, and lives withdrawn into social and sexual incompetence.

Cocaine Intoxication (305.60)

DEFINITION

Cocaine Dependence and Intoxication now constitute a major threat to child mental health. Especially the free-based, dried-paste form called "crack," which is ordinarily smoked in pipes, has become a lethal but widely used, addicting drug among young Americans. Cocaine Intoxication of children is not rare, late in the 1980s.

CLINICAL DESCRIPTION

This is identical to that described for Amphetamine Intoxication, since cocaine has always been sought for its anesthetic and sympathomimetic properties, both in the clinic and on the streets. Consequently, the differential diagnosis, the diagnostic workup, treatment, and prognosis follow along the same lines as described for Amphetamine Intoxication.

Phencyclidine or Similarly Acting Arylcyclohexylamine Intoxication (305.90)
DEFINITION

Phencyclidine (PCP) is an animal tranquilizer that does not calm children and indeed may prompt them into dyscontrol episodes during which they may commit murder. It is used mainly by older boys rather than by girls or younger children. Often called angel dust, it can be taken by mouth but acts faster when injected intravenously, smoked (often lacing marijuana cigarettes), or insufflated ("snorted"). There are other illicitly marketed arylcyclohexylamines producing effects similar to PCP.

ETIOLOGY

The causative intoxicant is PCP or similar agent.

CLINICAL DESCRIPTION

(See DSM-III-R for its depiction of physical, mental, and behavioral signs and symptoms.)

1. PCP or a designer congener has been used recently.
2. Within an hour, or less if smoked/sniffed/injected, *at least two* of these physical symptoms:
   (a) vertical or horizontal nystagmus
   (b) tachycardia and hypertension
   (c) numbness or decreased pain sensation
   (d) ataxia
   (e) dysarthria
   (f) muscular rigidity
   (g) convulsions
   (h) hyperacusis
3. Within an hour *at least two* of these mental symptoms:
   (a) euphoria
   (b) psychomotor agitation
   (c) marked anxiety
   (d) emotional lability
   (e) grandiosity
   (f) sensation of slowed time
   (g) synesthesias

4. Maladaptive behavior—bellicosity, assaultiveness, impulsiveness, unpredict-ability, or faulty judgment.
5. This picture is not due to Delirium or other mental or physical disorder.

CASE 5-4   Who later proved to be an *11-year-old pubescent male* on summer vacation at the beach was brought to a local hospital by a policeman, in the company of two associates, one of whom was 13 and the other 15 years old. His name and address were unknown, the two companions stated. One of the lads offered a specimen of what the disturbed lad had "snorted," saying, "I took it away from him when he *started acting crazy.*" X, as the doctor dubbed the psychotic youngster, *looked panicky, moving restlessly and clumsily around* the examin-ing room, *trying to escape* and boastfully proclaiming in a *slurred phonation* that his *Colles fracture of the left radius did not hurt* and that *he refused to permit treatment.* He kept asking, "Why is nothing hap-nin? Time has shtopped. Why's *everything hap-nin so shlow?*" He had a *vertical nystagmus* and his pupils did not appear dilated.

Two days later, wearing a cast on his left forearm, X returned with his vacationing parents to get a referral to see a psychiatrist in their home state. The mother feared that Sylvester, the real name of X, might be having flashbacks because he was having episodes of fright two or three times daily, but only when a policemen walked towards him.

Comment. Young drug abusers often become anxious after an episode of intoxi-cation and, no wonder, particularly when an agent of law enforcement approaches them. The anxious episodes are probably not flashbacks unless the child has been a heavy and steady abuser of PCP or a related drug.

DIAGNOSIS AND DIFFERENTIAL DIAGNOSIS

The diagnosis can be made only by obtaining an accurate drug history; by toxicologic study of blood, urine, or a sample of the drug used; and by observing the clinical symptoms and course of the illness. The differential most often called for is the LSD bad trip, and that sometimes must await sufficient recovery of the informant in order to ascertain what the patient believed (s)he was using. Urinary drug screens earlier may be helpful for identifying the causative drug. The lifestyle and symptoms of mental disorder also have to be appraised because the chemical agent is less important than ego or milieu in the long run.

TREATMENT

Although we believe many cases of PCP Intoxication do not come to medical attention, it could be that the worse ones do; hence we believe a child should be hospitalized on pediatrics or child psychiatry until recovery has progressed and a mental evaluation has been completed. After leaving the hospital, the child may find himself or herself traversing a rocky road necessitating attention by members of the mental health team—for both child and other family members.

PROGNOSIS

The prognosis of identified but untreated cases is grave, of detected and briefly treated cases is guarded, while the prognosis of unidentified cases is not known by child psychiatry.

ORGANIC MENTAL DISORDERS

These are subtyped into the nine conditions we itemized at the start of this chapter. As noted earlier, we have chosen to highlight only

Organic Personality Disorder
Alcohol Intoxication
Alcohol Idiosyncratic Intoxication
Amphetamine Intoxication
Cocaine Intoxication
Phencyclidine Intoxication

These are exemplary of the Organic Mental Disorders usually causing episodic disorders of behavior—our offering, in a beginning text, of the more common problems of behavior. Naturally, the brain is all of one piece so it was arbitrarily decided to isolate into this chapter the episodic behavior disorders. Since the brain seems to be the master organ for behavior, cognition, and feeling, we have discussed some additional brain syndromes in Chapter 22 of the section on "Thinking and Central Processing Disorders."

Questions for Study and Action

1. If Sylvester ("X") had taken LSD laced with strychnine—instead of PCP—and had come in psychotic and assaultive, why would it be malpractice to give him chlorpromazine to calm him down? Look up in a pharmacology text what chlorpromazine does to a strychninized heart.

2. Since no cases of single-incident Explosive Disorder were found, early drafts of DSM-III-R decided to go with actual incidence *data* and drop the former class of

disorders. Discuss the advantages *and* disadvantages of a classification that relies on an empirical data base.

3. List six cardinal signs of organic brain damage. List four secondary signs.

4. Consult a neurology text to find out the usual cause of each of the following:
    (a) first seizure at age two years
    (b) first epileptic seizure at age five years
    (c) major cause of infantile delirium

5. How would you account for the probable reasons that Miguel (Case 5-1):
    (a) developed ideas of grandiosity and invulnerability;
    (b) developed paranoid ideation toward his sexually awakened father;
    (c) stayed up to grade level in classroom studies but could not participate in the special program for talented and gifted children;
    (d) changed so quickly to loving and accepting a new stepmother;
    (e) showed such brief bereavement when he learned of his mother's death;
    (f) used psychotherapy so well; and
    (g) could cope so well with organic deficits?

6. Discuss the pros and cons of this statement: "Psychological testing is of more value in assessing a brain-damaged child's cognitive and educational capabilities than in aiding the localization or extent of the brain disorder."

7. Is accident-proneness just accidental? What circumstances a) within a child *and* b) between a child and the parents could cause a child repeatedly to sustain accidental injuries or poisonings? Consider gender, age, availability of noxae, lack of protection, and socioeconomic class in your answer, but add others from your logic or knowledge.

8. Write down the items you would include in a drug-history interview with a child. Why is a drug-history-taking so vital with today's youth? What specific substances would you inquire about?

9. Discuss: PCP and hydrocarbon inhalants are deadly to neural tissue. Include a consideration of their toxicity, mode of action, pathophysiology, and actual effects on neural tissue.

10. It has been said that war as an institution and especially cold war's nuclear terror do more to influence children's violence than do religious preachments in favor of peace and nonviolence. How would you design the details of an experiment to test this hypothesis?

For Further Reading

Laufer, M.W., & Shetty, T. Acute and chronic brain syndromes. In J.N. Noshpitz (Ed.), *Basic Handbook of Child Psychiatry: Vol. III, Disturbances of Development*. New York: Basic Books, 1979, pp. 381–402.

Monroe, R.R. *Episodic Behavioral Disorders: A Psychodynamic and Neurophysiologic Analysis*. Cambridge, MA: Harvard University Press, 1970.

Reich, W. *The Impulsive Character and Other Writings* (Trans. B.G. Koopman). New York: New American Library (Meridian), 1974.

Rubinstein, B., & Shaffer, D. Organicity in child psychiatry: Signs, symptoms, and syndromes. In J.H. Beitchman (Guest Ed.), *Symposium on Child Psychiatry, The Psychiatric Clinics of North America, Vol. 8*. Philadelphia: W.B. Saunders, 1985, pp. 755–777.

6

Factitious Disorders

Factitious Disorders are diseases, physical or mental, produced by the patients themselves, by their own voluntary, conscious acts, with the specific and sole purpose of being sick or, rather, being patients.

These disorders have become notorious as "Munchausen syndrome." The best-known patients are the peregrinating "professional" patients or "hospital hoboes," with scores of hospital admissions in various parts of the country. These extreme cases are all adults. Peregrination is not known to occur in children, but Factitious Disorders do occur in children.

DSM-III-R defines Factitious Disorders for the general patient population, which means largely for adults. The basic definition is, nevertheless, applicable to children. We will, therefore, present the DSM-III-R definition as it applies to children.

DEFINITION

Factitious Disorders are self-induced physical or psychological diseases that are produced by the individual and are under voluntary control. The acts of producing the disease have a compulsive, repetitive quality, in that the individual is unable to refrain from them. The disease is, therefore, "voluntary" in the sense that the acts (of producing illness) are deliberate and purposeful, but not in the sense that the acts can be controlled.

Factitious Disorders are subdivided into three categories:

1. *Factitious Disorder with Psychological Symptoms (300.16):* This disease has not, to our knowledge, been described in children.
2. *Factitious Disorder with Physical Symptoms (301.51):* This is the category for the famous patients with Munchausen syndrome. While there may be some chronic factitious diseases in children, what we usually see is the acute or subacute form.
3. *Factitious Disorder Not Otherwise Specified (300.19):* According to DSM-III-R, this category would be suitable for factitious disease in many children since it includes "dermatitis artifacta," and probably most acute or subacute cases would be included here.

Not mentioned by DSM-III-R, but of importance nonetheless, is *Munchausen syndrome by Proxy*. This is a severe form of child abuse, but will be described later in this chapter as a factitious disorder produced by the mother.

CLINICAL DESCRIPTION

Because the production of illness requires a level of sophistication beyond the grasp of most children, factitious illness is rare in children and, when seen, occurs in later childhood, when the child's cognitive apparatus is sufficiently developed for the considerable forethought in setting up the illness and, unfortunately, for the mendacity required to maintain it. In the same vein, we can expect that more Factitious Disorders will be "grafted onto" an existing, true, organic illness—the more visible and medically simple, the better. Therefore, factitial dermatitis is probably the most common, followed by diabetes mellitus. Other injuries to the skin can also be done, as the following case will illustrate.

CASE 6-1   Mary was 10 years old when she got severely burned by a grease fire on the kitchen stove where she was cooking supper for her three younger siblings. During treatment in a specialized burns unit, the staff became concerned about the *lack of progress* in the healing of her burns: skin grafts seemed not to "take": they became infected in patches, suggestive of excoriations.

Mary *denied* "picking" at her skin and started *crying* when confronted. The child psychiatric consultant then started seeing her on a daily basis. In "open-ended" interviews, Mary described the misery of her daily existence at home: the family's marginal finances, earning a meager existence from their small farm. There were seven children, and Mary was burnt when she was babysitting and caring for her younger siblings, while everybody else was away doing chores.

She liked the hospital and the good things it offered: good and plentiful food, *kind and attentive* staff, no work for her. She wanted to *stay there* as long as possible. She felt *guilty,* however, about being here in the midst of plenty, while there were chores to be done at home and her two younger brothers and sister to be looked after. She continued to *deny* picking at her grafts, but when she was placed next to the nurses' station and *constantly monitored,* her grafts healed *better.*

Comment. The secondary gain (attention, good life) is so transparent here that we might at first call this malingering; however, the pain and discomfort of the repeated grafting procedures were such as to make malingering simply "uneconomical." The gain was not a material one; what the patient achieved was the prolongation of her status as a patient, at the expense of a great deal of pain and the interruption of all her age-appropriate activities. There was no available relief for the patient's guilt, either: she knew what she was doing but was unable to stop it. She did not "bind" or "convert" previous guilt into a *conversion disorder*—that would have been an unconscious mechanism and would not have involved purposeful actions such as picking at the grafts.

ETIOLOGY AND PATHOGENESIS

The cause and the pathogenesis of Factitious Disorder are unknown. A number of hypotheses have been advanced, but none of them has been able to answer the question, "Why does the patient choose this form of disease and not another?"

What has been found in these patients and may account for some of the symptomatology of Factitious Disorder is poor verbal communicative skills; therefore, these patients use more primitive modes of communication, i.e., actions, hence the action of inducing illness. The other salient characteristic is a strong need for dependency, which may account for their seeking to attain and prolong the patient role. These tentative hypotheses have been derived mainly from the course of psychotherapy, where verbal communication per se has been both difficult and unproductive, and insight either unattainable or, when finally arrived at, of no real value.

DIAGNOSIS AND DIFFERENTIAL DIAGNOSIS

When discussing the process of diagnosing factitious disease (and it is always a process), we need to keep only a few diagnostic facts in mind: the child denies causing the illness, the organic illness produced has atypical features—it does not quite make clinical sense—and hospitalization with around-the-clock supervision (usually necessitating the exclusion of parents) results in improvement.

A high index of suspicion is the clinician's best tool—plus expert familiarity with the "original" of the disorder that is being "reproduced" by design. This is why most Factitious Disorders are at least tentatively diagnosed first by non-psychiatrist physicians.

Fortunately for the practitioner, the clinical pictures that children produce are less sophisticated and less complex than those of adults, and their reactions of denial lack the manipulativeness of their adult counterparts. To the latter there is one particularly bothersome exception: children can exacerbate their parents' protective reactions into overprotective ones. The children's denial is then compounded by their parents' disbelief and hostility towards the physician who diagnoses the disease as factitial.

The differential diagnosis must be made against the organic disease on the one hand, and against other psychiatric disorders on the other. The latter should include:

1. *Malingering.* This is also the conscious production of illness, but it is for an obvious advantage or gain. Simply put, this is "faking" a disease. Moreover, it can be "turned on and off" at will, i.e., it does not have the compulsive quality of factitious disease. Factitious Disorder creates lesions; malingering mimics the symptoms of diseases.

If we were to define malingering very broadly and without moral censure, it would be frequent and normal in children—everyday excuses ("I have a headache, my stomach hurts, my feet hurt") would qualify. Strictly defined, with gain either material (e.g., monetary compensation for injury) or the easing of constraints (e.g., getting out from the custody of one divorced parent), malingering is rarely originated independently by children themselves. It is probably quite a different story when the greed or amenities of their parents enter the scene: children may be coached or otherwise induced to fake symptoms or claim injury, such as child abuse. The manipulation of custody through children's symptoms by warring divorced parents, in particular, has recently been increasing at an alarming rate, with a reported increase in false allegations of child sexual abuse, among other charges. When the parents are "fighting dirty," they will coach their children to help their battle.

2. *Somatoform Disorder—Conversion Disorder.* These are the somatic (physical) expressions of internalized conflict (neurosis) and not under the child's conscious, voluntary control; the child is not producing the illness by any purposive action. There is no destruction of tissue. Watching the child around the clock will not put a stop to the illness. In most instances, the clinician can expect rather typical clusters of symptoms, such as various pains, especially abdominal, or difficulties in locomotion (rarely, hysterical paralysis), or visual and auditory symptoms—none of which can be produced outright. An example of the differentiation would be the production of multiple skin abscesses, without claiming too much pain, in factitious disease, and complaints of excruciating abdominal pains without physical findings in Conversion Disorder.

Since conversion disorders are expressions of internalized conflicts, positive findings of such conflicts can be elicited; however, this is usually quite difficult to do in factitial disease.

Finally, treatment outcome is a diagnostic tool in some instances. Dramatic disappearance of the symptoms with hypnosis or fortuitous brief psychotherapy sometimes happens in conversion disorders; factitious illness, on the other hand, never responds quickly to any treatment, but seems to be embedded and ineradicable.

3. *Childhood psychosis,* functional or organic, can result in self-mutilation. The differential diagnosis must be made on the basis of the positive findings of the psychosis.

4. *Hypochondriasis* is a differential diagnostic consideration only in the first encounter, that of the patient and the child's parents bringing illness to the physician's attention. But after that, hypochondriasis is the very opposite of Factitious Disorder. In the case of the latter, the child makes an unspoken presentation of an objective illness.

5. *Dissociative Disorders* (Dissociative Disorder NOS, 300.15). The splitting of consciousness differentiates dissociation from Factitious Disorder, but Ganser's syndrome may give problems to the diagnostician. This syndrome was originally described in 1893 as a peculiar dissociative state in which an adult patient gave nearly correct answers. Therefore, its name of "syndrome of approximate answers" came into use. The approximate answers may also take the form of "talking past the point." These maneuvers are not quite without intent, as they have been observed in prisoners for, presumably, any secondary gain they could derive from appearing mentally incompetent.

This is a disputed syndrome even in adults and is not mentioned in the standard texts in child psychiatry. Nevertheless, it may be encountered in children in what we feel is a fairly benign form.

CASE 6-2   Amelia was a cute five-year-old girl who was caught in a custody dispute between her recently divorced parents. She was brought for a court-ordered psychiatric examination by her mother, and both Amelia and her mother presented themselves as utterly helpless to deal with the current stresses. Mother's style was hysterical and expressive but the child appeared dazed. When asked about father, to whom she had been close, the patient denied that he had left, maintaining that he was at home as always. When asked about her age, she raised *three* fingers; she consistently substituted colors; the female Barbie doll was referred to as father, and Barbie's sports car was a truck. When she played, the child moved about as if oblivious of her surroundings. Each parent was putting pressure on Amelia to declare herself in favor of that parent, and Amelia did not know which way to turn. Split by her parents, Amelia dissociated temporarily.

After two sessions of psychotherapy, the patient identified objects and colors correctly and acknowledged the fact that father was not living at home. When reminded of her previous statements, she could not remember them.

Comment. The diagnosis of Ganser's syndrome was based on Amelia's dazed and trancelike appearance, a stressful situation that offered no immediate emotional escape other than by the symptoms described, and consistently approximate answers—never too far off the mark, yet not correct, either.

The main issue in Ganser's syndrome is the differential diagnosis in two directions: one direction is towards factitious psychiatric disease and malingering; the other is toward organic (usually toxic) and functional psychosis.

Ganser's syndrome, unlike Factitious Disorder, has a good prognosis in children and subsides either spontaneously (especially with removal from the stressful emotional situation) or with brief psychotherapy. This is, probably, its main differentiating feature from other, rather similar, disorders.

TREATMENT AND PROGNOSIS

Factitious Disorders are among the most difficult to treat. When they occur in children, the outlook both for timely results of treatment and for the more distant future are relatively better than in adolescents or adults.

There are several circumstances that make treatment of Factitious Disorders so difficult: the often primitive emotional makeup of the child; the difficulty in arriving at an adequate working "blueprint" of the child's psychodynamics; the involvement of the parents; and the pressure to succeed because the child is hurting himself/herself and may have the medical staff up in arms because of their countertransference. For that matter, the therapist's own countertransference has to be closely monitored, because it has traditionally been a source of trouble, too.

Although there is no universally accepted common therapeutic approach or technique for Factitious Disorder, the following are "musts":

- Maintain close relationships and ongoing communication with all the other medical personnel. Support and educate them. They have been traumatized by the patient who has made a mockery of their efforts.
- Maintain regular contact with the parents and stay on "the right side" of the relationship—i.e., do not antagonize them; be patient.
- The mainstay of the treatment of the patient is the therapist/patient relationship. Confrontation should be avoided, except when the therapist is quite sure that the moment is right for it. Admission of the production of illness is *not* a goal of treatment, and the therapist should not be hung up on that issue. Improvement occurs without admission, or even direct discussion, of the patient's culpability.
- Follow-up is mandatory. After all, we may speculate that the patient "exchanges"

his factitial illness for the working relationship with the therapist, with insight playing a small role.

• In the last analysis, we do not know what exactly will produce, or be responsible for, the improvement, just as we do not know the precise etiology of this disorder.

• And, finally, most, if not all, cases of factitial disease should be referred to a child psychiatrist—a justified relief for most mental health workers.

"Munchausen by Proxy" Syndrome

This syndrome was first described by Meadow in 1977. It consisted of maternal falsification of the medical histories of the children, leading to iatrogenic illness in the children.

CLINICAL DESCRIPTION

An increasing number of case reports has given rise to the following description: the mother brings a child (age range described from four months to seven years) with an inexplicable, persistent medical illness that does not fit any known medical syndrome. The mother is oversolicitous of her child's welfare and looks for the best possible medical care. When the child is hospitalized, the mother often insists on staying with the child or shows other signs of extreme, nearly symbiotic, closeness to the child.

Although the children's clinical pictures defy accurate diagnosis, they are sometimes seriously ill; at other times, they become progressively sicker.

They are similar to adult Munchausen's syndrome in that, depending on who sees them first, they may have long medical histories, with multiple hospitalizations, many diagnostic procedures, and many consultations reflecting the involvement of several organ systems and, correspondingly, consultations from many medical specialists.

When the mother is kept away, these children improve. Some of them have a downhill course resulting in death, and the term "nonaccidental poisoning" has been used.

Various forms of abnormal bleeding have been the most frequent symptomatology; dehydration, coma, metabolic/endocrine disorders, seizures, and infections have been some of the other illnesses produced.

PATHOGENESIS

In all cases, the disease was produced by the mother. Several of these mothers have been studied and their psychopathology found to have one strong parallel to that of patients with Factitious Disorder: strong dependency needs. In addition, depression and severe marital difficulties were also found. The mothers dealt with their depression by becoming symbiotically involved in the production and "treatment" of their children's illness.

DIAGNOSIS

Diagnosis is based on a high index of suspicion and the willingness to believe that the mother, given the requisite psychopathology, can do this to her child. Familarity with this rare, but very dangerous, syndrome and using appropriate laboratory tests to rule the organic disorders out or in are needed. Briefly stated, knowing that this syndrome exists and doing one's medical homework thoroughly will help initiate the diagnosis that will be confirmed ultimately.

TREATMENT AND PROGNOSIS

If Factitious Disorder is difficult to treat because of the various reactions of the members of the treatment team, Munchausen by proxy is even more so: the multitude of medical team members must be joined by lawyers and representatives of child protective agencies. All must work together, and work effectively and promptly, to protect the child's life—against one of the oldest receptacles of human trust, that of motherhood. Society will side with the mother, unless the legal system is more effectively enlightened about this syndrome.

When the mother has received adequate psychiatric treatment, the prognosis is good, but the first goal must be the protection of the child. This can usually be done only through legal means. The usual procedures of child protective services, as in child abuse, should be followed.

Questions for Study and Action

1. What gains could there possibly be for a child who, like Mary in this chapter, wants to sustain and lengthen hospitalization and the sick role? Have at least seven gains on your list.

2. Which of the Darwinian structures to express emotion (phonatory apparatus, mimetic musculature, voluntary musculature, vegetative system, endocrines) does the child with a Factitious Disorder use? Comment in detail on the way each is used, underused, or overused.

3. Reexamine the case of Mary in this chapter in order to list the important objective *observations* and important *historical data* that were elicited to raise the index of

suspicion that her burn wounds now had a heavy factitious component. In your listing of them, which had a more numerous list, the observations or the history?

4. Describe your ideal diagnostic workup for a case such as Mary's. What role would a psychologist's consultation play in your diagnostic efforts?

5. Try to make a case for Mary's diagnosis as a Stereotypy/Habit Disorder (Chapter 13) instead of a Factitious Disorder. Which diagnosis would be more likely to please her parents?

6. Propose five behavior therapy strategies that would apply to Mary's treatment regimen, to reduce her "picking at" her healing skin grafts. Explain why each strategy sensibly could be selected to alter her behavior.

7. Propose five expressive (emotional/dynamic) therapy strategies to include in her treatment of her Factitious Disorder. Explain the rationale of each strategy chosen.

8. How would you differentiate the case of "Munchausen by proxy" from one of
   (a) Factitious Disorder or
   (b) Induced Psychotic Disorder?

9. How could the mother of a child showing "Munchausen by proxy" employ each of the following, as described in Chapter 34:
   (a) projective identification?
   (b) role reversal?
   (c) narcissistic identification?

10. What is the rationale for doing individual psychotherapy with a "Munchausen by proxy" child? Would it help to see mother and child initially and then assign each to a separate individual therapist? Explain. Would you suggest periodic sessions to include child, child's therapist, mother, and mother's therapist? Explain.

For Further Reading

Fras, I. Factitial disease: An update. *Psychosomatics*, 19:119–122, 1978.

Goldin, S., & MacDonald, J. E. The Ganser state. *J. Ment. Sci.*, 101:267, 1955.

Meadow, R. Münchausen syndrome by proxy: The hinterland of child abuse. *Lancet*, II: 343–345, 1977.

Waller, D. A. Obstacles to the treatment of Munchausen by proxy syndrome. *J. Amer. Acad. of Child Psychiatry*, 22:80–85, 1983.

Whitlock, F. A. The Ganser syndrome. *Br. J. Psychiatry*, 113:19, 1967.

7

Firesetting

Although DSM-III-R uses the term "pyromania" for this disorder, we will use the term "firesetting" for very specific reasons: as defined by DSM-III-R, "pyromania" is a disease entity which can be applied only to an exceptionally small number of children (only three cases having been seen in the combined life-time practices of both authors), whereas firesetting in some forms is both a disorder and a common, nearly universal, developmental phenomenon. In children, the Impulse Control Disorder may not be so well structured or ominous.

In children, the demarcation line between "normal" or generic firesetting and "abnormal" or pathological firesetting is often indistinct. We will, therefore, have to offer definitions of each based on a comprehensive understanding of developmental issues and the latest state of the art of research into childhood firesetting. The British call this behavior *fireraising*.

DEFINITION

Pyromania (312.33) is defined (in DSM-III-R) as the inability to resist an intense impulse to set fires. There is an irresistible fascination with fires, a buildup of tension leading to setting fires, and relief following the firesetting and/or witnessing the fire. Pyromania is not diagnosed when the firesetting is secondary to another disorder, such as Conduct Disorder, Antisocial Personality Disorder, Schizophrenia, or an Organic Mental Disorder.

An extensive review of the literature on childhood *firesetting* as distinct from *pyromania*, as well as our own experience, shows almost unequivocally that firesetting in childhood is different from that in adolescence and adulthood, and that childhood firesetting can be divided into two broad categories:

1. *Curiosity* firesetting (synonyms: "exploratory," "experimental," "normal"). This is a one-time episode of the child's experimentation with matches in an exploratory, learning way, telling his or her parent about it, and often being frightened by any extension of the fire (e.g., paper or garbage starting to burn). This experiment is undertaken within the context of the child's own home and without an accomplice. Either discussion in a context of alarm or urgent explanation of the realistic dangers to the child usually terminates the experiment and, typically, the trial is not repeated.

2. *Pathological* firesetting (synonyms: "recidivist" or "repetitive") is characterized by its dangerousness, repetitiveness, and imperviousness to ordinary disciplinary measures. This type may be either primary or secondary. It is done by the child either alone or in company, and, depending on his age, at home (younger age) or away from home (older children).

The buildup of tension prior to firesetting, with its subsequent release, is hardly ever described by firesetting children and rarely witnessed by the parents. One reason for this may be the child's inability to verbalize retrospectively about an intense, momentary experience, and another is the rarity of an occasion when any adult could observe the child "in its natural habitat," as it were, setting a fire without the adult's intervening.

The differentiation between "curiosity" and "pathological" firesetting is often difficult to make, especially on the first episode, because many "curiosity" firesetters incorporate some of the developmental and family characteristics of the pathological firesetters. The characteristics shared by both groups are immaturity and developmental disorders in the children, and lack of structure in the families. Usually, it is a matter of degree, i.e., the "curiosity" firesetters have these characteristics to a mild degree, just enough for the firesetting impulse to "break through."

Finally, pathological firesetting can be primary or secondary. The latter is a direct result of another disorder from which it can be separated: Schizophrenia or neurotic disorders. All the rest of pathological firesetting is primary, even though it often appears to be only a *symptom* of another disorder. As will be seen from our considerations of its pathogenesis and hypothesized etiology, as well as from its treatment, this is a useful categorization because it is so inextricably intertwined with the *associated* disorder. Therefore, when we refer to *"firesetting"* in this chapter, we refer to *primary pathological firesetting*.

ETIOLOGY

There probably is no single cause or pathogenetic mechanism for primary pathological firesetting. As a matter of fact, we cannot say that we know conclusively why certain children continue to set fires or make more than one attempt at firesetting.

This lack of knowledge is probably the main reason for the number of theories proposed over the years. Another reason lies in the methodological shortcomings of most studies; thus, no one study is completely convincing by itself. The oldest theories about the causation of firesetting were based on the "irresistible impulse" concept of the 19th century which, as we shall see presently, has been revived in much of contemporary thinking.

Sigmund Freud (1932) offered an interpretation of the myth of Prometheus which has influenced several psychoanalytic writers. He noted the similarity between the flame and the phallus, the erotic excitement that fire produces in many, and the homosexually tinged pleasure experienced by primitive man when he extinguished fire by urinating on it. In order to possess fire, man first had to suppress the homosexual wish to extinguish it. Freud's followers then theorized that firesetting was the result of fixation of sexual impulses at the urethral level; and they emphasized the connection between firesetting, water play, and bedwetting. Karl Marx earlier, and in less vulgar metaphor, had interpreted the legend of Prometheus very differently, i.e., as a progressive step economically, which freed man from relying on gods.

While Freud's ideas were being propagated by the psychoanalytic school of psychiatry, the organically oriented European school, as represented by Wagner von Jauregg (in Scott, 1974), spoke of a universal human impulse to set fires which all of us have to suppress.

More recently, psychoanalytic theories of firesetting in childhood have emphasized aggression more than sexual excitement and have produced better-fitting descriptions of the behavior and thinking in these children. Children who set fires believe in the magic power of fire to purify and redress wrongs. The firesetting is a symbolic or magical attack on a frustrating family member, the usurping of adult power, an expiation of guilt, or even an attempt to bring about a reunion with an absent parent.

Separation from a parent may be a frequent precipitant of firesetting. Other provocations are death of a close family member, estrangement from a parent, or events resulting in loss of self-esteem. The child then seems to retaliate symbolically with fire. Some post-Freud writers also pointed to general ego weaknesses in these children. As Karl Marx wrote, the wish to start a fire may be a primordial impulse that set man's ancestors on the road to civilization. Firesetting, therefore, has connotations of attaining power, of regulating a disorganized environment, and of showing a deep wish to bring into the child's environment the structure which this child needs and has been lacking.

The proponents of learning theory have asserted equally strongly that firesetting is learned behavior in a broader social context of delinquency, and that the wrong behavioral cues given by the child's caretakers (parents) to the child—when he either witnesses a fire or experiments with fire—act as a reinforcer for a behavior that is perceived as successful by the learning child.

Lauretta Bender (1953), and subsequent authors, too, have drawn attention to the high incidence of brain damage in these children. We believe that authors like Nurcombe (1964) or Fineman (1980) offer the most convincing view of pathogenetic factors which can be formulated into the following hypothesis: children who set fires have a constitutional deficit to begin with, in most cases of the minimal brain dysfunction type, with defective impulse control. When there is associated learning disability, that further impairs their judgment. Moreover, their early encounters with fire were such as to fixate fire in their minds. The same circumstances that were responsible for this fixation continue to allow for firesetting to be present and to give it psychodynamic meaning: a disrupted family which frustrates the child and does not give him sufficient limits to internalize the taboo against firesetting.

This is a "core" hypothesis around which the "ingredients" may vary. There appears to be an organic basis, or at least component, in all firesetters. The frustrations to which these children are exposed may vary: from severely disorganized families (the most common) to environmental conditions that are seemingly normal but actually expose a child to deprivations and frustrations that he can cope with only through invoking the primitive magic of fire, remembered as it is transmitted through folklore or personal encounters.

The question, "Why did the child choose firesetting rather than another expression of pathology?" is answered incompletely by any one theory. To set a fire and see it burn may be one of the most primitive and primordial longings of man since the dawn of civilization. Juvenile firesetters may regress to such a level when overwhelmed by the stress of frustration and insecurity in their families.

CLINICAL DESCRIPTION

We will present "primary pathological" firesetting in children since "curiosity" firesetting is self-explanatory and little can be added to the definition previously given. "Secondary" firesetting will be considered under the primary disorder that activates the symptom.

CASE 7-1   Jeremy was a seven-year-old boy who had set several fires both at home and in the neighborhood. The last two fires he set did extensive *damage* to the apartment where he lived and *endangered* the lives of his mother and his younger sister, since he had set fires under their beds while they were sleeping.

He was described as a *hyperactive* and unmanageable child who *had difficulties both at home and at school.* Besides setting fires, he had been *stealing* from mother's purse and *lying* about it. He was *enuretic* about half the nights. At school, he was *distractible* and *constantly out of his seat,* and required *remedial reading* because of a *developmental reading disorder.* He was *aggressive* towards his peers.

The mother had her hands full with raising the two children and holding down a job. The children's *father had deserted* the family about two years earlier, approximately three months before Jeremy had set his first fire. The *mother* was still *depressed* and *discouraged* over this, and was *quite unable to set the firm limits which Jeremy required.*

Examination showed Jeremy to be *immature*-looking, *restless, verbally not very communicative,* and quite unable to explain why he had set the fires. In response to questions, he stated it was perhaps fun to see the fires; he had seen a couple of big fires in his life. But he denied any great excitement in connection with either witnessing the big fires or setting his own. He denied tension or nervousness before the firesetting, nor did the firesetting provide him with any noticeable relief.

He missed his father and appeared to have a mixture of feelings of anger towards father for his abandonment and of longing for his return.

Comment. This case illustrates a number of the characteristics of firesetters:

- male (there is a high male to female ratio, up to 10:1);
- hyperactive, aggressive, and difficult to manage;
- associated stealing and lying;
- learning-disabled;
- disrupted and inadequate family circumstances, including abandonment by father and lack of structure by a distraught mother;
- no evident external or psychodynamic reason for the firesetting;
- enuresis (associated with firesetting in some, but not all, cases). The triad, in clinical lore, of firesetting, enuresis, and cruelty to animals was not present in Jeremy's case.

DIFFERENTIAL DIAGNOSIS

Although DSM-III-R specifies that pyromania must not be due to certain other disorders, this distinction is impossible to maintain for childhood firesetters. At the same time, firesetting is usually *associated with* other disorders, *not due to* them. The exceptions are Schizophrenia and neurotic disorders which produce firesetting secondarily as a result of delusions (in Schizophrenia) and neurotic needs (in certain neuroses).

Firesetting is most frequently associated with Attention–Deficit Hyperactivity Disorder (ADHD), or rather, the entire group of disorders falling under the broad title of minimal brain dysfunction (MBD) and severe developmental disorders, which would include various learning disorders. Firesetting is also very frequently associated with Conduct Disorders. If we consider the overlap among ADHD Disorders (MBD), developmental learning disabilities, and Conduct Disorders, we can state that probably some 90% of firesetters show one or more of the above conditions.

In clinical practice it is of immediate practical importance to diagnose the type of firesetting, and then immediately proceed with treatment.

TREATMENT

The vital principle of treatment is the establishment or reestablishment of inner controls against the firesetting impulse through the imposition of external or environmental controls. Controls have to be internalized by the child; this internalization is achieved by the natural route of identification with or modeling on the controlling adult (parent) and sometimes facilitated by behavior modification. The latter can be administered in a variety of ways but one way (somewhat controversial) is the aversive conditioning of "preventive punishment."

CASE 7-2   Earl was seven years old when he set a series of fires, first in the kitchen, and then in his sisters' bedrooms. His mother became alarmed and took him to the local mental health center. She had considered this measure several times previously because of Earl's unmanageability and "lack of response to any punishment," but had vacillated because she did not want Earl to have "a record." However, the danger from his repeated firesetting ultimately overrode all of her other considerations.

Earl had been born out of wedlock and only rarely saw his father. Mother was divorced and lived on public assistance with occasional work as a housecleaner. She had relatively little difficulty raising the two girls, but viewed Earl as "always willful," "hyper," and given to "temper tantrums." His teacher reported similar troubles with obstreperous Earl.

The mother was instructed to remove all flammable materials from the household (she herself was a cigarette smoker) and to punish Earl every time she found any such materials *in his possession* or *very close to him*. It was made clear to her that Earl *need not have started a fire in order to learn*—by that time it might be too late. Instead, he should be *prevented,* by her punishment, from starting the fire. The type of punishment was left up to the mother—she was told only that it should be an effective form that felt right to her.

This time Earl responded to mother's management because mother followed through with her punishment—strongly motivated by the fear that the next time she and everybody else might go up in flames.

Earl was seen again six years later for aggressive behavior and trouble with the law; however, he had never set another fire after age seven, when his mother had, several times, taken away all privileges and once spanked him severely for appropriating a lighter and some matches. His other behavioral difficulties had not diminished, however.

Comment. The technique employed with Earl was behavioral modification running along the lines of "guilty until proved innocent." The aim was to suppress or extinguish the act or symptom of firesetting, *not* to achieve a psychodynamic working through or understanding of the dynamics of firesetting. As we have seen from previous discussions, the majority of children who set fires cannot come up with any information suggesting specific psychodynamics of firesetting; therefore, one need not look long for them in treatment. Physical punishment is *not the only means* of response stopping, it must be noted.

The most important reason for a symptom-suppressive approach is the dangerousness of firesetting for the child and others. The fastest elimination of firesetting is so desirable that all other considerations seem secondary. Some parents question an approach which does not give "self-understanding" or does not address the entire spectrum of the child's difficulties. This is usually a reflection of the parental pathology that helped to bring about the firesetting in the first place. It should be considered as a barrier or resistance to treatment.

In summary, treatment of childhood firesetting involves family counseling techniques and consists of the following steps:

- obtaining agreement with the family that firesetting is the main and foremost problem;
- obtaining agreement with the parents that punishing the child (by chastisement, deprivation of rewards, and the like) *before* a catastrophe happens, i.e., before the act, is not "cruel and unusual punishment," but a necessary and perhaps lifesaving measure;
- instructing the parents to stop the child if he is found to have, or to be near, any flammable substance (matches, lighters, etc.). The choice of punishment modality may be left up to the parents, as long as it is effective;
- modeling, reasoning, rehearsal, and implosion or flooding may be added to response-stopping techniques;
- direct treatment of the child is not necessary, but may help to promote better acceptance of these measures by the child and to spare the child from the parental wrath of a whipping.

When present, Attention–Deficit Hyperactivity Disorder should be treated pharmacologically and otherwise as described in Chapter 21; this facilitates the specific behavioral treatment of firesetting. The overall treatment approach that we have outlined can be practiced not only by all health care professionals, but also by firemen and law enforcement officers.

Needless to say, more comprehensive treatment of all associated disorders is highly desirable, but it cannot be stated often enough that stopping the firesetting is a meaningful and necessary goal in itself. Stopping the firesetting may not solve any of the other problems that the child has, but it keeps him and others from suffering serious injury.

Ambulatory treatment may at times be insufficient, especially when the family cannot be rallied. In that case, residential treatment of the child, along similar lines, promises success as described by Gruber and co-workers (1981). The great majority of children who have set fires do not set fires at an institution where they are adequately supervised and taught.

COURSE AND PROGNOSIS

The closer the approximation of primary pathological firesetting to "curiosity" firesetting, the better the prognosis, since the prognosis essentially reflects presence or absence of recidivism.

In our experience, it is the child's family who provide the single most important prognostic factor. As we have seen, most of these families are disrupted. However, if there is enough healthy cognition left in them to recognize the danger that firesetting poses, and they therefore take serious and unambivalent measures against it, then the chances of extinguishing this behavior are excellent. There appears to be no connection between childhood firesetting and pyromania in adulthood or arson in later life, but there may be a correlation between childhood firesetting and other forms of later antisocial behavior.

Questions for Study and Action

1. A three-year-old looks with fascination and excitement into the living-room fireplace, where a fire is roaring, while clutching his penis. His anxious mother wonders if her firstborn is in danger of becoming a "pyromaniac," especially since he has even tried to ignite some of the large fireplace matches. Write down, as if you had laryngitis and could not speak, the questions you would ask the mother and the information you would impart to her.

2. An eight-year-old boy is being admitted to a residential treatment center because of a long life of transgressions and ungovernable behavior, including setting his sister's bed on fire, with both children narrowly escaping burning and smoke inhalation. Should he be refused admission because of the firesetting? Why not? If not, write down the part of the treatment plan that should be devoted to firesetting.

3. A child psychiatrist advised father in the following terms: "First, read the riot act to your nine-year-old son against all unpermitted attempts to start a fire, while giving him supervision in starting the charcoal fire for the family barbecues." Give a full critique of this advice.

4. What does it mean that so many five-year-old firesetters have the expressed wish to grow up to be firemen, and delight in toy fire trucks? Do not hesitate to be imaginative and speculative.

5. Comment on this: the mother of a seven-year-old who had almost burned the house down asked the fire marshall to "talk to the child" about his dangerous behavior. However, the fire marshall noted that a cigarette lighter was lying on the coffee table and another on a lower shelf of the bookcase.

6. The 10-year-old only son of a prominent and successful businessman has repeatedly set fires. He tells the child psychiatrist that he does not want to do it, but that the tension becomes unbearable until he sees flames, which delight him and give him a sense of relief. His father has always paid for all the damages incurred but is now desperate. Write out all the diagnostic steps to be taken.

7. The caseworker for a family whose trailer has been burned by their six-year-old child refers him to a child psychiatrist for "in-depth" and "uncovering" psychotherapy. She believes his actions call for long-term psychoanalytic treatment. How would you deal with her request, before you have seen the child? after you have seen the child?

8. There has been an epidemic of fires set at an elementary school by a suspected group of 10 children. You are the mental health consultant to the school. Write out a consultation report after you have done all necessary interventions.

9. What projective tests would help you determine if the child in Question #6 was on the way to Pyromania? Incidentally, would you include projective tests at all?

10. Interview three family therapists in your community to find out what specific techniques they would employ with a family that includes a child who is a chronic firesetter. Do you wish to interview more than three?

For Further Reading

Bender, L. Fire setting in children. In L. Bender, *Aggression, Hostility and Anxiety in Children.* Springfield, IL: Charles C Thomas, 1953.

Fineman, K.R. Fire-setting in children and adolescence. *Psychiat. Clin. N. Amer.,* 3: 483–500, 1980.

Fras, I., & Saeger, D.L. The treatment of fire setters. Presented at the 29th Annual Meeting of the American Association of Psychiatric Services for Children, Washington, D.C., November 16–20, 1977.

Fras, I. Follow-up of childhood firesetters and factors predicting recidivist firesetting. Presented at the 54th International Meeting, Mayo Alumni Association, Orlando FL, March 25–26, 1987.

Freud, S. The acquisition of power over fire. *Int. J. Psychoanal.,* October 1932.

Gruber, A.R., & Heck, E.T. Children who set fires. *Amer. J. Orthopsychiatry,* 51: 484–488, 1981.

Kuhnley, E., Hendren, R.L., & Quinlan, D.M. Fire setting by children. *J. Amer. Acad. of Child Psychiatry,* 21:560–563, 1982.

Lewis, N.D.C., & Yarnell, H., (Eds.), *Pathological Firesetting (Pyromania).* Nervous and Mental Disease Monographs (No. 82). New York: New York Coolidge Foundation, 1951.

Meeks, J.E. Firesetting. In J.N. Noshpitz (Ed.), *Basic Handbook of Child Psychiatry, Vol. 2* (pp. 508–510). New York: Basic Books, 1979.

Nurcombe, B. Children who set fires. *Med. J. Australia,* 1: 579–584, 1964.

Scott, D. *The Psychology of Fire.* New York: Charles Scribner's Sons, 1974.

Yarnell, H. Fire setting in children. *Am. J. Orthopsychiatry,* 10: 272–286, 1940.

8

Functional Enuresis

DEFINITION

Functional Enuresis (307.60) has been defined as the involuntary voiding of urine, after an age at which continence is expected, that is not due to physical disease. There is some variation in defining the age in question: DSM-III-R defines it as five years; others as low as three or four years, and most practitioners as the age of beginning school. In other words, the diagnosis of enuresis is usually not made before the child has started school.

DMS-III-R further delineates the frequency of Enuresis as at least twice a month between five and six years of age, and once a month for older children.

Enuresis can be nocturnal—at night only (by far the most frequent—80%), diurnal—during the day only (15%), or both nocturnal and diurnal (5%) (Pierce, 1985). It is termed *primary* if there has been no urinary continence for at least one year, and *secondary* if there has been continence of at least one year and then a resumption of wetting. Histories given by parents in this respect may be unreliable, and primary enuresis is much more common than secondary enuresis.

129

ETIOLOGY AND PATHOPHYSIOLOGY

Although psychological factors play precipitating roles and, infrequently, appear to be the only cause, the prevailing contemporary view is that Functional Enuresis is not caused primarily by psychological factors. One of the most interesting facts supporting this thesis is the "democratic" nature of this disorder (an expression used by Chester Pierce [1985]): it occurs with equal frequency in every socioeconomic stratum, regardless of race or creed. Enuresis is considered a disorder of bladder physiology in a developmental sense: the bladder capacity itself, or the structures involved in micturition (levator ani, bladder, and abdominal muscles), or the sleep-waking cycle and the rate of urine production, are insufficiently developed and controlled. The basic cause for this neuromuscular insufficiency is probably genetic or maturational.

We will address each of the above factors again when we discuss treatment methods.

CLINICAL DESCRIPTION

CASE 8-1   Charlie was eight years old when his mother brought his bedwetting to the attention of the physician. He was wetting the bed at least *once or twice a week*, and mother's tolerance for these "accidents" was rapidly diminishing. Moreover, Charlie himself was not only becoming *ashamed and embarrassed* by it but also beginning to feel the *social implications*. He could not stay overnight with a friend, nor could he contemplate campouts with boy scouts once he "graduated" from cub scouts for fear of wetting the bed.

Family history showed that Charlie's father had been a bedwetter until age 14. *Past history* showed that Charlie always was considered an immature child with severe *temper tantrums* between ages three and five and, subsequently, *reading disabilities* diagnosed by the school. His *parents* were *divorced* when Charlie was four. Toilet training had been generally difficult because of Charlie's overall stubbornness, but he was trained for bowel and daytime bladder control by age three years. However, nighttime enuresis persisted, in spite of his mother's attempts to awaken him. As a matter of fact, Charlie proved to be *"impossible to arouse from sleep* on most occasions!"

Comment. This case shows the most common, typical features of enuresis:

- Boys outnumber girls roughly by a ratio of 2:1.
- Family history shows a high incidence of enuresis in first-degree relatives (parents, often both parents, and grandparents).
- The frequently associated features of immaturity: developmental lag, manifested

by generally immature behavior, temper tantrums, hyperkinesis, and learning disabilities.

- Sometimes conflictual family circumstances, such as those preceding divorce.
- One group of enuretics is characterized by exceptionally deep sleep and inability to be aroused from it by almost any stimulus, including that of a full bladder.
- The case cited is, of course, an example of primary Functional Enuresis.

CASE 8-2   Sheila was seven-and-a-half years old when she *started wetting the bed again. She had been fully toilet trained* at age three, although this was accomplished with some difficulty; her parents were permissive and therefore loath to be "too authoritarian" with her. When a *sibling was born,* Sheila's position of being the special, only child was threatened. Her parents *responded* with a mixture of *solicitous concern and anger,* which left them perplexed and ineffective for dealing with the problem.

Background history showed that these *parents* were highly intellectual, *neurotic* people who immediately seized upon Sheila's enuresis to stabilize their own disputes over it.

Comment. This case shows a relatively uncommon *secondary enuresis.* The sharp clinician hears all such reports with skepticism, for parents often assert that the child has been completely toilet trained for a year or more prior to the episode in question, but careful inquiry reveals episodes of enuresis in those periods as well.

Both primary and secondary enuresis may serve the parents' neurotic needs: their relationship is stabilized around the child's behavioral symptom. The child and his or her symptom of enuresis are often used by one parent to fight the other parent; the family thus becomes "triangulated."

DIAGNOSIS AND DIFFERENTIAL DIAGNOSIS

The diagnosis is, obviously, easily made once the child is wetting after a certain age (three to six years). However, the physician then needs to undertake two more steps:

1. The "refining" of the diagnosis

- Is it nighttime or daytime?
- Is it primary or secondary enuresis?
- Is the child an exceptionally deep sleeper and one who cannot be awakened?
- Is the child immature and perhaps even hyperactive?

- Have the parents noticed that he cannot hold his urine for over an hour, suggesting small bladder capacity?
- Has toilet training been inconsistent, or have the family circumstances generally been chaotic?

2. The differential diagnosis

The important aspect here is to differentiate between functional and organic enuresis. The latter is defined as enuresis due to an organic cause other than sociogenic, developmental (maturational), or genetic ones. Such causes are:

- Obstructive uropathy, especially congenital abnormalities such as bladder outlet and urethral abnormalities, stricture, and stenoses. The combination of nocturnal and diurnal enuresis, and/or dribbling by day (incomplete emptying of the bladder) are symptoms especially suggestive of organic causes.
- Urinary tract infections, especially cystitis.
- Convulsive disorder (less frequently). Micturition may be part of a seizure not otherwise suspected and of sickle-cell anemia.
- Spinal cord tumors (rarely), in which case the loss of bladder control is progressive and combined with loss of other functions.

The main consideration to keep in mind is that we must not assume any enuresis to be functional until organic causes have been ruled out.

TREATMENT

This is one disorder in psychiatry for which treatment can often be aimed at the underlying cause and, when this is not possible, at least treatment can be directed towards the general underlying mechanism. The physician should therefore correlate a detailed history (the "refined" diagnosis presented earlier) with the causative mechanisms and choose the treatment accordingly.

Before we get into specifics, however, there is one principle of treatment that must be emphasized: a good doctor–patient relationship is an integral part of the treatment and sometimes it literally works wonders. The rapport established from a detailed evaluation, or early in the course of psychotherapy, or even through a placebo intervention has been known to have stopped enuresis there and then! Unfortunately, those miracles are not predictable and deception should not be part of the clinician's armamentarium.

Since genetic factors are the main cause in a number of enuretic children, their recognition alone, in the face of obdurate persistence of the disorder, may be one therapeutic approach. If no treatment is effective, the parents' and the child's minds can be relieved of guilt, unnecessary recriminations, and punishment through the realization that, for example, father and grandfather wet the bed till age 14. This is sometimes called the "nihilistic" approach.

The immaturity and developmental lag so often found to be associated with enuresis have provided an "approximately" causal or etiological treatment, especially if associated with Attention–Deficit Hyperactivity Disorder: pharmacotherapy with stimulants (e.g., methylphenidate [Ritalin] or amphetamines). This has indeed proven therapeutically effective in some cases, but not in others, and is therefore not a standard approach to enuresis, *except* when the physician wants, in all events, to treat the Attention–Deficit Hyperactivity Disorder. In that case, an evening dose of the stimulant should be tried.

However, when the developmental lag is found to be more narrowly circumscribed as a disturbance of circadian rhythm, then treatment becomes more predictable: tricyclic antidepressants affect the ratio of REM to non-REM sleep and are effective in those enuretic patients who are described as heavy sleepers. Most Functional Enuresis occurs during non-REM sleep, or rather at the point of transition from REM to non-REM sleep, and tricyclic antidepressants may "even out" the EEG phases of sleep, although this is a controversial point, and peripheral adrenergic (anticholinergic) or local neuromuscular effects may be more likely to operate here (Rapaport et al., 1980). Imipramine (Tofranil) is the traditional agent, but there is no reason why other antidepressants cannot be used. Recently, actions of tricyclic antidepressants other than on sleep in enuresis have been postulated and the rationale for their use has been broadened to include cases other than "heavy sleepers." Administration is either one dose in the evening, or one dose in the afternoon and one in the evening. For dosage information, the reader is referred to our section on pharmacological agents (Chapter 2).

Of similar etiologically bound efficacy are bladder training exercises: the child who is reported not to be able to tolerate larger amounts of urine without great urgency is trained to retain gradually larger amounts of urine for longer periods of time. Perhaps the most effective nonspecific treatments for enuresis are conditioning devices. The principle of their action is to establish a conditioned reflex of waking up when micturition occurs or is about to occur. The efficacy of this method depends on parental acceptance of it and on the specific subtype of enuresis. The subtype associated with exceptionally deep sleep is not likely to respond to this conditioning device, although most other subtypes have a good chance to do so.

A number of other treatment methods have been used, but the only one still practiced is cystoscopy with urethral dilatation or meatotomy. This method once enjoyed great popularity among urologists; it was quite successful in that it, too, established a conditioned reflex because of the postoperative pain produced by a full bladder. The rationale was that a urethral meatal stenosis, reportedly found in most enuretics on endoscopy, had to be cut and dilated. This rationale, a matter of controversy, is used far less frequently now, and meatotomies are rare.

Atropine and other parasympathomimetic (anticholinergic) medications were used with varying success in the past, but have been replaced by the newer pharmacological approaches already described.

Psychotherapy must be viewed in a special light, since a psychotherapeutic relationship is always necessary and helpful in treating enuresis. Psychotherapy is indicated in enuresis secondary to psychiatric problems. It may take the form of individual psychotherapy, with parent counseling nearly always necessary. As pointed out in the discussion of Case 2, the family may need the child's symptom (in this case, enuresis) to stabilize itself neurotically, or the parents may have simply been remiss, inept, or otherwise handicapped in toilet training the child. In all these and similar circumstances, parents need support and guidance. Such situations should be referred to the specialist.

PROGNOSIS

Prognosis, too, is to a great extent developmentally–genetically determined. Statistics generally show that 16% of children are enuretic at age five years; by seven, 7% are enuretic; thereafter, a rule of thumb is that one-quarter (25%) of those still enuretic remit spontaneously each year, giving an incidence lowered to about 2% by age 18.

The age of spontaneous remission often parallels that of the parent's remission if there is a positive family history. Despite this 25% chance of spontaneous remission each year, it is advisable to treat enuresis, since the suffering and secondary emotional sequelae may be considerable.

Most modern treatment methods have at least some positive effect. Pharmacotherapy and conditioning devices are the most effective for selected subgroups. Psychotherapy contributes at least some relief and may be a necessary palliative approach in those patients who do not respond to any other treatment method.

Questions for Study and Action

1. List three practical reasons for asking the mother of an eight-year-old male bedwetter for her "gut level" responses to the child's enuresis, who puts the sheets into the dirty laundry, and what she thinks her attitude and behavior mean to her son. Be able to justify your logic.

2. How would you interpret an eight-year-old girl's telling you that she awakens briefly when her bladder is full, wants to get up and go to the bathroom but, since she is afraid of the dark, she urinates and resumes sleep in her bed? What would you prescribe for her?

3. How would it help you to refine your diagnosis if you elicited each of the following pieces of history for a seven-year-old male enuretic?
    (a) He shares a bed with a 10-year-old enuretic brother.
    (b) He never wets the bed when he "sleeps over" with an agemate.
    (c) He only wets the bed when he sleeps in the bed with his mother, when father is out of town on business trips.
    (d) He never wets except when he goes to bed feeling unhappy.
    (e) He wakes up feeling groggy and unrested, thinks he is dry, but always discovers he has already wet the bed.

4. Of what value is the finding of pus cells in the urine of a 10-year-old who was dry by age five years but recently reverted to bedwetting? Explain your supposition.

5. Of what psychiatric relevance is it that a seven-year-old child recently started bedwetting, school refusing, and talking like a baby?

6. Ask a pediatric resident to describe two or three cases of children of four or five years of age who reverted to bedwetting during their hospital stay. Also ask him/her to give you an estimate of how many such cases (s)he has seen in the past year.

7. What could it signify that a child wets only when she lives with her mother in New York City and not with her father in another state? What questions would you have?

8. Outline your treatment plans for a nine-year-old boy who resumed bedwetting three years ago when a sister (the parents' darling) was born. He refuses to swallow imipramine; he will not talk about his bedwetting; he mastered the electric conditioning device, became dry quickly, and then disconnected the device and resumed bedwetting. What treatment steps can be taken now?

9. An eight-year-old child with nocturnal seizures is humiliated about her bedwetting. What diagnostic and therapeutic measures would you employ in helping her overcome her enuresis and shame?

10. Contrast the situations of a 10-year-old enuretic whose father was an enuretic with a boy whose father was dry by age two.

For Further Reading

Bemporad, J.R. (Ed.). *Child Development in Normality and Psychopathology.* New York: Brunner/Mazel, 1980.

Foxx, R.M., & Azrin, N.H. Dry pants: A rapid method of toilet training children. In A.M. Graziano (Ed.), *Behavior Therapy with Children, II.* Chicago: Aldine, 1975.

Pierce, C.M. Enuresis. In H.I. Kaplan & B.J. Sadock (Eds.), *Comprehensive Textbook of Psychiatry* (4th Ed.). Baltimore: Williams & Wilkins, 1985, pp. 1842–1847.

Rapoport, J.L., Mikkelsen, E.J., Zavadil, A., Nee, L., Gruenau, C., Mendelson, W., & Gillin, C. Childhood enuresis I. and II. *Arch. Gen. Psychiatry,* 37:1139–1152, 1980.

9

Functional
Encopresis

Encopresis is both a symptom and a childhood disorder of elimination in its own right. This distinction is of more than academic interest for it will dictate the treatment, and clinicians are once more reminded to be diligent and circumspect in the diagnostic process.

DEFINITION

Encopresis is the repeated voluntary or involuntary passage of feces after the age when continence is expected (usually four years or older). It may include the additional smearing of feces in inappropriate places.

Encopresis can be functional or organic. The list of organic encopresis is short: aganglionic megacolon and anal fissure and similar painful anal or rectal diseases are organic conditions that precipitate or otherwise lead to encopresis. Various systemic diseases can lead to changes in bowel habits, and occasionally to encopresis. When no demonstrable physical cause can be found, the encopresis should be diagnosed as functional. This functional or "psychogenic" category is the most frequent and will be the subject of consideration in this chapter; when referring to encopresis, it will be understood that we are discussing

Functional Encopresis (307.70) only, unless otherwise specified. The concomitant medical disorder can be specified on Axis III.

It is useful to distinguish between "primary" or "continuous" and "secondary" or "discontinuous" encopresis. Secondary encopresis can be "retentive" (the usual) or "nonretentive" (infrequent for secondary encopresis) depending on the presence of constipation.

Primary Encopresis

CASE 9-1   Peter was five years old when he was seen by the child psychiatrist for *persistent encopresis* as well as *nocturnal enuresis*. He was brought to the office by his foster mother who complained that *"nothing worked"* to induce Peter not to soil. Peter simply *never was toilet trained*. This was not surprising during his first two years of life since he had been *grossly neglected* by his natural mother who was mentally retarded, lived in squalor herself, and made few attempts to toilet train him. There was no father in the home. After several transient foster-home placements, he was finally placed in his current foster home at about age three and a half. During the first year in the present foster home, Peter continued not only to soil himself but also to *smear feces* on the bathroom walls.

Examination showed a *pale, poorly developed, immature* youngster whose attention span was short and who had speech defects. The foster mother had *difficulty controlling him.* His handling of toys and play materials suggested strong *aggressive and destructive* impulses.

Comment. Primary encopresis is defined in DSM-III-R as fecal soiling occurring after the child has reached the age of four years without having fecal continence for at least one year. Primary encopresis occurs more in lower socioeconomic families and is usually associated with a significantly unstable environment. As Anthony (1957) has termed it, this is "a dirty child from a dirty family, burdened with every conceivable sort of social problem" (p. 613).

These children show delayed maturation in a number of areas, notably speech and impulse control. Attention–Deficit Hyperactivity Disorder, Conduct Disorder, and developmental disabilities (learning disorders) are frequently diagnosed upon complete examination. Toilet training may or may not have been attempted; at any rate, the child's own deficient perception of his gastrointestinal reflexes as well as the environment's haphazard habit training combine to make the learning of toilet habits unusually difficult for the child. Moreover, some of these children appear to have diminished reactions both to their gastrointestinal reflexes and to the social effects of their soiling.

Secondary Encopresis

CASE 9-2   Brian was an eight-year-old child of *upper-middle-class* parents who was referred to a child psychiatrist by his pediatrician because the treatment attempted for encopresis was unsuccessful. The pediatrician had tried *laxatives, stool softeners,* and a *simple reward system,* all of them to no avail.

The soiling had started two years previously, *coincident* with the *birth* of a *baby sister.* Up to that time, the patient had been toilet trained—as a matter of fact, he had been toilet trained at the *unusually early* age of 14 months by his *perfectionistic mother.* Indeed, the child had grown up to be as neat, compulsive, and constipated as his mother. He was well liked by adults but had periodic difficulties with *peers;* he was usually *demanding, domineering,* and tended to *victimize* some of his younger peers. He was unusually *compliant* towards his parents—except for occasional *temper outbursts* and "inexplicable," rare *"accidents"* when he could not make it to the toilet from the playground and *soiled* his underwear. He was then very embarrassed.

Since the *birth of his sibling,* however, the patient soiled his underwear regularly: this occurred either as *formed stools* about once or twice a week, or, more typically, going *without any* formed bowel movements for as long as 10 days until the child finally passed a *very large* bowel movement, usually in the evening (in his pants), or he had to be taken to the pediatrician for fecal impaction. During the 10 days or so of fecal retention, there was *leakage* of soft fecal matter into his underwear. The patient was *ashamed of it in school* but showed little shame at home, especially with his mother.

Examination showed a thin, *inhibited* child who at first acted in an excessively *serious, pseudo-adult manner.* Later, *teasing, passive-aggressive* attitudes could be seen. Although superficially verbal, he was "retentive" in his communications, i.e., he would *withhold* information about his feelings from the examiner. His drawings reflected themes of *retaliation* against *threatening, domineering* adults. He portrayed his *mother as extremely controlling,* and his *father as passive, uninvolved,* and ultimately rejecting.

His parents, especially his *mother,* were *preoccupied* with his toilet habits to the *exclusion* of any *other* aspects of his adaptive functioning.

Comment. The central and typical feature of this case of secondary encopresis is the *obsessive, controlling mother,* an almost universal ingredient in secondary encopresis. There is, as a rule, early, coercive toilet training. Often we find a precipitating event, although previously everything had not been so calm.

Constipation may or may not be present (although some authorities consider constipation to be central to the problem). We would suggest the differentiation "retentive" and "nonretentive" on the basis of constipation. The retentive type is more common.

ETIOLOGY AND PATHOPHYSIOLOGY

In primary encopresis, there are a number of organic contributory factors, such as various forms of developmental delays. In both primary and secondary encopresis, diminished sensitivity to both the gastrointestinal sensations and, perhaps, the social consequences are possible contributory factors. However, the basic etiology in encopresis is environmental—it is the toilet training. To oversimplify: in primary encopresis, there is not enough of it, and in secondary encopresis, there is too much of it. The details are amplified in the clinical descriptions and case histories that follow.

Whereas the psychodynamics in primary encopresis are simple, the entire scenario is one of neglect and primitive impulses. The psychodynamics of secondary encopresis are often more complex. The primary caretakers (mothers) are the central psychodynamic figures, often cast in the light of toilet-crazy martinets: "feminine dictators who expect their children to respond with the alacrity of soldiers" (Lehman, 1944). In orthodox psychoanalytic terms, they are "anal personalities," and the children are cast in the same characterological mold. However, the overcontrolled personality has a crack or an imperfection—the encopresis. Toilet training is described as so perfectionistic that it transmits the basic hostility of these highly ambivalent mothers. The children get back at their mothers by encopresis, which may also bridge their sense of rejection by forcing the mother to pay attention to the child. The fathers have been too detached (sometimes by divorce) to be an effective counterbalance to the mother's pathology. Interestingly, encopresis often ceases when fathers become involved in an empathic, helping way.

TREATMENT

Treatment will depend on the clinical subtype:

1. Primary Encopresis

The basis of all treatment is toilet training or retraining, usually involving the restructuring of the child's environment. At the least, this means helping the child to be aware of bowel sensations and reeducating the parent(s) about toilet training; at the most, it means removing the child from a grossly neglectful environment.

CASE 9-3   Tommy was six years old when mother complained to the pediatrician that he was still soiling his pants. She had "taken it very easy" with toilet training since the boy was hyperactive and the family was preoccupied with their upward economic mobility. Mother had found it easier to grant the child a great deal of freedom. Tommy simply kept too busy playing to go to the toilet.

The pediatrician decided to treat both the hyperactivity and the encopresis. For the latter, he advised the mother to put the child on the toilet every morning and every evening for half an hour. He was to receive random rewards for any bowel movements he produced, but mother was to insist on the child's sitting on the toilet regardless of negative results. A psychostimulant relieved the hyperactivity and attention deficit.

After less than a month, Tommy had become "habituated" to this toileting routine and ceased being encopretic.

Comment. This is the simplest treatment situation, facilitated by two factors: a cooperative parent with lack of specific "encopretogenic" pathology and the successful treatment of a concomitant, but predisposing condition, i.e., the hyperactivity.

CASE 9-4   Jeremiah had almost reached his 11th birthday when he was seen at the mental health clinic because of a long list of transgressions in school and at home, notably fighting, throwing food in the cafeteria, lying and stealing, and being unresponsive to discipline. In addition, almost as an afterthought, the mother mentioned Jeremiah's encopresis—"never has been fully trained." Mother looked exhausted. She was almost 50 and had already raised five older siblings with little help from her husband.

Jeremiah's treatment was multifaceted. He was seen in supportive, regular sessions by a male therapist with whom he could identify; his parents were counseled by a female social worker with a view towards greater involvement of the father; the school was encouraged to pursue more aggressively the remediation of Jeremiah's developmental learning disorder. Only when all these approaches were "in place" and looked promising was the encopresis tackled.

It transpired that Jeremiah had developed a pattern in his encopresis. He would hold his bowel movements all day and finally soil his pants in the evening. He had become so adept at hiding his soiled underwear that he was even able to go on overnight visits without being "detected." As the relationship with father improved, the patient responded better to social demands, and mother experienced some relief, the parents were advised to "schedule" the patient to sit on the toilet every evening for half an hour, at the time that he usually "filled his pants." The procedure eventually proved successful in stopping the encopresis.

Comment. Just as the encopresis here existed and continued in the context of a Conduct Disorder and inadequate parental relationships, so the treatment could be undertaken only in this context. Without improved intrafamilial relationships and a different outlook for the patient himself (identification with his therapist), the simplest program of bowel retraining could not have succeeded.

CASE 9-5   Alicia was six when she was brought to the attention of the department of social services for being physically abused by her mother's alcoholic boyfriend. At that time, she was enuretic and encopretic and given to severe temper tantrums. After placement in a foster home, her enuresis was brought under control, but she continued to have bowel movements in her bed, behind furniture, and even beside the toilet, in addition to smearing them on the bathroom walls. She was equally inappropriate with her food, eating out of the garbage cans and smearing food on walls.

Her behavior continued to present such difficulty for the foster parents that she was moved to a residential treatment facility where she made slow but steady progress.

Comment. Severe neglect and abuse have produced a multi-handicapped child. The resources of a foster home were overstressed by this child, and ambulatory treatment was not even attempted.

PROGNOSIS

Encopresis usually ceases with the advent of puberty. Until that time, the prognosis varies with the subtype.

Primary encopresis, where lack of bowel training has simply "lingered on" through parental overpermissiveness in an otherwise "normal" family, has the best prognosis. Next there come those cases of secondary encopresis in which the pathology in parents and child is relatively light, and where there is an identifiable and remediable precipitating event. In that case, the encopresis is similar to other "reactive" psychiatric conditions, with a similarly good prognosis if the stressor is removed. It should be borne in mind, though, that the specific psychodynamic constellation making for this particular choice of symptoms is somewhat more pathological than in many other "reactive" syndromes, and that, therefore, even this type of encopresis is often prolonged and resistive to easy treatment.

It is safe to state that all other cases of encopresis have a lengthy course, with ultimate resolution through treatment or simply time and maturation (puberty). The long-term implications for character development vary more with the specifics of each case of encopresis than with the general condition itself, with

Passive Aggressive Personality Disorder a frequent complication of severe secondary encopresis.

2. Secondary Encopresis

In contrast to primary encopresis, toilet training is not the approach here. Many authors have recommended long-term psychotherapy and, in view of the complex nature of many of these cases, that seems sensible. We should bear in mind, however, that psychotherapy must include the parents. Depending on the age of the child and the specifics of the problem, the duration of psychotherapy will vary. In addition to psychotherapy, physical methods (stool softeners) may be of benefit if the encopresis is of the retentive type; their value has been debated.

CASE 9-6   James started withholding his stools for extended periods (seven to 10 days) when he was eight years old, at a time of severe marital strife between his parents, which was followed by depression in his mother for which she had to be hospitalized for a month.

The pediatrician prescribed stool softeners, which provided some relief to James but did not alter the fact that he was still encopretic. He was therefore referred to a psychiatrist. In James' psychotherapy sessions, his thoughts focused on themes of murder, retaliation, and fights between "revolutionaries" and the police. These were interpreted as conflicts between his own angry, rebellious drives and mother's repressive tactics before she became ill. James then continued to portray all-powerful leaders in his play—anything was possible for them, they "held the world in the palm of their hand." This again was interpreted as his wish for control and belief in magic and contrasted with his (postulated) fears of being abandoned.

And so on! Therapy of the dynamic-verbal variety continued for seven months, during which time both parents effected a rapprochement and were then able to employ more appropriate child-raising methods.

Comment. The treatment of complex secondary encopresis belongs to the specialist, for whom it is difficult enough. The dropout rate is high since the parents often are ambivalent about treatment.

We have considered encopresis in some detail because it is encountered relatively frequently but is treated like a stepchild in most textbooks. The health professional needs to sort out what he or she can treat, and what to refer to a specialist. The primary care physician must make the differential diagnosis between organic and functional encopresis, and can be expected to treat simple, "lazy" primary encopresis and mild, "reactive" secondary encopresis. Others can be directed to a child psychiatrist.

Questions for Study and Action

1. Following family group casework in a social agency, a nine-year-old boy was seen for a diagnostic interview by a child psychiatrist. As soon as he sat down, the lad said haughtily, "I guess you'll say I'm shitting on my mother, heh?" How would you proceed with that interview?

2. You are working in a well-child clinic and are asked by a mother of a 20-month-old girl, "Should I read a book about 'toilet learning' to my daughter? She seems to be getting interested in using the grown-ups' toilet and my mother bought her a potty chair. What should I do?" How would you respond? Remember that parent guidance is a vital part of the physician's role.

3. Why did a famous psychoanalyst refer to the mother and child, when the latter is learning toilet discipline (18–30 months of age), as "the potting couple?" Explain what kind of mother-child interaction would make for wholesome toilet learning.

4. Why would a stool softener, such as dioctyl sodium sulfa-succinate, be prescribed again by a child psychiatrist who is treating, in dynamic-verbal psychotherapy, Brian (Case 9-2), an eight-year-old boy with secondary encopresis? Recall that the pediatrician had tried a stool softener earlier.

5. Explain—for a child to understand you—how a stool softener may be an efficacious adjunct to psychotherapy when a chronically constipated child with an anal fissure becomes encopretic. Write out what you might tell the child about what caused the fissure, how the fissure added to retention and constipation and aggravated soiling with bypassing liquid feces. What would you recommend about water and diet?

6. Write, in a child's terminology, how you would endeavor to encourage his understanding of the physiology of defecation if he is six years old and has never been free of encopresis. Would you do this with his parent(s) present in the room? How so? How would you describe the gastrocolic reflex? the sensations felt in the levator ani and other pelvic muscles during defecation? How would a "Dulcolax" suppository before breakfast aid your teaching (his learning) efforts?

7. If there are twice as many poor people as upper-middle-class people in your
    medical practice, interpret this clinical research finding: Neglected children and
    those with both parents working make up two-thirds of the encopresis cases; the
    affluent account for only one-third. Would you conclude that encopresis is
    disproportionately a lower-class disorder?

8. Try to build a case for the unconscious linkage of all the following:
    (a) Mother is constipated, takes laxatives regularly and worries about bowel functions.
    (b) Child soils and then stows his underwear in the piano bench.
    (c) Mother plays the piano rather well technically but without much feeling.
    (d) The child showed both murderous rage and fear of being killed on projective
        testing.
    (e) Mother feels that males are not only biologically inferior but also messy, dirty,
        and smelly creatures.
    (f) Mother spanks child on his buttocks when he misbehaves.

9. What questions would you ask of a psychological consultant during your diagnostic
    workup with a 10-year-old who first became encopretic four months ago?

10. List five markers or indices of a "chaotic family" when a child has primary encopresis.

For Further Reading

Anthony, E.J. An experimental approach to the psychopathology of childhood: Encopresis. *Brit. J.
    Med. Psychol.*, 30:146–175, 1957.

Baird, M. Characteristic interaction patterns in families of encopretic children. *Bull. Menninger
    Clinic*, 38:144–153, 1974.

Bemporad, J.L., Pfeifer, C.M., Gibbs, L., et al. Characteristics of encopretic patients and their
    families. *J. Amer. Acad. of Child Psychiatry*, 10:272–292, 1971.

Hoag, J.M., Norriss, N.G., Himeno, E.T., & Jacobs, J. The encopretic child and his family. *J. Amer.
    Acad. of Child Psychiatry*, 10:242–256, 1971.

Lehman, E. Psychogenic incontinence of feces (encopresis) in children. *Amer. J. Dis. Child*,
    68:190–199, 1944.

Levine, M.D. Encopresis: Its potentiations, evaluation and alleviation. *Ped. Clin. N. Amer.*, 29:315–330,
    1982.

Ohatawura, M. Encopresis: A review of thirty-two cases. *Acta Paediatr. Scand.*, 62:358–364, 1973.

Pierce, C.N. Encopresis. In H.I. Kaplan & B.J. Sadock (Eds.), *Comprehensive Textbook of Psychiatry*
    (4th Ed.). Baltimore: Williams & Wilkins, 1985, pp. 1847–1849.

10

Eating Disorders

Anorexia Nervosa (307.10) and Bulimia Nervosa (307.51)

We shall discuss these two disorders jointly, for the simple reason that in children we occasionally see Anorexia Nervosa, but rarely see Bulimia Nervosa in its pure form or separate from Anorexia Nervosa. Nevertheless, Bulimia Nervosa may be a precursor or a fluctuating accompaniment of Anorexia Nervosa and will, therefore, simply be mentioned alongside Anorexia Nervosa. Since this book deals with children only, all our references are to *prepubertal* or *premenarchal* Anorexia Nervosa. Prepubertal Anorexia Nervosa is still quite rare, and many clinicians do not agree that this category even exists (A.R. Lucas, personal communication, 1987). However, this is a rapidly changing clinical and social scene.

DEFINITION

The central definition of both Anorexia Nervosa and Bulimia Nervosa is that they are based on a disturbance of body image so severe that a morbid fear of gaining weight and becoming obese develops, and, in turn, the normal function of eating becomes steeped in pathological signs and symptoms. In Bulimia Nervosa, appetite becomes episodically excessive, and the patient then gets rid of the ingested food by inducing vomiting or purging (laxative abuse). In

146

childhood, Bulimia Nervosa used to be seen almost only as part of Anorexia Nervosa, and therefore has not qualified as a DSM-III-R diagnosis in this age group. However, isolated, informal case reports of prepubertal Bulimia Nervosa have come to the authors' attention recently. The five criteria necessary for the diagnosis according to DSM-III-R are: intense fear of becoming obese, disturbance of body image, weight loss of at least 15% of expected weight, refusal to maintain body weight over an age-appropriate minimum, and weight loss not due to a known physical illness.

ETIOLOGY AND PATHOGENESIS

First of all, there are several "short cuts" to pathogenesis: an "eating phobia" or "weight gain phobia" has been postulated, on the psychodynamic side of reasoning. A "forme fruste," or incomplete, form of Depression has been suggested on the organic side, particularly since the resultant endocrine disturbances in Anorexia Nervosa are the same as those in Depression. These hypotheses should be borne in mind when discussing treatment. However, we can attempt the following, more complete, composite hypothesis of etiology and pathogenesis, based on presently available data.

A genetic factor may be present, as suggested by twin studies, which predisposes the child to dysfunction in the hypothalamic-anterior pituitary-gonadal axis (Holland et al., 1984). This axis regulates the onset of puberty; in addition, the hypothalamus regulates appetite and weight gain, and the anterior pituitary secretes growth hormone, as well as gonadotrophins under the influence of the hypothalamus. The entire axis is susceptible to psychological influences, mediated primarily via the cortex to the hypothalamus, to the latter's own feedback (hormonal levels), and to nutrition (growth-sexual development, etc.), all of which are increased or decreased depending on the adequacy of food intake.

As the child approaches puberty, biopsychosocial changes occur. The child's changing perception of her body, and her emotional reactions both to this and to the social and cultural pressures of her age may become exaggerated. Why this is so is probably multiply determined: by the specific dynamics in the child's family, combined with social and cultural conditions brought to bear on her by the school, her peers, the culture around her, and chance events. Some even see the anorectic as emblematic of the convention-ridden female, fearing to be her natural self.

The candidate for Anorexia Nervosa has not been encouraged in her previous attempts at self-expression and is thus quite dependent on others for her self-concept. She tries to measure up to the expectations of her environment in a rigid, obsessive manner. As she grows, demands increase; "switching off" the growth and maturation (including sexual maturation) process by not eating is easily discovered in our diet-oriented culture. As her food intake is curtailed, her metabolism changes and the normal hunger mechanisms no longer operate under negative nitrogen balance. Moreover, abstinence from food is reinforced by the psychic relief of "switching off" the demands for growth on the one hand and overcomplying with parental demands for perfection on the other; again, obsessive-compulsive mechanisms take over. The patient is in an altered emotional and cognitive state, mentally, and is also in an altered physical state, metabolically. The latter reinforces the abnormal mental state, just as it stunts both somatic growth in general and sexual growth specifically. The anorectic child has thus created her own world and is in charge of it, helped and supported by this altered mental and metabolic state, rather akin to an organic brain syndrome.

CLINICAL DESCRIPTION

Prepubertal or premenarchal Anorexia Nervosa usually starts insidiously and is noticed after a longer course (usually realized in retrospect) than its adolescent/adult counterpart, because weight loss may at first be reflected only as a *lack of weight gain*. If the girl (most of these patients are girls) is near pubescence, the initial signs of pubescence simply do not occur.

The child may be given to obsessive rituals of excessive exercise. She skips meals, especially school lunches. She is generally compulsive and a high achiever. When confronted, she insists she is working towards an ideal, very slim body image and low weight.

CASE 10-1   Shortly after her 11th birthday, Celeste weighed 85 pounds but *took that down to 65 pounds* over the next year, upsetting her parents in the process and becoming "the odd one" of their five children. An older brother and two older sisters preceded Celeste in birth order and when Celeste was three a younger sister had been born. Her sisters remained solicitous but her older brother became an unmerciful teaser and bullier, telling Celeste she was ugly because she wore glasses, calling her "Brains" and "the Christian martyr," and warning her sarcastically when she ate a morsel of food, "Now, don't overeat or you'll have to exercise for four or five hours."

Celeste had often commented that she felt that she was *too fat* when obviously she was too skinny. She lived *in terror of becoming "more" obese*. She seemed to be healthy despite her *weight loss* and *her birdlike lankiness*. At Lent she *gave up soft drinks, candies, and sweets, and offered to wash all the dishes for the family and make up her bed each day.* After the Lenten season was long past, she continued in self-denial. Her father said, "She's more conscientious about religion than any of the others. *She seems to persist religiously in avoiding food, like a ritual.* At times, I see her *cry because she wants to eat but feels she must not.*" Like her nearly 14-year-old sister, Celeste had never menstruated and showed few signs of pubertal development.

Comment. Celeste had some features of Depression, Obsessive Compulsive Disorder, and Anorexia Nervosa. When she ate and felt she had broken her religious vows, she vomited her gastric contents, so she also showed some tendency to Bulimia Nervosa. She met criteria for Anorexia Nervosa and Obsessive Compulsive Disorder. A low dosage combination of perphenazine and amitriptyline was begun three weeks following initial interview and continued for about six weeks thereafter in her treatment as an outpatient. Two years after her expressive psychotherapy began, she was completely well, of normal weight, and had been menstruating regularly since she was almost 13 years old.

DIFFERENTIAL DIAGNOSIS

This is really not difficult, although Anorexia Nervosa and Bulimia Nervosa in the initial stage may be confused with Attention–Deficit Hyperactivity Disorder. The latter shows random hyperactivity, whereas the anorectic child imposes compulsive exercise programs on herself.

Depression in children may include loss of appetite, together with anhedonia and hopelessness. The anorectic child insists that her appetite is "normal," and overregulates it, to a ridiculous degree.

Naturally, the clinician must inquire about associated physical symptoms, such as gastrointestinal problems, endocrine difficulties (e.g., hyperthyroidism) or even malignancies. Infectious processes, especially in neglected children, should be borne in mind. Space-occupying lesions of the central nervous system are a remote possibility, but should not be completely overlooked, either.

Obsessive Compulsive Disorder (OCD) may coexist with Anorexia Nervosa and some writers consider *primary* Anorexia Nervosa to be OCD. Anorexia Nervosa may be *secondary* to Conversion Disorder, Schizophrenia, or Depression.

TREATMENT

The foregoing description of the patient's altered state, in charge of the world inside and around her, explains the resistance these patients put up to any change, i.e., treatment. Children seldom exert great efforts to avoid treatment, but children with Anorexia Nervosa go to great lengths of manipulations, dissimulation, and emotional "arm twisting" of their parents, to get out of treatment. Therefore, the first step in treatment is to establish a clear and solid working relationship with the parents and the child.

From that point forward, several paths may be chosen, but they should all lead to the same minimum goal—weight gain. Therefore, medical management is always necessary. Without weight gain, the altered emotional, cognitive, and metabolic state will be an effective barrier against the age-appropriate growth of a healthy ego that is aimed for so assiduously in psychotherapy.

Weight gain is exactly what the word means: increase in the child's weight as measured by the scales. It is a mistake to look for insight and psychological change before weight gain. This would be tantamount to treating a toxic brain syndrome with insight psychotherapy alone.

If the child is seriously underweight and/or growth has already suffered, hospitalization is the preferred first step. The clinician has a variety of approaches to choose from when it comes to increasing the child's weight; some form of conditioning or "bribery" underlies the majority of them, i.e., the child earns privileges, or even freedom from tube feeding or intravenous feeding, *not* by eating *alone,* but by gaining weight.

Once the child has gained weight, there are three main therapies applicable, usually in multimodal combinations: family therapy, individual psychotherapy, and pharmacotherapy. These can be started in the hospital and continued in the office after discharge from hospital.

Family therapy became almost a religious obsession a few years ago; it was touted to be the preferred and consequently the obligatory treatment for Anorexia Nervosa (not necessarily Bulimia Nervosa). This has yielded recently to saner views, and family therapy has been given its appropriate place, which is a very important one but not an exclusive one. Family therapy aims at resolving those psychodynamics that may have brought about the rigid, perfectionistic, compulsive misperception of the growing body image. However, this is not the only role for family therapy. An equally important role stems from the realization that some of the family pathology is secondary to the child's pathology. Helping the family, especially the parents, with their anger, guilty fears, and insecurities towards the anorectic child is a necessary part of any treatment.

Individual treatment is usually a necessity, but it may be administered in small amounts, i.e., in a supportive and directive framework, often conjointly with instruction to the parents in a behavior modification schema. Psychodynamic psychotherapy is useful to understand such psychodynamics as the emotional aspects of body misperception and of the "eating phobia" but it is not an effective solitary treatment tool.

Pharmacotherapy with prepubertal Anorexia Nervosa has consisted mainly of the use of tricyclic antidepressants (TCAs), because of the physiological parallels with depression and because of the TCAs' side effect of stimulating appetite. Moreover, the use of this class of medications may also be rationalized on the basis of the clinical experience showing some success for TCAs in behavioral, phobic, and avoidance disorders. The action of tricyclic medications is thus either directly antidepressant or behavior-modifying; in either case, weight gain can be expected to result, and does result, in a number of cases. However, whether pharmacotherapy can be expected to help in any particular case is uncertain. Nevertheless, pharmacotherapy is worth trying, especially in combination with other therapies.

PROGNOSIS

This is generally good in prepubertal Anorexia Nervosa and does not usually carry the serious foreboding of the adolescent or adult version. In this particular disorder, it is generally agreed that the younger the onset, the better the prognosis. We would add that the sooner treatment is initiated, the better the overall outlook, too, as puberty and growth will then proceed normally.

Obesity (Eating Disorder Not Otherwise Specified [NOS] [307.50])
DEFINITION

There is no universally accepted definition of what constitutes obesity in childhood. "Weight for height" charts or measures of skin-fold thickness can be used, but in the last analysis it is the appearance of gross obesity and the desire to change that define pathological or problematic obesity.

The pathological body image and need to lose weight significantly below the normal weight, so characteristic of Anorexia Nervosa, seldom occur in obese children. As a matter of fact, many obese children will not spontaneously acknowledge any discomfort about their obesity, in spite of the fact that their peers lose no opportunity to bring it to their attention.

ETIOLOGY AND PATHOGENESIS

Obesity from primary, demonstrable organic disorders will not be considered here. "Functional" obesity (by far the most common) is multiply determined. Some children are presumed to have a constitutional predisposition towards obesity; this is often associated with familial occurrence, i.e., most family members are obese and have had obese parents. Metabolic and other organic factors are probably operative in most obese children, but whether these are primary, causative factors or secondary ones (i.e., sequelae of the obesity) we cannot say, given the present level of our knowledge.

The most consistently demonstrable etiological factors, in the last analysis, are psychical ones. There is no one nucleus of specific conflict; there are a number of psychodynamic conditions that result in the final common pathway of obesity.

Psychological trauma, such as significant object loss, separation, or failure resulting in loss of either self-esteem or security, are examples of the psychodynamic conditions arising, at least seemingly, within the child. Unresolved parental problems, resulting in their covert attempt to control the child or keep him/her dependent through being overfed, are examples of conditions arising primarily outside the child. Even here, however, it should be remembered that we may need to postulate a physiological factor of compliance for obesity to occur, instead of some other disorder.

Finally, there also appears to be a socioeconomic factor. In our industrialized society, the lower socioeconomic strata and the disadvantaged tend to be more obese because carbohydrates are less expensive and easier to handle and prepare than are proteins, fresh vegetables, and fruits.

CLINICAL DESCRIPTION

From a psychodynamic point of view, according to Hilde Bruch, (1973) two types of obesity can be distinguished: (a) the reactive type and (b) the developmental type. The reactive form responds to psychological traumas, such as significant object loss (e.g., loss of a parent through death or divorce), loss of self-esteem, academic or repeated social or athletic failures, or post-traumatic stress disorder following sexual abuse. A combination of some or all of the above can also occur. An example is loss of a parent through that parent's incarceration for child sexual abuse.

1. The Reactive Type

CASE 10-2   Derek was eight years old when his parents *separated*. Shortly thereafter, his father was *jailed* for *theft and bigamy*. His mother, always an *anxious and depressed* person, became *oversolicitous* of Derek's *food intake*, always insisting that he *eat* "the right food." She chided him for sneaking sweets, of which she nevertheless replenished a *constant supply* at home. As his *peers* found out about his father, they called Derek "jailbird" and other *derogatory names*. Derek, never one to stand up for himself, *withdrew* from games and other activities and started spending *long hours* in front of the television set—and *eating*. He became visibly overweight and was teased about that as well. At this point, Derek *showed less chagrin* over the negative social consequences than he did previously.

Comment. The stressors in this patient's life were the loss both of father and of social status with his peers. His mother may have directed him towards overeating as a projective defense against her own preoccupation with food. She used food to keep Derek close to her, and Derek obliged—he withdrew towards eating. His obesity acted as if it were a stabilizing factor or armor and, additionally, a psychological "wall" against further outside stresses.

2. *The Developmental Type*

Precipitating stresses are not as prominent as are familial-genetic predispositions. The obesity is of longer duration and has started insidiously, usually earlier in childhood. One or both parents are obese or have strong tendencies towards obesity, and consuming food has always been an important ingredient of their family life.

Unlike the reactively obese children, these children have a greater lean (basic) body mass, starting with being large at birth. Bruch (1973) postulated that obesity is determined by family style, starting with mother's inability to respond to the infant's needs with any measures other than feeding. The child then internalizes this mechanism (resolution of discomfort through food), especially since the child is often targeted as the object of vicarious gratification by a dominating mother.

CASE 10-3   Danielle, at the age of six, was referred by her pediatrician who had noted her attitudes of *helplessness,* and even *despair,* over being teased and ostracized by her *peers* because she was grossly overweight. *Obesity ran in the family,* but Danielle was apparently the most conspicuous. Mother *admitted* to having *"a soft spot"* for her because Danielle *resembled* mother's younger sister, who had died before reaching adolescence. Mother, wanting to make sure that Danielle had a good life, expended a great deal of effort to prepare very fancy desserts for her. *Mother* explained that she would *bake or cook* for family or friends whenever she wanted to show them *special favors, recognition, or appreciation.* When the pediatrician hospitalized Danielle in order to initiate a regimen of weight reduction, *mother* was repeatedly "caught" by the nurses *sneaking "goodies"* to Danielle.

Comment. The patient was being singled out for "special treatment" because of a resemblance to her mother's dead sister. The only way that mother could carry out her distorted perception or identification was by overfeeding the child.

TREATMENT

Treatment should follow diagnosis and, in keeping with this reasoning, should be directed at the precipitating stress in a case of reactive obesity. The way to treat it will depend on the nature of that precipitant. In most, if not all, cases it will become evident that a program of reduced caloric intake and increased activity will be indispensable, no matter how impressive the psychodynamics of the precipitating factor may be.

Although the clinician can generally sort out and plan treatment more rationally in this type of obesity, that does not mean that treatment is necessarily easy. Depression in particular may become intricately linked with obesity.

Moreover, when treating childhood obesity of either type, we must recall that obesity is multiply determined, and therefore multiple treatment approaches are necessary: reduced calories, parental counseling, increased peer sports, helping with dietary plans, improving self-regard.

This multimodal option is even more appropriate when we treat developmental obesity. A regimen of caloric intake reduction is combined with therapy of the child and his or her parents. The therapy is not necessarily a dynamic-verbal psychotherapy; it can be behavior modification and may even be predominantly educational or exhortative. This is a disorder where "many roads lead to Rome."

In both types of childhood obesity, it is the authors' view that a great deal can be gained by encouraging and following up on a reasonable regimen of exercise. Exercise is relatively easy to prescribe for children, who have a natural tendency towards activity and towards expressing themselves through physical activity. The weight reduction therapy therefore "hitches a ride" on a normal impulse towards health.

The indications for pharmacological treatment are only those of the underlying disorder (Depression, Attention–Deficit Hyperactivity Disorder). Appetite suppressant drugs have no place in the treatment of childhood obesity, except for the incidental side effect of appetite suppression by the psychostimulants when used in Attention–Deficit Hyperactivity or Conduct Disorders. Unfortunately, the anorectic effect of these agents on children lasts only a week or 10 days, occasionally a little longer.

PROGNOSIS

This is likely to be somewhat better in reactive obesity, although it is really a highly individual matter, depending on the multiplicity of causative conditions and our ability to gain access to many of these patients in treatment. The prognosis is probably best when the entire family adopts a different philosophical outlook on life and food.

EATING DISORDERS OF INFANCY AND EARLY CHILDHOOD

Pica (307.52)

DEFINITION

This is defined in DSM-III-R as the persistent ingestion of nonnutritive substances, usually dirt, flakes of paint or plaster, clay, laundry starch, paper, or soil. The derivation of the word is from Latin, where it means "magpie"—an appropriate appellation.

To qualify for Pica, the child must be at least one year old, since indiscriminate ingestion of various substances may not be specific or conspicuous enough before this age is attained. The disorder rarely lasts beyond adolescence. It is most frequent in preschool children.

ETIOLOGY

Although the hypothesis that Pica is caused by a specific nutritional deficit is held by many, we find the "interactional" hypothesis more plausible: an inadequate relationship with the mother leaves a child's oral needs unmet and the child forages. Both the cause and the effect of this eating disorder resemble the etiology and phenomenology of the other eating disorders, in our view. We can thus see a logical continuum of interactional causation from nonorganic failure to thrive to psychosocial dwarfism and Pica, and even obesity.

CLINICAL DESCRIPTION

CASE 10-4   Jedediah was a five-year-old boy well known to the staff of the local general hospital because of his *multiple admissions* for severe *anemia, malnutrition,* and several instances of *lead poisoning.* The department of social services had had their hands full with him and his siblings because of recurrent situations of *neglect* by his single, highly *irresponsible, and manipulative* female parent. The family lived in a *run-down tenement,* and Jedediah was frequently *left unsupervised* or in the care of a seven-year-old sister. Jedediah and his siblings had had short placements in foster homes, but were invariably returned to mother's care after she convinced the court that henceforth she would look after them better. Jedediah was described as *stuffing everything into his mouth* practically from birth. He found ample opportunity to put *flakes of paint and plaster into his mouth* because they were "sugar to him," his mother stated.

Comment. Pica is not difficult to diagnose given a high index of suspicion in cases of children with anemia, malnutrition, especially combined with adverse socio-economic and emotional circumstances (especially neglect). Lead poisoning, correctable by the landlord, should require the diagnosis of Pica until proven otherwise.

TREATMENT

Remediation consists of preventing the child from ingesting nonnutritive, especially noxious, substances around him. Two vital measures are to be applied simultaneously: removal of noxious substances, especially lead paint, and adequate supervision of the child. It is sad to note that in environments where Pica occurs most, it is often impossible to institute these measures quickly or effectively enough, as our case vignette has shown.

Whenever Pica occurs, or continues, in socioeconomically better advantaged circumstances, direct treatment of the child, using behavior modification strategies, is undertaken with usually beneficial effects.

Rumination Disorder of Infancy (Merycism) (307.53)

This interesting disorder is not limited strictly to infancy or childhood, but occurs in adults as well.

DEFINITION

As defined by DSM-III-R, Rumination Disorder of Infancy consists of repeated regurgitation of food. The disorder starts between three and 12 months of age; prior to its onset, eating behavior will have been normal. There is no nausea or retching; the infant apparently uses a voluntary maneuver of straining and bringing partially digested food into its mouth, which is then chewed and reswallowed, accompanied by an expression of pleasure.

ETIOLOGY

Recent radiographic studies have shown that a large number of these infants suffer from gastroesophageal reflux; other instances of this disorder are thought to be due to autonomic nervous system dysfunction. Difficulties in the mother–child relationship were usually found. The etiology is therefore most likely an inopportune combination of somatic and interpersonal factors.

CLINICAL DESCRIPTION

CASE 10-5   Baby Jane was eight months old when her mother complained to the pediatrician that she was *disgusted* by the *half-digested* milk and cereal that the baby brought up into her mouth, as if she were *"a calf chewing her cud."* Moreover, the repetitive nature of this maneuver produced an offensive *smell* which alienated the mother. The infant *looked miserable while trying* to regurgitate the food; this was followed by an expression of *beatitude* once the maneuver was successful.

TREATMENT

Treatment follows from the combined etiology: surgery for gastroesophageal reflux and hiatus hernia, where demonstrated, and management of the mother–infant relationship, with special attention to feeding technique. Behavior modification with aversive stimuli to extinguish the regurgitation maneuvers has also been used.

PROGNOSIS

This is good when treatment is pursued vigorously; when it is not, malnutrition may become severe, leading to death. The disorder, even when successfully treated, is often associated with failure to thrive and developmental delays.

Questions for Study and Action

1. Why has Anorexia Nervosa been called "nervous consumption" by many writers since Morton gave it that appellation in 1689? What are its features that make it resemble tuberculosis? What features could clearly distinguish it from tuberculosis for a physician in the 20th century?

2. Hilde Bruch (1973) described a primary Anorexia Nervosa that was the same as Obsessive Compulsive Disorder. To what other primary disorders could Anorexia Nervosa be *secondary*? Describe the anorectic picture that develops secondary to at least three other mental disorders.

3. Discuss this statement: Anorexia Nervosa is the curse of the affluent whites of the United States. Give the pros and cons.

4. Hispanics in the United States, even when poor, do not suffer from the malnutrition and obesity seen in other ethnic groups, it is said. What is there about a diet heavy in rice and beans that provides better nutrition than fatback, cornmeal, and molasses?

5. Why is lead poisoning from Pica said to be "correctable by the landlord"? Why do campaigns against lead poisoning in many major cities receive opposition from landlords? Explain fully.

6. Examine the logic of this statement: Obesity runs in families, thereby proving the genetic and constitutional basis of this condition. What really *proves* that a disorder is genetic (genogenic)?

7. Aside from identifying Danielle (Case 10–3) with mother's dead sister, show how the following could have represented even graver distortions if mother had shown them:
   (a) projective identification
   (b) identification with the aggressor
   (c) role reversal
   (d) narcissistic identification

8. Argue that *developmental obesity* is only *reactive obesity* perpetuated over two or more generations.

9. Discuss this statement: Holding to an interactional or interpersonal viewpoint of eating disorders leads to therapeutic optimism.

10. Explain why hematological studies should be done in any case of early childhood Pica.

For Further Reading

Bruch, H. *Eating Disorders: Obesity, Anorexia Nervosa, and the Person Within*. Basic Books: New York, 1973.

Bruch, H. *The Golden Cage: The Enigma of Anorexia Nervosa*. Cambridge, MA: Harvard University Press, 1978.

Holland, A.J., Hall, A., Murray, R., Russell, G.F.M., & Crisp, A.H. Anorexia nervosa: A study of 34 twin pairs and one set of triplets. *Brit. J. Psychiatry*, 145:414–419, 1984.

Lippe, B.M. The physiologic aspects of eating disorders. *J. Amer. Acad. of Child Psychiatry*, 22:108–113, 1983.

Maloney, M.J., & Klykylo, W.M. An overview of anorexia nervosa, bulimia, and obesity in children and adolescents. *J. Amer. Acad. of Child Psychiatry*, 22:99–107, 1983.

Russell, G.F.M. Delayed puberty due to anorexia nervosa of early onset. In P.L. Darby et al. (Eds.), *Anorexia Nervosa: Recent Developments in Research*. New York: Alan R. Liss, 1983.

Sours, J.A. Depression and the anorexia nervosa syndrome. *Psychiat. Clin. N. Amer.*, 4:145–158, 1981.

Swift, W.J. The long-term outcome of early onset anorexia nervosa. *J. Amer. Acad. of Child Psychiatry*, 21:38–46, 1982.

11

Sleep Disorders

S leep disorders provide a meeting ground for different "ideologies": developmental, psychodynamic, constitutional–genetic, and neurophysiological concepts and approaches. Moreover, all are needed to understand and treat sleep disorders. Here, also, is an area where accurate diagnosis may call for the emphasis of one approach over the other. All told, sleep disorders are an etiologically heterogeneous group with a final common pathway—different sources feeding into the one river, disturbed sleep. The circumspect clinician is, moreover, often rewarded for his or her painstaking effort with a predictable outcome: accurate diagnosis leads to effective treatment.

Sleep disorders range from "normal" or "variations of normal" (i.e., age-related fluctuations of sleep patterns) to "symptomatic" or "traumatic" sleep disorder and, finally, to specific, psychodynamically or neurophysiologically determined, definitely pathological syndromes. There is no fully accepted classification of disturbed sleep, despite the great advances made over the last decade in sleep laboratory research and the existence of the diagnostic classification of the ASDC (Association for Sleep Disorders Center). We shall adhere to the latter for its scientific basis, but abbreviate the whole process of classification for clinical relevance and manageability.

DSM-III-R lists many sleep disorders. That classification pertains to adults' sleep laboratory research and cannot be meaningfully applied to children.

159

We propose the following practical clinical classification based on the disturbance of arousal:

1. Sleep disorders without disturbances of arousal—the "dyssomnias"
   (a) Normal and developmental sleep adjustments
   (b) Reactive sleep disorders
   (c) Nightmares
   (d) Sleep disturbances associated with other psychiatric illness
   (e) Narcolepsy
   (f) Sleep apnea
2. Sleep disorders with disturbances of arousal—"disorders of arousal" or "parasomnias"
   (a) Night terrors *(pavor nocturnus)*
   (b) Sleepwalking
   (c) Sleeptalking
   (d) Sleep-related enuresis

We shall describe each of these clinical entities, considering the symptomatology, etiology, and treatment for each.

SLEEP DISORDERS WITHOUT DISTURBANCES OF AROUSAL (DYSSOMNIAS)

Normal and Developmental Sleep Adjustments

ETIOLOGY

We have termed these phenomena sleep adjustments because they are normal developmental symptoms reflecting the "modal" and expected transition points in the child's mental and emotional development. When the child has to give up less mature mental mechanisms and operate with new ones, there may normally occur a period of time when the new mechanisms are not yet "firmly in place." At such times, the overall relaxation and regression that occur during sleep may be disconcerting, since aggressive and sexual impulses during sleep are the usual etiologic mechanisms.

CLINICAL DESCRIPTION

These sleep disturbances consist of refusal or procrastination about going to sleep and/or nightmares. Refusal to go to sleep may take the form of bedtime rituals, inability to "settle down," and excessive use of or hassle over transitional objects such as furry animals and blankets. Rocking and thumbsucking may be associated symptoms. The child may cling to the parents and demand to sleep with them. These sleep disturbances are usually encountered in the preschool child.

TREATMENT

"Easy does it" and "Don't panic" are probably the primary ingredients in treating this sleep disorder. The clinician's primary job is to rule out other psychopathology in the child or parents and to be sure there are no emotional problems calling for more specific intervention. Parents can be made aware of the normal hurdles in the child's mental development, and what they can and cannot do to help. A judicious amount of tolerating of transitional objects or engaging in calming activities at bedtime facilitates the child's return to better sleeping patterns. Overdoing such measures, on the other hand, only creates new rituals. Allowing the child in bed with the parents is never a good idea, as it is almost invariably difficult to get the child to "move out" subsequently. When the clinician is sufficiently certain of the diagnosis, but the parents continue to be in doubt about what to do, "benign neglect" is probably the best overall approach to this self-correcting developmental problem.

Reactive Sleep Disorders

ETIOLOGY

These disorders are secondary to other illnesses, both psychiatric and medical. Depression and various anxiety disorders, on the one hand, and reactions to psychological trauma, on the other, are the main examples of psychiatric underlying disorder. Although the number and range of medical conditions that can interfere with sleep are legion, there are actually only a few categories that are typically associated with sleep disturbance. The most common are the various manifestations of allergy: asthma, upper respiratory problems, and especially the ear–nose–throat problems of allergies, such as enlarged tonsils and adenoids. Pulmonary and cardiovascular (usually congenital) disorders are another source of insomnia or dyssomnia. The alert clinician will keep in mind toxic causes, and commonly used pharmacological agents, such as antihistaminics and decongestants, affect sleep in many ways.

Children with Attention-Deficit Hyperactivity Disorder are a special category in this sample: the syndrome itself often entails shorter sleep time overall; the pharmacological treatment with psychostimulants additionally alters sleep either by making it easier for the child to go to sleep and enabling the child to sleep longer, or by interfering with sleep. To date, no predictive factors have been identified to help the clinician to time the administration of the medication.

CLINICAL DESCRIPTION

CASE 11-1   Samantha was a seven-year-old girl who was referred to the specialist because she *could neither get to sleep at night nor get up in the morning*. In addition, she kept *feeling sleepy* in school.

Samantha described *her difficulty in settling down after an exciting day* (she was indeed an outgoing and active child) and that she dreaded the *darkness* of the bedroom because of her *fears* of burglars or similar intruders who would hurt her and kidnap her. *Nightmares* of a similar content made sleep itself less than appealing to her.

Background information revealed that Samantha's parents had *divorced* about six months earlier. The patient herself had always been close to father, and she felt a lot of *resentment* against mother whom she *blamed* for the divorce.

Comment. This child's inability to go to sleep reflects a neurotic conflict: her aggressive wishes against mother and the feared punishment for them become accentuated in darkness and in sleep, with the result that the inception of sleep is interfered with. The polarization of family alliances of the oedipal phase has been reactivated by the trauma of the divorce.

The clinical picture is usually in the realm of "initiating and maintaining sleep," to use the ASDC terminology, with "excessive somnolence" during day-time as a sequel.

TREATMENT

This must, obviously, be directed at the underlying cause. Therefore, it is nonspecific for the sleep disturbance, but specific for the underlying disorder.

Nightmares (Dream Anxiety Disorder [307.47], Anxiety Dreams)

DEFINITION AND CLINICAL DESCRIPTION

Nightmares—simple "bad dreams"—are prolonged dreams whose content causes anxiety, often to the extent that the child wakes up. Physiologically, such night-mares occur during REM (rapid eye movement) stages of sleep, not at the beginning of a nocturnal sleep period. They are not associated with significant autonomic arousal; i.e., respiratory and heart rate, blood pressure, penile erection, vaginal lubrication, muscle tone, and skin resistance are not greatly altered. The child can usually recall the contents of the dream, and, if sleep has been interrupted, the child can be pacified and returned to bed.

CASE 11-2   Alfred was five-and-half years old and had just started kindergarten. This had not gone smoothly, so Alfred continued to show *separation anxiety* and frequently *woke up* at night, was *scared*, and *came to his parents' bedroom*. He related scary dreams in which *Frankenstein*-like figures *took all his toys* and *chased him* out of his house, so that he could not find his way back. Usually he would awaken then and proceed to *make sure his parents were still there* for he was afraid the Frankenstein monsters might have harmed his parents. His parents were *almost always able to reassure him* and put him back to sleep.

Alfred was *an only child* who was somewhat overindulged, but not to excess, and who had had occasional, moderate difficulties with peers and his parents because he always tried to "be the boss." These difficulties had not impaired his day-to-day functioning, but the *advent of kindergarten* brought about some *separation anxiety* not previously noticed, accompanied by the nightmares just described.

Comment. The nightmares are part of the anxiety disorder based on "unfinished business" from Alfred's previous developmental phases. His aggressive impulses have not been quite resolved, and have carried over into the oedipal phase. The destructive wishes against his parents are reflected in his separation anxiety, both in waking and in sleep. Moreover, there is the fear of retaliation (toys will be taken away) and loss of his parents.

DIFFERENTIAL DIAGNOSIS

This encompasses mainly night terrors and convulsive disorders. Night terrors are characterized by autonomic arousal, and upon awakening the child is confused, dazed, and unable to recall any dream content. Roughly the same criteria can be applied to distinguish nightmares from epilepsy, with motor convulsions indicating grand mal, and EEG abnormalities diagnostic of other types of seizures, whereas the EEG is normal in both nightmares and night terrors.

Associated sleep disturbances, such as difficulty falling asleep, are often encountered with nightmares.

TREATMENT

This depends on the etiology and will usually encompass a number of psycho-therapeutic possibilities—from crisis intervention to long-term psychotherapy. Benzodiazepines are effective pharmacological agents, although they are rarely used in children. Their rarity reflects not so much any greater danger in using these medications with children, but rather that most clinicians are more familiar, and comfortable, with almost all other approaches, especially psychotherapy.

PROGNOSIS

Parents can be reassured that the prognosis is usually excellent. Interestingly, while nightmares (dream anxiety attacks) are benign disorders, they correlate, according to some statistics, with adult psychopathology.

Sleep Disturbances Associated With Other Psychiatric Illness (Dyssomnia NOS [307.40])

This is a heterogeneous group of disorders which in children involve mostly disordered initiation and/or maintenance of sleep, and only rarely excessive daytime somnolence. The sequence of the physiological stages of sleep remains unaffected, except in depression, where there is shortened REM latency (i.e., REM sleep starts sooner after the child falls asleep).

Classically, Depression has been associated with sleep disturbances, especially early morning awakening. In children, difficulty falling asleep is the most common form, but, because of changing criteria for the diagnosis of Childhood Depression, the incidence of sleep disturbance is still a matter of clinical uncertainty. Either insomnia or hypersomnia may be present in Childhood Depression. In our experience, mild to moderate difficulties initiating sleep occur in about one-fourth of depressed children.

A child with Obsessive Compulsive Disorder (OCD) appears to have more difficulty in sleep initiation and maintenance than a child with depression, but it is sometimes difficult to estimate how many of these children are depressed.

Of all the childhood disorders, Post-traumatic Stress Disorders probably have the highest incidence of sleep disorders, usually nightmares (dream anxiety attacks).

Difficulties initiating sleep occur in many children with childhood onset schizophrenia. Older children occasionally have sleep disturbances associated with personality disorders.

Treatment is, of course, geared to the underlying psychiatric illness.

Narcolepsy

DEFINITION AND CLINICAL DESCRIPTION

Narcolepsy is defined as a syndrome of excessive daytime sleepiness and abnormal manifestations of REM sleep. Clinically, it consists of a tetrad of symptoms: sleep attacks, cataplexy, sleep paralysis, and hypnagogic hallucinations. The diagnosis hinges on the presence of sleep attacks *and* cataplexy. Although the disorder usually affects adolescents and adults, it often starts in late childhood (age 10 years or older) and is therefore pertinent to child health care professionals, especially since a few cases start before age 10 years.

CASE 11-3   Archie was a 10-year-old boy, a fourth-grader who was referred to the school psychologist for *"excessive laziness"* and *falling asleep* in class. He had never been an outstanding student, but this was quite *out of keeping* with his usual habits. The school psychologist found the child bewildered and unable to explain what was happening, except to state that he *could not resist going to sleep,* even if he was standing up or moving about at the time. Archie then complained that not only did "his knees feel weak" when the sleep episode came on, but he had this feeling of *complete weakness* and *going limp* at other times as well, and had twice *injured* himself because he *fell* down a flight of stairs. As the school psychologist paid attention to the child and showed concern rather than incredulity or criticism, Archie confided that sometimes he had "terrifying dreams" as he lay in bed at night, just before dropping off to sleep. He described *seeing* gory figures and *hearing* threatening voices and sounds, while at the *same time* he felt an *utter inability to do anything about it* since he was *quite unable to move. Rarely,* he had the same experiences on *awakening* in the morning. He knew, he said, that the ghosts and sounds were not real.

The school psychologist conferred with the parents who also had become concerned and remembered *"something similar"* in Archie's paternal grandfather.

Archie's pediatrician referred him to a medical center. There, polysomnographic and daytime multiple sleep latency tests (EEG recordings of several of Archie's sleep episodes) showed REM onset sleep episodes, i.e., REM periods which *began immediately* upon falling asleep. This *established* the diagnosis of narcolepsy.

Comment. This case history shows the "perfect" *tetrad,* seldom present in all its aspects. It also reminds us of the greater incidence in males and the likelihood that genetic (genogenic) factors play a role.

Cataplexy is the indispensable diagnostic feature of narcolepsy and consists of muscular weakness and/or paralysis identical to that which occurs during REM sleep. It often follows strong emotions, e.g., laughter and delight.

ETIOLOGY

The cause of narcolepsy is now generally assumed to be a central nervous system defect in the regulation of REM sleep and of alertness, entailing bursts of REM sleep occurring during wakefulness. Narcolepsy occurs in other animal species as well, and from our ability to breed dogs with narcolepsy we can surmise that the disorder is inherited. Psychological factors appear to play no causal role, but do serve as precipitants of particular episodes, most visibly of cataplexy.

TREATMENT

Two types of medications are used: the psychostimulants and the antidepressants. The choice depends on the extent of the cataplexy, for which the tricyclic antidepressants are more effective. Combinations of the two may be necessary. Narcolepsy shows no spontaneous recovery. The prognosis is good as long as the attacks can be reasonably controlled by medication. Supportive psychotherapy is indicated in the majority of children to forestall or treat low self-esteem or depression arising from the attacks.

Sleep Apnea

Many clinicians tend to consider any child who shows excessive daytime sleepiness as being a victim of narcolepsy. But there are other sleep disorders that produce daytime somnolence, the sleep apneas, usually subdivided into the primary and secondary apneas, being important ones. Primary sleep apnea refers to both nonflowing airways and absence of abdominal or thoracic thrusts to breathe lasting more than 10 seconds. Secondary apneas are those in which breathing motions are made during sleep but because of upper airway obstruction (from adenoids or tonsils or soft palate malformations) there is no successful air flow. The supposition is that central apneas reflect abnormal CNS respiratory mechanisms and secondary ones reflect upper respiratory obstructions. In mixed apnea, a third form, there is no muscular thrust early in the apneic episode but respiratory efforts resume later in the attack.

By the definitions given, about nine out of 10 episodes of sleep apnea recorded in childhood are secondary apneas. In most cases tonsillectomy, adenoidectomy, or surgical correction of an overelongated soft palate will effect cure, but in a small percentage of cases a tracheal valve may be required.

Children with sleep apnea appear to have cardiac sinus arrhythmias, augmented stages 1 and 2 non-REM sleep, reduced stages 3 and 4 deep sleep, and a slightly reduced total REM, along with the dramatic excessive daytime sleepiness—all shown by adults with sleep apnea.

SLEEP DISORDERS WITH DISTURBANCES OF AROUSAL— "DISORDERS OF AROUSAL" OR PARASOMNIAS

Night Terrors or Sleep Terror Disorder (307.46) (Sleep Terror, Pavor Nocturnus, Incubus)

DEFINITION AND CLINICAL DESCRIPTION

DSM-III-R describes night terrors as recurrent episodes of abrupt awakening from sleep, usually beginning with a panicky scream.

Night terror is a nonrapid eye movement (NREM) arousal disorder that occurs in sleep stages 3 and 4, and is characterized by intense anxiety, motoric agitation, adrenergic autonomic activation, and retrograde amnesia ("4 As").

CASE 11-4   Teddy's parents became concerned when they were awakened by a *piercing scream* from his bedroom in the middle of the night. When they got there, they found Teddy *sitting up* in bed, *wide-eyed and dazed,* and the expression on his face was one of *terror.* The parents tried to comfort him, but Teddy took *no notice* and seemed *totally unaware* of their presence. Not only was he unresponsive to their attempts to quiet him down, but also he attempted *to get out of bed* and head towards the door. Teddy *did not speak* but uttered a few moaning sounds. This went on for several minutes. Eventually, the child quieted down and went back to sleep.

The following morning Teddy *could not remember* anything, but two nights later the same sequence of events occurred. When the night terrors kept recurring at the rate of two to three per week, the parents sought professional help.

Teddy was *six years* old at the time and his first-grade teacher considered him *immature* and *easily distractible.* A month earlier, the entire family had been involved in an *auto accident.* Teddy was not injured but was quite frightened, as he had "seen it all coming." The accident involved collision with a large truck and cuts and bruises on his mother's face and arms; mother was bleeding from them, and Teddy at first thought she was going to die.

Comment. The preceding is a "classical" case: the precipitating event is traumatic, there is developmental delay as a "substrate" in the child, and the child has the "4 As," as well as associated attempts at somnambulism.

ETIOLOGY

The paradigm of the etiology is a precipitating psychological event in a genetically predisposed individual. The psychological event may be either real or threatened loss of a parent or the anticipatory anxiety about such a possibility. The predisposition, linked to a family history of somnambulism, is in the general area of developmental delay. Since the psychological conflict triggers definite physiological changes in the autonomic nervous system, night terrors can be regarded as a psychophysiological (psychosomatic) disorder.

DIFFERENTIAL DIAGNOSIS

The main differential diagnostic consideration is of a convulsive disorder. Above all, the clinician should ascertain whether any episodes suggesting convulsive disorder occur while the child is awake. That information, plus the presence or absence of psychological precipitants and sleepwalking, can provide sufficient grounds to exclude epilepsy. In doubtful cases the routine daytime electroencephalogram can give fairly adequate evidence about petit mal and psychomotor epilepsy, whereas the presence or absence of convulsions and especially of biting the tongue will confirm or rule out grand mal seizures. If we want to be quite certain, however, special EEG leads (e.g., nasopharyngeal) and a period of prior sleep deprivation may be necessary.

The differentiation from dream anxiety attacks is easy: the child is scared but oriented, can be communicated with, and can remember his or her dream when a dream anxiety attack (nightmare) has occurred, but not with night terror. The ultimate differentiation—proof of REM or NREM period at the time of the episode—is for research purposes only; both disorders have a benign prognosis and are treated similarly.

TREATMENT

To treat or not to treat depends on several factors, such as the nature of the psychological trauma or psychological stress which the child is experiencing now; the child's record of strengths in dealing with past stress; his/her environment and the kind of support his/her parents can give him or her; and the child's general developmental maturity.

Therefore, the decision to treat is quite similar to most other situations in which the clinician finds symptoms of anxiety. The decision must be based on a comprehensive assessment of the overall psychosocial scene. In the rare instances that this is necessary, pharmacological treatment with benzodiazepines (especially diazepam [Valium]) is effective.

COURSE AND PROGNOSIS

Unlike in the adult, night terrors in children do not carry an unfavorable prognosis and are not predictive of any future psychopathology. As a matter of fact, most are "outgrown" (i.e., simply disappear through the normal course of maturation) or subside in time without psychiatric help.

Sleepwalking Disorder (Somnambulism) (307.46)

DEFINITION AND CLINICAL DESCRIPTION

Sleepwalking Disorder consists of repeated episodes of complex behaviors that frequently, though not always, progress to leaving the bed and walking about (see

DSM-III-R). The child is not conscious of these actions and does not remember them afterwards.

The *physiological* parameters are identical to those of night terror, i.e., sleep-walking occurs 30–200 minutes after onset of sleep during sleep stages 3 and 4, which are NREM stages. An episode usually lasts from a few minutes to half an hour.

There are also a number of *clinical* similarities to night terrors: the episode starts with the child suddenly sitting up in bed, with a dazed expression, lack of response to attempts to communicate, few (if any) intelligible utterances, and subsequent amnesia for the entire episode (retrograde amnesia).

The dissimilarities are in the absence of screaming and of terror, and the somewhat greater ease with which the child can be awakened. There is also much less autonomic arousal.

CASE 11-5   Tammy was seven years old when her parents first found her out of her room in the middle of the night. Tammy had a *staring expression* on her face, was *moving about clumsily,* and *did not respond* to her parents' efforts to awaken her or to communicate with her. Eventually, however, Tammy awoke from the state she was in; she *did not know* where she was at first, but finally told her parents she knew how to find her way back to her room. However, Tammy *could not remember* anything about the sleepwalking itself.

During the following weeks, there were more sleepwalking episodes. Tammy would get into her stepbrother's room, *open drawers,* rummage among his things, and then either try to *return to her bedroom* or go on to her parents' bedroom, where she would curl up in a corner and *go to sleep.* On one occasion, Tammy surprised her family by *awakening on her own,* and after a few minutes of disorientation, going back to bed.

Her stepbrother, Eric, had heard that one should "never awaken a sleepwalker," but his parents told him this was an *old wives' tale.* When the parents told Eric that *not only would he not harm* Tammy by *waking her up,* but also it was a *myth* that a sleepwalker was safe, Eric awakened Tammy and escorted her back to her bedroom.

Tammy had just joined the family "full time," custody having been switched from her mother to her father and stepmother. Eric was three years older than Tammy and she thought that her father spent too much time coaching Eric in sports, in which Eric excelled. She felt that she did not have nearly the same talents to capture her father's attention and felt quite insecure because her natural mother seemed to have chosen a new marriage over her.

When the sleepwalking persisted, Tammy's parents brought her to the child guidance clinic. Individual *psychotherapy* with Tammy and *family sessions reassured* Tammy that both father and stepmother cared a great deal for her. Eric, too, joined in the general support system, and the sleepwalking stopped.

Comment. This case shows a relatively easy course and fairly transparent dynamics. There are no typical psychodynamic patterns in somnambulism, and the above is one of many possibilities. However, its clinical picture is typical. Often, sleepwalking is associated with night terrors.

DIFFERENTIAL DIAGNOSIS

As in night terrors, the main differential diagnostic focus is on epilepsy. It is psychomotor epilepsy particularly that may mimic sleepwalking. Children with psychomotor epilepsy almost never return to their beds; they show repetitive automatisms, such as chewing or swallowing movements. Moreover, unlike sleepwalking, epilepsy finds children unresponsive to attempts to awaken them. Electroencephalography usually provides the definitive answer.

A "long shot" differential consideration is Psychogenic Fugue (a dissociative anxiety disorder), where the person leaves his or her usual place of residence. However, the similarity ends there; fugue is rare in children, occurs during daytime, and the person appears fully conscious and alert, i.e., awakening is not necessary as the person appears wide awake. Moreover, fugues involve long periods of time and more complex actions than are found in somnambulism.

TREATMENT

The indications for psychotherapy, as well as the need to individualize the treatment according to the underlying psychodynamics, are the same as those described for night terrors. The one additional consideration is the danger of injury during sleepwalking.

There is, however, a difference in the pharmacological response. The benzodiazepines are effective in both nightmares (dream anxiety attacks) and night terrors, but not in sleepwalking. Instead, tricyclic antidepressants (e.g., imipramine) have been found to be effective in reducing the frequency of sleepwalking in some cases.

Sleeptalking (Somniloquy) (Parasomnia NOS [307.40])

This is a disturbance that is usually closely associated with sleepwalking, and when found, should make the clinician look for sleep-related enuresis, as there may be a more-than-coincidental link between the two. The verbalizations are usually poorly articulated and often difficult to understand. Treatment and prognosis are the same as for sleepwalking.

Sleep-Related Enuresis

Enuresis has been covered in a separate chapter. We will focus here only on enuresis that is demonstrably related to arousal from stage 4 (NREM) sleep. It occurs during the first few hours of sleep, actually during the phase of relative motor and autonomic calm that follows the stage 4 arousal. The child at that point is difficult to arouse from sleep, and the subsequent REM period often incorporates the wetting (and wetness) into a dream. The importance of defining this type of enuresis lies in the fact that treatment with tricyclic antidepressants is the most effective modality.

SUMMARY

Apart from narcolepsy, which definitely requires treatment, all other sleep disorders may or may not need treatment. However, if the clinician is not knowledgeable in their diagnosis, a number of associated difficulties may be missed, on the one hand, and opportunities for realistic reassurance, on the other. In many respects, sleep disorders may be likened to the symptom of fever; as in the case of fever, sleep disturbances that are presented to us have to be appropriately noted and their causes explored, and, where necessary, treated.

Questions for Study and Action

1. Try to explain why two-year-old Joanne's pediatrician told the girl's mother that she could not dream. Explain also why she disbelieved the pediatrician. In your answers, include terms such as: a preverbal child; REM sleep in the infant under two years old; stage I REM sleep; proportion of REM sleep in infants.

2. Interview a five-year-old child about her dreams, asking *if* she dreams, what was the plot of her most recent dream, and what her scariest dream was about. Also, ask her if she knows what her dreams mean. Take notes. Later, go through the same exercise with older children. Are children's dreams useful, as imaginative productions, to the clinician?

3. Why do preschool children, more than adults, believe that they can control their dreams' content, feelings, and occurrence? What does that say about the preschooler's cognitive development, position in family and society, and wish to gain mastery?

4. The term *nightmare* is a popular one covering both Sleep Terror Disorder and Dream Anxiety Disorder. List the distinguishing characteristics of one from the other, putting them into a phraseology you might use in eliciting a history and in explaining these characteristics to a seven-year-old child's parent.

5. What four features distinguish childhood-onset idiopathic insomnia (Primary Insomnia, 307.42) from the insomnia that may appear as a biological concomitant of Depression?

6. What health and mental health professionals may be called on for the teamwork needed to help a child with both Dream Anxiety Disorder and Sleep-induced Respiratory Impairment, an Axis III diagnosis (from an upper airway obstructive apnea)? Did you include a surgical subteam within your listing?

7. Assume that Archie (Case 11–3) did not doze during the day, did not have cataplexy or abnormal sleep lab findings, *but* had the same "terrifying dream" experiences on both falling asleep and awakening that are described in Case 11–3—seeing gory figures and hearing threatening voices and noises. What would the diagnosis likely be in a child with frequent anxiety dreams, sleep paralysis, hypnagogic and hypnopompic states?

8. What might we say about the developing self-criticism that is displayed in the case of a five-year-old girl who occasionally bites her older brother and has frequent anxiety dreams about crocodiles, large dogs, and biting monsters pursuing her?

9. Differentiate between narcolepsy and petit mal epilepsy, giving at least four ways to contrast their clinical pictures.

10. Account for the common observation that a sexually abused child, aged two years, responds mainly with disorders of sleep and eating, and separation anxiety.

For Further Reading

Anders, T.F., & Weinstein, P. Sleep and its disorders in infants and children. A review. *Pediatrics,* 50:312, 1972.

Kales, J.D., Jacobson, A., & Kales, A. Sleep disorders in children. In L.E. Abt & B.F. Reiss (Eds.), *Progress in Clinical Psychology.* New York: Grune & Stratton, 1968.

Keith, P. Night terrors: A review of the psychology, neurophysiology and therapy. *J. Amer. Acad. of Child Psychiatry,* 14:477–481, 1975.

Williams, R.L., & Karacan, I. *Sleep Disorders: Diagnosis and Treatment.* New York: Wiley, 1978.

Zales, M.R. *Eating, Sleeping and Sexuality: Treatment of Disorders in Basic Life Functions.* New York: Brunner/Mazel, 1982.

12

Gender and Sexual Disorders

Sexual dimorphism is the source of many "individual differences." Male or female conceptuses are detectable in early embryonic life, and the Y-chromosome, whether by its presence or its absence, is a forceful inducer (at least) of the genitourinary system *in embryo* and probably of the entire body and brain during fetal life. Babies may be born with erect penises (males) and with vaginal lubrication (females), denoting a sexual readiness that is a natural function of being human and a recurrent vital function during sleep and wakefulness throughout the life cycle. Consequently, the disorders of gender, sex drive, and sexual expression may be manifest in childhood. Therefore, we shall consider three groups:

    gender identity disorders
    paraphilias and dystonicities
    sexual dysfunctions

Gender Identity Disorder of Childhood (302.60)

DEFINITION AND ETIOLOGY

By age 30 months a child acquires a core gender identity, even if stereotypic masculine or feminine patterning may not appear until age four and a half or

173

five years. Masculinity and femininity or androgyny are acquired in varying degrees as we grow up, reflecting our life experiences. Also, our preferred modes of sexuality are learned. But the core identity as male or female is more likely innate, or else learned early in postnatal life. In reality, gender assignment is hardly a problem for most children: they are what they are, and everyone accepts that, so the child does, too. But in cases of pseudohermaphroditism (a male with severe hypospadias and undescended testes or a female with a hypertrophied clitoris) in the era before we readily could do chromosomal studies, children who were chromosomally female might be assigned (by pediatrician and mother) to male gender and vice versa. After age 30 months that ascription was accepted by the child in question and thereafter it was virtually immutable. Hence, some modeling and mirroring of caretaker attitudes must be involved in the gender identity of every child but in most cases it is done unconsciously and without ado and quickly fades into amnesia. Gender identity is complicated; it includes an acceptance of one's gender, integration of one's genitalia, genital structures and sensations into the body image, and self-definition as having one's chromosomally determined and socially assigned gender. Gender identity disorders are early and fundamental disturbances in one's sense of self and may be based on frankly delusional thinking.

Many schemata of self-regard are laid down by the age of 30 months: the body image, the core gender identity, and the self-concept as a good or bad person.

CLINICAL DESCRIPTION

In Gender Identity Disorder of Childhood the main symptoms are strong and persistent distress about one's assigned gender before reaching puberty. For the chromosomal female before puberty, there are two diagnostic criteria other than age, according to DSM-III-R:

1. Persistent and extreme distress about being a girl and an explicitly stated desire to be male or an insistence that she is or will become a male.
2. Either (a) or (b): (a) aversion to "girlish" dressing with an insistence on wearing what boys wear; (b) repudiation of her female anatomy with one of the following: 1) asserting she has or will develop a penis, 2) refusal to urinate in a sitting position, 3) asserting she does not want to menstruate or grow larger breasts.

For the prepubertal male the criteria are:

1. Persistent, extreme dysphoria about being a boy and a stated desire to be female or an insistence that he is or will become female.
2. Either (a) or (b): (a) aversion to boys' dressing, games, or pastimes with a preoccupation about "girlish" attire, toys, games, and activities; (b) repudiation of his male anatomy with one of these assertions: 1) that he will grow up to be a

woman, 2) that his male genitalia are disgusting or that ulimately they will disappear, 3) that he would prefer not to have penis, scrotum, and testes.

CASE 12-1   Cleeta was brought to a child psychiatrist by her father and step-mother shortly after she became eight years old, and three months after coming to live in their reconstituted family. "She wants to be a boy. Her mother always wanted to treat the boy and girl just alike. But now Cleeta refuses to wear a dress and wants to play football when she grows up." Indeed, Cleeta did announce to the child psychiatrist that she *was* a boy. When the doctor said, "Boys have penises and those sacs with testicles inside," Cleeta assured the physician that *she had* all that was needed to fill that bill—specifically, *penis, scrotum, and two testes.* On physical exam these were not present but instead a normal female's external genitalia. Yet Cleeta *wore boys' jockey shorts,* chose her clothing from the boys' sections of department stores, and seemed male-identified in every way, although on projective testing she was female-identified.

She was seen twice-weekly for some 30 weeks in dynamic–verbal psychother-apy that focused on her envy of her brother and stepbrother, her oppositional behavior at home and at school, her loud and agitated boisterousness, her desire to be reunited with her addicted biological mother, and her resentment of her wealthy father and stepmother. Gradually, Cleeta became sexually enlightened, cathected her clitoris, labia, and vagina, and was able to have visits with her biological mother who played the decisive role ultimately in Cleeta's self-acceptance as female. By the time she was nine years old she displayed little of the demeanor of a compulsive tomboy.

DIFFERENTIAL DIAGNOSIS

The major conditions requiring discernment are five instances of cross-dressing: 1) for play or experimentation; 2) for facilitation of homosexuality; 3) for relief of tension; 4) boys who do female impersonation; and 5) transvestism. A boy, for example, who is determinedly feminine will not have a gender identity disorder if he knows that he is male and generally accepts his maleness. Only when he deludes himself into feeling that he is a female does he qualify for the Gender Identity Disorder diagnosis. For simplicity, all cross-dressing instances in chil-dren may be classified as Gender Identity Disorder Not Otherwise Specified. DSM-III-R assigns the code of 302.85 to Gender Identity Disorder NOS for cross-dressers who do not meet all the criteria for 302.60, Gender Identity Disorder of Childhood. For all intents and purposes, a child who has met all the criteria for Gender Identity Disorder throughout the past two years might be regarded as being a child transsexual. However, that diagnosis, by convention, is reserved for adults only.

Those who impersonate females are, like their adult counterparts, actors. Those boys who are male-identified but for the past six months or more cross-dress for sexual arousal are pretransvestites, or transvestites, or transvestic fetishists (302.30).

TREATMENT AND PROGNOSIS

There is truth in the familiar call for early treatment for, as indicated in the foregoing, a child who has been misassigned in gender after age two-and-a-half years is no longer able to change over to acceptance of the chromosomally correct gender. The treatment of the very young child is done primarily by that chief caretaker, the mother, who has for millenia borne, reared, and shaped little boys to be male and little girls to be female. If the caretaker is too finicky, hysterical, or narcissistic to observe and respond to the child's genitals and gender, then surrogate caretakers or psychotherapists may be helpful. Most boy children are not regarded as effeminate nor girls as too masculine or "butch" until they approach puberty, but some parents have sensitive antennae, as in the case of Cleeta cited earlier. Usually, it is not only the gender identity that is at issue but also other matters of relationship and selfhood within and between parents and children.

PARAPHILIAS AND DYSTONICITIES

DEFINITION AND CLINICAL DESCRIPTION

Children are seldom established and patterned in any specific channel of sexual activity. This has led some writers to characterize them as polymorphously perverse, while others have said that children are not sexual. Since sexual experimentation is not governed and administered, provided children are granted privacy and freedom, it seems absurd perhaps to characterize a child as suffering from paraphilia. The term was *perversion*, formerly, and our word still denotes a deviance *(para)* in the person or thing to which one is erotically attracted *(philia)*.

Indeed, both authors have known children who masturbated in private (formerly regarded as a cause of insanity) or got aroused as they peeked at nude siblings and parents (Voyeurism 302.82), or unzipped and exposed their genitals to a sometimes-shocked observer (Exhibitionism 302.40), or engaged in sex play with household pets (Zoophilia 302.90), or cross-dressed (Transvestic Fetishism 302.30), or indulged in fondling and rubbing of another (Frotteurism 302.89), or made a fetish of the mother's wig or underpants (Fetishism 302.81), or smeared feces (Coprophilia [Paraphilia NOS 302.90]) and urine (Urophilia [Paraphilia NOS 302.90]) on their own and/or a playmate's body. Children, then, do show paraphiliac tendencies but not so much in rigidly fixated, exclusive perversions as can be seen in adults. In fact, many regard the "perverse experimentations of childhood" as good preparation for a "joyful and resourceful foreplay and lovemaking in adulthood."

Ego-Dystonic Homosexuality (302.90) is a disorder that is rarely described for children. When homosexual activities occur (as they do) among child age-mates, they are usually ego-syntonic but not advertised indiscreetly, particularly to adults.

TREATMENT AND PROGNOSIS

Paraphiliac tendencies of children may upset the child's parents more than the clinician, since the latter is generally not easily alarmed by the sexual involvement of others' children! Treatment may be mainly parent counseling or family therapy. The clinician has several options available if parents note "deviant" sexuality in their children:

1. *Reassurance* of its normality in a generic trial-and-error approach by the child can be attempted but usually will not assuage parents' anxieties. They may see, though, that they and the child have more than sexual problems in their marriage and family relations.

2. *Advising* the parents to provide sexual information to the child can be done. This, too, is usually fruitless because the child often clings to sexuality as the one zone to be preserved as inaccessible to parents. At least, such advice can be consciousness raising so the parents will not see curiosity and experimentation as "perverse" but human.

3. *Reviewing* with the parents their own sexual biographies can help them to be more empathic towards the child. Empathy helps.

4. *Asking parents what they can condone or recommend in the way of childhood genital pleasure* is much more productive; for that challenges them at least to "lay off" the child's sex play and at most to be candid about their own limited experiences.

5. *Negotiations to permit the child psychiatrist to aid in the child's sexual enlightenment* may be necessary because many parents, even after considerable exploration of their own views and values, choose to be shy and let the expert educate. This option gives more work to the child and the doctor but permits parents to model their sexual information giving on what they observe from behind a one-way mirror, for example.

6. The context of the child's life is larger than genitality alone, so *treatment should not be so narrowly focused* that the child perceives his or her sexuality as the only hot topic of interest to a psychiatrist.

We have endeavored to state that little needs to be done in direct therapeutic work with children who display trends towards paraphilias or have dystonic sexual orientations, and that most work should be done with the parents, the gatekeepers and family powerhouses. Children are not believed to require direct therapy for their sexual problems, which rarely meet the diagnostic criteria for adults.

Parents often misinterpret all of these statements to be tantamount to "There is nothing wrong here," and they do not hear the admonition that there may indeed be something definitely wrong in the child's life, but that the recommended treatment focus is not one of "sex therapy."

SEXUAL DYSFUNCTIONS

DEFINITION

Disorders of sexual desire, sexual arousal, orgasm, and sexual pain (dyspareunia and vaginismus) are specified for adults but generally not for children. An ambivalence reigns. Prudishness dictates that grown-ups, even if sensually pre-occupied themselves, do not take note of the child's genitality even when logic and data convince them that children do have normal desire, arousal, and orgasm (for the male, prior to ejaculation). That ambivalence described may include the framers of diagnostic manuals who also may not wish to believe that disorders of desire, arousal, and orgasm can befall young children.

CASE 12-2   Frances was a case of improperly diagnosed gender who had been *reared as female* and only at the age of 11 years, in her early puberty, was a chromosomal study performed. Her referral was to a child psychiatry clinic at that time because of her *physical violence* towards her mother and her *misconduct* at school, where the teachers found her to be *militant, prone to hitting* at agemates, and *difficult to control* or discipline.

Physical examination showed mesomorphic and muscular Frances to have *a small clitoris but within the range of normal size* for a girl of 11; the labia (excepting a *small lump* thought to be a hernia) and vagina were also normal and Frances had a "marital introitus," as gynecologists depicted the introitus of coitally experienced women in a former era. After *biopsy* of the small herniation of one labium presented male gonadal tissue, without any admixture of ovarian tissue, chromosomal study showed Frances to have a normal XY chromosomal configuration. Frances had been predestined to be male but, understandably, she had been *reared and experienced as female.*

When the child psychiatrist revealed to the treatment team that Frances had been involved pleasurably in coitus with several boys dating from age nine, the team decided to take several appropriate steps: to extirpate, with parental consent, the remnant male gonads from the labia bilaterally, to administer hormones that would facilitate her biological feminization, and to advise Frances that she would not be able to have children but would have to adopt if she wished that at a later age. Frances truly did not know all that her surgery and medications and advice entailed but with her formalized consent added to the approval of both her parents, the plan was carried out with good results then and in later years.

Comment. One male member of the medical school faculty who was consulted about this treatment plan was unabashedly horrified that anything would be done to demasculinize someone who had been genetically endowed with male chromosomes! A male resident in psychiatry (who had evaluated Frances and her parents initially and who adhered to the cult of virginity) was dumbfounded that Frances was eroticized by her male companions and had been their sex partner at such a young age; but he conceded that it was her having had coitus that served to clinch his notion that Frances should be helped to be as feminine as desired by her and be confirmed as female. Many of the team members expressed their feelings that ethical and professional quandaries grew out of the case of Frances, but the endocrinologist said she was not fazed by the case. For the endocrinologist, the fact that gender assignment had been so fully female and that with hormones the necessary task was "doable" was all that counted. Frances—with less than full comprehension—felt good about herself and stopped beating up family and friends.

Questions for Study and Action

1. Discuss why a Swiss Protestant clergyman would have wanted Sigmund Freud to soften some of his early views about childhood sexuality. For example, show how it evolved that such a pastor would be so pleased when Freud began to emphasize *pregenital* phases of libidinal development. What *difference* does it make if a psychiatrist blatantly says children are born with the capability of genital sexual arousal? Would the public care one way or another?

2. Discuss the impact of findings by child analysts (such as Herman Roiphe and Eleanor Galenson) recently showing that young children have some genital awareness at least by eight months of age, and that they enter "an early genital phase" between 15 and 18 months of age when they display touching or grasping of the genitalia, while becoming flushed, perspiring, and kissing another person, for example.

3. Why does the case of ambiguous genitalia that has reached age three years provide us with a kind of "natural experiment" for testing whether gender identity is established before age three? What did the case of Frances show about the role of genetic versus postnatal conditions in determining core gender identity?

4. Make out a case for Frances's (Case 12-2) belligerence towards her mother being a consequence of her mother's brisk corporal punishment of her when Frances was a toddler. Why would that history be more decisive than Frances's onrush of testosterone at age 11?

5. Define and distinguish between *sex drive, sexuality, sexual orientation,* and *sex-role differentiation.* Harry Stack Sullivan meant which of the terms when he spoke of *lust?*

6. What is the difference between advocating sexual freedom for children with their agemates and the contention by the pedophiliac person or group that pedophiles should be given leeway to "educate" children about sexuality?

7. What treatment plan would you devise for a girl like Cleeta (Case 12-1) who seems to be straining a point to insist to her new stepmother and father that she is a boy? Be specific and include every part of the comprehensive plan, such as schooling, family therapy, topics to cover in her sexual education, and medications. Would you ask the custodial parent to allow you to meet with the noncustodial parent? Explain.

8. What do you make of the fact that a boy who has had heterosexual relations will dream of what he has done, although perhaps with a different girl, while a boy who has had homosexual contact will dream only of that? What do you make of the fact that when both boys are grown they may be exclusively heterosexual but both will have occasional homosexual dreams?

9. What would you tell a mother and father who complain that a boarding school teacher has "had sex with" their 11-year-old son? How would you question them? Would you tell them to report this? to take it seriously? or to relax because it may have no serious sequelae? What line of questioning and information giving would you take with the 11-year-old boy, if brought to see you by the parents in question?

10. List five each of arguments pro and con sex education being carried out in public schools.

For Further Reading

Money, J., & Ehrhardt, A.A. *Man & Woman, Boy & Girl.* Baltimore: Johns Hopkins University Press, 1972.

Pillard, R.C., & Weinrich, J.D. Evidence of familial nature of male homosexuality. *Arch. Gen. Psychiatry,* 43:808–812, 1986.

13

Tic and Habit Disorders

Tic disorders are subdivided into specific and atypical movement disorders. Specific stereotyped movement disorders all involve *tics*.

There is no agreement as to how frequent tics are among children. The incidence of all tics in children has been variously estimated to range from 1%-23% of the general child population (Silver, 1985, p. 1711). Most tics are transient, a small number are chronic, and a minority of the latter may develop into Tourette's Disorder.

DEFINITION

Tics were defined by Arthur and Elaine Shapiro (1981) as "involuntary contractions of functionally related groups of skeletal muscles in their normal synergistic relationships, and involuntary noises and words" (p. 193). A similar definition has been adopted by DSM-III-R.

Although tics are purposeless and inappropriate, they often look as if they have a hidden symbolic meaning. For instance, squeezing the eyes shut or blinking may represent a defense against seeing something terrible or forbidden; tics around the shoulders may represent shrugging; those making slapping gestures with hands may represent an inhibited aggressive act, and so on.

The clinician should realize that inferences about the tic's symbolic meaning only facilitate our differentiating them from other abnormal movements and do not imply that such symbolic meanings are causative. Symbolic causes may or may not enter into the development of transient tics and practically never do so in Tourette's Disorder.

Further characteristics of tics are: the patient's ability to suppress them voluntarily for varying periods of time; their frequent disappearance during sleep and hypnosis; and their direct relationship to anxiety. By the same token, when the patient's attention is distracted away from the tics, they may temporarily remit. These characteristics should therefore not be taken as indicating malingering or that the child is "merely seeking attention."

ETIOLOGY

The pendulum of etiological opinion has swung twice in the organic direction: 19th century psychiatrists considered tics to be the expression of hereditary/ degenerative disease, 20th century psychiatrists were led by psychoanalysis to look for exclusively psychodynamic explanations; and again, contemporary theory gives either an exclusive or at least substantial role to organic factors. Many authors view all tics as on a continuum, from the transient tics of childhood to Tourette's Disorder, the latter the most severe and most organically determined of all. The pathophysiological mechanism of tics is not clarified, but the impressive response of many tics (especially Tourette's Disorder) to neuroleptics, which block dopamine receptors in the nigrostriatal areas of the brain, strongly suggests that dopamine excess or hypersensitivity to dopamine in those structures plays an important role. The tiqueur's response to neuroleptics is in direct proportion to the neuroleptics' dopamine-blocking action. Haloperidol is a most potent dopamine blocker as well as the most effective agent for controlling the symptoms of Tourette's Disorder.

Transient Tic Disorder (307.21)
CLINICAL DESCRIPTION

This tic disorder is characterized by limited duration (less than one year) and reversibility. Many are not brought to the physician's attention, being considered "bad or odd habits" by some parents. Others are incidental findings requiring differential diagnosis and monitoring but usually remit without treatment. At times, however, short-term treatment is necessary, as illustrated in the following case.

CASE 13-1   Rudy, age six, was brought to the doctor because he had developed a tic consisting of frequent eye blinking *following his experience of an auto accident.* He was sitting on the front passenger seat when his mother's car had collided with a motorcycle. Rudy was uninjured, but his mother had suffered facial cuts when the motorcyclist was thrown against the car's windshield. Rudy had always been a shy boy who was very close to his mother; as a matter of fact, he was considered overprotected. The *accident* brought many of his *inner conflicts* to the surface: he expressed concerns about his mother's safety, had difficulty sleeping, and feared being driven anywhere, especially by his mother. His tic increased *in intensity* when he became anxious, and *disappeared* when he finally fell asleep at night. He could also *stop it by conscious effort* for several minutes, at the end of which tension became so high that the tics reappeared.

This child required *short-term psychotherapy* because of the *exacerbation of previous difficulties* and the probability of this complex of symptoms becoming *fixed behavior* ("fixated").

Chronic Motor or Vocal Tic Disorder (307.22)

The characteristics are the same as for transient tic except for longer duration (over one year at least). Instead of the visible muscular tics, vocalizations may occur accompanied by only the necessary contractions of thoracic, abdominal, and diaphragmatic muscles. But both vocal and motor tics do *not* occur; it is either one or the other.

The most important differential diagnostic features are the unvarying intensity of the tics over periods of weeks or months. Differential diagnosis will be considered jointly for all tics. Treatment is long-term, both pharmacological and, where indicated, psychotherapeutic. Haloperidol is considered the most effective pharmacological agent for this chronic group.

Prognosis is relatively guarded since Chronic Motor or Vocal Tic Disorder does not respond readily to treatment. Yet the long-term prognosis in children is good, provided the disorder is not an early heralding of Tourette's Disorder.

Tourette's Disorder (307.23)

DEFINITION

This disorder is defined by its symptoms, their course, and its associated features.

The symptoms consist of multiple tics affecting multiple muscle groups, including multiple vocal tics. Central to the diagnosis are the *vocal tics.* In 60% of cases, coprolalia is present and confirms the diagnosis. *Coprolalia* is an irresistible urge to utter obscenities. The nonverbal tics usually involve the upper half of the body and, most frequently, the head, but may be manifest in the lower extremities as well. The course of the symptoms is fluctuating since the symptoms vary in intensity, frequency, and location over weeks or months. The associated features can be organized into two groups.

(a) One consists of specific symptoms: mental coprolalia (obsessive thinking about obscene words), echokinesis, palilalia (repetition of one's own last words or phrases), obsessive thoughts, and compulsive acts.

(b) The other group includes entire symptom *complexes,* such as those of Attention-Deficit Hyperactivity Disorder with marked neurological findings, also of developmental disorders.

CLINICAL DESCRIPTION

CASE 13-2   Jim was seven years old when his parents first noted his *facial tics,* predominantly on one side; they involved grimacing (pulling up the corner of the mouth) and eye blinking. Neither the parents nor the pediatrician were particularly alarmed since the child was in constant motion anyway—he was "kind of *hyper,*" as his mother put it. This was considered "just another of his quirks" at first, and the parents were not worried since the *tics disappeared during sleep* and *"when he really tried."* Their theory appeared justified when the tics nearly vanished after six weeks. Alas, they were followed by *jerking of the left arm and shoulder.* Jim found this quite embarrassing at school and barely was able to keep it from happening whenever he was with his peers.

By this time, his inability to keep still in school and pay attention had dawned on everybody and the pediatrician prescribed methylphenidate (a *stimulant*), since he was considered to be hyperactive and the jerking of his arm and shoulder were thought to be part and parcel of Jim's hyperkinesis. The *medication* improved his ability to concentrate somewhat, but the *arm jerking became worse,* and besides, Jim started making *grunting noises.* Moreover, the *facial tics reappeared.*

Although Jim's overall behavior, apart from the hyperactivity, had never been a problem, his language presently became one: he started interjecting four-letter obscene words seemingly out of context. These words came out *as if under pressure;* he would feel very bad and assure everybody that he *did not mean* to say them *(coprolalia).* This previously happy-go-lucky youngster now *became preoccupied, compulsively watched his every move,* and eventually became depressed. The methylphenidate was discontinued and this diminished the intensity of his symptoms, but they did not disappear altogether and his distractibility worsened. Jim's pediatrician concluded that Jim was suffering from Tourette's Disorder and started him on haloperidol, in slowly increasing doses, until at a daily dose of

3 mg both the *tics* and the *explosive uttering of four-letter words (coprolalia)* disappeared. His parents were relieved.

Comment. The preceding case history is a special case: the symptoms of Tourette's Disorder appeared, at least in clinically recognizable form, following Jim's treatment with stimulant medication. Although the issue is disputed, to prescribe stimulant medication for a child with a history of tics is contraindicated.

DIFFERENTIAL DIAGNOSIS

This can become a very involved process, for purposes of clinical relevance.

Differential diagnostic step I

Tics vs. other movement disorders. First, we should keep in mind that tics are stereotypic contractions of *functionally related groups of muscles.* These movements often carry symbolic meaning. Ruled out by this definition are disorders involving less than one muscle:

(a) *Fibrillations:* twitchings of muscle fibrils.
(b) *Fasciculations:* twitchings of groups of muscle fibrils.
(c) *Myokymia:* twitching of muscle fibers of eye muscles.
(d) *Synkinesis.*

These disorders may or may not be found in organic disease.

The following disorders involve groups of muscles but the "shape" and direction of the movements are different from what we see in tics:

(a) *Chorea:* jerky, random and irregular movements of trunk and limbs, the latter directed away from the body.
(b) *Athetosis:* by contrast, has slow, continuous, writhing movements in the distal parts of extremities (fingers and toes).
(c) *Hemiballismus:* flinging, "throwing," wingbeating, unilateral movements of the limbs.
(d) *Dystonia:* slower, twisting movements. They are focal (e.g., spastic torticollis), segmental or generalized. A salient feature of the dystonias is that general muscular tensions are present even when there are no movements.
(e) *Myoclonic* movements are sudden shocklike contractions affecting only one muscle, not a group of muscles. They may be organic or functional.

The foregoing movement disorders are expressions of organic disease. None of these five disorders carries a hidden or implied symbolic meaning. However, symbol makers as we are, organic disorders may acquire symbolic meanings.

Differential diagnostic step II

This separates Tourette's Disorder from the other tics. The onset of the disease up to age 15 years, multiple and varying tics, and coprolalia make the diagnosis of Tourette's Disorder practically certain. When coprolalia is absent, the differential diagnosis is based on the first two conditions, with the understanding that in Tourette's Disorder the tics wax and wane slowly and that vocal tics are practically always present. Echolalia, echopraxis, and palilalia, although relatively rare, add a lot of weight to the diagnosis of Tourette's Disorder. By contrast, Chronic Motor or Vocal Tic Disorder shows *steady* symptomatology confined to the same part of the body. This is important since vocal tics may occur in this disorder. Transient Tic Disorder is acute in onset and fluctuates, usually more abruptly than Tourette's Disorder, rarely involves vocalizations, and can often be traced to a traumatic event.

The tics of Tourette's Disorder never look as if they have a hidden meaning. Further, Tourette's Disorder must be differentiated from childhood psychosis, because of the psychotic child's frequent bizarre posturing, and from severe obsessive neurosis, wherein the child may be preoccupied with foul language and "bad thoughts." Obsessive neurosis and Tourette's Disorder often coexist and the two are then diagnosed concomitantly. The association of Attention–Deficit Hyperactivity Disorder with Tourette's Disorder is rather frequent. Tourette's Disorder should not be confused with the choreoathetoid movements of Attention–Deficit Hyperactivity Disorder with a strong organic component (minimal brain dysfunction), since a missed Tourette's Disorder may have negative consequences if it is treated with stimulants, as was shown in the Case 13-2. By contrast, the pharmacological agent for Tourette's Disorder (haloperidol) will not make Attention–Deficit Hyperactivity Disorder worse (it will help moderately). However, the psychological consequences of "wrong labeling" are worth avoiding.

Differential diagnostic step III

This encompasses the side effects of neuroleptic medication:

> *Tardive dyskinesia*—This may confuse the clinician because there may be tic-like movements in the face, neck and upper extremities. Vocalizations do not occur, and there is the history of neuroleptic use.

> *Withdrawal emergent syndrome*—The signs are very similar to those seen in tardive dyskinesia (the two may actually be the same disorder), with additional autonomic symptoms of nausea, vomiting, and elevated temperature.

Neither of these syndromes exhibits obscene vocalizations to the extent found in Tourette's Disorder. Clearing of the throat and other expressions of dystonia extending to the larynx can occur, but can easily be distinguished from the repetitive and definitive vocalizations of Tourette's Disorder.

Appropriate history will usually finalize the differential diagnosis.

TREATMENT

Conforming to the etiology, psychotherapeutic treatment helps whenever emotional trauma and/or intrapsychic conflict are in evidence, and organic treatment is called for whenever the etiology is organic. Thus, Transient Tic Disorder is treated psychotherapeutically and behaviorally when treatment is necessary. Occasionally, antianxiety medications can be used adjunctively, oxazepam or lorazepam being appropriate for short-term use.

The treatment of Chronic Tic Disorder should be left to the specialist, who will weigh the psychological versus the organic factors and proceed accordingly. Treatment is often lengthy and difficult. Besides dynamic-verbal psychotherapy, behavioral therapy has been used: relaxation techniques try to minimize the use of motor function for the discharge of tension and "negative practice" uses voluntary repetition of the tic as fast as possible.

Tourette's Disorder is primarily treated pharmacologically and secondarily, psychotherapeutically. The standard pharmacotherapy is haloperidol in slowly increasing doses (e.g., in 0.25 mg increments) until an effective dose has been reached. The clinician should not aim for 100% control, since this pushes the dose of haloperidol to levels where its side effects outweigh the benefits of total control of symptoms. Fortunately, total control of coprolalia can be achieved before total control of the tics. It is usually preferred to have occasional tics rather than to have the child so drowsy that schoolwork and other activities are impeded, even after extrapyramidal side effects have been controlled. Tardive dyskinesia, although very rare in children, has to be borne in mind as a delayed ill effect. Examining the child's tongue for fasciculations is an easy and effective way of detecting them early. Any suspicion of haloperidol-induced dyskinesia should prompt referral to a specialist, since this then involves a careful weighing of the risk-to-benefit ratio in close cooperation with the parents and child.

Several additional pharmacological agents have been introduced recently. Pimozide (trade name Orap) is a phenothiazine neuroleptic whose effects and side effects are similar to haloperidol; it is reputed to cause less sedation and may be the alternative when a peculiar side effect of haloperidol, viz., a sudden upsurge in separation anxiety, is encountered. One untoward effect of haloperidol in Tourette's Disorder is to produce a Separation Anxiety Disorder that outlasts cessation of haloperidol. For such events, pimozide may be very welcome.

Clonidine (trade name Catapres) is an antihypertensive agent which has been found effective in a variety of organic movement disorders—in a limited number of cases. It is administered in increasing doses, starting with 0.1 mg; hypotension is an occasional side effect. It should be discontinued slowly and gradually to avoid sudden increase in blood pressure. Chlorimipramine (trade name Anafranil) is available only for research in the United States, but is being tried elsewhere, a partial rationale being the overlap between Tourette's Disorder and Obsessive Compulsive Disorder; chlorimipramine has shown promising results with OCD.

Psychotherapy of varied duration and "depth" may become necessary for reactions of frustration, anger, depression, or conduct disorders associated with both the social consequences and the effects of the tics on the child's self-image and self-esteem. For the family, support and guidance, including explanations of the latest "state of the art" in the treatment of this disease, are necessary.

PROGNOSIS

The outlook for Transient Tic Disorder is excellent, often even without treatment. For Chronic Motor or Vocal Tic Disorder forecasting is more guarded because of its tendency sometimes to resist almost all treatment approaches for a long time; yet the outlook is not hopeless in children. Resolution and diminution of anxiety and depression have been associated with good outcome in chronic tic disorder. Tourette's Disorder is lifelong in most instances, although spontaneous remissions occur. The need for medication usually fluctuates in the long term, so that adjustments are always necessary; however, with conscientious follow-up, the vast majority of patients can lead satisfactory lives.

Stereotypy/Habit Disorder (307.30) (Includes Thumbsucking)
DEFINITION

DSM-III-R defines this disorder as "intentional, repetitive, nonfunctional behavior" (p. 95). Examples are body rocking, head banging, nailbiting, picking at the skin, etc. That definition also postulates that the disorder "either causes physical injury to the child or markedly interferes with normal activities" (p. 95).

The usual habit disorders of childhood are thumb (or finger) sucking, and nailbiting. Their exact place in nosology has not been determined: many consider them to be time-limited developmental disorders. We have chosen to attach them to stereotyped movement disorders because of their descriptive resemblance to tics and the others.

ETIOLOGY

There is probably no uniform etiology underlying these disorders. The mild, transient habits may be based on chance learning, imitation, or response to organic irritation such as allergies. It appears that immaturity of the central nervous system may be the most common and perhaps necessary ingredient in all these disorders, with head banging and rocking being known to be associated with definite brain damage.

The entire spectrum of these disorders may, therefore, represent the expression of one of two mechanisms: either the inability of the central nervous system—because of damage or immaturity—to contain excitations, or the need of such a central nervous system for stimulation. The former may be viewed as a "spillover" phenomenon and is exemplified by the many types of excessive movements such as waving, shaking, or flailing of extremities. The latter comprises most of the habit disorders and many of the stereotypies, and has been considered a self-stimulating phenomenon.

Habit disorders are both symptoms of underlying anxiety and idiopathic disorders wherein a normal phenomenon (especially finger/thumbsucking) continues beyond its normal phase, serving the function of tension reduction. Psychoanalytic theory views finger/thumbsucking as a regressive, oral phenomenon; nailbiting is viewed in more severe terms, as a reflection of competitive strivings toward parent(s), and even as a murderous or suicidal equivalent. In line with the greater severity of psychopathology that *may* be associated with nailbiting, there is a stronger link between this disorder and self-mutilation. Nailbiting that is quite destructive may be seen in children with organic or functional psychosis.

Proponents of learning theory offer simpler explanations—these habit disorders are learned experiences, the rewards being a feeling of comfort and relaxation (tension reduction). Maternal deprivation has been considered a predisposing factor in the persistence of finger/thumbsucking from infancy into childhood.

Habit disorders become an issue because of their social, physical, and, to a smaller degree, emotional consequences. The social consequences are general opprobrium and ridicule from peers when finger/thumbsucking is carried over into the school years. Emotional problems consist of becoming secretive and of preferring the self-stimulating, immediately gratifying escape of the habit; as time goes on, the child avoids detection by peers by increasing his/her social isolation and further increasing the need for the gratification offered by the habit, and a vicious cycle results. The physical damage is to the teeth and development of the maxilla and the palate, and may be considerable whenever thumbsucking goes past the age of permanent dentition, which coincides with the beginning of school (the incisors are the first permanent teeth and the most vulnerable because of their position). Severe damage to the thumb or fingers is rare, but infection may result from both fingersucking and nailbiting. Probably the most frequent sequel is an overbite giving prominent front upper incisors.

Thumbsucking is probably the most notorious of all habit disorders and is both a self-stimulating and a regressive act. Head banging and rocking are probably combinations of "spillover" and self-stimulating acts, classically seen in patients with definite brain pathology. Other stereotypies are associated with "minimal brain damage," i.e., Attention–Deficit Hyperactivity Disorder (ADHD) or Schizophrenia.

CLINICAL DESCRIPTION

Habits or stereotyped movements are frequent. Many of them are transient, especially in the preschooler; they come and go as "bad habits," such as nose picking, nail biting, thumbsucking, or picking at various other projections of their bodies.

More severe stereotypies are head banging or rocking of the upper part of the body or head. These are usually of long duration. All stereotypies or odd habits are exacerbated by overstimulating, which is usually nonspecific.

DIFFERENTIAL DIAGNOSIS

Stereotypies are to be distinguished from the various organic movement disorders, the choreas and hemiballismus. Overall neurological evaluation, appropriate history and family history, and the presence or absence of volitional control over the habit disorders help in the differential diagnostic process.

Tic disorders have just been described in the preceding sections as fairly distinct from habit disorders. Excessive movements, such as picking of skin, may occur as a side effect of stimulant medication.

TREATMENT

Treatment aims at the underlying causative pathology. Thus, many stereotypies respond to appropriate pharmacological treatment (e.g., stimulants for ADHD). Behavior modification has been successful as well. Thumbsucking, finger sucking, and excessive nose picking often become self-perpetuating gratifications and are treated with simple suppressive measures (e.g., applying a bitter-tasting or -smelling preparation on thumb or finger). The regressive "pull" in some of the foregoing habits may need to be explored psychotherapeutically. Neuroleptics are sometimes the only effective treatment modality in otherwise intractable stereotypies.

PROGNOSIS

This depends on the underlying cause. It is excellent in mild, though highly visible, habit disorders such as thumbsucking. Rocking and head banging that are of long duration reflect pathology which may have to be treated aggressively, depending on its nature, and the prognosis, although guarded, hinges on the compliance with appropriate treatment.

Trichotillomania (Hairpulling) (312.39)

DSM-III-R defines trichotillomania as a repeated failure to resist the impulses to pull out one's own hair. Hence, this Impulse Control Disorder results in noticeable hair loss by the affected child. An increasing sense of tension immediately precedes the act, which is relieved by pulling out the hair.

Although DSM-III-R lists this disorder among disturbances of impulse control, we feel that it is more closely related to the Stereotypy/Habit Disorders, probably sharing with them a common etiology or at least pathogenetic mechanism.

CASE 13-3   Joanie was a 10-year-old girl who was referred to the child psychiatrist because her hair had been thinning over several *areas of the scalp*. Her parents found tufts of hair on her pillow at various times.

Joanie *denied* pulling her hair, and her parents had at first wondered about a disease causing her hair loss. Multiple medical investigations by her pediatrician yielded only *normal* results. Her mother finally *observed* the patient *pulling her hair by twisting it around her fingers* just as she was *about to fall asleep*.

Psychiatric examination *failed* to pinpoint any mental disorder, except to raise the likelihood that Joanie may have had difficulties with her *attention span* and was generally *immature*. As a young child, she would often *"go spas"* [*spastic*] *when excited*, i.e., she would *flail* her arms and shake her hands.

The hairpulling did not seem to bring *any primary* or *secondary* emotional *gain*, and did *not* respond to attempts at psychotherapy. Finally, bedtime administration of a neuroleptic (thioridazine) arrested the hairpulling, after stimulant medication failed to do so (although *it caused her attention span to improve*).

Comment. The above is a case of trichotillomania or hair pulling. The symptom seems to be "free-standing," i.e., it is not the outcome of any other disorder. Pathogenesis and etiology are unknown, but may be the same as in Stereotypy/Habit

Disorder. Treatment is symptomatic, usually with neuroleptics, although tricyclic antidepressants may be tried.

Questions for Study and Action

1. Realizing that a tiqueur's mother may have read some early psychoanalyst's doctrine about symptom-substitution, how would you deal with her question, "Doctor, if the boy's tic is suddenly taken away, won't some phobia or other symptom take its place?"

2. How would you answer a mother's question, "Will Tourette's Disorder be passed on to my child's offspring?" How can you tell a mother a disorder *may be* inherited but that its mode of transmission is not known? that females seem more likely to transmit the disease? How will you deal with urgent questions that require confessions of ignorance and tentative answers?

3. Darwin (1871) listed these bodily structures as available for expressing emotions: muscles of phonation, mimetic musculature, voluntary muscles, involuntary muscles of the vegetative nervous system, and hormones. Which of those could be involved in a child's transient and psychogenic tics? Explain fully and indicate how we can *measure* emotional responses in children.

4. If Rudy, the six-year-old boy with transient tics (Case 13-1), gave a history of sexual abuse by a grandfather (*not* of an auto accident), how would you proceed with your examination, interviewing of him and his mother, and planning a treatment and protection program for Rudy? Give details.

5. Knowing what you do about dopamine in Tourette's Disorder, would you prefer amantadine or benztropine to control the extrapyramidal side effects of haloperidol? How so?

6. When Jim's (Case 13-2) Tourette's Disorder had been diagnosed and effectively treated with haloperidol, what would you have done for him if his attention deficit had persisted but without hyperkinesis? Explain.

7. If a child's tics and coprolalia have lasted for two years before being eliminated by haloperidol, what emotions other than fear (anxiety) would the child be likely to experience? Make a list of at least five troubling emotions that you can imagine the child would feel.

8. What cognitive (academic, learning, reasoning) impairments might accompany the motor disorder in a child with Tourette's Disorder? List at least seven.

9. Describe three ways in which a child's social or interpersonal development would be affected by having Tourette's Disorder.

10. Give a plausible accounting, in psychodynamic terms, of a throat-clearing tic in an eight-year-old girl who had acceded to her older cousin's request that she fellate him during a family visit six weeks earlier.

For Further Reading

Darwin, C. *The Expression of the Emotions in Man and Animals.* London: D. Appleton, 1871. (Available in University of Chicago Press paperback, 1965.)

Ferre, R.C. Tourette's disorder and the use of clonidine. *J. Amer. Acad. of Child Psychiatry,* 21:294–297, 1982.

Fras, I., & Karlavage, J. The effects of methylphenidate in Gilles de la Tourette's Disease. *Am. J. Psychiatry,* 134:195–197, 1977.

Shapiro, A.K., & Shapiro, E.S. Do stimulants provoke, cause or exacerbate tics and Tourette Syndrome? *Comp. Psychiatry,* 22:265–273, 1981.

Shapiro, A.K., & Shapiro, E.S. The treatment and etiology of tics and Tourette's Syndrome. *Comp. Psychiatry,* 22:193–205, 1981.

Silver, L.B. Stereotyped movement and speech disorders of childhood and adolescence. In H.I. Kaplan & B.J. Sadock, (Eds.), *Comprehensive Textbook of Psychiatry* (4th Ed.). Baltimore: Williams & Wilkins, 1985.

Slaughter, W.G., & Cordis, C. Covert maternal deprivation and pathological sucking behavior. *Am. J. Psychiatry,* 134:1152, 1977.

Tobrack, C., & Rajkumar, S. The emotional disturbance underlying alopecia areata, alopecia totalis, and trichotillomania. *Child Psych. & Human Development,* 10:114–117, 1979.

SECTION B

FEELING AND
MOOD DISORDERS

The following section of Part II is concerned with so-called emotional disorders. The ancient Greeks knew that our feelings have two main dimensions—breadth and depth—and that temperament was a shorthand term for appraisal of feelings in both of the dimensions. Although the Greeks postulated humors (*black bile* to give one a melancholic rut of deep but narrow-range feelings, *phlegm* to give one both narrow and shallow feelings, *blood* to make one sanguinely shallow but broad-ranged in affective expression, and *yellow bile* to give one a choleric depth and range of emotional expression), we do not agree with their humoral psychology but do find ourselves impelled to compliment them for their astute observational skills. In expression of emotions, children, too, develop disorders.

The feeling disorders that we consider in this Section are: Reactive Attachment Disorder of Infancy or Early Childhood, which looks highly similar to a deep melancholy; the various "mood disorders" along the depression-mania spectrum; Separation Anxiety Disorder and even the Panic Disorder that accompanies that disorder for some children; Anxiety Disorders; Phobias; Dissociative Disorders; Somatoform and Psychophysiological Disorders; concluding with the Adjustment Disorders and their prevailing mood states. As we stated previously, disorders of feeling spread over into cognition and behavior, but we group them together because there is something awry, or at least arresting of our attention, in the feeling states that are so intimately bound up with signs and symptoms of mental disorders in each condition that we consider here.

195

14

Reactive Attachment Disorder of Infancy or Early Childhood

This disorder is more generally known as "failure to thrive" (FTT) or "non-organic failure to thrive" (NFTT). The two terms are interchangeable, except for the fact that "Reactive Attachment Disorder" is the DSM-III-R term. Oddly, this is one of the rare disorders that specifies a sociogenic cause or etiology.

Psychosocial dwarfism (PSD) is a disorder not included in DSM-III but which will be described here in our extension of the concept of "failure to thrive" into "failure to grow." It is coded on Axis III. Both disorders have a common etiology and identical treatment. Indeed, a quick reversal of the clinical picture when caretaking is adequate is one of the seven diagnostic criteria cited by DSM-III.

DEFINITION

Reactive Attachment Disorder of Infancy or Early Childhood (RADIEC) (313.89) is defined in DSM-III-R as poor (faulty or inadequate) emotional and physical development, with onset before the age of five years, because of lack of adequate caretaking (formerly, "mothering") (abuse, neglect, repeated change of caretakers).

DSM-III-R offers no specific definition of psychosocial dwarfism (PSD); however,

197

PSD is quite similar to RADIEC except for the failure to gain in length despite actual gain in weight and the active seeking to ingest food (bizarre feeding patterns or ingestion of inappropriate food).

Both disorders characteristically improve with adequate parental care, which, in most instances, means removal from the environment in which the infant or child had been raised inadequately theretofore.

ETIOLOGY

Lack of proper caretaking of the infant is the undisputed *cause* of RADIEC. "Grossly inadequate care" is, uncommonly enough, given as one of the diagnostic criteria in DSM-III-R. There is theoretical dispute whether the mechanism is primarily by way of lack of weight gain with resulting stunting of all other functions, or whether it is primarily by way of inadequate stimulation, with cognitive and emotional malfunction resulting in psychosomatic lack of weight gain. We favor the theory that the disturbance in the mother-child relationship is both the cause and primary mechanism, as it explains the entire symptomatology of the disorder.

The role of the mothering person is vital for the disorder and its alleviation. The causes for her inability to take care of her child are usually severe psychiatric disease, e.g., Schizophrenia or Depression, or a pairing of psychopathology and environmental factors. The most common example of this pairing is severe socioeconomic deprivation throughout the mother's life, resulting in significant immaturity and an inability to form sustained relationships. Reliability was not learned from her own unreliable parents, in many cases. Often, drug and alcohol abuse and delinquency compound this maternal picture.

The child may play an interactive role if he or she has the characteristics of the maternally perceived "difficult" child described by Thomas and Chess (Thomas, Chess, & Birch, 1968). The "difficult child" has the following characteristics: irregularity in biological functions; withdrawal responses to new stimuli; slowness in adapting to changes in the environment; and frequent expressions of negative mood and intense reactions. What this often means is that these children sleep, feed, and eliminate irregularly and unpredictably; they cry and spit out new food; no matter what the mothers do to induce quieting down, it does not work, and so on. These children are known to be the source of considerable exasperation, but do *not* develop RADIEC *unless* there is severe neglect by the mother. This neglect, in turn, is caused by factors outside the child, but the "difficult child" may tip a precarious balance towards RADIEC.

Children with physical handicaps including those showing brain damage or "minimal brain damage" are also at greater risk for RADIEC when faced with a marginal or less than adequate mother.

CLINICAL DESCRIPTION

Historically, the first comprehensive description of the infantile disorder was made by René Spitz (1965), who called it "hospitalism." Within three months of total emotional deprivation (no mothering) after the third month of life, the infants of a foundling home lay supine in their cots and their faces became vacuous; when movements of the upper extremities did finally occur, they were reminiscent of decerebrate or athetoid movements.

CASE 14-1   Baby Ronald, age six months, was admitted to the general hospital in a *dangerously emaciated* state. He was *dehydrated, malnourished* to the point of marasmus, and his *protruding abdomen* and thin extremities were reminiscent of the publicized pictures of victims of *famine* in Ethiopia. Ronald's face was that of a *sad* adult, suggesting profound, indeed painful, *depression.*

He *reacted sluggishly* to all stimuli, despite giving an occasional impression of alertness due to a *roving gaze* by which he seemed to *"scan"* the environment as if his eyes were a *"radar"* set.

When admitted, Ronald *reacted with indifference* to any person trying to interact with him. His *mother* visited once, and his reaction to her was *no different* from that to strangers.

Ronald had been removed from his mother's apartment by the department of social services because of *neglect.* The department had been involved on several occasions before, but it had taken several weeks to obtain the court order since the *mother* almost violently *resisted* all contacts by the caseworker—when she could be found. The mother led a highly *precarious existence,* frequently moving from one place to another. She had had several hospitalizations for *schizophrenia* at the state psychiatric hospital and had also been jailed for brief periods of time for her *prostitution.*

The caseworker had become concerned about the baby soon after his birth: the *mother rarely sensed the infant's needs* and even more *rarely fulfilled* them. She fed the child in a *perfunctory* manner, usually *"propping up his bottle."* She resisted, and resented, the caseworker's attempts to induce her to hold the infant, to cuddle him, or to play with him. She saw her baby as devoid of any capability to learn, to respond, or to demand.

The baby responded in kind, as it were, and *did not pay attention to the mother,* did *not respond to her approach with a smile,* and *never cooed or "gurgled"* even when six months of age. On the rare occasions when the caseworker was able to take mother and child to the well-baby clinic, the pediatrician was concerned about the *lack of weight gain* and the increasingly *delayed developmental landmarks.*

Comment. Ronald's case is a severe example of RADIEC, showing the physical and mental stunting of the child's development. Physically, the main effect is of malnutrition and failure to thrive and gain weight; developmentally, it means delay; and emotionally it is one of lack of bonding, of attachment. It is a failure to learn that, being human, one's survival needs will be important to others.

CASE 14-2   Charlton was six months old when he was seen in consultation on the referral of the mother's psychiatrist, who had been treating her for *postpartum depression*. The mother, now improved, had just started to take care of Charlton and had expressed her concern about him to the psychiatrist. The baby simply *did not respond* to her sufficiently: Charlton *did not maintain eye contact, never smiled at mother's face, did not respond to her voice,* and in general did not anticipate or enjoy her presence. He *could not sit up* yet and rarely turned from supine to prone position. However, he was *not totally disinterested* in his environment: he followed the objects on a mobile, and occasionally grabbed or pushed the toys strung across his crib. His weight was four pounds below the norm. Charlton had been cared for by relatives during the five weeks of mother's psychiatric hospitalization. Her husband and relatives continued to help take care of him for another month after mother's return from the hospital. Both Charlton's parents and the extended family were strapped economically, and Charlton's *care had to be parceled out among a number of people,* according to their work and time-off schedules.

Comment. This is a milder, but much more common example of RADIEC, showing moderate deceleration of weight gain without any loss of growth in height, however. The main symptoms were Charlton's lack of emotional responsiveness to the caretaker (mother).

DIFFERENTIAL DIAGNOSIS

RADIEC (and subsequently psychosocial dwarfism) must first be differentiated from *organic* failure to thrive. The most common causes of organic failure are: renal pathology, including renal abnormalities and infections; congenital heart disease; various neurological disorders (usually congenital); and the gastrointestinal malabsorption syndromes. These must be differentiated by appropriate physical and laboratory investigations and by a comprehensive clinical assessment which will usually, but not always, show the absence of the special emotional features of RADIEC.

Among the psychiatric disorders to be distinguished from RADIEC is, first of all, Pervasive Developmental Disorder—Autistic Disorder. Although autistic children do not relate well and may show developmental delays, the latter are uneven, and autistic failure to relate is not at all like the sad, depressed, apathetic attitude of the RADIEC infants. Moreover, generally autistic infants usually are physically well developed.

Mental Retardation shows similarly retarded developmental landmarks, but without the lack of emotional responsiveness.

An early major affective episode has been postulated: this develops after eight months of age, the infant's development having been normal up to that point. This syndrome's documentation awaits future research.

Infants with sensory deficits may show some difficulties relating to their caretakers as well as delay in mental development, but weight gain and facial expression are normal.

As infants with RADIEC become older, they may show Pica and Rumination Disorder as part of the total clinical picture.

TREATMENT AND PREVENTION

The essence of treatment is to provide to the child what he or she is not getting: adequate emotional and physical care.

The specific modes of treatment will depend on the severity of RADIEC.

CASE 14-1 (continued)   The department of social services *obtained a court order to remove* Ronald *from his mother.* He was *hospitalized,* in intensive pediatric care at first, and then on a general pediatric unit. He made increasingly rapid *progress,* both in *weight, developmental landmarks,* and in *relating to his caretakers.* He was discharged from the hospital after six weeks and placed in a *foster home.* Two months later he had achieved normal weight, his motor landmarks were "on target," and he responded, often with anticipation and pleasure, to the foster mother.

However, Ronald developed "habits" that were trying to his new caretakers: he *ate everything in sight, including garbage,* and *drank water out of the toilet bowl* when he could reach it. He occasionally even *tried to eat his own feces* and often smeared the feces on the walls; he was now so *active* that he got into everything, causing material damage and damage to himself. When frustrated (and this happened often) he would sometimes *beat his head* on the floor, or bite himself, or get into a frenzy of screaming and kicking.

Comment. Severe cases of RADIEC require *hospitalization.* The hospital staff are instructed to provide as much personal interaction (play, cuddling, etc.) as the child can tolerate at that particular stage. Even though this means that care and interaction are provided by a number of different individuals, hospitalization is an eminently successful procedure but is best when followed by stable, attentive parental care.

This patient's hospitalization was followed by foster-home placement—the only effective residence, given the severity and poor prognosis of mother's psychiatric illness and her poor past track record of mothering. This entire treatment approach was enabled and eased by the authority of court interventions.

CASE 14-2 (continued)   Charlton's treatment was undertaken *at home.* It was realized that mother had nearly recovered from her postpartum depression and could take care of her child. The psychiatrist, in consultation with the child specialist, provided ongoing psychotherapeutic support to the mother for several more weeks to help her tolerate Charlton's lack of response. At the end of this time the child started reacting to mother's verbal and nonverbal cues. This, in turn, *encouraged* mother and gave her new assurance.

In addition to *office psychotherapy* and frequent follow-up visits by a child caseworker, a homemaker was provided by the department of social services.

Three months later, Charlton was "on track" developmentally; his previous lack of responsiveness was eventually *superseded by outright attention-seeking behavior.*

Comment. Where there is an identifiable and remediable cause or set of causes for the RADIEC, the mother should be helped towards greater proficiency in childcare. In Charlton's case, mother's postpartum depression was treated successfully, and there would have been little advantage in placing the child away from her. However, support systems had to be set up in this case—primarily aimed at preventing the development and fixation of negative reactions in the mother because of the frustrating clinical picture of RADIEC.

While most of the clinical aspects of treatment of RADIEC are clear and we definitely know how to treat RADIEC, the reality is often very discouraging: many such infants either remain in their original, inadequate circumstances, or are returned there following successful hospitalization. Sometimes durable foster home placement is achieved only after delays due to legal wrangling about the parental rights. By then, the consequences for the child may be irreversible.

RADIEC is thus closely linked with the larger issue of child abuse and neglect. Some of the RADIEC patients are abused directly, but all are abused indirectly by neglect.

Treatment can never be completed by only one professional or group of professionals. This has to be a community effort, with cooperation among several different professionals and agencies.

COURSE AND PROGNOSIS

The sequelae and long-term effects of RADIEC are what child psychiatrists and many other mental health professionals see more frequently in their practices than RADIEC itself (which is more likely to be seen by the pediatrician).

It is one of the characteristics of RADIEC that it is reversible with appropriate care. This statement has to be tempered by including an assessment of the extent and the duration of the neglect. It is conceivable that if adequate care is established quickly, no adverse sequelae occur. However, work in a child psychiatry clinic that treats children from all socioeconomic strata will convince most students that few children escape RADIEC without some scarring. The lack of emotional input at a very early age leaves the child with intellectual, cognitive, behavioral, and affective deficits. One sequel, the "affectionless character," has been described; many of these children show difficulties in establishing lasting bonds of affection and are quite vulnerable to any rejection, all of which they tend to perceive as major stresses and thus react with aggression or depression.

Psychosocial Dwarfism (PSD)

This disorder (coded on Axis III) may be viewed as *an extension of RADIEC* beyond infancy and early childhood.

Children with PSD usually come to the attention of the pediatrician because of failure to grow in height. Endocrinological workup then shows diminished levels of growth hormone and occasionally other findings of pituitary insufficiency. Hospitalization almost invariably results in the normalization of these laboratory findings within a few days, indicating that it is not improved nutrition, but rather the change in interactional climate that brings about the changes.

The clinical picture can be seen from the following case vignette.

CASE 14-3   Anthony was a four-year-old boy who was brought to the pediatrician by the caseworker for evaluation of his *failure to grow.* Examination showed a height and weight appropriate for half his chronological age (i.e., two years). Because of a previous history of neglect charges, abuse, and malnutrition, the child was hospitalized. He was noted by the hospital staff to be *withdrawn, apathetic,* yet given to *temper tantrums when some of his behaviors were interfered with.* This applied especially to his *eating behaviors:* he seemed *never to get enough,* would take *other children's leftovers* and *voraciously stuff them into his mouth,* and he would sneak into and raid the corner of the nurses' station where soft drinks were kept. Moreover, the nurses were horrified to find him *drinking water out of the toilet bowl* and *rummaging through the garbage pails,* the object of his search being food.

Comment. None of these *behavioral* symptoms is found in genuine pituitary dwarfism. Moreover, the differential diagnosis from the latter is aided by the fact that growth-hormone levels do not return to normal by the simple expedient of hospitalization.

ETIOLOGY

PSD is thought to have the same causative factors as RADIEC. Although there may be contributions by the children themselves, neglect (both emotional and nutritional) is the main cause. This is substantiated by the rapid normalization of the endocrine abnormalities.

TREATMENT

It follows that treatment is quite similar to that of RADIEC, i.e., provision of adequate emotional and material care. As with RADIEC, there are social and economic obstacles in the path of treatment, and a significant number of these children "fall between the cracks" of social services and legal networks. Even when placed in foster care, the persistence of their minimal habits and difficult behavior makes it hard for the new caretakers to provide them with the consistent emotional support they need, and they may move from foster home to foster home. Nevertheless, prolonged foster care is usually the treatment of choice, which offers a fair-to-good prognosis.

THE EMOTIONAL DEPRIVATION OR ATTACHMENT DISORDERS

A BRIEF OVERVIEW

The disorders just described—Reactive Attachment Disorder of Infancy or Early Childhood (nonorganic failure to thrive) and psychosocial dwarfism—can be viewed as a simple entity with a common etiological denominator: severe deprivation of parental care, both emotional and physical. As a result, bonding and attachment do not take place, or take place haphazardly or insufficiently.

The recognition of these disorders is important, because they are preventable. Their prevention and treatment give psychiatric and medical workers a brisk challenge, to be sure, but constitute an even greater sociopolitical issue.

The prevention of these severe, and physically and emotionally crippling, disorders should be the concern of everybody, especially those whom our society has entrusted with the welfare of our children. The workers in our social service and law enforcement agencies might be remiss in their duties at times because of their insufficient knowledge. Their ignorance is preventable. Removing a child from his or her mother may look like "the treatment is worse than the disease," but the fact is that the disease is potentially lethal and that we all, especially professionals, have a duty to work in the best interests of the child.

When confronted with the unpleasant duty of removing a child from his/her mother, the professional can derive at least some comfort from the fact that caretakers other than the child's mother can give the necessary bonding. The need can be filled, for a while, by a combination of several caretakers. The child's survival may depend on adequate parenting.

In some countries, attachment disorders are exceedingly rare, it should be noted. In the United States they are not rare among the very poor.

Questions for Study and Action

1. Abraham Maslow wrote that he would not have survived his infancy had it not been for an uncle who cared for him, loved him, and saved his life. Do you know an infant whose caretaker is anyone other than the mother or mother surrogate? Do you know a male who serves as an infant's primary caretaker (often called a house-husband)? Try to interview at least three such men to learn what their joys and sorrows are.

2. Argue the case that it is perfectly appropriate to have a category such as RADIEC included in a psychiatric diagnostic manual, holding as it does caretaker neglect and abuse as the responsible etiology. Note that some critics of DSM-III-R opine that the etiological condition does not belong in a diagnostic manual.

3. Why do many authors of any matter pertaining to neglected infants get accused of sexism? Would we have been well advised to remove all words like "mother" from our writing about RADIEC? Can we be gender-neutral when dealing with very young children?

4. Given the treatment examples of Ronald and Charlton (Cases 14-1 and 14-2), which of the two plans tended to neglect the mother, leaving her incompetent and unsupported? Write a better scenario of ways to help Baby Ronald's mother realize her assets and strengths. Would your new scenario be prohibitively expensive?

5. Does calling a child "difficult" say more about that child or about the child's caregiver(s)?

6. Map out a plan to change the behavior and socioeconomic circumstances of an unwed mother whose child suffers from RADIEC. Be specific about what you would show her, tell her, rehearse with her, and advise her about contacting diverse community resources.

7. What remote effects on parenting might you expect when the RADIEC infant or young child grows up? Name at least five effects.

8. Since there is a presumption in RADIEC that both physically and emotionally inadequate care leads to the impaired social relatedness, what would you say if the child's impaired social relatedness *preceded* the grossly inadequate care? Is an autistic child vulnerable to receiving grossly inadequate care, as an example?

9. Knowing what you know about attachment disorders, would you expect them to increase or decline under the following conditions?
    (a) rapidly mounting impoverishment of women and children
    (b) cutting of federal and state funds for maternal and infant care
    (c) growing numbers of vocational and childcare training programs for adolescent mothers
    (d) instituting a family allowance to be given for every child born
    (e) reduction of food stamps, housing assistance, and income assistance to the poor

10. Is it "nonmedical" to consider RADIEC, poverty, and public health and welfare in a beginning textbook on child psychiatry? Can you summon any counterarguments to your immediate response to this question?

For Further Reading

Spitz, R.A. *The First Year of Life.* New York: International Universities Press, 1965.

Thomas A., Chess, S., & Birch, H.G. *Temperament and Behavior Disorders in Children.* New York: New York University Press, 1968.

Woolston, J.L. Eating disorders in infancy and early childhood. *J. Amer. Acad. of Child Psychiatry,* 22:114–121, 1983.

15

Mood Disorders

The mood disorders that we discuss in this chapter are Depression and
Mania.

CHILDHOOD DEPRESSION

DEFINITION

Only recently has there occurred some resolution of the long-standing dispute
over the diagnostic criteria for and indeed the very existence of childhood
depression. Depression is now considered a relatively frequent disorder of
childhood and most child psychiatrists now diagnose depression in children on
the basis of symptoms that also characterize a major depression in adulthood.
We must remember, however, that childhood depression more often is associated
with behavioral disturbances, especially aggressiveness, and various combinations of somatic complaints than would be typical for an adult major depressive
episode. Yet this association does not justify our using the term "masked depression,"
a concept currently disfavored by the specialist and often regarded as highly
misleading to the nonspecialist physician.

Therefore, childhood depression must be diagnosed on *positive* evidence, i.e., the presence (unheralded by Mania) of five or more of the following cardinal symptoms lasting for at least two weeks:

1. dysphoria = depressed affect
2. anhedonia = lack of pleasure
3. self-deprecatory ideation
   - low self-esteem
   - guilt
   - suicidal ideation
4. social withdrawal and loneliness
5. decreased concentration
6. impaired school work; general indecisiveness
7. change in psychomotor functioning
   - usually, retardation
   - occasionally, paradoxical hyperactivity
8. aggressive behavior
9. morbid ideation, including suicidal ideation and attempts
10. somatic/vegetative complaints: sleeping (insomnia), eating (loss of appetite), failure to gain weight, various aches and pains, easy fatiguability

The foregoing list should be used according to the age-appropriate guidelines set forth in the section on the clinical description of depression.

ETIOLOGY

No definite cause or causes have been established for depression; moreover, it is hard to distinguish between psychosocial precipitants, biochemical mechanisms, and true causes. These putative and partial causes can be divided into psychosocial and organic or psychobiological causes and mechanisms. (See Table 15–1.)

Some instances of psychogenic causes are separations from or losses of important persons, relationships, self-esteem, or sources of emotional nurturance. The loss of, or rejection by, a parent is the most important. The resulting feelings of emptiness, guilt, lowered self-esteem, and general loss of well-being lead to depression. Parental rejection and depreciation can be overt or subtle; a special case of rejection or abandonment is a mood disorder (depression) in the parent, who, when depressed, may be unavailable to make a child secure.

The main biological causes of childhood depression are genetic or genogenic. There is a high concordance rate for depression among monozygotic twins, whether reared together (76%), or apart (67%); this compared to only 19% among dizygotic twins reared together (Tsuang, 1978). Higher rates of depression have also been found in children of depressed inpatients as compared with those of healthy parents (Welner et al., 1977). Looking at the family histories of depressed children, we find a higher incidence of depression in their families (Frommer et al., 1972; Puig-Antich et al., 1978).

Table 15-1
Etiology and Pathogenesis of Childhood Depression

A. *Genetic* (genogenic)
  1. Family history of mood disorder
    (a) depression
    (b) suicide
    (c) alcoholism
    (d) trouble with law
  2. Biological parameters
    (a) cortisol and DST
    (b) Insulin-induced hypoglycemia, lowered growth hormone, and desipramine response
  3. Depressed adoptees ($3\times$ higher concentration of depressed relatives than of adopting families)

B. *Sociogenic* (learned)
Incidence up with
  1. Increased age
  2. Concurrent parental depression (single mothers, especially)
  3. Family stress and disorganization
  4. Parental abuse, abandonment, neglect, rejection
  5. Protestants, whites, of European derivation; boys > girls (but reverses later on)
  6. Physical illness (see *Note* below)
  7. Uprootings

C. *Maturational* (developmental)
  1. Incidence varies by cognitive age
  2. Also age-specific norms:
    (a) Terrible twos
    (b) Sulky sevens
    (c) Trying teens

Note: Clinicians often say depression occurs "secondary to" chronic renal disease, lung disease, liver disease, or neoplasms. However, if the diagnostic criteria are met, the disorder is a major depression, pure and plain. (Too dogmatic?)

Psychobiological aspects of childhood depression (they should be considered mechanisms rather than causes) closely parallel those that appear in adolescents and adults; thus, cortisol hypersecretion is similar to the disturbance of the circadian rhythm of cortisol secretion in depressed adults. Decreased REM sleep latency is also found in children and adults, though less often in children. However, sleep continuity measurements taken on children (i.e., sleep latency, early morning awakening, and total sleep and wakefulness) do *not* resemble those of depressed adults. Although some investigators claim that drug response to antidepressants and lithium in depressed children resembles that in adults, there are divergent views on this matter and caution is advised in the practical application of complex and controversial pharmacological findings.

Finally, one special approach to the psychosocial etiology of childhood depression is that of emphasizing the parallel with the "learned helplessness" of experimental animals who found themselves in situations of unavoidable aversive consequences (Seligman & Maier, 1967).

In addition to "primary" or "functional" depression, there is depression secondary to or associated with other medical illnesses: thyroid disorders, brain tumor, asthma, chronic renal and lung diseases, ulcerative colitis, and diabetes mellitus. Such secondary depressions are similar to a primary major depression in terms of clinical picture, outcome in response to treatment, and other aspects.

PATHOPHYSIOLOGY

What is known has been covered under Etiology, since we have few, if any, leads to real causality. As in adult depressed patients, the amounts of urinary metabolites of neurotransmitters are diminished in depressed children. This strongly suggests decreased levels of the neurotransmitter substances in the body in general and, particularly, decreased MHPG (3-methoxy-4-hydroxyphenylethylene glycol) in the central nervous system. The precise pathophysiology of the cortical-hypothalamic-hypophyseal-adrenal axes may soon be more fully spelled out because of current research.

CLINICAL DESCRIPTION

For very practical purposes, childhood depression can be divided in two directions: 1) according to whether acute or chronic, and 2) according to the age and developmental stage of the child, into preschool, early school age, and mid-latency to preadolescent years. The incidence of depression increases especially after age 10 years and becomes a serious public health issue by late adolescence, when suicide becomes a major cause of death.

Acute Depression

CASE 15-1   Stacy, a seven-year-old girl, was referred by her teacher because Stacy had exhibited progressive *withdrawal* from peers and from school activities; her *schoolwork* had shown a marked *decline*. What bothered the teacher was the girl's general expression of *sadness and apathy* and a totally *"negative view* of the world." Even if she happened to do something well, there was *no pride of achievement* in it. Whenever the teacher reprimanded somebody, Stacy would feel it pertained to *her* and would feel *guilty* that she had, in some way, contributed to classroom disruption. All this started about *three months* prior to referral and was quite different from the child's usual disposition to show some joyous involvement with her life.

Stacy had been raised mainly by her maternal grandmother, with mother taking erratic care of her. The father was rarely present since the parents' divorce years ago. Four months ago, grandmother became gravely ill. This, and the fact that the mother had remarried and settled down, resulted in Stacy's move to mother's home and a de facto *loss* of grandmother, although fortunately the patient remained in the same school system.

After two months of individual psychotherapy with Stacy and counseling with mother (who fortunately had indeed settled down), Stacy was *considerably better* and *remained so* for the next two years of follow-up.

Comment. Acute depression is characterized by a precipitating or traumatic event (loss or object loss), relatively rapid emergence of characteristic symptoms, and good recovery. Premorbid adjustment is usually fair to good; at any rate, the history shows no previous depressive symptomatology.

Chronic Depression

CASE 15-2   Josh was nine years old when he came to the attention of the child psychiatrist, but his personal psychiatric history *extended all the way back* to preschool age. He was described as *always having been a moody, withdrawn* child, his *general apathy* being rarely punctuated by *occasional aggressive* outbursts, about which he indirectly acknowledged *guilty feelings* by stating it was *bad* of him to have been fighting. His *schoolwork* was *lackluster*, as he always appeared to *lack drive* and *motivation;* the same lack of energy characterized his involvement in *peer group* activities. He was often *called names* and responded either by withdrawal or by whining and complaining. Generally, he seemed *unable to derive any pleasure* from the activity at hand: in summer, he would talk about sledding, in winter about baseball. His teachers further noted *poor concentration* in that he seemed to be preoccupied—often revealed as ruminations about how he could *be better but really was not.*

His family was superficially intact, but the father had severed almost all emotional ties to the family except to provide for them materially and to complain bitterly about (and put all the blame onto) mother, who suffered from recurrent bouts of major depression for which she had had several hospitalizations.

The patient felt closer to mother than to father, but mother's hospitalizations and *inability to function adequately* as a parent because of her depressed moods made this a *tenuous relationship.*

Review of systems revealed that Josh had *anorexia, insomnia,* and frequent *stomachaches.*

Comment. Chronic depression is of long duration, often without any *one* clear precipitating event. A long history of withdrawal, listlessness, apathy, lack of ambition, and inability to take advantage of opportunities for success is typical. Anhedonia and low self-esteem follow, and nonsupportive, often interrupted, relationships with abuse and primitive attitudes result in insecurity and guilt. School reports are marked by underachievement, or by withdrawn or aggressive behavior. Somatic symptoms are usually present.

The examiner must bear in mind that childhood depression, especially the chronic type, is the one disorder in child psychiatry for which the history, as given by the child's parents or caretaker, may be noncontributory. The parents may miss the insidious onset and the gradual worsening of the child's mood. The child himself or herself has to be carefully examined, with the affective state determined by the examiner, both by observation and by age-appropriate communication of thought content. The section on treatment will provide further details.

Since cortisol levels are elevated in both depressed and nondepressed children, the dexamethasone suppression test, which measures cortisol suppression, is sometimes helpful in the diagnosis of cases of depression which may not be fully apparent to the clinical observer. It is important to note that depressed children may be suppressors, but nonsuppressors are highly likely to respond favorably to treatment with tricyclic antidepressants.

DIFFERENTIAL DIAGNOSIS

The first "cut" in differentiation should be between organic and functional disorders. As already mentioned, depression may be part of the symptom picture of an organic medical disorder. Even when organic illness is found, the depression may have psychogenic aspects, e.g., the depression in diabetes mellitus, where some of it is primarily related to the organic factors, while other portions are functional or psychogenic.

The second "cut" is between simple sadness or grief and the full clinical syndrome of depression. Simple sadness lacks the low self-esteem, guilt, anhedonia, and recurrent morbid thought content of a major depression. In other words, depression cannot be diagnosed on the basis of sad affect *alone*. A more comprehensive clinical picture with several positive findings (five or more of the 10 cardinal symptoms of depression) has to emerge. Grief reaction can carry over into depression if unresolved for a longer period, in children any-time after three-to-six months, especially if accompanied by self-blame and self-depreciation.

To label a disorder "masked depression"—i.e., to diagnose aggressive, antisocial, or acting-out behavior as masking an underlying depression—is controversial, even for the specialist, in view of recent doubts that such an entity as "masked depression" exists; for the nonspecialist, it may be outright disastrous, since the treatment of Conduct Disorder is different from the treatment of depression. Depression may coexist with Oppositional or Conduct Disorders, so it is impera-tive to make the positive diagnosis of depression in all cases.

Occasionally, the question of depression versus Attention-Deficit Hyperactivity Disorder arises, since some children express depressed affect, guilt, and an inner sense of loss by displaying random activity and poor concentration. Referral to a specialist is usually indicated, unless the primary care physician is able to convince himself of one or the other diagnosis on the basis of the child's depressed thought content or lack thereof. Occasionally, response to medication is diagnostic: the depressed child with random overactivity will respond better to antidepressant medication than to stimulants.

TREATMENT

The child's way of formulating and expressing depressive thought content is a function of the child's cognitive developmental level, but the firsthand, observable behavior (general appearance, psychomotor retardation or occasional hyperactivity, facial expression, social withdrawal) tends to be fairly constant throughout childhood. Therefore, the amount of verbal interaction with the physician therapist and the latter's use of the child's cognitive skills in psychotherapy will be influenced by the child's developmental level, while the need to give basic support and increase the child's self-esteem will not vary so much by age.

CASE 15-3   Janice was a six-year-old girl with a history of repeated parental rejections, who became exceedingly *aggressive* towards a foster sibling when she thought the foster mother "catered too much" to that child and not enough to her. Examination showed a *sad-looking, shy* youngster who *could not explain* her feelings or *justify* or explain her recent actions, but who presented the same themes in *her doll play:* children were *beaten, punished, and abandoned.* The children *tried to be "good,"* but were nevertheless shouted at and *punished.* Parallel with individual sessions for Janice, the clinician worked with the *foster parents to find activities* in which Janice could be *successful* and for which the *foster parents could* then *realistically praise and reward her.* Janice's mood and self-esteem improved forthwith.

Comment. The six-year-old child was able to convey her depressive condition in play but could not conceptualize it verbally. Understanding of the message and *parental* counseling *towards realistic improvement in self-esteem* resulted in relief from depression. At this age, most of the child's self-esteem is dependent on *parental* input and reflects parental valuations.

CASE 15-4   Jason was 11 years old when he was brought for child psychiatric evaluation following a *threatened suicide* attempt (he had threatened to jump out of a third-floor window but was restrained by peers). He had been *brutally beaten* by his alcoholic stepfather following a fight with his 12-year-old stepbrother. *His mother was a weak, passive-dependent person,* who considered herself *helplessly stuck* with this husband and *took no action to protect Jason against him.*

Jason had been described as a *morose, chronically brooding* and *often depressed* individual who had a *learning disability* and was *picked on by peers.* He spent most of his time watching horror or war movies on television and indulged in seemingly endless *fantasies of breakouts from prison camps,* all of which somehow ended unsuccessfully, with the patient stopping the fantasy just before he was captured and presumably shot or severely punished.

Discussion with Jason revealed not only anger and despair, but also very low self-esteem *expressed* as *severe disappointment in himself. He thought of himself as stupid and inept,* and even *blamed* himself for not being able to "outsmart" his stepfather and stepbrother.

Therapy with Jason consisted of the *involvement* of the county social services department to protect him, counseling *with mother,* and *individual sessions* to explore with Jason the sources of his self-depreciation and self-blame.

Consultation with the school produced a "tightening" of his *special help* in reading. He was referred to a boys' club where a *counselor* worked with him to *find areas in which the boy could become successful;* he turned out to be a good sprinter and did quite well on the football team. While all this was implemented, the patient continued to *assimilate these changes into his thinking* with the help of the psychiatrist.

Comment. In the older child, self-esteem depends not only on parental input but also on realistic achievement in such important extrafamilial areas as school and sports. Psychotherapy, therefore, involves those areas as well as the patient's own concepts of low self-esteem, guilt and helplessness, and their verbal expression.

Treatment of depression thus has several components: age-appropriate individual psychotherapy, environmental manipulation or guidance, usually counseling of parents, and recommendations for interventions by other adults or agencies. A full package is designed to provide areas of success and support for the child. Pharmacotherapy, too, is of help in treating a depression in childhood.

PHARMACOTHERAPY

Recently, this modality of treatment has gained an increasing number of advocates. The clinician must make sure that the diagnosis is positively made, i.e., that there is good reason to use medication, since the antidepressants are not without danger.

The tricyclic antidepressants are the agents used mostly to date. Imipramine (Tofranil) has been the standard medication in this group. The daily dose is in the range of 1.5 to 5 mg/kg/day, given orally, the total daily dose not to exceed 150 mg/day, with the admonition to use the lowest effective dose. Desipramine (Norpramin, Pertofrane), the active metabolite of imipramine, is now being used with increasing frequency, at the same dosage as imipramine. Amitriptyline (Elavil), nortriptyline (Aventyl, Pamelor) and (one of the least cardiotoxic tricyclics) doxepin (Adapin, Sinequan) have also been used in similar dosages.

As in adults, children may take up to a month to show noticeable beneficial responses to antidepressants, while side effects are usually apparent as soon as the agent is absorbed.

The initial antidepressant effect that we expect is *not* a subjective feeling of elation or euphoria, but rather the progressive disappearance of the depressive symptoms. The somatic symptoms of depression are often the first to respond: appetite and sleep improve; there are fewer aches and pains to complain about. Next comes discontinuation of crying, followed by lessened irritability and better socialization. Better attention span and improved schoolwork, as well as greater interest in work and participation in potentially successful activities, usually complete the course of improvement.

Side effects can be divided into *central nervous system* side effects, chiefly drowsiness, dizziness and weight gain, and *overall* side effects, of which the peripheral ones are the most important and, in turn, are mainly the anticholinergic effects of tricyclics. These are important to remember, since they include cardiovascular effects with tachycardia in mild cases and increase in cardiac conduction time with resulting increase in the QRS interval. These manifest themselves with initial bradycardia followed by arrhythmia and are the side effects to be watched carefully. The simple expedient of taking the patient's pulse on every recheck visit (and these should be frequent) is the best safety measure. EKGs should be ordered before treatment is instituted if there is any doubt in the clinician's mind about the integrity of the child's cardiovascular functions and during the treatment if there are changes in the pulse rate. Whenever in doubt, the doctor had better discontinue the medication, as the risk–benefit ratio of tricyclics is not excellent.

Full discussion of all these pharmacological effects with the parents is a prerequisite for the proper practice of pharmacotherapy; fully informed consent by parents should be obtained prior to initiating treatment.

Dry mouth and mydriasis are the most common anticholinergic side effects. The former can, on rare occasion, predispose to throat infections. A rare central side effect is deterioration of the child's behavior, with hyperactivity, aggressiveness, and lack of consideration for others (reminiscent of Conduct Disorder). The rare movement disorders occasionally reported in adults have not been observed in children.

The chief danger of tricyclic antidepressants lies in the relatively narrow therapeutic range, so that overdoses are very easy but dangerous; if overmedication is not discovered early enough for quick and vigorous treatment to be undertaken, tricyclics can be lethal. It follows that the physician should write prescriptions ordering only such quantities as are not likely to be lethal if consumed all at once and should warn the parents to lock up the medication and never allow the child to be in charge of administering his/her own medication. Since many of the parents of depressed children are not functioning optimally themselves, the clinician should not assume that they will use good judgment.

PROGNOSIS

This is generally good if the disease is promptly treated and environmental circumstances are improved so that the child's subsequent long-term development is towards positive self-esteem and a sense of security and well-being. A poor prognosis characterizes those children whose depression goes unrecognized and therefore untreated.

The relationship between childhood depression and adult depression or other adult psychiatric disorder is as yet unknown, since reliable criteria for diagnosis of childhood depression have only recently been established.

SUICIDE IN CHILDHOOD

Although considered very rare in the past, suicide has been found more frequently in this age group in the last decade. Certainly the number of suicidal threats is now relatively large, although successful childhood suicide attempts are still rare.

The clinician is well-advised to pay careful attention to *every* suicidal threat. Most children threaten suicide in order to draw attention to some problem area. Not all suicidal children are depressed. If, however, depression is diagnosed, the danger heightens. The depressed child contrasts with the otherwise healthy child who has learned that, by talking about killing himself or herself, he/she can obtain certain superficial, often material, benefits. If one finds a component of impulsivity and aggressiveness, the danger of suicide is increased, especially if these traits are combined with symptoms of depression. An environment of abuse, violence, alcoholism, or severe medical or psychiatric illness, holding little chance for change, will make it more likely that the child will feel impelled to go through with the act, either because of intolerable mental pain or because only drastic action will provide relief from an oppressive environment.

As with adults, there is no reason why the clinician should not ask the child about suicidal ideation and intent. The technique should be tactful and sensitive, but it can be direct: "Is all this so bad that you feel you want to hurt yourself, kill yourself?" Also, questions that respect the child's need for security are okay: "Do you need the protection of the hospital to keep you from hurting yourself?" If a child does not deny this need, it is probably there, and hospitalization, even if brief (no more than two weeks), is indicated and may be lifesaving.

In summary, the danger of suicide is increased significantly in impulsive, angry children with low frustration tolerance, especially when these children become depressed and when they live under conditions of abuse, violence, chaos, or significant psychiatric or medical problems—situations with "no way out" for the child.

As soon as the clinician suspects danger of suicide, consultation with a child psychiatrist is called for: if there is delay in obtaining the consultation, hospitalization of the child on a pediatric ward usually is adequate protection wherever a child psychiatric inpatient facility is not available.

QUESTIONS LIKELY TO BE ASKED BY PARENTS

Q. My son's paternal grandmother was treated for manic–depressive (bipolar) disease; does this have anything to do with his depression? Will he also develop manic–depressive disease?

A. Manic–depressive disease is an inherited disorder and his grandmother's disease may have something to do with his depression; however, the diagnosis of manic–depressive disease, to date, has not been reliably made in children.

Q. You are saying my child is depressed, but all I see is that he is mean. Is he really depressed?

A. Sometimes the depressive content comes through only on thorough, structured interviewing. You may try to ask him directly and repeatedly about feelings of dejection, sadness, and lack of feeling successful or liked.

Q. Will he become addicted to antidepressant medication?

A. No.

OTHER MOOD DISORDERS

CLINICAL PRESENTATION

Depressions are called "the American disease" but other prominent mood difficulties, while less common in children than even depressive conditions, require our brief consideration now. Loneliness as a primary affect is often elaborated into suspicion and self-aggrandizement, which are seen in all the paranoid conditions. Sexual exploitation of a child may lead to the child's having feelings of being a powerless victim and, oddly for the casual observer, may lead to sexual aggression by that child against other children so that, in fact, a child's suddenly emerging anger and sexual sadism becomes a suggestive sign that the child has been molested. As a consequence, an affect of anger and sadism can come to dominate that child's life, producing both affective and behavioral disorders—and compromising cognition, too.

Euphoria, another form of self-expansion, also occurs as a prevailing mood disorder. Euphoria may develop historically out of feelings of joy (as in apocryphal stories of a boy who became elated when he discovered that he could bend enough to suck on his own penis) but in ordinary practice elation seems to come out of a blue sky of blissful ignorance and self-deception, not joy. Indeed, the child manic—like adolescents and others—is more often rather "defensively manic," i.e., very volatile and easily tearful when underlying sadness can be tapped by another.

Mania of any form, whether of the suspicious, euphoric, or angry–belligerent subtype, is a rarity but when it is considered by an alert, clever clinician, it can be found in children. When a detailed family history over three generations is elicited of the family's (a) suicides, (b) trouble with the law (often for fights and brawls), (c) major depressions, and (d) alcohol and other substance abuse, the index of suspicion is raised. Moreover, when the child has been depressed but becomes hypomanic when given a trycyclic antidepressant, the probability increases of a bipolar disorder in that child. Many young people, if asked, will report experiencing a week or so of elation, "feeling pepped up," prior to worsening depression—and that nudges the diagnostician seriously to consider Cyclothymia or Bipolar Affective Disorder as the true condition.

CASE 15-5   Marlon was described as usually an outgoing and exhibitionistic lad, 10 years old when he was brought to a child psychiatrist, but his clinical condition at the time was one of *sadness, psychomotor retardation, self-depreciation, loss of appetite, school work that had halted, inability to concentrate, crying* and *morbid ideation* for the preceding five weeks.

At first, Marlon disclaimed any *feelings of elation* preceding his "getting down in the dumps" but later he recalled that he had been quite pepped up "for days" before he became depressed. Also, as a period of about four months elapsed, he became *hyperalerted,* felt his *thoughts racing,* became *overly talkative* and *energetic in doing sit-ups,* was *distractible,* made it *difficult for parents to get him to bed,* was *insomniac,* and *made obscene and erotic remarks* to his mother's twin sister (for the first time in Marlon's life). The loss of sleep was the parents' main worry.

Comment. Marlon was 10 years old when he saw a child psychiatrist, and his diagnosis of mood disorder was considered virtually an impossibility; but by the time he was 30 he was diagnosed as manic depressive (Bipolar Disorder) and successfully treated with lithium salts and tricyclic antidepressants. Since he cycled at least twice yearly, many doctors who saw his wildness first believed him to be schizophrenic and schizoaffective. His drug abuse only muddied the waters for some diagnosticians. His father and paternal grandfather had both abused alcohol, led stormy marital careers, and been high-pressure salesmen; his father was also a lithium responder when he had a hyperalerted, psychotic episode at age 40.

DIFFERENTIAL DIAGNOSIS

Any hyperalerted child should be considered a possible manic if the prevailing mood for more than a week has been euphoric, angry, or suspicious. In that mood state, if the child has shown four of the following: increased activity, talkativeness (pressured speech), flight of ideas, inflated self-regard, insomnia but needing less sleep, distractibility, and poor judgment—the diagnosis is nearly confirmed. But there cannot be: bizarre behavior or mood-incongruent delusion or hallucination.

To be ruled out are:

1. *Schizophrenia or Schizophreniform Disorder*—often confusedly misdiagnosed in manics of all ages because American psychiatrists readily think, Schizophrenia! The schizophrenic has mood-incongruent delusions and hallucinations and shows profusion of thoughts, perplexity, thought insertion, thought broadcasting, blocking (thought deprivation), oddities in affect (blunting), and so on. The manic is not a productive thinker but lacks the formal thought, or thinking, disorder of the schizophrenic.

2. *Delusional Disorder*—again an easily misapplied label to a young manic. The delusions of the paranoid are not as consistently mood-congruent as those of the manic, and whereas the paranoid is lonely and socially withdrawn, the manic who is suspicious makes a better case for his overall sociability, even while he may imagine he is the center of a great conspiracy originated by Very Important Persons. In a manic the affect has a crispness and the delusion has mood congruence.

3. *Organic Mental Disorder*—the manic is unlikely to show disturbed orientation, memory, speech or handwriting, and the faulty judgment present is in an expansive mode. The manic expands and enlarges his world while the patient with an organic brain syndrome constricts and simplifies his milieu.

   Amphetamine Intoxication may mimic a manic episode but the incidence of both in children is very low. Toxicology and eye exam (dilated pupils) would differentiate one from the other condition rather readily.

4. *Attention-Deficit Hyperactivity Disorder*—Both are highly distractible but the manic has a more consistent heightened affect, seems more purposeful in his or her overactivity, and gives a history more often of a definite onset of an episode of hyperalertedness.

TREATMENT AND PROGNOSIS

Some manics do not give a favorable response to lithium; some will respond partially and need to have an antipsychotic drug added to the regimen when they are in an up-phase, with a tricyclic antidepressant added when they are in a depression. Occasionally, carbamazepine will help when lithium is not an effective agent.

The prognosis for the young manic is grave—even a lifetime of taking lithium (with a risk of tremors, renal damage, hypothyroid disorder carried by lithium) is not optimistic. Fortunately, Mania is rare among children.

Questions for Study and Action

DEPRESSION

1. Discuss the meaning of the fact that the suicide rate increases for each year of age advancing beyond 15 years through age 35 at least. Why are suicides typically quite low in children under 12 years of age? In your discussion, invoke Freud's theories on conscience development, Piaget's views on cognitive development, and Erikson's views on psychosocial development of children.

2. Make a list of nine groups of children whom you might see in any public school who would be at risk for a major depressive disorder. Include in your list those who are not identified as the children of parents who suffer from mood disorders.

3. How would you account for the fact that some children with acute anxiety episodes, phobias, obsessive compulsive symptoms, and even Anorexia Nervosa can, on careful diagnostic evaluation, be found to be depressed and be treated successfully with a tricyclic antidepressant? Does the concept of primary and secondary symptoms make sense? Or the concept of treating depression wherever it exists in spite of the presence of other disorders?

4. What conditions other than Dysthymia, Cyclothymia, Major Depression and Bipolar Disorder need to be ruled out in a thorough differential diagnosis when a child has shown symptoms of depression for as long as two weeks? Think of all the "organic" and "reactive" disorders that should be listed in such a complete differential.

5. Discuss persuasively the relative weights that you would assign to the Dexamethasone Suppression Test (DST) and the clinical picture presented by a child when:
   (a) the DST shows nonsuppression when the clinical picture is one of a Major Depression during childhood;
   (b) the DST shows suppression when the clinical picture is consistent with Major Depression;
   (c) the DST shows nonsuppression when the clinical picture is not that of a Major Depression or Atypical Depression;
   (d) the DST shows suppression and the clinical picture is that of a child with severe Obsessive Compulsive Disorder;

(e) the DST shows suppression and the clinical picture is that of a child with Anorexia Nervosa.

In each of the foregoing instances, be certain to explain what course of treatment should be embarked on.

6. In order to facilitate the bereavement of a child whose parent has died, the psychiatrist has recommended that the child see the corpse, attend the memorial services and burial of the dead relative, and be encouraged to cry and talk about feelings of loss and sadness. What reasoning could you muster to justify each of those psychiatric recommendations?

7. What is to be made of the fact that many five- and six-year-old school phobics suffer from a major depressive episode by the time they are 40 years old? Does that mean that a school phobia should be regarded as merely a premonitory form of affective disorder? Give a plausible and convincing justification for your position, whether your original answer was negative or affirmative.

8. A child whose parents have divorced becomes more withdrawn, harder to manage, sulky, adopts a negative outlook towards life, becomes brutal to his little brother, and begins to show academic failure mainly because he will not do his homework for school. List two or three other symptoms that would be required in order to clinch a diagnosis of a depressive episode.

9. A 10-year-old child has developed early morning awakening, becomes generally listless and apathetic, does not like formerly enjoyed games and other play, and has taken on the characteristics of a loner both at school and in the neighborhood; she began complaining about two weeks ago of easy fatigability and sleepiness by 3–4 P.M. every day, including weekend days. Indeed, she comes home from school, retreats to her bedroom, and naps for one or two hours each day. Of what is her sleep pattern almost pathognomic, considering her age? Explain.

10. How would you evaluate the fact that an 11-year-old who achieved menarche last June still has scanty and irregular menstrual periods when she comes for a medical consultation the following October? This young woman presents a family history (alcoholism, substance abuse, depression and suicide, trouble with the law) of mood disorder and the physician wonders if her menstrual situation can be attributed to depression. What kind of additional diagnostic information would be required in order for you to give a positive answer to the physician's question? What is an anovulatory cycle?

MANIA

1. List six important things to ask *both parents* if you are taking a history of mood disorder in *their* parents and siblings, and in themselves.

2. What four laboratory studies are needed before a child, having met all the criteria for Mania, is begun on lithium salts? Justify each item.

3. How would you evaluate the observation that a child whose diagnosed Mania is under control with lithium salts has shown delusions and hallucinations now and these have been unshakeable for the past three weeks? What is going on? Consult DSM-III-R if you cannot figure it out.

4. Explain, as if to a third-year medical student, this statement: "Mania is not all elation. Mania has two other faces."

5. Why was it said, by an experienced general (for adults) psychiatrist, "Bipolars more than any other patients need to have the doctor give them a patient, detailed and clear drug education"?

6. Of what value was the NIMH-sponsored Epidemiologic Catchment Area (ECA) five-site study of mental disorders in discovering the prevalence of Mania in children? Hint: You can read about the ECA study in the entire issue of *Archives of General Psychiatry*, Vol. 41, October 1984.

7. How would you clinically differentiate a distractible Mania from Attention–Deficit Hyperactivity Disorder? What are the key points in differentiation?

8. Explain how parents do not detect pathology in a manic child but do so readily when the same child becomes severely depressed. Why would they think the child is recovering when he begins to cycle up into a hypomanic state?

9. Why do children with Obsessive Compulsive Disorder show an increase of family history positive for mood disorders?

10. Why do untreated cases of Bipolar Disorder join, in adult life, their schizophrenic agemates on skid row? What in their lifestyle makes for a "downward socioeconomic drift?"

For Further Reading

Bemporad, J.R. Childhood depression: Developmental considerations. *Psychosomatics*, 23:272–279, 1982.

Frommer, E., Mendelson, W., & Reid, M. Differential diagnosis of psychiatric disturbance in preschool children. *Brit. J. Psychiatry*, 121:71–74, 1972.

Petti, T.A., Depression in children. *Psychosomatics,* 22:444–447, 1981.

Puig-Antich, J., Blau, S., Marx, N., Greenhill, L.L., & Chambers, W. Prepubertal major depressive disorder. *J. Amer. Acad. of Child Psychiatry,* 17:695–707, 1978.

Seligman, M., & Maier, S. Failure to escape traumatic shock. *J. Experimental Psychol.,* 74:1–9, 1967.

Tsuang, M.T. Genetic counseling for psychiatric patients and their families. *Am. J. Psychiatry,* 135:1465–1475, 1978.

Welner, Z., Welner, A., McCrary, M.D., & Leonard, M.A. Psychopathology in children of inpatients with depression: A controlled study. *J. Nerv. Ment. Dis.,* 164:408–413, 1977.

16

Separation Anxiety Disorder and School Phobia

Separation Anxiety Disorder (309.21)

GENERAL COMMENT

The only disorders of feeling that get specific listing in DSM-III-R under "Disorders Usually First Evident in Infancy, Childhood or Adolescence" are Separation Anxiety Disorder (309.21), Avoidant Disorder of Childhood (313.21), and Overanxious Disorder (313.00). Childhood is a time for many other anxieties, or for other anxiety disorders, but general psychiatric nosology has developed mainly through studying adult populations and probably that is the reason why other "official feeling disorders" are not consigned to disorders of childhood. Avoidant Disorder and Overanxious Disorder will be discussed in Chapter 17. Once an adult disorder is named and described, it can be applied only with some awkwardness to most suffering children who, as Leo Kanner wrote, do not "read the books" and consequently wind up presenting some syndromes that are mixed or will not meet adult-based criteria! Children may have symptoms of multiple disorders and symptoms that are incapacitating without constituting a complete clinical picture as seen in adults. Children's psychopathological situations are full of *formes frustes,* surprises, and incompletely structured or "atypical" pictures. Children are indeed immature, compared to adults, and not quite matching of adults in their disordered behavior, thinking, and feeling. Thus it is that child psychopathology will have to emerge in the future; for now it is an imperfect science.

Separation anxiety has intrigued many students of psychopathology, along with others who have considered the human condition. It certainly deserves a prominent billing for a species *(homo sapiens)* that has evolved a unique place for anxiety and fear *and* for relatedness. The human animal was born to be social, interrelated, and interdependent, not independent and alone. Attachments to others are vital and, perhaps, the fear of losing them is inevitable. That kind of fear can mount to such a degree that it irritates others and cripples the victim of separation anxiety.

In our lexicon, the most crippling episode of fear (or anxiety) is a state of *panic*. If a child undergoes three or more panic attacks during a three-week period and dreads having another for another month, and otherwise shows the relevant symptoms (dyspnea, palpitations, sweating, feeling faint and dizzy, fear of dying, etc.), it would seem logical that that child has a genuine Panic Disorder. Yet some experts rule out the diagnosis, Panic Disorder, for children. We shall give examples later in this chapter of attacks of fear, in connection with children who refuse to go to school, surrounding separation anxiety that may or may not be coupled with even "Limited Phobic Avoidance" (see DMS-III-R). It will soon be evident that we employ an old and rather unsatisfactory term, "School Phobia," to depict these catastrophic reaction states occurring so often among school children with Separation Anxiety Disorder. This is controversial but not unreasonable, nor lacking an empirical base.

DESCRIPTION OF CLINICAL APPEARANCE

Conceding that Separation Anxiety Disorder can exist without reference to school attendance (a common and often difficult occasion for the child's separation from family members), let us now describe the generic Separation Anxiety Disorder as DSM-III-R characterizes it. First, at least three of the following nine symptoms should be present: unrealistic worry about attachment figures being harmed or leaving; fear of being lost/hurt/killed/kidnapped; reluctance to go to school in order to stay with attachment figure; unwillingness to sleep away from attachment figure; avoidance of being solitary; anxiety dreams about separation; physical symptoms; emotional distress when separation is anticipated; inability to work and play when not with attachment figure. Second, the disturbance has gone on for two or more weeks. Third, it is not present during the course of Pervasive Developmental Disorder or psychosis. That portrayal gives an excellent surface picture of what goes on at the outset when a child suffers a Separation Anxiety Disorder. But we hasten to add that neither of us has seen those overt behaviors lasting as briefly as two weeks. The reason is that most parents can wait longer before they feel unable to help their child solve such problems and then consult a specialist.

ETIOLOGY AND CLINICAL DESCRIPTION

There is more to Separation Anxiety Disorder than DSM-III-R spells out. From the standpoint of the child's attachment, in addition to its being truly infantile in character, it has an interesting double edge of ambivalence. The child lacks the total trust in the parent (read, attachment figure) that might be expected from one with such clinging and longing. Doubt and mistrust appear to be necessary ingredients in the disorder. The parent usually senses some anger, vindictiveness, and desire to enslave or control the parent by the child. One such mother said, "This tremendous attachment is no compliment, doctor!" Beyond the child's longing for a welding attachment, there are some features of the relationship between child and adult that warrant some comment. The relationship is often a sadomasochistic one in spirit, and some have aptly labeled it a hostile dependency. Moreover, the very parent who angrily pleads to the child, "Give me a break!" may derive some secret delight from the exaggerated dependency shown by the child. Or the adult may also harbor fears of being deserted and abandoned (that happens to many adults), may be depressed or anxious and actually want to lean on the child for comfort and companionship (role reversal), and may still refuse to move out of the grandparents' neighborhood. Hence, if a grandparent dies, it is not the child only who feels bereft of an "attachment figure," for the child's parent has a resurgence of earlier separation fears and that gets communicated to the sensitized child.

CASE 16-1   Eddy, aged eight years, was the son of a working father and a rather *shy, housebound mother*. Eddy's parents lived in the working-class section of a small American town and within two blocks of both sets of grandparents and numerous in-laws. At age eight, Eddy had entered a school further away from home. Both his mother and father were apprehensive about his being so distant, so father offered *to drive him* to spare him riding a school bus. The *mother cried daily* as Eddy and father drove away. Soon Eddy had a spiralling *longing to be with his mother;* he *worried about her, felt he would die* if he did not reunite with her at once, and *ran home* from school—about one mile. His mother clutched him to her bosom on that day and Eddy *refused to go* again for over six weeks. When the time came for school each day he became *hoarse, short of breath, sweated profusely,* complained of *nausea* and *numbness and tingling* in his hands, and told his parents he was *going to die*. He *refused to go out to play* with his cousins after school. *A mere mention of school would precipitate panic, even on weekends* when he also *refused to attend Sunday school.* He became *withdrawn* and *"pitiful,"* his mother said.

Comment. Eddy's symptoms qualified his case for a diagnosis of a Panic Disorder as well as Separation Anxiety Disorder, because of his symptoms that the child psychiatrist (pre-DSM-III) diagnosed as "school phobia." His entire family discouraged separation, thereby promoting the boy's anxiety.

DIFFERENTIAL DIAGNOSIS

Truancy in a Conduct Disorder would probably find Eddy leaving school to go elsewhere but not home. Autism would have had earlier onset of pervasive developmental difficulties. Post-traumatic Stress Disorder, had Eddy been sexually abused without informing the parents, would not carry so much resistance to separation in a child as old as Eddy. Other diagnostic alternatives would include Simple Phobia, a Somatoform Disorder, or the beginning of childhood Schizophrenia, but those diagnoses are truly farfetched.

TREATMENT

Ultimately, a child like Eddy must go to school, so that is a primary goal to be attained. It is discussed subsequently under the heading School Phobia. But the inner anguish over separation, anger, mistrust, and death is not as easily abated as the overt behavior and may require emotional therapy. The cognitive distortions need more attention, so perhaps direct cognitive therapy is needed. Certainly, a child withdrawn to home misses out on academic work and may need some remedial tutoring. Some work encouraging the parents to hatch their offspring is helpful, work that can be done with the family group, helping them to accept their emotions and differences from each other. In Eddy's case the mother learned to drive an automobile and reduced the amount of time she spent showing filial piety towards her own parents. Getting the family halfway reoriented towards some individuation and separation may take several months after the outward behavior has been changed.

CASE 16-2   Winnie, 11 years old, developed Separation Anxiety Disorder when mother divorced her second husband. Winnie showed five of the nine symptoms contained in DSM-III-R, one of those being school refusal, when the summer had ended. She returned to school promptly with help from the psychiatrist and when her mother had to seek employment outside the home. Winnie called her mother at work during every lunch break at school. Since Winnie had no way to come to see the child psychiatrist, a once-weekly telephone conversation was arranged and seemed to reassure and support Winnie, who seemed only precariously stabilized.

Because Winnie had never been to summer camp and was not inducted into the world of her peers, the child psychiatrist encouraged her to enroll in a two-week summer camp and a summer recreational program. As it evolved, Winnie derived pleasure from the recreational program and developed two shy girls as confidantes. But leaving home for summer camp "threw" her, she said. The evening before she was to leave for camp, she called the psychiatrist.

> Dr. X, you don't know how I feel. I am very sick and you don't take it seriously. I'll die if I go there. My heart is hurting right now. I am sweating all over and am about to throw up. My hands and feet are numb all over. I can't possibly sleep away from home; being able to sleep with mom every night was all that made me able to go to school all this year. You don't understand. It is cruel to force me to do something that I know will kill me.

Comment. Parents of a child with Separation Anxiety Disorder often withdraw the child from treatment as soon as resumption of school attendance comes about, even if the basic disorder persists and pervades the child's life with separation fears. Winnie shows how acceding to school attendance could be achieved only when her desire to sleep with mother was gratified. The juggling of symptoms through bargaining and threatening is a good example of how older children with Separation Anxiety Disorder begin to take on some features of Oppositional Disorder or Conduct Disorder.

School Phobia

School phobia is a time-honored, clinically valid term. It is not included in the official *Diagnostic and Statistical Manual of Mental Disorders* (DSM-III-R) under this name; nevertheless, we do not consider it, clinically or conceptually, a valid maneuver completely to split this syndrome into independent parts such as separation anxiety disorder, social phobia, or other anxiety disorders. The reason for this categorical statement is simply that whatever the dynamic background, the result is the same: fear of "going to school," resulting in school absence that cripples a child socially and academically. Fear is the characteristic feeling, so we are prompted to include it under the disorders of feeling.

The term *school refusal* is often used synonymously in as comprehensive a sense as school phobia. However, a few authors include "truancy" with school refusal, i.e., willful, manipulative absenteeism from school without anxiety. Truant behavior is not included here but under Conduct Disorders and other categories. Therefore, we prefer the term *school phobia* even though we realize that only a relatively small portion of school phobias are "true phobias," showing the typical mechanisms of displacement.

DEFINITION

School phobia is a disorder with refusal to go to school resulting from anxiety. If the child is forced to go to school the child's anxiety increases to the point of panic. An addendum to this part of the definition is the fact that the panic often, but not always, subsides upon the successful conclusion of the maneuver to return the child to school. As with many true phobias, response stopping and flooding (see below) should be done gradually.

ETIOLOGY

At the present state of the art and science, no organic cause or causal mechanism can be pinpointed with any accuracy, although encouraging basic experimental research into the organic mechanisms of anxiety is just beginning.

The cause of the disorder is to be sought—and found—in intrapsychic, i.e., neurotic, conflicts both within the child and often within the relationship between the child and the parents. The specific conflicts and psychodynamics will be discussed with the clinical description of each subtype.

EPIDEMIOLOGY

Incidence varies with the "peak period": school entry, third and fourth grades, and junior high school entry. However, Hersov (1985) estimates the overall incidence of school phobia to be 5% of all children referred for psychiatric intervention. The "peak periods" will be explained as they coincide with each subtype of school phobia.

CLINICAL DESCRIPTIONS

1. Separation anxiety disorder (309.21)

This is the characteristic disease process underlying school phobia that is earliest in onset. It occurs most frequently during the first "peak period" of school phobia, i.e., when the child first enters school or at least in the first or second year of school attendance.

Separation Anxiety Disorder is classified as a disease in its own right and defined as an exaggerated distress when separation from parents, home, or other familiar surroundings becomes necessary. *Not all separation anxiety disorders* manifest *themselves as school phobias; a high proportion* of them do.

CASE 16-3   Five-year-old Jenny was brought to the specialist because five weeks into the beginning of the school year, no way had yet been found to keep her in kindergarten. Her mother dutifully brought her to school every morning, after protracted *crying and imploring by* Jenny not to do so. In front of the school building, the *child hung onto mother* with every fiber of her body and with every ounce of her strength, which turned out to be considerable (as the staff found out when they tried to help mother and child separate). As a matter of fact, this was only tried once or twice, because *the mother turned out to be as anxious and as clinging to the child* as Jenny. Of course, mother *did not admit* that she could not bear to separate from her daughter; she stated that she needed to comfort and reassure her daughter and "explain" to her that she would be all right.

Jenny was the only child. Her father *had died* in an accident at a time of considerable strain in the parents' marriage, during which the mother was actively planning to leave father, whom she had come to hate. Following his death, the *mother felt very guilty* and became depressed and anxious. She became *overprotective* of her child, *fearing that if she did not constantly watch over her,* serious harm, comparable to that of her late husband, would befall Jenny. As a result, the *child felt helplessly exposed to unending dangers, especially when mother was not around, and neither could let go of the other.*

Comment. This is an almost "pure culture" Separation Anxiety Disorder, with transparent dynamics: mother had hated her husband, conceivably wishing him dead; he then actually died and her death wishes seemed to have come true. This made mother guilty because, on an unconscious level, she felt it was the power of her negative, hateful thought that had brought about her husband's death. If her hostile thought could kill one person, it could do so to another close to her—her daughter. Granted, the negative side of her ambivalence to her child was not quite as intense as it had been to her husband; nevertheless, mother was by now "sensitized" and needed to counteract whatever negative feelings she had towards the child. Her defensive mechanism was excessive but appropriate to the magic power attributed to her thought: if I keep the child close to me, I can make sure the magic thought will not harm her.

The practitioner should always remember that these are psychodynamics, i.e., *unconscious* processes, and that suddenly confronting anybody with their interpretation will produce very strong resistance, usually manifested in total rejection of the physician. The working through of dynamics must be left to the specialist and should *not* be undertaken by anybody else.

CASE 16-4   Fred was a bright nine-and-a-half-year-old fourth-grader who was brought to the specialist's attention because of several problems, the chief being a progressive increase in the number of days missed from school. The usual reason given by the patient was that he could not go to school because of *headaches or abdominal pains.* These typically *clustered around the Sunday evenings and Monday mornings.* As a result, Fred had had *many diagnostic studies,* including several brief hospitalizations, all of which produced *normal results.*

Once the parents were told by their pediatrician that a psychiatric consultation would help, they brought up additional problems: *Fred had also developed fears of being by himself at night* and insisted on *sleeping in his parents' bedroom.*

Fred's problems had started about a year earlier, when his *mother was hospitalized* for a long period because of a complicated illness Prior to that, Fred had practically *never been separated from her,* since they had been *very close.* He was an only child, born after years of childless marriage and several miscarriages. There had been overt separation anxiety when Fred first entered school, but this was overcome thanks to the concerted efforts of the school staff and the father.

Nevertheless, this was accomplished only after overcoming great resistance on the part of the mother, who for weeks afterwards would drive up a hill overlooking the school and observe her child's classroom through binoculars.

When interviewed, the *parents admitted their helplessness* to deal with the sleeping problem; they had fortunately stopped insisting that there must be something *physically wrong. They were divided* as to what to do about the school. Father was in favor of a "strong arm" policy, i.e., forcing the child to go to school. Mother (almost predictably) was against it and her view prevailed—no pressure was brought on the child to attend school.

Review of the school situation showed good overall acceptance of the child by his peers and no difficulties with his teachers, either behavioral or academic.

Interview with the child revealed a child who was quite verbal and *cooperative initially, as long as his denial was not questioned.* He denied any fears or anxieties except nocturnal fears and dreams of monsters, which he minimized. When confronted with his frequent absences from school, he explained them on the basis of his *physical symptoms.* When the patient was asked about concerns he may have had about his mother's health, he first *denied* them, then wanted to leave the session. He subsequently told the parents that the examiner was making him worse by "putting problems into my mind." The parents, especially mother, were quite eager to use this as a basis for questioning the entire approach to the child's problems and for being ready to *project* their difficulties onto the psychiatrist.

When this was forestalled by discussion with the parents, the child was seen again. He was brought back to the session after trying to *stay away from it with physical symptoms similar to those used to stay out of school.* After supportive but persistent questioning of and "guessing about" his feelings by the doctor, he acknowledged that he was indeed *quite worried about his mother and feared that something would happen to her while he was in school* and *thus unable to come to her rescue.* It further transpired that he was especially *anxious after being angry at her.*

Comment. In this case (16-2), the child is older and the separation anxiety is denied, but manifests itself, instead, through somatic symptoms.

The corresponding parental (usually maternal) separation anxiety is usually handled by that parent through the use of the psychological defense mechanism of denial and projection: everybody else is blamed for the child's difficulties, or causes are sought in physical illness. As a result, frequent medical investigations, "doctor shopping," or visits to consultants or different medical centers are typical.

In summary, school phobia on the basis of Separation Anxiety Disorder is most frequent and most obviously due to separation anxiety at the beginning of the child's school career. In addition, it occurs in subsequent years as well, up to the beginning of adolescence. Most of these cases are a continuation and final eruption of previously marginally controlled separation anxiety. The older the child, the more the separation anxiety is mixed with age-appropriate conflicts which may initially make diagnosis difficult.

Social phobia (300.23) and school phobias

This group of school phobias is likely to cluster around the third or fourth grade.

CASE 16-5   Danny was 10 years old and in fourth grade when he was brought for psychiatric evaluation. About two months after the start of fourth grade, he had begun to use every means he could think of to *stay out of school;* he complained of *feeling sick* to his stomach, to the point of vomiting; *headaches, sore throat, stomach cramps* were prominent on *Sunday evenings* or on the eve of a *test in school*—he invariably felt fine on weekends until Sunday evening.

In addition, Danny complained that the *teachers were "mean" to him* and too *strict and critical of his work.* He *was afraid of what they would say and do to him* if his work was not good and, as a matter of fact, his work had been getting progressively worse.

Danny was the youngest of five siblings and had always been treated as the *baby of the family,* often literally so. Everything he did was found to be cute, especially by his mother, but also by his siblings who were considerably older than he and who had few feelings of rivalry towards him. When he started school, his natural giftedness allowed him to *do well without much effort.* Supported by an *indulgent family,* he became *self-assured, cocky, and occasionally unruly* in third grade and felt it was all right to tease peers mercilessly, although his innate intelligence and a rather permissive teacher enabled him to do relatively well academically.

His fourth-grade teacher was different; she insisted on honest work and did not look kindly on Danny's transgressions, which up to now had been regarded as "boyishness." Danny *could not abruptly stop his customary teasing* and "smart-alecky" ways, since for so long adults, especially mother, had seemed to like it. But now he was singled out for criticism and punishment, and *combined with stricter standards for academic work, it all turned school into a place where there was no success;* even more painfully, school became a place where Danny felt that his innermost *self,* his way of dealing with life and people, was being *attacked and degraded.* He became *angry* and at the same time *frightened to expose himself to school.* He was not aware of his contributions to his misery but felt it was solely due to a mean teacher.

Comment. The central issue here is the loss of self-esteem, although Danny was eager to emphasize the Social Phobia (300.23) aspects of his dilemma. The patient had not been given the opportunities, guidance, and indeed appropriate pressure in his home environment to mature at the usual and expected rate. Instead, he had stayed at the level almost of a preschooler, experiencing ready tolerance for all his aggressive acts and lack of academic effort until, in fourth grade, the demands of the world at large caught up with him. Rather than face the pain of loss of self-esteem, the child avoided the situation where the painful confrontation took place. In addition, the child displaced the causes onto the school: it was not he who was deficient in development and adaptation; it was, instead, the fault of the teacher. In the same way, the child dealt with his feelings of anger: "The teacher hates me, I am not angry at her."

The first maneuver—avoidance—suggests this type of school phobia as a Social Phobia and the second, displacement onto the teacher (and/or the peers), reinforces its being a "phobia." School phobia is embedded in a longer history of difficulties, although these are often *latent* and become overt only with the school phobia.

The junior high school phobia

As the made-up name implies, this type of school phobia occurs in junior high school, i.e., sixth or seventh grade (depending on the school system).

CASE 16-6   Marjorie was 11 years old and had started *junior high* this year. From the very beginning, everything seemed to go wrong: the school was *farther away from her home* than the grade school had been; in fact, this was the first year in which Marjorie had to be *bussed,* having walked to a neighborhood school before. It meant being thrown in with *new peers, from different areas* of the city, from *different socioeconomic backgrounds* than her peers from her rather homogeneous neighborhood had been. She soon found that many of the peers on the bus were much *more streetwise* and were much more overtly *aggressive;* they also talked openly, even crudely, about things Marjorie had fantasized a great deal about but never discussed directly, i.e., sexuality.

Marjorie found the *academic* side of this new life equally unsettling. The once familiar figure of the one teacher teaching all the subjects was replaced by *half a dozen teachers, each concerned with his or her own subject only.* Whereas Marjorie could—and did—*depend on her grade school teacher,* this was *not* the case now.

The patient had always been quite *close to her parents* and her older sister. Her life was relatively *sheltered.* The development towards *pubescence* and witnessing her older sister's dating and hearing her accounts of her romances *intensified her sexual fantasies.* She *felt overwhelmed* by them and developed a number of obsessive rituals and phobic mechanisms to deal with them.

Losing the support system of her neighborhood grade school upset the precarious balance between her drives and the psychological defenses against them. Overstimulated as she was, the *greater worldliness* of her new peers was a threat *to be avoided.* There were no "safe," comforting adults.

The only solution to Marjorie was to *avoid* this *new* situation with its dangers of *sexual acting out* and the *demands for self-sufficiency,* both in *impulse control* and *academic performance.* She was *not up to those demands yet. Returning to the dependency* of home life, i.e., staying out of school, was a solution, but at the same time a step backwards. Physical symptoms were a *face-saving compromise.* The patient became ill with a number of complaints which were eventually diagnosed as Conversion Disorder: attacks of dizziness (vertigo) and, at other times, a hacking dry cough. These symptoms *clustered* around the time of greatest anxiety about school: *Sunday evenings* and the evenings preceding gym classes, since the patient dreaded to *take showers,* where overt comparisons about bodies and sexual characteristics were often being made.

Comment. The preceding case history portrays the conflicts of a pubescent girl and her loss of environmental supports. She lost the familiar, supportive school and the one teacher on whom she became dependent for adult reinforcement of her psychological defense mechanisms against her burgeoning sexual and aggressive drives. In addition, she lost the group support of familiar peers. Instead, she became exposed to an overstimulating peer group combined with an impersonal school system, which left control up to the patient, who was not quite ready to assume so much responsibility.

The way out was not to go to school, but her self-esteem could not tolerate this overt regression. Instead, she developed physical symptoms which made absence from school legitimate in the eyes of her own conscience, i.e., conversion symptoms.

In essence her problems showed partial features of a Simple Phobia along with a mixture of phobic, conversion, and obsessive compulsive symptoms.

OVERALL SUMMARY OF CLINICAL MANIFESTATIONS

1. Separation anxiety can occur at any time but is most common at the beginning of the school years: kindergarten or first grade. It is based on the child's need to counteract hostile impulses by staying close to the person whom the hostile impulses might harm, usually the parent and vice versa, since the separation anxiety is a two-way interaction between parent and child.
2. Avoidant disorders and genuine phobias are most frequent around the fourth grade and are related to the need, at that phase of the academic process, to do independent work and take on responsibility.
3. School phobia in junior high school is based on the child's inability to keep a balance between impulses (sexual and aggressive) and defenses against them. This inability is due to the child's being abruptly faced with a new and much less supportive environment where the burden of repression of unacceptable impulses is on the child. Identity conflicts and issues of dependency versus independence also enter into the mechanism of this type of school phobia.

DIAGNOSIS AND DIFFERENTIAL DIAGNOSIS

School phobia can and should be diagnosed on positive grounds, i.e., the symptomatology should strongly suggest this disorder. The positive symptoms are panic when taken to school; significant increase in anxiety before return to school, especially late on weekends and on evenings and mornings of school days; disappearance of anxiety in its various manifestations, including physical symptoms, when the pressure to go to school is off.

When the underlying mechanism is separation anxiety, separation anxiety from significant caretakers (usually the mother) may arise on other occasions as well. However, many older children separate from home for social occasions (such as sports, sleepovers at a friend's house, and the like), the explanation being that these separations are not so consistent and qualitatively, in the sum total of time away, not nearly as significant as going to school.

Since complaints about physical dysfunction are so frequent, appropriate diagnostic evaluation is necessary. A thorough history and physical examination and appropriate laboratory tests are a must, but repeated and unrelated diagnostic procedures are not only unnecessary but usually counterproductive as well. Some parents may insist on increasingly complex and esoteric diagnostic procedures and additional consultants to be drawn into the ever-widening circle of physical examinations. This is usually an expression of their own psychological defense mechanisms of denial and projection of their hostility and guilt. If such requests are complied with, the child is eventually firmly convinced that he or she has become an invalid and a new posture of helpless dependency is thereby created.

In the differential diagnosis, the first consideration must be given to truancy. This is a willful staying away from school not based on anxiety ("playing hookey"). While school-phobic children are either good students or at least would like to be, truant children usually are not. In addition, the latter generally have histories of behavior disorders and of an absence of anxiety and guilt. They tend to come from families that are more seriously disrupted than those of school-phobic children.

On the other end of the differential diagnostic spectrum are severe anxiety disorder where almost anything will provoke the child's anxiety. Waxing and waning school attendance is but a part of the disorder, without any specific anxiety related to school.

Childhood psychosis with anxiety encompassing all interpersonal relationships will affect peer and school relationships, too, but can be distinguished by the other positive signs of childhood psychosis and the indiscriminate involvement of all relationships.

Finally, we must not forget that problems may indeed exist in school, either between the child and peers or between the child and the teacher. Usually (but not always), these factors have already been explored by the parents prior to bringing the child to the physician.

TREATMENT

There is a simple and proven rule about treating all school phobias prior to adolescence: acute school phobias (two weeks' duration or less) are best treated by speedy return of the child to school. Thus, school phobias represent one of the emergencies in child psychiatry—not so much because of danger, but because of missed opportunity and altered prognosis, if the problem is not promptly addressed.

An otherwise benign school phobia can become fixated if left unattended for too long (again, the rule of thumb is two-to-three weeks). The younger the patient, the more likely this measure is to succeed. It follows that Separation Anxiety Disorder in a young child will respond best, whereas a complex conflict in a junior high school student approximates the adolescent type of school phobia requiring very different treatment.

Needless to say, the above procedure will apply mainly to simple, mild cases. Not all cases can be treated in this manner, but, unless it is immediately apparent that the amount of pathology in both the child and the family is severe, most acute cases should at least have benefit of an attempt at prompt return to school.

A prerequisite for this approach is a thorough medical evaluation. Every effort should be made to make it definitive—the physician should feel comfortable that there is reasonable certainty of absence of organic pathology. All reasonable lab work should be done, preferably while the child is being returned to school, but the parents' pleas for repeated and increasingly complex diagnostic procedures should be resisted on the basis of the probability of the disorder being a school phobia being much greater than that of being an esoteric disease.

The circumspect clinician will never fight with the parents over absolute certainty of diagnosis; the parents are ultimately responsible for the child and the physician can only advise them as to the most likely diagnosis and recommend appropriate treatment. If the parents, usually because of their own psychopathology, choose not to accept the clinician's diagnosis and treatment, he or she should keep in mind the reason for their refusal and not react to it as if it were a personal attack upon his or her professional competence—although it often takes that form, since the parents project their anger as well as self-doubts onto the clinician who advises a painful treatment (separation).

It further follows that a great deal of tact and delicacy is required when discussing with the parents return to school. The clinician should always consider school phobia as a *family* problem, although technically it helps to start with the child since the parents are usually not ready to work on their part of the problem right away. Nevertheless, it is the parents who hold the key to the success of any therapeutic intervention in school phobia. Therefore, the therapeutic alliance must be primarily with the parents—their healthy egos. The relationship with the child is secondary—desirable as a good relationship may be.

Once the most opportune time for intervention has passed, i.e., after the first two-to-three weeks have passed without successful intervention, treatment of school phobia should be handled by the specialist. Several techniques have been used:

- Behavior modification—"desensitization" techniques, where the child is gradually exposed to greater "doses" of school.
- Psychotherapy, where the child shares his or her magic thoughts with the psychiatrist and is helped to recognize the fact that his or her anger does not destroy people.
- Exploration and guidance of the child's strengths and special talents in order to enhance the child's self-esteem.
- Judicious manipulation of the environment for the child's benefit, such as excusing the child from participation in physical education (especially in junior high school) if body image difficulties are the main issue.

Most commonly, a combination of the above techniques is used.

In addition, as already emphasized, work with the parents *must* accompany whichever technique is used with the child. The child's symptoms may help stabilize an emotionally brittle parent, or the parents' marriage, where bilateral separation anxiety is the psychodynamic wellspring. Rehabilitating one partner of the dyad (the child) may precipitate exacerbation in the other (the parent), with resulting sabotaging of the treatment. Thus, parallel treatment is necessary.

Involvement of the school in the therapeutic process varies: a gradual reintroduction of the child into the school will obviously have to be explained to the teacher. However, in most instances, the parents can constructively be given the task of providing a bridge between doctor and school system. Not only is such a move economical, but it is also simultaneously a safeguard against parental projections of anger ("the doctor and the school are banding together against us"). Although most teachers are very eager to help, some of this eagerness is not tempered by knowledge of the complex issues at play and excessive, though well-intentioned, "therapeutic" activity on the educators' part can be counterproductive.

Severe school phobia, especially in older children, may require hospitalization, sometimes as the initial phase of treatment, sometimes as longer-term treatment. Separation anxiety, genuine phobias, and especially depression over unresolved identity conflicts may have escalated to an unmanageable extent where office treatment simply cannot be effective. When child psychiatric inpatient facilities are unavailable, hospitalization on a pediatric ward can accomplish the purpose of initial separation from the parents in a supportive environment. When that is done, support and guidance must be given to the hospital nursing staff. However, severe identity problems in preadolescents must be treated in specialized psychiatric hospital facilities.

Pharmacological treatment is sometimes a helpful adjuvant, both in office and hospital treatment. After thorough evaluation and the setting up of *all* the psychological interventions, a short-acting benzodiazepine, such as lorazepam (Ativan) or oxazepam (Serax) can be administered prior to attempted return to school. For dosages and other information, refer to the chapter on Psychopharmacology. A tricyclic antidepressant (e.g., doxepin [Adapin or Sinequan]) can be used in children with severe phobic and obsessive disorders and, of course, in those with depression. However, too great a reliance should not be placed on any pharmacological agent, and if the child is refractory to outpatient treatment even with adequate doses of an appropriate agent, a change in overall psychotherapeutic strategy is usually required, often in the form of hospitalization.

School-phobic children with severe neurotic problems of any of the subcategories may make statements that are highly frightening to the parents but are usually reflective of dissociative or hysterical symptomatology. However, a small number of these patients turn out to have childhood psychosis and must be hospitalized in appropriate psychiatric facilities.

PROGNOSIS

All school phobias can serve as examples of the clinical wisdom that prognosis depends on the extent and severity of the underlying causes and the extent and efficacy of treatment. One more point can be added, and that is time elapsed from onset of school refusal to the return to school: the longer that interval, the more opportunity and likelihood of the psychological defense mechanisms to become fixated, sometimes to the point of personality disorders; at the same time, the physical symptoms may, during prolonged absence from school, develop into psychosomatic illness and become a difficult problem in themselves.

Generally speaking, Separation Anxiety Disorders at the kindergarten or first grade level, without serious corresponding problems in the parents, have an excellent prognosis and often do not even come to the attention of the physician.

Persistent Separation Anxiety Disorders carry a variable prognosis, generally good with treatment for both child and parents, but increasingly cautious when treatment is started late. If the disorder persists into preadolescence, the psychiatric outlook is quite guarded.

Long-term prognosis in terms of later, adult functioning of all forms of school phobia is fair to good, with the exception that severe school phobia with persistent refusal to attend school, carrying over from preadolescence into adolescence, has a guarded and sometimes poor long-term outlook.

Recently there has been mounting evidence of a significant correlation between Separation Anxiety Disorder of childhood and Panic Disorder in adulthood, as reflected in the histories of separation anxiety in many patients with Panic Disorder on the one hand, and the more than threefold risk of separation anxiety in children of parents with Panic Disorder (Taylor, 1986).

Questions for Study and Action

1. Make the case, in writing, for dropping the term "school phobia" from a diagnostic manual for mental disorders. Give at least *four* arguments for that position.

2. From Winnie's (Case 16-2) scanty history, give a dynamic (meaning *motivational*) *formulation* of how her disorder arose. Would it help you to know that an older sister suffered from obesity and bulimia? or that her mother had separation anxiety as a child? or that her stepfather when in the family had been an excellent provider and showered Winnie with material gifts?

3. Danny (Case 16-5), in addition to the history already given, had received corporal punishment when he was uncooperative at school. How would that datum affect your differential diagnosis?

4. Discuss: Stranger anxiety in the child eight months old is an early, developmentally

normal expression of separation anxiety. It contains both dysphoria and positive attachment.

5. Otto Rank, an early psychoanalyst, said themes of separation and individuation were in a lifelong struggle with themes of merging, fusing, and not being different. Can you see, among persons your own age, signs of that struggle? Give three examples.

6. Margaret Mahler, a later (than Rank) analyst, postulated an elaborate separation-individuation phase of infantile development. She also described a later-onset (after 30 months of age) "symbiotic psychosis" of childhood that appeared overtly similar to autism. What were the *mirroring* and *rapprochement* subphases according to Mahler?

7. Why do many asthmatic children show Separation Anxiety Disorder? Do you see "parentectomy" as a rational therapeutic step with such children? Explain.

8. Describe how you'd explain to a child with a school phobia that the experiment of going back to school will help him/her to grow, to learn about fears, and to see surely that what is feared will not come to pass. What behavioral strategies would you use to get the child to monitor behavior, precipitating stresses, fantasies, and success?

9. The childhood histories of adult depressives show a concentrated high incidence of school phobia. Does that mean that children with school phobia may be depressed children? What else could it mean? Be detailed and specific.

10. In the Oriental culture, children are taught that their adult goal will not be to become *independent* of others but to become *dependable* to others. How does that compare, in its healthy realism, to the "Horatio Alger" Western goal of fierce autonomy and independence? Explain fully. Which goal—Eastern or Western—is more conducive to family concord?

For Further Reading

Atkinson, L., Quarrington, B., & Cyr, J.J. School refusal: The heterogeneity of a concept. *Am. J. Orthopsychiatry,* 35:83–101, 1985.

Bernstein, G.A., & Garfinkel, B.D. School phobia: The overlap of affective and anxiety disorders. *J. Amer. Acad. of Child Psychiatry,* 25:235–241, 1986.

Hersov, L. School refusal. In M. Rutter & L. Hersov (Eds.), *Child and Adolescent Psychiatry. Modern Approaches* (2nd ed.). Oxford, England: Blackwell Scientific Publications, 1985, pp. 385–386.

Kanner, L. Childhood psychosis: A historical overview. *J. Autism Child. Schizophrenia*, 1:14–19, 1971.

Reich, J. The epidemiology of anxiety. *J. Nerv. Ment. Dis.*, 174:129–136, 1986.

Taylor, G.J. The psychodynamic aspects of panic disorder. Paper presented at the Annual Meeting of the American Psychiatric Association, Washington, D.C., May 1986.

Waldron, S., Jr., Shrier, D.K., Stone, B., & Tobin, F. et al. School phobia and other childhood neuroses: A systematic study of the children and their families. *Am. J. Psychiatry*, 132:802–808, 1975.

Weissman, M.M., & Merikangas, K.R. The epidemiology of anxiety and panic disorders: An update. *J. Clin. Psychiatry*, 47:11–17, 1986.

17

Anxiety, Phobic, and Dissociative Disorders

his chapter will focus on the "neuroses" of Anxiety Disorders, Phobic Disorders, and Dissociative Disorders. In its earliest days, private child psychiatry concentrated mainly on children with inner conflicts, while public-sector child psychiatry tended to deal mostly with delinquent and brain-damaged children. Both of those groups are still in existence, but the neurotic disorders are either not as frequent or not as highly acclaimed as they were earlier. Still, Anxiety, Phobic, and Dissociative Disorders occur in childhood and some of the rudiments of their psychopathology will be described here. The emotion of fear is the main feature of these anxiety disorders, hence we include them in this section on Feeling and Mood Disorders. In reality, fear and anxiety today may be less gripping, dysphoric emotions than anger, loneliness, sexual unrest, shame, sadness, feelings of inadequacy, or meaninglessness.

The Anxiety Disorders discussed in the first section of this chapter will be Generalized Anxiety Disorder, Obsessive Compulsive Disorder, and Post-traumatic Stress Disorder, to be followed by a discrete section on Phobic Disorders, and another on Dissociative Disorders.

Generalized Anxiety (GAD) (300.02)
Overanxious Disorder (313.00)

DEFINITION

Generalized Anxiety Disorder includes or is interchangeable with Overanxious Disorder and describes a child persistently (more than six months) fearful, apprehensive, and tense. The child will worry and be excessively preoccupied about life circumstances such as accidents, school or athletic or social performances. It must be proven that the state of fear has no organic condition (hyperthyroidism, Caffeine Intoxication, pheochromocytoma, etc.) to sustain it. Furthermore, it has to be shown that it is not a secondary revelation of a more serious underlying disorder (e.g., a psychotic or mood or pervasive developmental disorder). It is *not* separation anxiety, or any other clearcut symptom picture that has a separate diagnostic code assigned to it.

CLINICAL DESCRIPTION

Generalized Anxiety Disorder can be diagnosed when a child has at least six of the following 18 symptoms, well elicited by a standardized interview (but note DSM-III-R for the fewer criteria for Overanxious Disorder):

Motor tension:
1. trembling
2. muscle tension
3. restlessness
4. easy fatigability

Autonomic hyperactivity:
5. dyspnea or feeling choked
6. palpitations/fast heartbeat
7. perspiration
8. dry mouth
9. dizziness
10. nausea, diarrhea, or other abdominal distress
11. chills
12. urinary frequency
13. various symptoms of the digestive tract, from throat to colon

Vigilance and scanning:
14. feeling on edge or tense
15. having exaggerated startle responses
16. difficulty concentrating

17.   difficulty sleeping
18.   irritability

Such a child appears to be, and attests to being, decimated by anxiety. Such children beg for reassurance and encouragement, earn a reputation from adults of being highstrung and from children of being a "nervous Nellie." They are children lacking emotional security. Either GAD or Overanxious Disorder may be found in children.

CASE 17-1   Wenona, a nine-year-old girl, was the older child, with one five-year-old brother, of an alcoholic father and a mother who worked as a waitress. The father was a housepainter who used alcohol for its anxiolytic effects; the mother had a morbid preoccupation that she would lose control and be abusive towards her two children but particularly dreaded doing bodily harm to her sometimes unruly son. Gentle scratching turned up a marriage full of discord and lack of sexual fulfillment for both partners. Wenona was the *family's fear barometer.* When her mother or father worried or became upset, her symptoms were aggravated.

After seeing her parents for a marital and family history, the child psychiatrist saw Wenona. She was *tight as a wire* and her *speech was pressured* and with overtones of *whining* as she told of counting her father's disulfiram tablets every day for the past year. She had learned that, when he got uptight and would not eat properly, his next step would be to stop taking the disulfiram and third would be a binge in which he would insult his wife and then stay passed out for a couple of days. Wenona counted the tablets *in dread,* hoping he would not stop taking them.

Wenona was in a *heightened state of anxiety.* She appeared bright but showed a *scattered and inconsistent deficit in her performance on the WISC-R subtests.* Especially on coding and digit span, she showed *poor concentration* and *impairment by excess anxiety.* She endorsed all of these items on a diagnostic interview for children: *feeling keyed up* most of the time, *unable to do school work* or *enjoy her peers,* *overreaction to sudden noise, tired* before she got to school each morning, felt *as if she'd jump out of her skin, akathisia* both at home and school depending on her state of *worrying, tachycardia, dyspnea,* and *globus.*

Comment. With the whole family at the lowest edge of the working class, economic insecurities were real but heightened by the parents' pervasive anxieties, conflict, and worries. The mother "tightened up her disciplinary act" with both children and soon lost her fear of hurting them. The father was treated with a tricyclic antidepressant for a recurrent endogenous depression and stopped being a drunk when anxious secondary to depression. Her little brother stopped calling Wenona a "scaredy cat" and Wenona improved when she found her parents more trustworthy. Wenona's Generalized Anxiety Disorder diminished, without a complete cure being attained, as she became able to talk about her fears, play them out in psychotherapy, and resume her growth as a happier child. She was an example of how uncertainty and worry can be communicated from parents to child, and how positive emotions too can be transmitted in that same channel.

DIFFERENTIAL DIAGNOSIS

Separation Anxiety Disorder is distinct from GAD in the former's focus on separation. Panic Disorder is distinguished by its recurrent panics and worries that a future panic will befall the victim. Obsessive Compulsive Disorder can be differentiated by its obsessions and compulsions that make it more structured than GAD. Anorexia Nervosa has an explicit and specific focus on getting fat, repulsive, and inhuman, unlike GAD. Underlying Depression and Pervasive Development Disorder or Psychosis can be ruled out by different age of onset and the dominance of depressed mood or thinking deficits or anomalies in the clinical picture.

TREATMENT

It may not be necessary for health professionals to intervene directly with a child who suffers from GAD *if:* 1) the child is not truly incapacitated socially or academically; or 2) the child's parents feel capable of taking help given to them and using it to help their child; or 3) the parents do not agree to bring the child into treatment. Yet if the parents seek help for their offspring, at least a brief course of family-plus-child treatment is indicated.

Behavior therapy—e.g., social skills training and training the child in relaxation techniques—can be used. Hypnosis has also been used for these purposes. Cognitive therapy designed to mute and moderate intense feelings can be undertaken in conjunction with behavioral and other modalities.

Emotional, expressive therapy can be used to clarify and interpret the target symptoms, the defenses, the basic unrest, and to obtain insight in order to restore good morale to the child.

Family group therapy, especially combined with individual therapy for the child, can be useful, or child-focused family group therapy can be helpful just by itself in some cases.

Drug therapy has little place with GAD in the experience of the authors. There are clinicians who use anxiolytic agents (hydroxyzine, diazepam, or alprazolam) and like them, claiming their efficacy. We believe they should be used with caution and that the way to unseat a GAD is not by drugs but by helping relationships.

Remedial tutoring and other special educational techniques are needed if the child's anxiety picture has interrupted academic learning.

Outpatient occupational therapy groups provide solace and increased feelings of competence to some children with Generalized Anxiety Disorder. There they can work meaningfully in a relaxed atmosphere devoid of competitive rushing, achieving mastery on both solitary and group projects.

Other forms of peer group therapy may be efficacious but too many acting-out, unruly children in a group can unhinge a child with GAD, so caution in composing the group is warranted.

PROGNOSIS

Given worthwhile individualized treatment, the forecast for GAD is good. Some of the best follow-up studies (reviewed by Casey & Berman, 1985) show these neurotic children to be improved in some degree. Compared to Conduct Disorder, for example, the prognosis is bright. It is important to bear in mind that a misdiagnosed case, for example one with underlying Schizophrenia or Depression, will carry the prognosis of the underlying but undiagnosed disorder.

Obsessive Compulsive Disorder (OCD) (300.30)

This disorder is traditionally lumped with the Anxiety Disorders, although it shares—in a sizeable number of cases—a common biological substrate with Major Depression. For our purposes, the feeling disorder aspect is prominent enough to allow us to group it with Anxiety Disorders as a subgrouping of Feeling Disorders. When there is an underlying Major Depression, that is what must be confronted, *not* the secondary OCD, which will usually disappear when the depression is adequately treated.

OCD is not a patrician illness, nor is it as rare as previously thought. In the general population, the prevalence may be higher than 10%, although in clinic populations the incidence rarely goes over 2%. Formerly, it was believed that children could not develop "caseness" with OCD but indisputably young children can have episodes of OCD that do not, and do, prompt parents to seek help for them.

DEFINITION AND CLINICAL DESCRIPTION

The required features of OCD are:

1. Intrusive impulses (compulsions), images or fantasies, and ideas (obsessions).
2. A feeling that these intrusions are forced upon one—compulsion, anancasm, ego-dystonia.

3. A desire to resist the compulsive and ego-dystonic intrusions, with inner distress resulting from the inability to succeed in the resisting.
4. The child ultimately relents and gives up to the obsessions and compulsions so that school and peer relations are impaired.

In summary, DSM-III-R states that OCD is characterized by obsessions or compulsions that cause distress to the individual or interfere with social or role functioning, and that are not due to another mental disorder.

Although labeling the necessity (to a child) to step on imaginary toxic "dots on the floor" *ego-dystonic* or *ego alien* or *subjectively exogenous* catches the quality of forced labor, it does not convey the child's subjective agony of unnaturalness and nonspontaneity in the thrall of obsessions and compulsions. Or hours may be consumed in hand washing, brushing teeth, saying silent prayers to a feared parent, and playing magical mind games as if desperately seeking to ward off annihilation. The child with OCD suffers greatly, is unhappy, is insecure and tense, and never feels fully human in the obsessive compulsive maze. Interpersonal relations are impeded and the mother as chief caretaker usually senses the partly disguised battle for autonomy that the child is engaged in. Some writers stress the diphasic quality of compulsive thinking in the clinical situation and describe *the compulsive maneuver* to be one in which a child's communications go from powerlessness to omnipotence, guilty fear to rage, sin to perfection and vice versa.

DEVELOPMENTAL CONSIDERATIONS

Although most children may relieve tension or anxiety by magical acts or thoughts of undoing, they do not come to suffer the full-blown disorder of OCD. Two- or three-year-old children frequently engage in rituals as do pubescent children, but they do not impede development very seriously. The same is true of elementary-school children who in groups play jump rope and hopscotch for hours, with great attention to rules and details and much ritualized chanting and jumping about; it is also true of solitary children who persist in ritualized play of solitaire or with string figures or mechanical toys. Perhaps a bit more serious is the fanatical collecting—as if self-esteem or survival were the issue—of sports cards, stamps, rocks, coins, or match covers that may be seen in some preadolescent children. Preadolescent children with "circumscribed interest patterns" seem even closer to OCD as they become experts in astronomy, rockets, meteorology or memorize call letters of television and radio stations all over North America. They lose friends because they have "gone nuts" over a special interest and they are often alone and lonely, unable to make new friends. Such a clinical picture as circumscribed interest patterns could develop into OCD but may not. Not every transitory compulsive act or notion becomes fixed, for some are transitory, developmental, and are transcended.

CASE 17-2   Sherry was a pretty fifth-grader, aged 10 years when she was brought to the child psychiatrist by her mother who also wanted help (and obtained it from a social worker). Sherry was preoccupied with the thought *(fear) that she or her mother might die of some incurable disease.* She had become *sickly,* suffering *nightmares* almost nightly, and had *adopted several ritual acts:* closing doors repeatedly, touching the table five times with her glass before putting it down, tracing over every "r" that she wrote 15 times, and looking "intense" when sitting staring into space—she said, "A thing is spinning in my head and I try to make it go in the opposite direction." There had been some OCD *symptoms since she was seven* but only six months earlier had they grown to paralyze her. The present episode had *followed the death* of her brother's playmate whose funeral Sherry had attended. She promptly *graduated from being uptight to being crazy,* her parents noted. She complained of "being tense" all the time and *asked repeated questions* about death, sex, and life after death.

Sherry had been *molested sexually* at age three by a 12-year-old male neighbor and her *parents had been unable to comfort her* then or subsequently. History also showed an older sister with recurrent Depression, an uncle with Paranoid Schizophrenia, and an older brother with brain damage and frequent psychotic episodes. Sherry's father was a conventional and superficial man who, when anxious about them, would make a joke about his wife's separation panic and Sherry's rituals. The mother said, "Sherry drives herself and everyone else crazy with her rituals. I have to shut myself in a vacuum to keep my sanity."

In expressive (dynamic-verbal) psychotherapy, Sherry revealed that her death obsession was only her reaction to her *mother's fears of death and separations,* that she had high *anxiety about her own sexual feelings,* and she had formed *a hostile dependency* on her mother from which she could not extricate herself through ritual making. Her fears of a vague terror that would be fatal was both a result of her seeing an infanticidal gleam in her parents' eyes and her own fear of her inner emotions. She had strong emotions that she tried to deny, disown, and undo.

Comment. Sherry had obsessions and compulsions that enslaved her and interfered with school achievement, family interactions, and peer relations. She tried to resist those intrusive ideas and urges but could not, so she relented and made rituals; but that gave only temporary abeyance in her state of siege by anxious tension. Her symptoms were not too dissimilar from her mother's, father's, and older sister's.

DIFFERENTIAL DIAGNOSIS

Adjustment Disorder with Anxious Mood, unlike OCD, does not show obsessions and/or compulsions but can mimic OCD's anxious tension. Post-traumatic

Stress Disorder, which could be important in a case like Sherry's, where she had been sexually abused, can be differentiated by its symptoms of reexperiencing and focusing on the traumatic event, having a heightened startle response, and so on, but not showing obsessive compulsive symptoms. Tourette's Disorder can be distinguished by the presence of vocal and motor tics. Schizophrenia shows a more severe thinking disorder than does OCD. Major Depression shows a more profound biological picture that may not be too easy to differentiate at times, and an Organic Mental Disorder shows definite signs and symptoms of "organicity" not seen in OCD. Anorexia Nervosa may need listing of OCD as a second diagnosis but is distinguished by its *eating* obsessions and compulsions.

TREATMENT

Biological treatments most employed are tricyclic antidepressants, especially chlorimipramine, which appears to bring both antidepressant and antiobsessional relief to the child. Individual psychotherapies for OCD have traditionally been emotion-focused (child analysis, dynamic-verbal-insightful psychotherapy) but in the past 15 years many modalities have been tried that are behavior-focused or cognition-oriented. One of us (PLA) has found that cognitive repair is required, although the child with OCD seldom complains of a cognitive problem. Emotional repair through concentrated working with a child's dreams is mainly a liberation of some strong affects that the child experiences but is not aware of and conceals by repression and denial. Group psychotherapies, which are usually adjunctive, include peer-group therapy, milieu therapy, occupational therapy and family group modalities. When the OCD has wrought school failure, special educational help is needed. In general, a multimodal (biological, psychotherapeutic [both group and individual], behavioral-feeling-thinking) approach works best to restore the child to healthier development as a human person. The earmarks of improvement with treatment are diminished symptoms, i.e., greater naturalness, spontaneity, and freedom.

Post-traumatic Stress Disorder (PTSD) (309.89)

DEFINITION

The DSM-III-R definition of Post-traumatic Stress Disorder (PTSD) encompasses all ages, and we will edit it for what pertains to children. PTSD is defined by DSM-III-R as a *syndrome* following a psychologically traumatic event that is outside the range of usual human experience. Hence, it is a *reactive disorder* to an unusual fright.

The *stressor* is more severe than common traumatic experiences and would evoke distress almost universally. These stressors include accidental, natural, and man-made disasters (natural catastrophes and various accidents), as well as intentional (deliberate) disasters (bombing, terrorism, kidnapping, or torture).

The mainstay of the symptomatology is the reexperiencing of the traumatic event. In children, this takes the form of recurrent dreams or nightmares during which components of the event are relived. Anxiety, in various forms, is frequent. Other typical symptoms are clinging, crying, withdrawal, and symptoms of excessive autonomic arousal (exaggerated startle response and difficulty falling asleep).

DSM-III-R further states that intense mental distress is often intensified when the individual is exposed to acts and events that resemble or symbolize the original trauma. Although anxiety and depression are associated features in adults, they are an integral part of PTSD in children.

The chronic or delayed subtype is specified if it develops more than six months after the trauma, or lasts six months or longer.

ETIOLOGY AND PATHOGENESIS

PTSD and all synonymic disorders ("traumatic neurosis," "shell shock," etc.) are a normal response to an abnormal situation. They represent the child's adaptive response, or attempt to adapt, to overwhelming danger or threat of harm. Of course, PTSD is not the immediate response to the danger, but its subsequent elaboration. Strictly speaking, therefore, PTSD is both the continuation of the initial response and the adaptation to the child's internalized mental picture of the traumatic event.

It is because the child is dealing with an internalized, frightening mental representation that we see the characteristic reexperiencing of the original event—the "repetition–compulsion" in order to master the internalized trauma—just as Freud (1920) originally described it in "shell-shocked" soldiers during the First World War.

CLINICAL DESCRIPTION

Some of the most dramatic features of PTSD in adults, such as psychic numbing, amnesia, and intrusive flashbacks (intrusive recollections), are rarely encountered in children, yet enough typical symptomatology is present to give the clinician a "core" to work with. This "core" is represented by the "repetitive phenomena" (Terr, 1981). Recurrent nightmares about the traumatic event are probably the one symptom common to all PTSD in children. Fearful focusing on, or preoccupation with, the trauma and fear about its recurrence are common, often shown in "post-traumatic play" and "reenactment" (Terr, 1981). Reactions of fear or panic can be triggered by events that remind the child of the original trauma, and many children suffer from somatic, especially autonomic, complaints. Depending on the outcome of the terrifying episode, guilt, including survivor guilt, is present.

Around this "core" are built the "usual" reactions, a multitude of forms of anxiety and depression, as well as regressive phenomena (enuresis, encopresis, self-stimulating behaviors, etc.) and exaggerated dependency and clinging and looking for reassurance that the child's needs will be met.

We now present a brief list of examples of terrifying situations and describe the resulting PTSD. There is a sliding scale of specific symptomatology according to the extent of the human causality of the stressor. Purely natural disasters produce symptoms which are the least typical of PTSD. Those natural disasters that have been precipitated by man produce symptomatology more typical of PTSD, and the most characteristic syndrome is seen after direct terror of human origin and instigation.

Therefore, the clinician can generally expect to see PTSD on a continuum of severity and specificity, ranging from the least specific in natural disasters to the most severe and most specific when children have been subjected to direct terror or have witnessed terror perpetrated on their families.

In war and terrorism, the severity and extent of PTSD depend on the presence of family, the parental reactions, and what happens to family members. In addition to the previously described nightmares, withdrawal, clinging, and feelings of insecurity and survivor guilt, the children traumatized by these situations have subsequent difficulties with aggression. A small but tragic group are those children who suffered the ultimate abuse by their parents—attempts by their psychotic parents to murder them; others witnessed the murder of one parent by the other (all of this is referred to as "familicide"). These children exhibit all the typical symptoms of PTSD in their greatest severity: repeated nightmares about the event, hyperalertness, and anxiety; reminders of the episode cause depressive states, somatic symptoms, and an overall decline in functioning (poor concentration, poor school performance).

Children who *witness harm or death to a parent* by perpetrators outside the family show very similar symptoms: reiteration of the event in play and behavior, intrusion of and preoccupation with thoughts about the event, intrusive thoughts, depression, poor school work, and difficulty with aggression.

DIFFERENTIAL DIAGNOSIS

There is no difficulty in diagnosis when PTSD is *acute,* since the relationship to the traumatic event is obvious. The major differential diagnostic consideration is Adjustment Disorder. This is differentiated on two parameters: one is the stressor, which is less severe and "within the range of common experience," to quote DSM-III-R, in Adjustment Disorder. The other is the nature and severity of the symptomatology: PTSD is always characterized by the reexperiencing of the traumatic event, and sometimes by the emergence of symptoms when a similar set of circumstances occurs.

Differential-diagnostic difficulties may arise in the chronic or delayed subtype of PTSD, since the syndrome can arise years after the stressor. This is best exemplified by children who survived the Nazi Holocaust (usually concentration camp survivors), where chronic PTSD has had to be differentiated from Anxiety Disorder, Depression, or Adjustment Disorder of later origin, both for clinical and forensic purposes. The forensic aspect concerns compensation, as it does with victims of other disasters and accidents, none of which, however, approached the Holocaust in either overall horror or length of time elapsed between event and possible litigation.

Since compensation may be an issue, *malingering* must be considered. This is very rare in children in its true form, but may happen "by proxy," i.e., parents coach their children to report symptoms. Malingering means the conscious production or reporting of symptoms for material gain.

CASE 17-3   Seven-year-old Bernard was *tied up to a post* by his *psychotic* father and *threatened* with shooting if he cried or otherwise "misbehaved," while father beat and nearly killed the mother. For *weeks afterwards*, Bernard not only suffered from *severe nightmares*, with the recurrent theme of being chased, held down, and choked; but he also exhibited typical *night terrors* (without memory of dream content) and simply would *not go* to sleep because "something might happen" or because of the scary dreams.

TREATMENT

These considerations of pathogenesis provide a rationale for the treatment. The child is treated along the same lines that the syndrome has evolved: reexperiencing the trauma is encouraged, and then the child is helped to change his or her concept of what happened, towards a greater sense of realism, and subsequently to achieve a greater sense of control.

This increases the child's self-esteem and counteracts the pervasive feelings of total helplessness. A psychodynamic treatment philosophy is basic to most approaches, although there are many modifications, as well as combinations with other approaches (such as group interactions and behavior modifications). Eventually, all treatment strategies have one common final pathway—mechanisms of survival and coping, particularly coping with losses of family or relationships and answering the basic question of childhood: Who will take care of me?

PROGNOSIS

If there is one area where the original dream of child psychiatrists—that of preventing adult psychopathology through intervention in childhood—may come true, this is it: treatment of PTSD in childhood may indeed forestall later psychiatric disturbance, or, in other cases, lessen the person's vulnerability to later stress.

PHOBIC DISORDERS

Although Sigmund Freud, observing the ubiquity of phobic reactions in four-year-olds, called phobia "a normal neurosis of childhood" and "quite extraordinarily frequent" (Freud, 1909, p. 283), an episode of a phobic disorder is not happy or normal for the suffering child. Moreover, not all phobias are fleeting and transient, for some become fixed and crystallized into a thoroughgoing childhood neurosis, with very serious decrement and constriction in a child's social functioning.

With regard to the Phobic Disorders, we have already discussed school phobia; we do not consider Agoraphobia here, since it is mainly an adult syndrome; and we are left with Social Phobia, Simple Phobia, and Avoidant Personality to consider here.

Social Phobia (300.23)

DEFINITION

A social phobia has ingredients of shame, timidity, terror, and anticipated humiliation. A specific context or situation is singled out for a special dread: being seen naked, being ridiculed for one's ineptness in sports or schoolwork, being robbed and bullied by other children, being punished physically by an adult, being called "a bastard" by one's playmates, and so on.

CLINICAL DESCRIPTION

The hallmark of Social Phobia is a fear of being observed and humiliated that exceeds the bounds of moderation or reasonableness, which the child understands but cannot modify. The situation that will put the child onstage is dreaded and avoided with a vengeance. If the child is suddenly exposed to the situation, anxiety of great dimensions will immediately ensue. What the child might do when he or she is the center of attention will cause no trepidation when done in solitude: for example, undressing, learning math, learning to read.

CASE 17-4   Wendy was still seven years old when she heard her third-grade teacher announce, at the beginning of school, that there would be *examinations* for all the third-graders early in the school year. Wendy, whose mother had chastised her for immodestly stroking her labia and clitoris during that summer, believed that she would have to undress at school in front of her entire class. The only examination she had heard of was a physical one. The ones in school were tests, according to Wendy. Although her teacher told her not to worry about the examinations for they were "just something new to see how you have developed during kindergarten and your first two grades," Wendy was more terrified and asked each day if it was the day for the examination.

Less than a week later, Wendy *refused to attend school,* and when pressured to do so she became *panicky—sweating, complaining of dying, having stomachaches, and locking herself in her room.* The school teacher knowingly and unabashedly reassured the mother that Wendy had a "school phobia" that had nothing to do with school but reflected only her immaturity and fear of separating from her anxious mother. To that, the mother reacted with perplexity because mother worked outside the home and had to hire a sitter for Wendy when she stayed home and refused school.

Comment. What her teacher did not know was that Wendy had no separation anxiety–school phobia but a true Social Phobia. Wendy had displaced her fears of *her own sexual feelings* and *exhibitionistic trends* from inside herself and onto the school examinations that she misidentified with being naked. To support her displacement, elaborations of dread of humiliation and public display of nudity had been added, and a fear that others would ridicule her (for her unconscious longings). The spread of her avoidant fear of exposure had meant that any talk of school or thought of school was sufficient to precipitate intense and unreasonable dread. It interfered with her schooling and her peer relationships. Adults did not understand her symptoms at all.

DIFFERENTIAL DIAGNOSIS

Separation Anxiety Disorder is ruled out by definition. Fear of repeating a Panic Disorder is ruled out because the incident feared is not a panic attack but an imagined scene of being the center of others' attention and being humiliated. The Social Phobia lacks the content of an Obsessive Compulsive Disorder, too.

TREATMENT

The most salutary event for the child with a Social Phobia is to be put in touch with an adult who can empathize with the child's unconscious wishes even while listening attentively to her or his "displacement symptoms." Hence, the therapy of choice is individual psychotherapy that is flexible in combining behavioral, cognitive, and emotional foci. Anxiolytic medications are rarely called for. Parental and sibling involvement in the psychotherapy can also enhance the efficacy of this multimodal approach to helping a phobic child.

Simple Phobia (300.29)

In some senses, a Simple Phobia is a residual category for those phobic disorders that are not centered on panic or humiliation in certain social contexts. DSM-III-R Code 300.29 can be applied to children with episodes of *persistent fear—a* fear recognized by the child as *excessive or unreasonable—of a circumscribed stimulus. Exposure to the phobic stimulus precipitates immediate anxiety* and as a result the phobic object or situation becomes even more *dreaded and avoided.* The phobia causes *marked inner distress* or *interferes with social or role functioning.*

While claustrophobia and fear of elevators, stairs, heights, and bridges may be seen as Simple Phobias of Childhood, there are others to be labeled for the etymologically inclined student of the displacement mechanism:

Beards	pogonophobia
Bees	apiphobia
Being buried alive	taphophobia
Blood	hematophobia
Blushing	ereuthophobia
Cats	ailurophobia
Choking	pnigophobia
Death	thanatophobia
Fear	phobophobia
Frogs	batrachophobia
Germs or contamination	mysophobia
Insects	entomophobia
Light	photophobia
Men	androphobia
Mirrors	eisoptrophobia
Nakedness	gymnophobia
Night and darkness	nyctophobia
Number 13	triskaidakaphobia
Pleasure	hedonophobia
Ridicule	katagelophobia
Sharp objects	belonophobia
Slime	blennophobia
Snakes	ophidiophobia

Strangers	xenophobia
String	lininophobia
Women	gynophobia

The objects of phobic dread in childhood are much more numerous than those mentioned.

DIAGNOSTIC WORKUP

The most important things to do in understanding the Simple Phobia are history taking, observation, mental status examination, and clinical interviewing. Rarely required are special laboratory studies or consultations from colleagues. In making the diagnosis it is important to determine in detail how crippling, or generalized to produce social incompetency, the disorder is. Only when adaptive functioning is impeded is it necessary to treat a Simple Phobia. If the phobias are numerous, the skittish child is likely to need treatment.

TREATMENT

This condition, formerly called anxiety hysteria, responds well to individual psychotherapy. The behavioral therapy approaches used include classical or respondent conditioning; systematic desensitization with flooding or implosion and negative practice; and operant conditioning. Classical conditioning would simultaneously present the feared object and a pleasant stimulus; desensitization would pair the anxiety-provoking stimulus with a response antagonistic to anxiety (such as the relaxation response); operant conditioning would look mainly to environmental reinforcers of non-fear responses to a phobic stimulus.

Cognitive therapy would encourage the child to talk about the irrational and excessive aspects of the phobia, to reason out strategies to alter the fear response, and to use adaptive thinking to help mute and moderate the fear response. Cognitive therapy can be used along with behavioral and emotive techniques.

Emotive or expressive therapies dwell on the affect of fear, encourage other affects, and usually depend on both emotional and cognitive insight. Witness psychoanalysis, Gestalt therapy, transactional analysis, play techniques, psychodrama, guided imagery, and many other techniques.

Drugs are rarely used for Simple Phobia in childhood. Also, group psychotherapies are seldom employed as the basic treatment thrust.

Avoidant Personality Disorder (301.82) (Axis II)

This was DSM-III's Avoidant Disorder of Childhood or Adolescence carried over to DSM-III-R. Deleting the category of Avoidant Disorder from DSM-III-R, as earlier planned, and subsuming it under the adult Avoidant Personality Disorder would have made sense nosologically and clinically. For that reason, we drop Avoidant Disorder of Childhood because we believe that Avoidant Personality Disorder better serves our clinical needs. It would then be on Axis II, as we formulate it, and would have to meet criteria that would be much closer to a neo-Freudian concept of *phobic character*. Here are the seven attributes, according to DSM-III-R, of which four are needed, to make this Axis II diagnosis of persons, either young or old, who are timid, have social discomfort, and fear negative evaluations by others:

1. No close friends or confidants outside of home.
2. Feels easily hurt by disapproval and criticism.
3. Reluctant to interact with anyone who is not certain to like him/her.
4. Avoids all activities that will require more interaction.
5. More fearful (than most others) of novelty, new experiences, or fearful (s)he will look foolish or get embarrassed.
6. Fearful of losing control of emotions or impulses.
7. Exaggerates the dangers or risks inherent in everyday living, or avoids everyday activities because (s)he says (s)he is fearful of exhaustion or physical discomfort.

As defined, these are seven signs of a very constricted and unsatisfyingly unsociable and phobic lifestyle, but they are not indicative of a clearcut mental disorder such as one recorded on Axis I. Some emotionally coarcted and avoidant children would fall conveniently into this category. Their treatment follows the same lines as that of milder Phobias.

DISSOCIATIVE DISORDERS

CLINICAL FEATURES

The well-structured Dissociative Disorders such as Multiple Personality Disorder are more often adult phenomena, hence they will be omitted herein.

DSM-II, to recall our past, considered the hysterical neuroses to be divided into conversion and dissociative subtypes. All together, the Dissociative Disorders comprise around 5% of childhood neuroses and only a tiny portion of the total of mental disorders affecting children, so we will comment briefly on them as a group.

The Dissociative Disorders have had a special appeal for hypnotists, partly, we surmise, because of the disorders' combining psychogenic disturbances in consciousness, personality disorganization, and certain odd motor acts. The combination means that a dramatic split or dissociation of consciousness appears, with the "unaware" part surprisingly greater than the "aware" part. Amnesia, twilight states, pseudodelirium, trances, and stupor may show the dissociation in consciousness. The personality disorganization is a crackup of the self, self-concept, and formerly functioning personality—ranging from derealization and depersonalization to multiple personality. The bizarre motor behavior seen in Dissociative Disorders ranges from aimless pacing to "running fits" and fugue states, with, along the way, psychogenic catalepsy, narcolepsy, cataplexy, and somnambulism.

SUBTYPES OF DISSOCIATION

1. *Multiple Personality Disorder* (300.14) is a seldom looked-for rarity in children; it is a disorder in which two or more distinct personalities exist and assert full executive control at some time. Most adult cases were abused physically and/or sexually in childhood.

2. *Psychogenic Fugue* (300.13) is also rare in children but one of the authors has observed two cases. It is a disorder in which a child leaves home, becomes amnestic about her or his identity, and takes on a new identity at least in part for a few days at a time.

3. *Depersonalization Disorder* (300.60) is rather more common. Following sexual abuse the child may show repeated episodes of depersonalization: Who am I? What is my name? Why do I feel unreal? With derealization that often accompanies depersonalization, the child asks: Are you real? Is this room real? Why has the world changed so?

4. In a *Trance Disorder* (300.15) the child has altered consciousness with a marked diminution in awareness of and response to the surroundings. This has to be independent of any other severe mental disorder or physical disorder and also independent of any religious ritual or culturally prescribed ceremonial behavior. It may be easy to differentiate, under amobarbital injection, from the stupors of catatonia, depression, or mania.

5. *Possession Disorder* (300.15) is also not religious, not culturally sanctioned, but shows a conviction that one is possessed and taken over by another—a spirit, a dead relative, an enemy, a friend. Missionaries' descriptions of *leopard men* in Gabon illustrate this state well. In a frenzy of anger the victim of the mental disorder would leap upon and bite an adversary, a highly dangerous act because the human bite is so lethal.

6. *Dissociative Disorder NOS* (300.15) is a residual category for Ganser's syndrome, variants of Multiple Personality Disorder, abused children who show incomplete trance or amnesia or derealization/depersonalization, and brainwashed individuals. This perhaps would be the most frequently used code for children with symptoms of dissociation that have not congealed into a full and discrete disorder.

DIFFERENTIAL DIAGNOSIS

Organic Mental Disorders can be differentiated by their showing "organicity" and a less variable (with stress) picture in the delirium, dementia, amnesia, etc., which Dissociative Disorders may exhibit. A Brief Reactive Psychosis may be difficult to distinguish at first blush, but that disorder shows more turmoil, loose associations, delusions, and hallucinations than does the Dissociative Disorder. Temporal lobe epilepsy or complex partial seizures may mimic a trance state but its automatisms help to distinguish it from a dissociative state and its sleeping EEG also helps to differentiate it further. Eventually, Schizophrenia, Mood Disorders, and Anxiety Disorders can be ruled out by their respective symptom contents.

TREATMENT

As we stated previously, hypnosis has been much celebrated in Dissociative Disorders, for they are most frequently found in "nonstandard" subcultures of suggestible, noninsightful, vicariously living, so-called "primitive" persons, the same persons who are easily hypnotized. Hypnosis is most useful in making the diagnosis and of some utility in treatment through posthypnotic suggestion and in combination with other modes of individual psychotherapy. It would seem to most observers that sodium amytal interviews are as valuable as hypnosis. The most accepted form of individual psychotherapy is combined work with the child and the parents to build some structure and respect for saner behavior and to aim towards integration and "synthesis," not more dissociation. Hence, both family and individual child are treated.

Questions for Study and Action

1. In the pathogenesis of Anxiety Disorders, Phobic Disorders, and Dissociative Disorders, what is the role of frightful *worry, displacement,* and *splitting* in each? Explain. How does a child learn these maneuvers? Or is it all a matter of constitution and inborn temperament?

2. Outline a diagnostic workup for a child with Obsessive Compulsive Disorder, one that will rule out Organic Mental Syndrome, Tourette's, and Schizophrenia.

3. What qualities in a parent would lead the parent to bring a child with Generalized Anxiety Disorder or Overanxious Disorder to see a child psychiatrist?

4. What qualities of the GAD itself would prompt a parent to seek psychiatric help for the child?

5. What would you consider in the differential diagnosis of a nine-year-old boy who steals, reads at second-grade level, lives in slum housing and witnessed his mother's murder of his father? Be inclusive.

6. Which in each of these pairs shows more symptomatic structuring into a definite disorder?
    (a) Adjustment Disorder with Anxious Mood *or* OCD
    (b) Post-traumatic Stress Disorder *or* Psychogenic Fugue
    (c) Dissociative Disorder NOS *or* Psychogenic Fugue
    (d) Simple Phobia *or* Avoidant Personality Disorder
    (e) School phobia *or* Separation Anxiety Disorder

7. These were "actual neuroses" for Freud and his early followers: anxiety neuroses, neurasthenia, hypochondria, and depersonalization neurosis. Freud said of them that he "could find neither (intra) psychic causations nor psychic mechanisms." Explain what he meant by that.

8. Among the "symptom neuroses" that could be treated by use of transference, Freud included phobic, hysterical, and obsessive compulsive ones. Among those that were too "narcissistic" to be treated thus, Helene Deutsch included melancholic depression. What did these Freudians mean? Is it a useful distinction clinically? How so?

9. Wilhelm Reich distinguished between symptom neurosis and character neurosis, saying that the personality trait itself was like a neurotic symptom in the latter. How has that appellation carried over into DSM-III-R? Critique this statement: "Some children suffer from narcissistic wounds but lack the overt symptoms of psychoneurosis. They might nonetheless manifest partial internalization of external demands and develop *character neuroses* or personality disorders."

10. Can you make a case in support of Yale psychiatrist Robert J. Lifton's hypothesis that, in the nuclear terror of cold war following Hiroshima and Nagasaki, many children suffer a kind of indirect or vicarious Post-traumatic Stress Disorder? Outline a research project that would test the Lifton hypothesis.

For Further Reading

Adams, P.L. *Obsessive Children*. New York: Brunner/Mazel, 1973.

Adams, P.L. Psychoneuroses. In J.D. Noshpitz (Ed.), *Basic Handbook of Child Psychiatry*, Vol. 2. New York: Basic Books, 1979, pp. 194–235.

Casey, R.J., & Berman, J.S. The outcome of psychotherapy with children. *Psychol. Bull.*, 98:388–400, 1985.

Eth, S., & Pynoos, R.S. (Eds.). *Post-Traumatic Stress Disorder in Children*. Washington, DC: American Psychiatric Press, 1985.

Freud, S. Analysis of a phobia in a five-year-old boy (1909). *Collected Papers, Vol. 3, Paper II.* (Trans. by Joan Riviere.) New York: Basic Books, 1959.

Freud, S. Beyond the pleasure principle (1920). In J. Strachey (Ed. Trans.), *Complete Psychological Works, Standard Edition, Vol. 18*. London: The Hogarth Press, 1955.

Kluft, R.P. Childhood multiple personality disorder: Predictors, clinical findings, and treatment results. In R.P. Kluft (Ed.), *Childhood Antecedents of Multiple Personality*. Washington, DC: American Psychiatric Press, 1985, pp. 167–196.

Terr, L.C. Psychic trauma in children: Observations following the Chowchilla school-bus kidnapping. *Am. J. Psychiatry*, 138:14–19, 1981.

Waldron, S., Jr., Shrier, D.K., Stone, B., & Tobin, F. School phobia and other childhood neuroses: A systematic study of the children and their families. *Am. J. Psychiatry*, 132:802–808, 1975.

18

Somatoform and Psychophysiological Disorders

This chapter encompasses all the disorders presenting with physical symptoms for which no organic basis can be demonstrated and for which there is at least strong presumption of a psychogenic basis. The psychogenic impetus for these disorders derives from unconscious psychic conflict and is, therefore, not under voluntary control.

All the subdivisions of Somatoform Disorders may occur in children. However, it is extremely difficult to diagnose Somatization Disorder (300.81) and Hypochondriasis (300.70) in childhood, because these disorders require the patient to have a backlog of knowledge and experience, as well as a level of cognitive development, that are rare before adolescence. Somatoform Pain Disorder (307.80) frequently occurs in children but is usually diagnosed as Conversion Disorder (300.11), since the dynamics are the same and pain is one of the most common symptoms of Conversion Disorder. Therefore, we shall describe the latter in detail, while advising the reader that Somatoform Pain Disorder follows the same course and prognosis and calls for the same diagnostic and treatment approaches as Conversion Disorder.

Conversion Disorder (or Hysterical Neurosis, Conversion Type [300.11])

As far as its symptomatology is concerned, Conversion Disorder is the classical "hysteria" that physicians have diagnosed in adults and children for centuries. The name is derived from the Greek "hyster," meaning uterus. Medieval theory explained hysteria as a "wandering uterus." Remnants of this myth persisted to the end of the 19th century along with the belief that hysteria could occur only in females. It was Sigmund Freud who put an end to this misconception, proving that hysteria could and did occur in males as well, and he was reviled for that by his male colleagues (Freud, 1925). It was Freud, too, who elaborated the psychodynamics of this disorder (Freud, 1893, 1905); indeed, hysteria (i.e., Conversion Disorder) was the original clinical case material for psychodynamic research, and Conversion Disorder continues to be understood primarily in psychodynamic terms.

DEFINITION

Conversion Disorder is defined in DSM-III-R as a somatic (physical) dysfunction which is the expression of repressed psychological conflict. The name is due to the psychological mechanism of converting psychological conflict into somatic (physical) symptoms. The physical symptoms often appear to express the psychological conflict symbolically through the voluntary musculature or the somatosensory system, as if the symptoms were a symbolic solution to the inner conflict; yet the physical dysfunction is not under voluntary control, but is the external manifestation of unconscious mechanisms of repression and conversion.

At one time, clinicians were inclined to exclude from Conversion Disorder those syndromes in which the autonomic nervous system and smooth muscle were involved, maintaining that Conversion Disorder should be limited to symptom clusters involving the striated muscles and the motor and sensory parts of the nervous system. This distinction is no longer made, although DSM-III-R considers involvement of the autonomic or endocrine systems to occur more rarely among the cardinal signs of Conversion Disorder.

ETIOLOGY AND PATHOGENESIS

We do not yet know what role is played by "somatic compliance," i.e., an organic substrate that lends itself to be acted upon by psychic factors. We are keeping it "on hold" for future discoveries. What we do know is that psychic factors are of paramount importance in causing Conversion Disorder. However, in spite of the fact that any overview of the etiology of hysterical symptoms reads like the history of psychiatry, and especially that of psychoanalysis, there is no agreement as to the mechanism.

The classical theory is that of the mechanism of repression of conflict, and the channelling or "conversion" of that conflict into somatic symptoms. This provides two "gains" to the patient. The "primary gain" means that the internal conflict is kept out of awareness, and anxiety is decreased. The "secondary gain" is the support from the environment. It means attention, sympathy, relatedness.

So far, everything has been simply explained—perhaps too simply. Why does one child develop Conversion Disorder, while most of his/her peers are either anxious, or develop phobias, or confront their conflicts by acting them out?

Several answers have been suggested. The unknown "somatic compliance" is one of them. Of more immediate relevance is the identification of the child with the "somatization" style of one or both parents, which encourages communication through somatic channels. These range from various nonverbal, histrionic lifestyles, to immature distortions of reality, to, finally, using illness as a medium of communication or leverage. The latter has been referred to as the "sick role," and the susceptible child learns to take on this role. The susceptibility is probably due either to lack of resolution of the oedipal phase with resulting persistence of unrealistic sexual and aggressive fantasies, or, if the oedipal phase is resolved, it is done so by identifying with a histrionic or sick parent, without an additional healthy dilution of the oedipal feelings through strong peer relationships.

These children are emotionally more dependent on their parents than is appropriate for their age. The greater the dependency and suffocating closeness, the greater the ambivalence and intensity of their feelings. Because they are so dependent and have not completely resolved their oedipal conflicts, their mental mechanisms remain primitive. The magical quality of their thoughts, so characteristic of the oedipal phase, is also perpetuated. In the extreme case, this leads to distorted reality testing and, in the average case, to a fluctuating perception of the world which varies from near-normal to that of a fairyland or make-believe. It is within the latter that Conversion Disorder is thought to originate.

Conversion symptoms have been thought to be symbolic of the underlying drive. For instance, the paralyzed arm is unable to strike, the drive having been to strike and hurt or kill an ambivalently beloved person (e.g., Case 18-2); in "hysterical aphonia," the child cannot shout the curse or accusation, and so on. However, many, if not most, conversion symptoms are devoid of such heavy symbolism.

Although Conversion Disorders arise preferentially in families where the style is one of overemotionality and histrionics and are more likely to arise in children with histrionic (hysterical) personality traits, such a family or such a personality is by no means a prerequisite for Conversion Disorder. In other words, Conversion

Disorders can arise in any type of family style, and a child does not have to "behave hysterically" before developing a Conversion Disorder.

CLINICAL DESCRIPTION

The most frequent conversion syndromes among outpatient pediatric patients have been pain, fainting spells, and pseudoseizures. The latter have been frequently associated with incest. In addition, sudden blindness and ataxia are also found. Syndromes involving paralyses of limbs, one of the classical symptoms of hysteria, are now less frequent generally but can still be seen occasionally.

Conversion Disorders have varied in their manifestations over time, depending on the prevalent culture and the age and sophistication of the involved children. We may expect more of the classical syndromes, such as limb paralysis and "glove-and-stocking" anesthesias, in isolated rural regions, bizarre patterns of pain among children of religious sects, and more "plausible" syndromes of vague discomfort, pain, and dysfunctions of various organ systems among middle-class urban children.

CASE 18-1   Xenia was a nine-year-old girl whose *surgeon* asked for a psychiatric consultation because of *abdominal pains* initially suggesting mesenteric adenitis. The surgeon became uncomfortable with the child's willingness to be in the hospital and *her blasé lack of concern* about her pain. The pain at times assumed *dramatic proportions,* and at other times *disappeared,* as if by magic. The waxing and waning seemed linked to the *presence of her parents,* but in a complex, at first unintelligible way.

Repeated sessions with the child and her parents revealed severe *marital* problems between the parents; they were actively *considering a separation* when Xenia *became ill.* While the child was hospitalized, the plans for separation were *held in abeyance,* but were discussed from time to time during parental visits to the child. Xenia's *symptoms* became *worse* during *such scenes;* thereupon, the parents showed concern, the subject of separation was dropped, and Xenia's symptoms abated.

Comment. The surgeon astutely called for psychiatric assistance, not because convincing physical findings were absent but because of the linkage of the symptoms to emotional conflict. The surgeon noted how the child's illness fluctuated with the state of her parents' marriage and *"secondary gain"* kept the parents' marriage going for Xenia to have an intact family to look after her. Moreover, the illness immobilized the child in the hospital, thereby precluding any contribution the child could make to her parents' difficulties, i.e., the illness prevented any guilt-provoking action and thus prevented anxiety—the *"primary gain."* These are explained more fully in the section on "Etiology and Pathogenesis."

CASE 18-2   Travis was a seven-year-old boy whose left hand became *limp* and *numb* from *the elbow down*. A few days earlier, his father had been hospitalized with serious injuries following a fall from a construction scaffold.

Background history revealed a family who believed in fundamentalist religious principles. Father wanted to raise his children according to strict "principles," i.e., he administered the rod to the point of abuse, denouncing "permissiveness" and "secular humanism." Travis feared the frequent *beatings* and felt a great deal of *anger* against his father. Yet, he also appreciated the good times he and his father had and *loved* him for it. From the intense indoctrination he received in Sunday school, he learned that it was *wrong* to resent his parents and felt guilty for his anger against his father.

Travis *felt terrible* when he learned of his father's accident; he *could not concentrate* on his work in school and hung by his mother's side, *anxiously* asking about his father's welfare.

Four days later, when he woke up, Travis was unable to move his left hand. Medical examination showed *no signs of injury* or changes in musculature. There was, however, an area of *numbness and insensitivity* to touch and pinprick extending from the elbow down. Travis's mother was overcome with anxiety at this second calamity, although Travis himself appeared quite *unconcerned*. As a matter of fact, not only was he not worried about his paralysis, but also his fears for his father were much diminished. He seemed to live in a dreamlike world.

Comment. This is a case of classic Conversion Disorder. The child was left-handed, and the conversion disorder represented a "way out" for him—a compromise, struck in the unconscious, between his angry feelings against his father and the demands of his conscience to love and respect his father. By this compromise, guilt was alleviated.

Contributing to the classic picture were special conditions of relatively archaic conditions: intense religious beliefs making for guilt over aggressive impulses and causing the magical quality of thought of a young child to persist into the grade-school years. The patient feared that his angry thoughts and murderous wishes against his father had caused father's accident. Perhaps he had had fantasies of pushing or hitting his father; the paralysis of his left (i.e., dominant) arm made this impossible and thus permitted him not to worry anymore. This indifference to the disability has been called "la belle indifférence."

DIAGNOSIS AND DIFFERENTIAL DIAGNOSIS

These two tasks are almost inseparable in Conversion Disorder: the diagnosis of Conversion Disorder is made concurrently with the differential diagnosis ruling out organic diseases. The clinician is immediately faced with the question: "Is this organic disease, or does it just look like organic disease?" That the clinician should *not* miss an organic disease goes without saying, but it is sometimes easier said than done: Conversion Disorder and organic illness coexist relatively frequently.

The time-honored rule is to diagnose Conversion Disorder on positive psychiatric and medical evidence. The positive psychiatric evidence is the incongruity between the complaints and the child's actions and attitudes. This usually means that the emotions are divergent from the physical complaints, e.g., despite complaints of severe pain, the child is not worried about it. If he or she is worried about anything, it is about other matters—peers, school, parents. Thus, the symptoms are treated with "la belle indifférence," or this indifference extends over the child's entire life (simultaneously with the onset of the physical complaints), or else there is anxiety, but it does not concern the symptoms that the child so loudly complains about.

The positive physical evidence is yet another divergence, or discrepancy, and that is between the signs and symptoms of disease as expected from human anatomy and physiology, and those described by the patient, which follow the child's concept of what a disease would be like. For instance, a child's numbness or insensitivity to stimuli does not follow anatomical nerve distributions; instead, these areas are mapped out according to the child's own concepts of anatomy or disability. The locations fluctuate and are characteristically vague and uncertain. Moreover, the child reacts normally during sleep or hypnosis.

When Conversion Disorder involves seizures, the child does not know about accompanying manifestations, such as postictal confusion. Paralyzed limbs can be made to work when attention is diverted, such as movements of the paralyzed limb when dressing; a paralyzed arm will not fall on the patient's face. Blindness can be differentiated by a number of relatively simple tests, such as response to a threatening gesture, pupillary reactions, involuntary tracking movements, and visual field mapping. The use of a striped drum to elicit optokinetic nystagmus is a very useful test. In general, the symptomatology in Conversion Disorder of children is less well defined than in that of adults and is more "transparently" linked to precipitating factors.

Apart from the ever-present need to differentiate Conversion Disorder from physical illness, it has to be differentiated from other psychiatric disorders as well. Malingering is a conscious attempt at deceit by claiming sickness where no sickness exists and no discomfort is felt. It is quite transparent when a child is trying to avoid a difficult situation, usually in school.

Factitious disorder is a product of unconscious conflicts, but with a conscious, purposeful effort to create real organic disease (see Chapter 6); as a result, real physical lesions exist. Conversion Disorder, by contrast, is the image of disease without demonstrable organic substrate to account for the symptomatology.

Psychophysiological disorder is a physical illness brought about or exacerbated by unconscious mental conflict. In practice, Malingering can be differentiated by the obvious gain. Factitious Disorder requires of the clinical worker a suspicious mind and, with older children, well-honed clinical acumen based on sound medical knowledge. Psychophysiological Disorders are diagnosable medically, i.e., physical examination is positive for organic disease.

In rare cases, childhood schizophrenia may present differential difficulties if the psychosis starts with somatic delusions. Acute brain syndromes (Delirium), especially of toxic origin, may be confused with Conversion Disorder if the clinician pays attention only to the confusing complaints and does not make an effort to check the child for neurological signs.

Again, we would like to point to the possibility of a coexisting organic disorder (Axis III) in the differential diagnosis; sometimes organic disorders present with an overall clinical picture that has both positive psychiatric components and missing organic substrate, only to reveal themselves as organic disorders years later. This is especially true of neurological disease which has presented with visual difficulties or disturbances of gait of insidious onset and long duration.

TREATMENT AND PROGNOSIS

Treatment should be psychodynamic, but not classically psychoanalytic, in most instances. What we mean by this is that we extend the treatment to the family, especially the parents, and get the help of "allies," such as schoolteachers. The treatment of the child varies in length and intensity according to the severity of the disorder and, again, the modern approach to Conversion Disorder is highly pragmatic.

It follows from the considerations just mentioned in the preceding section that the treatment of Conversion Disorder should be primarily psychodynamic, since the main causes and causative mechanisms are based on unconscious, internalized emotional conflicts.

The great variability of the disease and the importance of the environment have dictated a comprehensive treatment approach, rather than the narrow psychoanalytic treatment previously practiced. The clinician should reconstruct the conflict that has given rise to the symptoms and then relieve the pressure of those conflicts. This may entail reexamining the child's defenses, while rearranging some of the family dynamics that have contributed to or caused the child's conflicts.

The treatment will, moreover, vary with the course of each case, and this is highly individual. Depending on the psychodynamics of the child ("the inner network") and those of his or her family ("the outer network"), Conversion Disorders may be obdurate and ingrained for long periods of time, with disability and "secondary gain" becoming a way of life for the child and the child's family; or they may be short, and the symptoms "given up" almost spontaneously, with treatment providing an "out," an excuse to save face.

CASE 18-3   Ruth was a *lively, somewhat flirtatious* 11-year-old girl, whose parents had divorced when she was seven years old. For a year before her psychiatric consultation, her mother had been living with a man slightly her junior, who became *very close* to Ruth. One night, Ruth had a *seizure,* which consisted of convulsive movements of her back, waist, and all four extremities. There was *no postictal confusion,* she *did not bite* her tongue, and she *did not injure herself* when she fell. She did *not wet or soil* herself. Neurological evaluation, including waking and sleeping EEGs, was *normal.* The seizures kept recurring in the evenings, and psychiatric interview with the child revealed Ruth's fears of *strong sexual innuendos* by mother's boyfriend. Mother, who by then was ready to terminate the relationship with the young man, asked him to move out. However, the seizures *persisted.* Ruth then *suggested that she be treated by hypnosis.* The treating psychiatrist, who rarely practiced hypnosis, agreed and proceeded to induce what appeared to amount to a slight trance, in which she made the "posthypnotic suggestion" that the patient would no longer suffer from seizures. The patient continued in supportive psychotherapy at longer intervals and *never experienced another seizure.* Follow-up two years later showed Ruth to be doing well.

Comment. This is an example of the willingness of the patient to "give up" her symptoms, because the circumstances that necessitated them (as a way out) no longer existed. Nevertheless, the patient cannot just get better—it would negate the reality of her illness, to her especially, and would give the message of malingering to her environment, with resulting loss of self-esteem. A ritual—an official act—was needed, and the patient "responded" to the hypnosis that she requested.

In summary, the treatment of Conversion Disorder requires solid expertise on the part of the clinician, so that the therapist is not swayed by his or her own emotions. In particular, physicians should be warned against pejorative attitudes, such as "showing the patient that there is nothing wrong with her." We have seen neurologists make that mistake.

The prognosis in Conversion Disorders in childhood is generally quite good: most cases do not last nearly as long as similar cases in adolescence, and certainly are much more benign than their counterparts in adulthood.

Psychophysiological (or Psychosomatic) Disorders
(Psychological Factors Affecting Physical Condition [316.00])

The traditional time-honored term for this group of disorders is psychosomatic illness, although its successor, psychophysiological disorder, has also been well accepted, probably because of its greater accuracy.

The cumbersome DSM-III-R term (*mental* might have been better than *psycho-*

logical) aims at greater neutrality but cannot do away with the notion, in most clinicians' minds, that here is a special group of disorders which hang together on threads of psychodynamic and physiological theory. This perception of homogeneity has persisted in spite of changing research findings and changing fads and fashions in psychiatry. The fact that the concept of psychophysiological disorder has survived the glaring overinterpretations of the early psychosomaticists attests to its inherent humanistic and medical appeal. Here are demonstrable mechanisms of mind-body interaction, the undoing of the artificial mind-body separation, and a zone for holistic medicine to operate, potentially at its best.

DEFINITION

Psychophysiological or psychosomatic disorders are a group of *physical* disorders in which mental processes contribute to the etiology and the course of the disease by integrating cerebral cortex with hypothalamus and all other body parts.

DSM-III-R defines this group as consisting of those cases in which a close or proximal temporal relationship between psychologically meaningful environmental stimuli and the initiation or exacerbation of a physical disorder can be demonstrated.

ETIOLOGY AND PATHOGENESIS

The contemporary approach to psychophysiological disorders is biopsychosocial: an open systems model of biological vulnerabilities in the child, familial and extrafamilial environmental influences, and the mediating mechanisms of the mental mechanisms and nervous system substrate. Put more simply, there is no one cause for psychophysiological disorders; the causal complex consists of the biological predisposition, outside influences, and the inner mechanisms that react or overreact along certain physiological pathways. Rather than present the details of this model here, we shall use it in our subsequent description of the specific disorders.

CLINICAL DESCRIPTION

We will describe two psychophysiological disorders, bronchial asthma and ulcerative colitis, and only briefly list a few others.

Bronchial asthma

This is the most frequently encountered chronic illness, and most common psychophysiological disorder, in children. Pathophysiologically, it shows a diffuse narrowing of the entire bronchial tree (trachea, bronchi, and peripheral bronchioles) brought about by bronchospasm and increased mucus secretion. This "hyperactivity of the bronchial tree" is thought to be caused by a definite pathophysiological sequence, with the final result of overreactive vagal bronchoconstrictive reflexes. The clinical signs are wheezing, coughing, and shortness of breath due to expiratory obstruction.

Among the precipitating factors are physical and/or psychosocial stress, allergens, infectious agents, or irritants (e.g., tobacco smoke). The resulting anxiety in both the child and her or his environment sets in motion chain reactions of anger, frustration, conflicts of dependence and independence, hostility, and overprotectiveness that make the psychodynamic picture extremely complex as the asthmatic attacks repeat themselves over the years. To tease out which factor came first is impossible, and we are simply left to conclude that the etiology is multifactorial. The following case summary will illustrate some of these points.

CASE 18-4   Yvette was eight years old when first seen for psychiatric evaluation. The reason for the referral was that the child was simply "extremely difficult"; she was "hyperactive," "high-strung," "unpredictable," and moody. She was fairly difficult to manage at school, but not nearly so trying there as at home.

She *never fought physically* and was actually afraid of bigger peers (she herself was quite small), to whom she related at times *submissively*, at times provocatively. She was quite *demanding of attention* in almost all situations, again especially at home, and could not bear to see her older brother get any recognition, especially from mother. The brother, who was 11 years old, was a relatively quiet boy, quite popular with peers, and an excellent student.

Yvette had had bronchial asthma since age three and a half; she had frequent attacks of dyspnea, requiring numerous visits to the pediatrician's office and a number of hospitalizations. By the time she was seen by the psychiatrist, a measure of relief had been obtained by a desensitization program for respiratory *allergies*. Nevertheless, she required a great deal of *attention*, both preventive and interventive, from her parents.

Her parents were both professional people, father being an attorney and mother a physician. Father was an easygoing, but slightly detached person. *Mother*, by contrast, was *high-strung, hardworking*, yet *ambivalent* about her professional role versus that of mother, wife, housewife, attractive socialite, and daughter of her own ambitious mother. When the children were born, mother stopped practicing full-time in order to devote herself to raising the children, but by the time Yvette was two years old, mother had developed many *conflicting feelings about staying home*. Her attitude fluctuated between *solicitous care and resentment*.

When it became clear that Yvette had bronchial asthma, mother's *solicitousness turned to overprotectiveness* with a rather overt component of *resentment*. Yvette had become quite *dependent* on mother and her asthma seemed to follow a pattern of coming on in *anticipation of separation from mother* (e.g., when mother traveled to a medical meeting). However, that pattern was not consistent.

Shortly after starting psychotherapy, Yvette had a severe attack of asthma, for which she was hospitalized at a major medical center. A *"parentectomy"* (i.e., withholding all contacts between parent and child) was carried out with success while she was there: Yvette had no more attacks while in the hospital, but she developed *aggressive behavior* towards peers and staff.

Yvette continued in psychotherapy and her parents in parental counseling after her discharge from the medical center. The old patterns became evident again: mother attended to Yvette with *oversolicitousness* when Yvette had respiratory difficulties, and "made up" for missed professional work in between. Only slowly did they both gain a modicum of genuine insight into this pattern which helped to make Yvette's attacks of bronchial asthma emotionally rewarding—she obtained *dependency* gratifications from mother which she otherwise could not get. Unfortunately, the psychotherapy was pursued almost exclusively on the mother–child axis, because *father kept hiding* behind a façade of neutrality and lack of involvement. Nevertheless, Yvette became progressively *more self-sufficient* emotionally. She did not react with attacks of asthma whenever she anticipated *separation* from mother. She sought out *stronger peer* relationships, even though *overt aggression* was often a problem there, and finally she found several *activities in which she excelled* in her own right. She was especially successful in music, where she discovered both a talent and a surprising perseverance in playing the piano.

On follow-up at age 12, Yvette was an *active*, somewhat *overly assertive*, slightly overindependent, pretty and petite girl who led a somewhat idiosyncratic, but successful and largely happy existence. She continued to have episodic attacks of bronchial asthma, but these were fewer than before and were treated matter-of-factly by both patient and mother.

Comment. In this case we have a mother-child relationship based on ambivalent closeness; excessive dependence on the mother is gratified and overgratified through the leverage of illness (asthma). This dependence requires repression of normal aggression, which comes out when the child is placed in a supportive environment without the overprotective parent ("parentectomy"). The mother sometimes has an unresolved dependency relationship with her own mother (which was mentioned here) and a highly ambivalent feeling about her own role as mother made worse by the asthmatic child's chronic disease. Not all asthmatic children conform to the psychological model of overprotective mother-dependency-repressed aggression and "the cry for mother = the asthmatic attack."

The result of treatment in Case 18-4 was not a cure of the bronchial asthma but rather a strengthening of positive coping skills and a diminution of noxious patterns. The positive results may retain vestiges of pathology, but they work for the patient; Yvette perhaps became too assertive and independent in a compensatory way.

Since the etiology of bronchial asthma is multifactorial, so the treatment has to be multidimensional. If psychical factors are not significant, psychotherapy will obviously not be necessary. However, even though not all children with bronchial asthma have the "primary" psychophysiological ingredient, the anxiety and concern by the family may call for occasional psychiatric intervention. This is especially so in view of the fact that bronchial asthma may still be life-threatening and most parents fear that their child may die.

In general, the prognosis for childhood bronchial asthma is fairly good; there are studies that have shown that psychiatric intervention, both individual and family therapy, has improved the physical outcome of bronchial asthma (Alexander, Miklich, & Hershkoff, 1972; Lask & Matthew, 1979). Therefore, the clinician should be ready to offer psychiatric help, be it in the form of psychotherapy of the child with concomitant therapy or counseling for the parent or parents (as illustrated in our case example), or group therapy for asthmatic children, or behavior modification (relaxation, breathing exercises).

Ulcerative colitis

This is the most serious among the traditional psychophysiological disorders. As in the case of bronchial asthma, there are a number of instances where sociogenic factors have combined with organic factors in a primary causative role. In the majority of cases, the social/interpersonal component is a precipitating or exacerbating one. On the other hand, lymphocytes that are cytotoxic to bowel epithelium are also present. Therefore, immune suppressive therapy, steroids, and antimicrobial agents are useful empirically, especially in combination with focused psychotherapy. The following case history will illustrate some of the interplay between autoimmunological and psychodynamic circumstances.

CASE 18-5   Missy, a white girl of 11 years, developed loose stools shortly after her older sister left home to attend college and her younger sister began to share Missy's bedroom when her maternal grandmother had a stroke and came to live with Missy's family. Missy had been born weighing just over five pounds following a pregnancy characterized by maternal depression, nausea, and vomiting. At the time of her birth, the family lived in relative poverty and the mother returned to work shortly after Missy was born, leaving her in the care of a series of black servants. She was a superior student in school and developed in a healthy fashion until age 10. She then became constipated for several days. This resulted in an abdominal swelling about which "the doctors said that it made them think that I was pregnant." The constipation was relieved, as well as the abdominal swelling, and Missy had no remarkable gastrointestinal complaints for almost a year when the bloody diarrhea commenced. Menarche was established when she reached 11 years of age. After the onset of bloody diarrhea, Missy had lost weight, developed arthralgias, and shown little improvement on a strict medical regimen. The referring pediatrician adopted the "comprehensive pediatrics" approach: he recommended hospitalization for hematological study, proctoscopy, stool cultures, psychiatric evaluation, review of the barium enema, and continuation of salicylazosulfapyridine.

Once hospitalized, it was established that Missy had idiopathic ulcerative colitis and that although she appeared passive she was teeming with suppressed rage. She was not preoccupied exclusively with her bowel complaints and indeed stated during her first interview with the psychiatrist that her main problem was difficulty "in getting along with others." Also during this interview she spoke realistically of her assets and accomplishments. She was aware that her mother's attention had been diverted away from her into taking care of the invalided maternal grandmother. Almost immediately, it seemed that improvement could occur only within the context of help to Missy and her parents.

Both of the parents were seen regularly by a psychiatric social worker who emphasized the desirability of having both of the parents committed directly to the therapeutic enterprise. The social worker's appraisal was that these parents resisted any dependence on the psychiatric social worker. They did not see any dramatic disruption in the family's patterns, claiming that it was only Missy who suffered. The social worker described the colitis as being "ego syntonic for the family ego." Indeed, the family's tension had lessened following the onset of Missy's colitis.

In the very first session with Missy, the therapist urged her not to be passive but to express her feelings in many ways. The therapist suggested that she needed to express anger—a human, justified, and often deserved affect—by means other than her colon. Furthermore, the therapist told Missy that expressing her feelings verbally and giving them muscle expression would be effective ways to serve her self-expression.

This augmentation of her expressive repertoire became then an announced, mutually accepted part of the goals of therapy. Since the contract was stated explicitly and early, and since it involved *adding on* (not taking away or giving up anything), it was more acceptable to the patient.

Following the initial interview the therapist could easily appeal to the patient to "show me anger with your face" and "now with your arms and legs" and "now talk some of your anger." Missy soon laughed and wept during the therapy sessions and became more expressive and fluid; her colitis improved; and her health improved rather radically.

The following changes were encouraged and advocated by the social worker and the psychiatrist: Missy began spending nights away from home and having more peers visit her at her home; she went to camp, engaged in community activities, went to dances, and joined a debating team. Early, she discovered that her diarrhea—which she called "being upset"—remitted while she was at camp but was exacerbated when she returned home. Her bodily concerns shifted from the GI tract to being too tall, but recognizing that Miss America was always tall, and to having hips that were too large, to adopting new hairstyles, and to wearing contact lenses instead of eyeglasses. Missy began receiving a regular allowance. She began eating an unrestricted diet.

Comment. The assumptions with which the child psychotherapist undertook treatment were stated to be:

1. The entire family is considered to be the relevant biosocial unit.
2. The child is viewed from a holistic standpoint.
3. The child needs a rebalancing and enriching of his or her expressive behavior repertoire, with the goal of more body pleasure.
4. The child is to be treated in his or her individual historical context, with an orientation towards health, not disorder.

Other childhood psychophysiological disorders

Atopic dermatitis has been viewed as the most "visible" psychophysiological disorder of childhood, since it seems to worsen in direct consequence to psychosocial stressors. The organic basis is allergy; the psychodynamics are thought to be based on a hostile-dependent mother-child relationship. When tension between mother and child rises, atopic dermatitis often gets worse, and vice versa.

By contrast, *neurodermatitis* is *not* based on allergy, yet can also be exacerbated by any emotional conflict between child and his/her environment.

Another psychophysiological disorder is *juvenile rheumatoid arthritis*. It is somewhat similar in parts of its etiology to ulcerative colitis in that it is an autoimmune disorder and fear of loss of parent (caretaker) is an important ingredient of the patient's psychodynamics, since feelings of helplessness contribute to exacerbation.

Similar to adults, children may also suffer from *tension headaches and bruxism*, with anxiety translated into muscular tension. What many of us tend to forget, until we are reminded by a young sufferer, is that *migraine headaches* occur in childhood and that many an adult sufferer started his or her calvary in childhood! In children, nausea and vomiting are at first more prominent than the headaches themselves. As in adults, the psychodynamics often involve perfectionism and repressed and suppressed anger.

Psychosocial dwarfism is an early-onset psychophysiological disorder and has been covered in Chapter 14.

Peptic ulcer and *hypertension* occur in children but are rare enough not to be discussed in detail, especially as their psychophysiological mechanisms have not been sufficiently worked out for the pediatric population.

Because of the importance of the limbic-hypothalamic pathways in psychophysiological disorders, one would assume that some endocrine disorders would be prime examples of psychophysiological disorders. This is indeed the case in psychosocial dwarfism, where we can substantiate both psychosocial factors (neglect) and measurable endocrine abnormalities (growth hormone releasing factor). However, such is not always the case, and *diabetes mellitus* is an example of how tenuous the primary contribution of psychosocial conditions may be. The only psychophysiological correlation that is reasonably well established is the role of intrafamilial psychosocial stress (of any nature) in both hyperglycemia and ketoacidosis. However, diabetes mellitus is an "almost psychophysiological" disorder, in that the disease makes such emotional demands on the child and the family that it sets up a reverberating circuit involving emotions, insulin production, and diet.

Faced with a child whose health and, indeed, life are often in precarious balance, the parents of a diabetic child are prey to conflicting feelings of extreme, yet realistic anguish about the child's safety on one hand and anger and frustration on the other. The question "Why does this have to happen to our child?" alternates with anger and overprotective attitudes. As a result, the child's normal reactions cannot always be taken as such or responded to normally. Normal oppositional behavior may result in refusal to adhere to the dietary regimen; therefore, the parents have difficulty in allowing typical assertion of independence and may smother the child with regimentation.

Behavioral difficulties may, however, simply coexist with diabetes. For example, the child may be hyperactive, and the parents may attribute this to the diabetes mellitus. Therefore, the consequences of the diabetes mellitus usually call for more psychiatric intervention than the issue of psychogenic factors that produce or exacerbate the diabetes.

PHYSICAL ILLNESS:
CHILDREN'S REACTIONS TO PHYSICAL ILLNESS
AND HOSPITALIZATION

We will address this topic in two phases: first a brief overview of children's reactions to physical illness and hospitalization, and then a detailed discussion of an example of an illness that has both acute and chronic features as well as hospitalization. That example will be congenital heart disease.

GENERAL OVERVIEW OF CHILDREN'S RESPONSES TO ILLNESS

Acute and chronic physical illness cause both disorganization of the child's life and reorganization around the illness. The latter is an adaptive process.

The disorganization finds expression in a variety of psychiatric symptoms, chief among which is regression. Regression manifests itself in the loss of previously acquired mastery, such as enuresis, encopresis, sleeping difficulties, and clinging or separation anxiety. Other common symptoms are generalized anxiety, hyperactivity, and depressed mood.

The reorganization or adaptation around the physical illness occurs in both acute and chronic physical illness, but is more pronounced in chronic illness because the need for adaptation is greater.

There are two healthy strategies for adapting to acute illness: withdrawal into illness, with resulting conservation of emotional energy, on the one hand, and a "healthy, transient, adaptive regression" or "regression in the service of the ego" (Kris, 1952), on the other. The child showing the latter becomes demanding and lets his parents fret and worry, almost so as not to have to do it himself or herself. Again, this supports the child's recovery by conserving emotional energy.

Adaptation to chronic illness takes the form of chronic adjustment disorders with varying manifestations, including Anxiety, Depression, Conduct Disorder and Conversion Disorder. Because of the chronicity of the underlying disease, the child's mode of adapting to illness may become incorporated into the child's personality—the least desirable form of adaptation.

Adaptive mechanisms also are called into play when the child is hospitalized. As with the adaptations to the illness itself, hospitalization results in regression with a variety of ramifications and in reactions to a strange and threatening environment, usually associated with separation from the parents.

All responses to physical illness and hospitalization are predicated on the child's basic reactivity pattern, past development with its fixations and vulnerabilities, and the reactions of the parents. Therefore, management of these responses is directed at the child and the parents, and the hospital environment needs to be in better harmony with the child's psychosocial needs. These needs are a function of the child's age, with the youngest children calling for the most radical modifications of hospital routines— for instance, allowing a parent to stay with the child almost around the clock.

THE CHILD WITH PHYSICAL DISABILITY

Physical disabilities can be divided into two categories: those that are present since birth (congenital) and those that occur at any other point in the child's life (acquired).

Generally speaking, adjustment to a congenital handicap is easier on every-body (child and parents) than adjustment to a suddenly acquired handicap. However, the most significant determinant of psychiatric sequelae is brain damage: physical disorders that cause damage to the central nervous system are more likely to result in psychiatric difficulties than those that do not. Meningo-encephalitis of infectious origin, brain tumors, and head trauma are prime examples of such disease.

Epilepsy is a disorder that causes psychosocial difficulties both because of the organic disorder and because of the child's altered self-image and parental reactions. The organic disorder probably accounts for the impulsivity and poor judgment frequently shown by these children; these difficulties may be precipi-tated and exacerbated by anxiety in the parents and by family disruption. These children frequently have severe Conduct and Attention–Deficit Hyperactivity Disorders. According to Rutter's (1981) Isle of Wight study, psychiatric disorder was twice as frequent in children with illness involving the central nervous system as in normal children or children with physical disorders not involving the brain.

A special case of a physical handicap is a sensory deficit, deafness, or blindness. Depending on the age of onset, and on whether the disease process causing the deafness or blindness involved damage to the rest of the central nervous system, the ravages of a sensory handicap may be grave. A case in point is the following:

Case 18-6   Rollo was three-and-a-half years old when he had severe *meningo-encephalitis,* which resulted in *total deafness.* He had acquired an age-appropriate amount of *speech* (words and short phrases) which subsequently deteriorated. When he was seen for psychiatric consultation, he was 11 years old and in fourth grade. He was a bright boy and fluently communicated with the examiner by writing. *His parents and the school system* were involved in a chronic *fight* over the *use of sign language:* the school urged the use of sign language, but the parents sided with Rollo's wishes to be *"like the other kids."* Rollo tried his best to read lips, but his *attention span was short* and he was *impulsive* and very *easily frustrated;* as a result, he kept falling behind academically, and everybody was getting more and more upset about him and with him. Rollo could not bear this: his temper tantrums became *destructive episodes,* and he alternated between *aggressive outbursts* against his parents, and regressive *clinging* to them. He became progressively more isolated from his peers.

Comment. The child's language development, interrupted by deafness, suffered. He was caught in a conflict between two approaches: the apparent "normality" of lipreading, and the visibly different, but more efficient and effective sign language, which facilitates communication, if not speaking. The illness that had brought on his deafness also produced an Attention–Deficit Hyperactivity Disorder, which made his adjustment even more difficult, and which made the lack of agreement between school and parents all the more counterproductive.

Similarly, blindness that strikes before solid acquisition of spoken and written language occurs will disrupt the child's development, but not as severely as deafness.

Both deafness and blindness are better integrated and less disruptive if they arise in a family in which both parents have the same handicap (i.e., both parents are deaf, or blind, respectively). It is as if the parents can help to instill the skills and compensations that their child needs; this is similar to ways in which sighted and hearing parents transmit coping skills to their children.

Parental attitudes and management are of paramount importance in all situations entailing children suffering from physical diseases and handicaps. Overprotectiveness, lack of normal structure and deficient limit setting are particular dangers for the child with cancer or equivalent disease, such as cystic fibrosis.

These and similar parental attitudes should be the prime focus of psychiatric intervention with physically handicapped children. Treatment of the child will vary with the underlying disease and the nature of the handicap, whereas the treatment of the parents is more uniform and follows this common denominator of attitudinal and behavior change. Parental counseling often needs to be combined with school consultation, so that teachers and other school professionals can mobilize their skills towards the child's overall development.

The goal of treatment, as in other childhood disorders, is to safeguard the child's development in spite of the handicapping disorder.

Questions for Study and Action

1. The consulting neurologist has made a diagnosis of "hysteria" and "nothing but hysterical symptoms" in your 11-year-old patient. The symptom picture is confusing and the neurologist is really quite pleased with himself for finally "solving the case" and proving that this patient has led you down the garden path. How would you deal with this situation?

2. An eight-year-old boy has had a sudden onset of aphonia (inability to use his voice), without previous hoarseness or other symptoms. As a matter of fact, the problem literally arose overnight. You feel you have made a good case for "hysterical aphonia" on the basis of the child's and the family's psychodynamics. Medical,

neurological, and ear-nose-and-throat evaluations have revealed no organic pathology. You want to proceed with treatment, but the parents insist that there must be something physically wrong. Outline several approaches you can take.

3. A 10-year-old girl has developed diplopia and occasional difficulties with gait, over the last six to nine months. She is seductive, and very dramatic about her symptoms. Outline a *complete* diagnostic evaluation plan. Suppose all neurological and other medical evaluations come back without organic findings, what would you do? Is one set of evaluations at one point in time sufficient? Should the patient be followed at regular intervals? If so, why? Would you have the same feelings about the case discussed in question #2? What is the usual age of onset for symptoms of multiple sclerosis?

4. The pediatrician of a nine-year-old boy with severe bronchial asthma suggests that the boy spend his entire summer vacation in a special camp for asthmatic children. The child resists the idea, the mother is ambivalent, the father says the boy should go. List the pros and cons of such summer programs of parentectomy.

5. The attending surgeon states flatly that psychiatry has no role to play in ulcerative colitis, especially in children. However, the family is worried about a partial colectomy that is being planned for their eight-year-old child with severe ulcerative colitis. Formulate several approaches to how you can help the child and his family—and how you can overcome the surgeon's negative attitude.

6. An 11-year-old girl has periodic attacks of nausea and vomiting, followed by hemicranial, throbbing headaches. She flees into a darkened room and protests loudly against the slightest movement of her bed, e.g., when a parent or sibling sits down on it. Outline the differential diagnosis and treatment plan. If you find psychophysiological connections, would you delve into "lines of petty authority" both at home and at school, and deal with compulsive, rigid, perfectionistic attitudes?

7. How strongly do you feel about the "psychophysiological connection" in diabetes mellitus? Should you look at it etiologically, or should you consider the secondary effects of the disease—interference with independence, self-image, and self-esteem, and family relationships? Review the latest information about the pathophysiological mechanisms in childhood-onset diabetes. Does the complexity of the pathophysiology call for more or less psychological support?

8. Is there a basic contradiction between autoimmune and biopsychosocial explanations of ulcerative colitis? Explain.

9. What sense was there, if any, in the contention by early psychosomaticists that patients with dermatitis had exhibitionistic tendencies? Explain their contention and your own.

10. Would you expect a six-year-old child who saw both her parents gunned down by a mass murderer to have had a Histrionic Personality Disorder prior to developing a Conversion Disorder's blindness? Explain fully.

For Further Reading

Alexander, A.B., Miklich, D.R., & Hershkoff, H. The immediate effects of systematic relaxation training on peak expiratory flow rates in asthmatic children. *Psychosom. Med.*, 34:355–394, 1972.

Allen, L., & Zigler, E. Psychological adjustment of seriously ill children. *J. Amer. Acad. of Child Psychiatry*, 25:708–712, 1986.

Barglow, P., Berndt, D.J., Burns, W.J., & Hatcher, R. Neuroendocrine and psychological factors in childhood diabetes mellitus. *J. Amer. Acad. of Child Psychiatry*, 25:785–793, 1986.

Bearison, D., & Pacifici, C. Psychological studies of children who have cancer. *J. Appl. Develop. Psychol.*, 5:263–280, 1984.

Burns, W., & Zweig, A. Self-concepts of chronically ill children. *J. Genet. Psychol.*, 137:179–190, 1980.

Cassell, S., & Paul, M. The role of puppet therapy on the emotional responses to children hospitalized for cardiac catheterisation. *J. Pediat.*, 71:233–239, 1967.

Delamater, A.M., Rosenbloom, N., Conners, K., & Hertwick, L. The behavioral treatment of hysterical paralysis in a ten-year-old boy. A case study. *J. Amer. Acad. of Child Psychiatry*, 22:73–79, 1983.

Freud, S. On the psychical mechanisms of hysterical phenomena (1893). *Collected Papers, Vol. 1, Paper II.* (Translated by Joan Riviere.) New York: Basic Books, 1959.

Freud, S. Fragment of an analysis of a case of hysteria (1905). *Collected Papers, Vol. 3, Paper I.* (Trans. by Joan Riviere.) New York: Basic Books, 1959.

Freud, S. *An Autobiographical Study* (1925). In J. Strachey (Ed. & Trans.), *Standard Edition, Vol. 20.* London: Hogarth Press, 1953.

Fritz, G.K. Psychosomatic illness review: Childhood asthma. *Psychosomatics*, 24:959–967, 1983.

Gath, A., Smith, M.A., & Baum, J.D. Emotional, behavioral and educational disorders in diabetic children. *Arch. Dis. Child*, 55:371–375, 1980.

Gayton, W.F., & Friedman, S.B. Psychosocial aspects of cystic fibrosis: A review of the literature. *Amer. J. Dis. Child*, 126:856–859, 1973.

Goodwin, J., Simms, M., & Bergman, R. Hysterical seizures: A sequel to incest. *Am. J. Orthopsychiatry*, 49:697–703, 1979.

Goodyer, I. Hysterical conversion reactions in childhood. *J. Child Psychol. Psychiatry*, 22:179–188, 1981.

Henning, J., & Fritz, G.K. School reentry in childhood cancer. *Psychosomatics*, 24:261–269, 1983.

Koon, R.E. Conversion dysphagia in children. *Psychosomatics*, 24:182–184, 1983.

Kris, E. On preconscious mental processes. In E. Kris, *Psychoanalytic Exploration in Art.* New York: International Universities Press, 1952, pp. 303–318.

Lask, B., & Matthew, D. Childhood asthma—a controlled trial of family psychotherapy. *Arch Dis. Child,* 54:116–119, 1979.

McDermott, J., & Finch, S. Ulcerative colitis in children: Reassessment of a dilemma. *J. Amer. Acad. of Child Psychiatry,* 6:512–525, 1967.

Meadow, K.P., Greenberg, M.T., & Erting, C. Attachment behavior of deaf children with deaf parents. *J. Amer. Acad. of Child Psychiatry,* 22:23–28, 1983.

Minuchin, S., Baker, L., Rosman, B.L., et al. A conceptual model of psychosomatic illness in children. *Arch. Gen. Psychiatry,* 32:1031–1038, 1975.

Ravenscroft, K. Psychiatric consultation to the child with acute physical trauma. *Am. J. Orthopsychiatry,* 52:298, 1982.

Rutter, M. Psychological sequelae of brain damage in childhood. *Am. J. Psychiatry,* 138:1533–1544, 1981.

Stores, G. School children with epilepsy at risk for learning and behavior problems. *Develop. Med. Child Neurol.,* 20:502–508, 1978.

19

Adjustment Disorders

As we have done throughout this text, we now take the DSM-III-R definition as our modus operandi, but, especially in this chapter, we will include as much as possible of the wealth of clinical and developmental knowledge accumulated by clinicians under labels other than "Adjustment Disorders." Therefore, a glossary of synonyms will be presented after the main definitions. We consider Adjustment Disorder in this section on Feeling Disorders because the emotional content of the disorder is often so conspicuous.

DEFINITION

Before we present the formal definition, here is an informal one: an Adjustment Disorder is a reaction to a stressor that is meaningful and specific to the child; the reaction, in turn, is specific to the stress. The reaction must have happened in sufficiently close temporal relationship to the stress and is more than an expected, "healthy" reaction; it temporarily interferes with the child's development and psychosocial functioning, but is ultimately reversible following removal of the stressor or following such further maturation of the child that enables the child to master it without being "derailed."

Therefore, the basic definition of Adjustment Disorder is that it is a maladap-

283

tive reaction to an identifiable psychosocial stressor occurring within three months after the onset of the stressor (DSM-III-R). The reaction must be causally related to the stressor (Group for the Advancement of Psychiatry, 1966) and has to allow ongoing, further, normal development once the stressor has been removed (Neubauer, 1972).

Many conditions can be stressors, and they may be single or multiple, recurrent or continuous. The stressor may arise internally in the child, such as illness, or externally, such as death of a parent or any event that has specific significance for the child's mental functioning.

The child's reaction to the stressor must be maladaptive, i.e., pathological, and not merely be any and every response. It is therefore reflected in impairment in social functioning or symptoms that are in excess of a normal and expected reaction to the stressor (DSM-III-R).

DSM-III-R has also continued the tradition of previous classifications which categorized Adjustment Disorders as "transient situational disorders": once the stressor ceases, the disorder will remit as well.

In 1966, the Group for the Advancement of Psychiatry (GAP) published a proposed classification of childhood disorders. There, adjustment disorders were by-and-large equivalent to "reactive disorders," most of which were considered transient; however, the GAP classification allowed for some of them to become chronic. One of the most important aspects of this classification is its emphasis on the child's endowment, his/her dynamic history, and the impact of the stressor on the child's *development.* Interference with the child's development is, therefore, one of the hallmarks in distinguishing reactive disorders, i.e., Adjustment Disorders, from healthy responses.

DSM-III-R adds the predominant symptom to the words "adjustment disorder," e.g., Adjustment Disorder with Physical Complaints.

OTHER RELATED TERMS

The following is a list of terms that may be considered as roughly synonymous with Adjustment Disorder.

Reactive disorder: This is the GAP (1966) term and is defined as "a manifestation of a predominantly *conscious* conflict between the child's drives and feelings and his social environment; . . . it does not include those disorders which have developed into a structuralized psychoneurosis, a personality disorder with fixed patterns, or a psychosis" (p. 222). The reactive disorder must be "*causally* related to the specific (emotionally traumatic) event, not just coincident with *it*" (p. 222) (italics added). This definition further clarifies these disorders from a psychodynamic point of view.

Situational disorder is defined as a reaction to environmental pathology in excess of that associated with normal development. This definition stresses the impact of life stresses or crises on development (Settlage, 1964).

Developmental interference: This definition deals with the impact of gross external interferences with certain needs and rights of the child, and the fact that the child may not have the developmental ability to deal with these interferences. The child then reacts with abnormal manifestations which in many instances resemble neurotic conflict (Nagera, 1966).

If we look at it further in a developmental light, Adjustment Disorder permits ongoing development once the stress is removed (Kessler, 1966; Neubauer, 1972), which brings us back to the definition emphasizing the transient nature of the disorder under salutary circumstances.

Some authors formerly included Post-traumatic Stress Disorders (PTSD) with the reactive disorders. Nowadays, DSM-III-R has made a distinction between PTSD and Adjustment Disorder. (See under "Differential Diagnosis" in this chapter and "Post-traumatic Stress Disorder" in Chapters 17 and 36.)

ETIOLOGY AND PATHOGENESIS

The pathogenesis of Adjustment Disorder is represented by the interaction of two etiological factors: the noxious psychosocial stressor and the vulnerability of the host child. Certainly, some stressors are traumatic for just about every child because of their nature or extent, e.g., severe deprivation, witnessing murder, severe abuse, massive bodily or psychic trauma. However, in most instances the traumatic or stressful nature of the event will be governed by the child's vulnerability. This means that a stressor that may not produce a disorder in one child will produce an Adjustment Disorder in another child because it means serious disruption in the child's equilibrium.

The child's vulnerability is predicated on constitutional–temperamental factors on one hand and experiential factors on the other. An additional issue is the phase and harmony of the child's development.

Constitutional factors consist of the degree of development of basic ego functions (perception, memory, mobility, etc.), ability to postpone gratification, and the extent of the "protective barrier." The latter is a concept, first proposed by Freud, of a constitutional barrier against stimuli. If this barrier is insufficient (if the child is "thin-skinned"), the vulnerability is greater.

Temperament is another aspect of the constitutional "given" of the child. Whether the child will withdraw from stressors, adapt well or poorly, preserve stable mood and the usual biological rhythm (e.g., eating, sleeping) are among the main characteristics of temperament contributing to vulnerability (these are among the criteria first described by Thomas and Chess [1968, 1977]).

Experiential factors are many, and include, among others, past trauma, the nature and extent of parental support or protection, and the quality and amount of gratification of impulses. Excessive protection from "ordinary" stress, for instance, leaves the child unprepared, "unimmunized," and thus more vulnerable. Too ready a gratification of the child's instinctual wishes may equally predispose the child to greater vulnerability.

Among experiential factors, the family holds a central place. Not only may the family be the direct cause of the Adjustment Disorder by providing the stressor (e.g., divorce, parental illness, parental psychopathology in general), but also the family is an integral part of the child's adaptive functioning and contributes in many ways to the formation of the Adjustment Disorder. It is impossible to list all these ways without creating an unwieldly confusing mass: the clinician will simply add his or her generic understanding of family dynamics to the formulation of the case and will find that the pieces will fall into place.

Whenever we think of vulnerability, we always have to keep in mind not only the level of development, but also the relationship of its different parts; discrepancy between them increases the vulnerability. An example is the child with advanced motor development but few restraints and immature judgment; immobilization by a cast for a fracture is more likely to lead to an Adjustment Disorder in this child than in one with a more harmonious relationship among his or her developmental components.

Our final statement on the etiology and pathogenesis of these disorders is that psychodynamically they are a coping act between the child's ego, on one hand, and a stressor that is external to that ego, on the other. Adjustment Disorders are *not* intrapsychic (i.e., internalized) conflicts. They are a "face-off" between the child's "equipment," (i.e., the child's ego) and the external world, with symptoms partially dictated by that ego's level of development.

CLINICAL DESCRIPTION

We shall present a series of case vignettes to illustrate the wide variety of the symptoms of Adjustment Disorder.

CASE 19-1   Steven, age eight, had become progressively more *listless* and *morose following the separation of his parents.* The father moved out and maintained sporadic contact with Steven. The child's *school performance deteriorated,* and he was often caught *daydreaming* or engaged in *disruptive* teasing of his friends.

This went on for *almost half a year,* at the end of which the parents, after marital counseling, reunited. However, Steven's problems did not remit right away, and he was brought for psychiatric consultation. This showed that Steven was not sure that the present state of relative marital harmonly between his parents would last, but he was *not hopeless.* He felt some guilt about his role in the parents' arguments, but generally did *not* feel that "nobody likes me" or that he had no friends or could not do better schoolwork.

He was seen in brief psychotherapy and *improved*.

Comment. The diagnosis here is Adjustment Disorder with Depressed Mood (309.00). Depression is present and has lasted for a considerable time (six months), but other, essential criteria for affective (depressive) disorder are missing or only partially present: guilt, low self-esteem, hopelessness, and helplessness. Improvement in the child's environment, i.e., removal of the psychosocial stressor, plus brief psychotherapy, reversed the disorder.

CASE 19-2   Billy was five years old when his mother sought help at the social services agency because he had "developed into a monster." Mother reported that the child's stepfather was becoming increasingly *harsh and abusive in disciplining* the child, especially when the stepfather was *drunk*, which was, by now, happening quite often.

Billy was *capriciously beating* on two younger siblings. He would also stage *destructive* battles with neighboring children in which he did considerable *damage* to *his own as well as a neighbor's house.* The neighbors were up in arms because Billy was showing a "Jekyll and Hyde personality," being friendly one moment and becoming *hyperactive, aggressive, and uncontrollable* the next, usually *when he did not get his way.*

The stepfather proved to be impervious to all attempts to induce him to stop drinking; the charge of child abuse resulted in *parental separation.* Billy spent several weeks attending a summer day camp run by a church group which emphasized the outdoors and getting along with each other. By the end of the summer, he had regained much of his previous, better disposition.

Comment. The Diagnosis in this case is Adjustment Disorder with Disturbance of Conduct (309.30). We see a clear violation of the rights of others, apparently in the typical psychodynamic attempt to turn passive suffering (of abuse by stepfather) into active mastery (aggression against siblings, destructiveness). All of this occurred in response to abusive handling and abated after removal of the abuser and then *environmental treatment* (summer camp).

CASE 19-3   Kimberly, age six, was brought to the child psychiatrist's office by a distraught and worried mother. The child had *fallen* off a ledge near her house while "fooling around" with several friends and had sustained a Colles' fracture. Although the fracture had *by now healed* and the cast been removed, Kimberly continued to be quite *fearful of* any situation where there existed the slightest chance of falling. She had become *generally anxious*, had developed *nightmares,* and kept *clinging and hanging* onto her mother when called upon to join peers, especially if the proposed activity looked "rambunctious" to her.

During her first two sessions with the psychiatrist, Kimberly recalled her *fear of getting hurt,* which both preceded and followed the incident. Her grandmother, who lived in a little "apartment" adjacent to her house, had plied her with horror stories of accidents that could befall people who are not cautious.

However, in subsequent sessions the child concentrated on more pleasant scenes: the *good times* she had with *her friends,* and the things they had gotten away with, after all, except for the accident. She was *not* afraid for her mother's safety when she clung to her, but for her own. Little by little, she rejoined her group of friends in their activities, and her anxiety subsided.

Comment. The diagnosis is Adjustment Disorder with Anxious Mood (309.24). The affective symptom is that of anxiety and there is a clear relationship to the precipitating stressor. The patient has been made vulnerable by her grand-mother; her clinging behavior is not separation anxiety, but rather an avoidance reaction based on anticipatory fear. Psychodynamic elaboration and fixing of the anxiety are lacking, and she is able to overcome the anxiety with brief psychotherapy. Her world, although shaken, remains intact.

CASE 19-4   Carl had just turned six years of age when he was *placed in a foster home.* His parents had led *disruptive* lives, with frequent episodes of *neglecting* Carl. Nevertheless, the child, surprisingly, did not appear to suffer from signifi-cant psychiatric difficulties with the exception of stealing, but mother's increas-ingly frequent *alcoholic* binges and father's *erratic* presence necessitated foster-home placement.

Carl *obviously resented this intervention.* The foster mother tried to make him feel at home, but *he kept mostly to himself.* The foster home was fortunately located in the same school district in which he had lived before. Carl had *related well* to his kindergarten teacher and had friends among his peers, although his forays into their lunches or other possessions had caused trouble.

Following his foster-home placement, Carl became *bad-tempered and played less and less* with his classmates in school. He made no attempt to strike up friend-ships with neighborhood peers and kept largely *aloof* from the other children in the foster home.

When this state of affairs continued for several weeks, the foster mother and the caseworker decided something was not right, and Carl was brought to the mental health center.

Carl's statements, and especially his play with a castle and an array of "Fisher-Price people," communicated his feelings *of anger* at having had his world disrupted and of the *loneliness* he felt. No significant feelings of sadness were found, nor was Carl hopeless about the prospects of ultimately living with his parents again. He protested he had been used to being left alone by his parents and he could manage all right, without being stuck into a foster home.

Comment. The diagnosis is Adjustment Disorder with Withdrawal (309.83). The absence of sadness and other aspects of affective response rules out the diagnosis of depressed mood, which would be the main differential diagnostic consideration.

The other subcategories of Adjustment Disorders are self-explanatory: either combinations of the preponderant symptoms or another predominant symptom such as academic inhibition. The latter is occasionally found in and of itself in children, but is more often part of the other dominant syndromes.

DIFFERENTIAL DIAGNOSIS

Put most simply, we have to distinguish between disorders that are milder than Adjustment Disorders, and those that are more serious.

Healthy Responses	Adjustment Disorder (Transient, Reversible, "Fluid")	Fixed Psychopathology (Anxiety Disorder, Depression, Personality Disorder)

The disorders that are "less" or milder than Adjustment Disorders are represented by healthy responses. These are usually divided into developmental crises and situational crises. The former do not enter into the differential diagnosis with Adjustment Disorders, since the psychosocial stressor is absent; developmental crises include such known reactions to developmental "nodal points" as the eight-month anxiety and the normal phobias of the three-to-five-year-old, but recovery quickly ensues and the child's overall response is wholesome and salutary.

Situational crises are normal adaptive responses that are expected reactions to a stressor which is generally recognized as a stressor. In other words, we would expect such a stressor to cause a reaction in every child. An example would be a grief reaction to the death of a parent: uncomplicated bereavement.

The feature that differentiates healthy responses from adjustment disorder is the lack of developmental impairment in the former: the child's social or academic or emotional functioning stays basically the same. Much of the research on how situational crises beset children is reported under the research categories of "stressful life events" or "life crisis units."

On the other side of the differential diagnostic balance (i.e., the more serious side), there are all the disorders listed as "Fixed Psychopathology," that is, the disorders are no longer transient or reversible, but have become internalized and part of the child's "fixed" psychic structure.

Consequently, the differential diagnostic process should mainly consist of ascertaining the inner structure and the completeness of the dominant symptom picture. Thus, to differentiate Adjustment Disorder with Anxious Mood from Anxiety Disorder, we address not only the extent and severity of the symptoms, not only the extent of interference in social functioning and development, but also, whenever possible, what primary and secondary neurotic gain and what symbolism have been caused by the neurotic compromise that underlies the Anxiety Disorder. As mentioned, the rule of thumb is that Adjustment Disorders do not represent internalized conflicts and show no primary or secondary gain and no symbolism.

A similar differential-diagnostic procedure can be adopted for other disorders by looking for what is typical for that particular disorder: helplessness-hopelessness and guilt in Depression, and pervasive difficulties in interpersonal respect and relatedness in Conduct Disorders.

Among the more severe disorders is also Post-traumatic Stress Disorder (PTSD), considered in Chapters 17 and 36. As in Adjustment Disorders, PTSD is the child's severe reaction to an external stressor; PTSD is not an internalized disorder even though it may be incapacitating. The differential diagnosis should be based on: 1) the difference in the stressor: it is universally acknowledged to be extraordinary and overwhelming in PTSD, but often subtle and highly personal in Adjustment Disorders; 2) the difference in the symptoms shown: PTSD is characterized by the reexperiencing of the traumatic event by the child, either in intrusive memories or in nightmares, in addition to the fear of recurrence of the trauma and a gamut of behavioral, somatic, and psychosomatic symptoms. In truth, other serious "reactive stress disorders" that we can diagnose (DSM-III-R) include Reactive Attachment Disorder of Infancy or Early Childhood (RADIEC), and Brief Reactive Psychosis.

Special note on Axis IV

Each estimate of the severity of psychosocial or biopsychosocial stressors can be recorded on Axis IV when we use DSM-III-R. The further we can go in giving a quantitative weight to the diverse stresses that we have specified, the better it is for our work. Using the Stressful Life Events scales for children, which have been devised by the child psychiatrist, R. Dean Coddington (1972), is one option to be taken, much benefiting our nosology and psychopathology. It would be wise to record the total score attained by any child on such an instrument, thereby giving the raw data from which one's overall estimate was derived.

The student should be mindful of the basic epidemiology of psychosocial stressors imposed on children. Not all individuals are equally vulnerable to stresses. For example, only the children in our society can be physically beaten with impunity (as will be dealt with in Section D of Part II, Being Victimized). Further, in childhood the male seems to be more often prey to stressors, yet during adult life it is the female. Other population groups (please note how often the groups include or describe children) who are at greater risk of morbidity resulting from psychosocial stresses would encompass:

- members of minority groups oppressed by discrimination
- lower-class persons
- persons with few social skills
- those with low self-esteem
- those with low sense of self-direction
- those with uncertain social support networks (Pearlin, 1982)
- those with genetic vulnerability (e.g., to alcoholism, sociopathy, mood disorders)

In short, the child's diagnosis should include considerable information concerning the child's stresses (rather more than less), recalling what the poet Gwendolyn Brooks wrote of Chicago's poor black child: "His lesions are legion, But reaching is his rule."

Adjustment Disorder is *not* a "wastebasket diagnosis," but a developmentally and psychodynamically defined entity. Properly understood, the categorization of Adjustment Disorder is highly useful for correct treatment planning.

TREATMENT

The foregoing consideration of pathogenesis is very important to the treatment of Adjustment Disorders. Again, here is an example of the need to diagnose a disorder "in depth and breadth": the developmental status of the child, the past track record of coping with stress, the overall meaning of the psychosocial stressor, plus the child's conception (or sometimes misconception) of the stressor and its context. Once this kind of diagnostic work has been done, the rest follows naturally (if not easily!).

The treatment frequently employed is some form of focused, brief psychotherapy. This should target the interface between the child's coping mechanism and the psychosocial stressor. The specific techniques will vary considerably, and the clinician should be eclectic and choose the most appropriate approach. Involvement of the family will similarly vary according to several factors, such as the child's age, the nature of the family's functions, their closeness, and their psychological assets.

It follows that the correct and effective treatment of Adjustment Disorders is a task often calling for considerable clinical maturity and expertise, underscoring the fact that these disorders cannot be taken lightly or considered easy to treat. Many, if not most, should probably be referred to a child specialist.

We will use the case examples in the preceding (diagnostic) section to illustrate the basics of individual psychotherapy.

CASE 19-1   *Adjustment Disorder with Depressed Mood:* Steven's treatment focused on his perception that "you can never tell what parents are up to" and the possible consequences, to him, of any potential future split between them. His natural wish to have both parents was recognized, but a series of "contingency plans" was introduced: "What if it happens again?" The attitude was taken, and Steven encouraged to consider it, that he was quite a capable boy who could deal with some adversity, utilizing his age-appropriate good functioning.

CASE 19-2   *Adjustment Disorder with Disturbance of Conduct:* Billy was a child who was neither aggressive nor basically vindictive and he had a fairly healthy ego. Therefore, his behavior was reversible with environmental manipulation (structure) only after the noxious factor (the abusive stepfather) had been removed.

CASE 19-3   *Adjustment Disorder with Anxious Mood:* The treatment with Kimberly, the six-year-old girl who had fallen off a ledge, focused on her fears of bodily harm and on the "natural" counterbalance to such fears: mastery of similar situations through her own skills, as well as the fact that good times could be had with peers without getting into trouble and without getting hurt. No attempts were made at environmental manipulations—the relationship with grandmother was not laden with pathology—and removing the old lady from the premises would have been a therapeutic overreaction.

CASE 19-4   *Adjustment Disorder with Withdrawal:* Play therapy with Carl concentrated on feelings of anger and what a child can do with them—just "sit there by yourself and stew and brood or mingle with the others, such as the little toy figures could do. Occasionally, they (toy figures) shouted and showed in other ways that they were angry, but they still talked to one another. . . . Perhaps just always staying by yourself, being alone, makes you miss mom and dad even more, and you get angrier at everybody who took you away from them, even foster mother. . . . "

The variations on psychotherapeutic techniques in cases such as the ones illustrated above are legion, and the practitioner must follow his own style. The principle is the appeal to the healthy parts of the patient's ego so that the child can master the psychological reverberations of the noxious stressor.

We have illustrated the individual brief psychotherapeutic approach and the approach of environmental manipulation based on thorough understanding of the child's strengths and weaknesses. Obviously, a disorder for which the role of the family is so important will lend itself to family or conjoint approaches, and the practitioner should feel encouraged to be pragmatic and inventive.

When a clinician is most skilled in, and comfortable with, behavior modification, he or she can apply this approach judiciously with both the child and the parents, as long as the technique is not used thoughtlessly and mechanistically.

In summary, the *goal* of treatment is to ensure that the child's further development is not significantly worsened by the stressor and that, indeed, the child learns by this experience and grows.

PROGNOSIS

Since most cases of Adjustment Disorder are transient (i.e., reversible), the prognosis is generally favorable—especially with skillful treatment. What will negatively affect the prognosis is any fixation and internalization of the transient Adjustment Disorder into a more permanent disease, such as neurosis or personality disorder.

The factors contributing to the "binding" of the adjustment reaction into more fixed and serious psychopathology are:

- *Age*—The older the child and the more his or her mental apparatus is developed, the greater the possibility of internalizing the "face-off" of the Adjustment Disorder.
- *The state of the "protective barrier" and vulnerability*—The implications are obvious.
- *The state of the family*—Neurotic or depressed parents or those with Personality Disorders that clearly *affect their parenting* will "cement" and solidify the Adjustment Disorder of their child.
- *The severity of developmental disorganization, arrest or regression.*
- *Acuteness of onset*—The sudden onset of a stressor does not give the child time to adapt.
- *The duration of the stressor*—If the stressor lasts beyond the adaptive capabilities of the child, maladaptive (i.e., *pathological*) defenses will be formed.

Once the Adjustment Disorder has been "internalized" or "structuralized," the prognosis is equivalent to that of the "fixed" disorder: Anxiety Disorder, Depression, Personality Disorder, and so on.

Finally, we would like to underscore once again the importance of the Adjustment Disorders. If they are attended to, i.e., fully diagnosed and treated early enough when necessary, their transient nature ensures a certain benignity of outcome—though never a freedom from suffering for the child.

Questions for Study and Action

1. Name three contributing conditions to these facts: children are more often reported by mental health workers to have suffered psychosocial stresses than are adults; many child guidance or child psychiatry clinics affix the diagnostic codes of Adjustment Disorder of one or another type to children more often than any other diagnostic label; Adjustment Disorders that are treated are less permanent than neuroses or personality disorders.

2. Name three "reactive disorders" that are nonpsychotic, one that is psychotic, and take care that all are more severe than Adjustment Disorders.

3. Outline the relevant components of a diagnostic workup for a child whose history and mental status point towards the diagnosis of Adjustment Disorder.

4. Why and how may each of the following predispose a child to Adjustment Disorder?
   (a) being adopted
   (b) moving to another state
   (c) a death in the family
   (d) mental retardation
   (e) having major epilepsy

5. Give the differential diagnosis of a child who witnessed his father murder his mother and now seems to meet the criteria of Adjustment Disorder with Mixed Emotional Features.

6. By what logic would you anticipate that most 10-year-olds diagnosed as Adjustment Disorder with Disturbance of Conduct and left untreated will be diagnosed as Antisocial Personality Disorder on 15-year follow-up? Explain.

7. Map out the several components of a comprehensive treatment plan for Carl (Case 19-4). Note especially environmental changes.

8. Outline a rational and comprehensive treatment plan for Billy (Case 19-2).

9. Can you make a convincing case that children are at greater risk of morbidity from stresses than adults? Attempt to do so.

10. What is the difference between a "psychosocial stressor" and "psychic trauma"?

For Further Reading

Coddington, R.D. The significance of life events as etiologic factors in the diseases of children, I: A survey of professional workers. *J. Psychosomatic Res.*, 16:17–18, 1972.

Group for the Advancement of Psychiatry (GAP). *Psychopathological Disorders in Childhood: Theoretical Considerations and a Proposed Classification.* Vol. VI, Report No. 62. New York: Brunner/Mazel, 1966.

Kessler, J.W. *Psychopathology of Childhood.* Englewood Cliffs, N.J.: Prentice-Hall, 1966.

Nagera, H.D. *Early Childhood Disturbances, the Infantile Neurosis, and the Adulthood Disturbances.* New York: International Universities Press, 1966.

Neubauer, P. Normal development in children. In B. Wolman (Ed.), *Manual of Child Psychopathology.* New York: McGraw-Hill, 1972.

Pearlin, L.L. The social contexts of stress. In L. Goldberger & S. Breznitz (Eds.), *The Handbook of Stress.* New York: The Free Press, 1982.

Settlage, C. Psychoanalytic theory in relation to the nosology of childhood disorders. *J. Amer. Psychoanalytic Assn.*, 12:776–801, 1964.

Thomas, A., Chess, S., & Birch, H.G. *Temperament and Behavior Disorders in Children.* New York: New York University Press, 1968.

Thomas, A., & Chess, S. *Temperament and Development.* New York: Brunner/Mazel, 1977.

SECTION C

THINKING AND CENTRAL PROCESSING DISORDERS

This section is devoted to disorders that permeate the child's styles of adaptation and coping in the world, sometimes constricting the child's competence rather severely and at other times (as in the Personality Disorders) seeming less grossly debilitating but creating a considerable unhappiness for the affected child and those who give care to the child. Hence, we have brought together in this section the mainly cognitive disturbances, all the disorders that have a thought disorder prominent in their symptoms, along with those disorders showing general developmental delays and derangements.

We are cognizant of the way that DSM-III-R deals with the Developmental Disorders of Children and find it appropriately sensible: all the Developmental Disorders, including Pervasive and Specific Developmental Disorders and Mental Retardation, are coded as Axis II diagnoses, along with the Personality Disorders. Personality Disorders are now applicable to children—all except Antisocial Personality that still requires a minimum age of 18 years. In essence, then, we have placed all these disorders under our rubric of Thinking and Central Processing Disorders, but in addition we have included Organic Mental Syndromes and the psychoses. We think that this way of treating these disorders makes sense, although we know that, at heart, diagnostic classification is rather arbitrary and based on convention and consensus. What we have done is not very startling and may have some merit, we hope.

20

Personality Disorders

ETIOLOGY AND PATHOGENESIS

Believing that human suffering, when it is in the form of psychoneuroses and personality disorders, and even in very partial forms or prodromes of neuroses and personality problems, was played down in DSM-III, many have clamored for a nosology that gives more attention to difficulties less gross than psychoses and mood disorders. DSM-III-R might have done that sufficiently to satisfy some of DSM-III's critics. In any event, there are nine types of Personality Disorders that we cover in a preliminary way in this chapter.

"A personality disorder is not a mental illness," some purists have always insisted, because they reason as Harry Stack Sullivan did when he said of the obsessional neurotic, *"He does not have a good time, but he could have a much worse time."* In truth, many who have neuroses *and* Personality Disorders have a horrible time.

DSM-III was reluctant to have a diagnosis of a Personality Disorder made on persons below 18 years of age, but DSM-III-R removed that age specification on all Personality Disorders except Antisocial Personality Disorder. If personality problems create problems for adult nosology, for child classifications they almost create nightmares. Childhood is a time of passage, not of staying put; thus children's psychopathology is often too fluid to fit categories that are useful with adults.

Most child psychiatrists would consider it foolish to diagnose a child under six or seven years of age as having a Personality Disorder. The incidence would increase, but very little, up to the time that childhood ends (at 11 or 12) and increase more noticeably during adolescence and young adulthood. How did these personality troubles worm their way into the nosology of childhood disorders? Mainly because they entail suffering.

Wilhelm Reich, despite his subsequent bad press, was well-received when, in the 1920s, he was the first psychoanalyst to describe and treat character neuroses (as he called Personality Disorders) in adults. They could be called latent neuroses because, in lieu of manifesting neurotic symptoms, they appear as overly rigid armoring of the personality (or character or personal lifestyle). They are like personal traits that have overshot their mark and, instead of being part of a comfortable ego-syntonic style as they formerly were, they become, like an illness, sources of inner distress and of impaired functioning at work or home. Since Personality Disorders are malfunctions of the entire psychobiological unit in its interpersonal context, we have included them with other disorders of higher mental functioning, "Thinking and Central Processing Disorders" (Section C), but it should be remembered that they are less severe than the psychotic, organic, and pervasive developmental disturbances also included in Section C. These exaggerated personal traits are all coded on Axis II in DSM-III-R, "Developmental Disorders and Personality Disorders," including Mental Retardation, Specific Developmental Disorders, Pervasive Developmental Disorders, and Personality Disorders. DSM-III-R holds out, as shared features of all these Axis II disorders, their childhood or adolescence onset, with stable persistence on into the adult years. Hence, according to DSM-III-R conceptualization, we are trying to consider Personality Disorders in their early forms—*in statu nascendi*—in this chapter.

Inadequate knowledge prevents our giving proper attention to various etiological aspects of Personality Disorders. Ideally, we should attend to 1) the readying or predisposing conditions, 2) the mobilizing or precipitating conditions, and 3) the finally necessary and sufficient conditions that lead to Personality Disorders. Practically, we cannot do so but can only assert in general terms that these etiological circumstances are plausible enough to account for many cases:

1. *Predisposing*—Biological conditions such as genetic endowments and temperament, physique, intelligence, and gender; environmental circumstances such as parental personality, temperament and parenting patterns, parental psychopathology and parents' communication patterns.

2. *Precipitating*—Physical ailments, deaths of relatives, parental discord and divorce, psychic traumata, and other disruptions and lacks.

3. *Necessary*—Both biological and social predispositions, added in with the child's maturational level to form the necessary or enabling conditions.

4. *Sufficient*—An added extra criticism, rejection, shock, or strong emotion, like the "straw that broke the camel's back," will be necessary to create the appearance of a Personality Disorder—an experience that upsets the preexistent equilibrium of personal strengths and deficits and, sometimes, suddenly turns happiness into unhappiness, subjective distress, and impaired schoolwork and interpersonal relations. The *sufficient cause* is hard to assess, to pin down, and is, alas, often left to mere guesswork, but not always, for a specific stress—in its timing and weight—can be implicated.

Histrionic Personality Disorder (301.50)

DEFINITION AND CLINICAL DESCRIPTION

The Histrionic Personality Disorder child is both highly expressive and dramatic in emotional responses and eagerly seeking attention in ways that turn off other children and adults. These dramatic expressions are sources of repeated distress to the affected child. The DSM-III-R definition is as follows:

1. a speech content of overstatement and hyperbole
2. constantly seeking praise and approval
[3. inappropriate sexual seductiveness (mostly adults)]
[4. overconcern with physical appearance (mostly adults)]
5. exaggerated emotional expression
6. discomfort whenever not center of attention
[7. perceived by others as shallow, not genuine (mostly adults)]
8. egocentric and self-indulgent

DSM-III-R "requires" at least four of the eight ways listed for a diagnosis of Histrionic Personality Disorder. Since three of those listed (see bracketed numbers) seldom apply to children, we are left with five of the specific behaviors generally relevant to children. It would be wise to make the diagnosis of Histrionic Personality Disorder only when four of the five are present in a child, in order to prevent overuse and misapplication of the label.

CASE 20-1   Gina, age 10, was brought by her six-times-divorced mother to a clinic that was the children's division of a general and family psychiatry clinic, in which the mother had been diagnosed with three different Personality Disorders. Gina was wearing *eye and facial makeup*. Her mother depicted her as "10 going on 25" since in the mother's eyes she apparently expected to be her *mother's equal in* catching men. (The interviewer let that pass, since mother's catches had not, according to the medical chart, been either notable or durable.) But the interviewer pursued the mother's saying *"10 going on 25."* The mother said she had meant that Gina *competed with the mother for mother's male companions' attention, threw "herself at them"* in ostentatious *flirting* and *seductiveness, dressed and made up like a 25-year-old* "woman *on the hunt,"* and *pouted if adult people did not talk mainly to Gina* when they came to see her mother. Gina always *felt that adults did not like her* if they did not focus on her with *praise and spoken approval.* It *did not matter if their praise was insincere,* because mother said Gina *herself was insincere* in her *use of superlatives* like "Awesome! Fantastic! Beautiful!" Nothing was ever "just so-so" but always overdrawn to be hideous or marvelous; and mother added, "And talk about narcissism, *with Gina it's me-me-me* and nothing else!"

On psychological testing Gina was found to be functioning with an *IQ of 85* on both performance and verbal tests, to be grossly *immature and impulsive,* and to be *overly concerned with femininity, sexuality, and bodily disease or deformity.*

Comment. Gina turned out to be more dependent than the average 10-year-old, insecure about her own worth, and unsure about how reliable her mother would be as her parent. She was tired of "having to act like a grown-up" in order to get her mother's attentive, grudging care. She had an array of the symptoms of Histrionic Personality Disorder.

DIAGNOSIS AND DIFFERENTIAL DIAGNOSIS

Both parents, whenever available, *and* the child must be interviewed and studied in order to arrive at the diagnosis. As with Gina, personality testing is an important diagnostic step. Information about developmental history, family history, and school behavior also contributes to the diagnostic process, as does the history of any neglect and sexual abuse in the child's life.

The main differentiae to be considered are:

Hysterical neuroses, but the child with Histrionic Personality Disorder does not have the symptoms of a Conversion, Phobic, or Dissociative Disorder;

Narcissistic Personality Disorder, but the child with a Narcissistic Personality Disorder is more grandiose, excessively self-involved, and devoid of empathy for others than the child with Histrionic Personality Disorder.

Erotization or molestation by adults, while not a disorder, can be at the roots of a picture of Histrionic Personality Disorder and can be elicited by history and brief treatment. Children who behave erotically towards adults have usually been stimulated by adults to behave in that way. Also, to some extent, "seductiveness is in the eye of the beholder" (see Chapter 28).

TREATMENT AND PROGNOSIS

Since children are so dependent on parent(s), and their recovery from mental disorders—episodic or characterologic—depends so much on what changes their parents can make, it becomes imperative to work with both generations.

Drugs are for target symptoms and not used in treating Histrionic Personality Disorder, so we are left with the prospect of reliance on one person (a therapist) helping another (the child with Histrionic Personality Disorder). We depend on that child's "significant others" in the process of understanding and modifying behaviors that emerged, initially, to be typical of the child and acceptable to everyone; but eventually those traits turned into a disorder in which the child is distressed and the others are annoyed, worried. A multimodal psychotherapy combining behavioral-cognitive-expressive individual approaches (yet heavier on cognitive and behavioral techniques) with family group therapy will have the best outcome.

The prognosis in most treated cases will be that the child is left with residues of Histrionic Personality Disorder but with some symptomatic improvement that may permit forward movement even though some vulnerability is retained. In the face of adequate stressors, the Histrionic Personality Disorder, according to the psychoanalytic hypothesis, will break into a Conversion, Phobic, or Dissociative Disorder (all three are "hysteroid"); but that hypothesis has not been proven to our knowledge.

Narcissistic Personality Disorder (301.81)

DEFINITION AND CLINICAL DESCRIPTION

Childhood egocentrism is a natural state of affairs for infants and toddlers but ordinarily lessens as the preschooler learns to play "together but not in common" with peers and, later, to engage in collaborative play with others. Only the boldly risk-taking would diagnose a child under six or seven years to have a Narcissistic Personality Disorder; the diagnosis is made mainly on adults.

However, children who are neglected and abused may develop personal traits akin to a Narcissistic Personality Disorder: greedy and imperiously demanding, expansive in their claims on others but returning nothing, devoid of empathy, feeling that they have special gifts and prerogatives, showing inordinate envy and covetousness, and outdoing a histrionic child in being the center of attraction and attention. Those are six of the nine diagnostic behaviors listed by DSM-III-R, with five of nine required to make the diagnosis. Several of the others are primarily adult phenomena: reacting to criticism with feelings of rage or humiliation, grandiose sense of self-importance, alternating between extremes of overidealization and devaluation of others in personal transactions, belief that one's problems are exceptional and need a specially gifted person to help them. Without help, they will suffer greatly and be unprepared for healthy parenting when they grow up.

CASE 20-2   Lester, at nine years of age, was a boy with an Expressive Writing Disorder (see Chapter 25) who ruled by his storminess over both parents and a younger sister. He received remedial tutoring at school for his specific reading disability but still substituted the letters B and D inaptly. His spelling, despite his high IQ (130), was so atrocious that his paternal grandfather remarked, "He cannot spell SH-- without putting a Q in it." Any mention the child psychiatrist made about his spelling and writing precipitated *rage* and reminders that he was *the smartest kid in his class.* He had learned a great deal about atomic structure and *made that his claim to fame. He rebuked his parents for being selfish* when they wanted to go anywhere without their son and daughter. Lester was *only interested in Lester* and did not care one whit if they took him and left his sister with the sitter. He *said insulting things* to his sister and openly regarded her as an annoyance beneath contempt. Covertly, he *envied* her with passion.

Lester was bright, had a rich vocabulary, and impressed the psychiatrist as a grand overcompensator who had underlying negative self-regard each time that he *spoke grandiosely* of his superior knowledge in physics and astronomy and his *ability to dominate and exploit his agemates* whom he called "dumb clods." He said, in a rather menacing tone, to the psychiatrist, "I'd prefer seeing a doctor who is famous in atomic physics and astronomy as well as in psychiatry. Have you written any books? *Are you famous* for anything?" *(overidealization or contempt).*

At home Lester *tried to take control of his parents' sex life,* not allowing them any privacy in their bedroom by *throwing screaming tantrums* outside the bedroom door, and trying to have knowledge of and control over the family budget, "always contending that *too little went to Lester the Great,* " his father reported. The parents vacillated between finding him obnoxiously bratty and suspecting he had a psychiatric disorder. They felt powerless to help him when they sought the child psychiatrist's consultation.

Comment. Lester's Expressive Writing Disorder made him feel inferior, but knowing he was otherwise intellectually superior, he overshot realism and balance, landing into the kind of expansive character trends that Karen Horney labeled "narcissistic-vindictive." He was well on the way to an unhappy state, to a Narcissistic Personality Disorder. By DSM-III-R's criteria he had arrived there— a position of self-defeat, frustration, insecurity, and instability.

DIAGNOSIS AND DIFFERENTIAL DIAGNOSIS

The diagnosis is given by the history and the clinical picture and confirmed by psychological testing. The differential diagnosis includes other Personality Disorders such as the Histrionic, Borderline, and Passive-Aggressive types, but each can be ruled out by the nonoverlapping behavioral items they list. Because of the greater number of overlapping items, the Borderline type will create more confusion, but in the borderline child the symptoms will be more severe and unpredictable than in the Narcissistic Personality Disorder.

TREATMENT AND PROGNOSIS

To improve the gloomy prognosis, treatment (individual, family group, and peer group psychotherapy) will need to be prolonged beyond what the Histrionic Personality, for example, would warrant, and will need to be carried out by a specialist in psychotherapy if any positive changes are to ensue.

Borderline Personality Disorder (301.83)

Borderline Personality Disorder has not been recognized sufficiently in children chiefly because there has been lack of agreement on uniform diagnostic criteria until DSM-III appeared in 1980. However, a source of difficulty has persisted since then because the DSM-III and DSM-III-R definitions address themselves mainly to adults, and do not reflect the changing and developing aspects of childhood. This is an unnecessary hardship for clinicians, because the overlap between the diagnostic symptoms of adults and those of children far outweighs the differences between them. What the clinician working with children needs are empirically validated diagnostic standards which emanate from the child's developing world, not from observations made in adults and whittled down to apply to children. Indeed, the criteria derived from work with children (Bemporad et al., 1982) bear a close resemblance to those in adults; this formal similarity of their symptoms helps to confirm the validity of the concept of Borderline Personality Disorder in childhood. These are children who generally appear neurotic or normal but who display psychotic behavior on occasion, usually responding promptly to adult care, interest, and reassurance.

DEFINITION

Originally, the term *borderline* referred to a person with a character disorder who showed mini-psychotic episodes. In effect, these people were *borderline psychotic*.

The core definition of Borderline Personality Disorder, according to DSM-III-R, is that it is a syndrome based on severe instability and fluctuation in the child's basic mental functioning, i.e., cognition, thinking, modulation of affect, control of impulses, and handling of anxiety. So defined, it belongs with pervasive psychosocial disorders, disorders of central processing, on Axis II, in this text.

The specific groups of symptoms of the disorder are cognitive, relational, impulsive, affective, and self-regarding, with some associated signs and symptoms.

1. Fluctuating deficits in cognition: "micropsychotic" episodes (Frijling-Schreuder, 1970), i.e., short periods of psychosis that are transient; bizarre ideation; concrete thinking. These symptoms wax and wane in response to interpersonal stresses.

2. Unstable relationships to others, which, moreover, fluctuate widely in intensity. Where their immense emotional needs are not met, these children disintegrate temporarily and may display panic or rage attacks even with familiar persons.

3. Poor impulse control: temper outbursts, intense overactivity, and severe behavioral difficulties.

4. Poor modulation of affect, and poor handling of anxiety. Depressed affect becomes utter despair, and anxiety is not "bound" with adequate defense mechanisms, so that terror and panic rapidly emerge. Some of these children are then given to self-mutilation.

5. Poor self-concept and poor identity which develop by indiscriminate imitation of adults who happen to fulfill psychological needs at a given moment.

6. Associated organic signs and symptoms of uneven development, such as neurological soft signs, developmental disorders (motor, language, learning disorders), hyperactivity attentional deficits, and electroencephalographic abnormalities.

CLINICAL DESCRIPTION

Unstable mood, unstable relationships, and unstable or insecure self-picture—unstable because of the sudden appearance of psychotic-like behavior—give the hallmarks of the borderline child's clinical appearance.

CASE 20-3   Sharwell, 11 years old, had reached puberty when he entered a children's mental hospital at the request of a Child Protective Services agency for *bizarre and aggressive behavior* in three different places: home, school, and neighborhood. He had been expelled from school for *assaultiveness* and ostracized in the neighborhood for physically beating and raping a six-year-old girl. The police threatened to haul him into juvenile court if Sharwell's parents did not get him into a psychiatric hospital. The police officers had noted well his *uncontrolled anger* and his *bizarre fantasies* about violence, death, and destructiveness, as well as his occasional lapses into baby talk. Sharwell had been seeing psychiatrists in three states since he was five years old but the parents said, "Nobody helped, they blamed *us*."

On admission to the children's mental hospital, Sharwell was ingratiating and overly complimentary to his therapist, whom he considered the only "good guy in this whole damned place," but was abusive and obscene in talking to most people. Later, he wrote off his therapist too, at times. He displayed marked shifts from *depression* and *complaints of boredom* to *an equilibrated mood,* and then at the drop of a hat he would get *restless* and *become enraged,* become *abusive* to other children, and *make threats to kill adult staff.* He was *impulsive* and had *no ability to back off or dampen his cravings.* He *overate* and had the table manners of a two-year-old; he became obese within two months of admission. He constantly *conned other children out of their belongings, turns at bike riding,* and their desserts at mealtimes. Unabashedly, he would *bully and manipulate* the others.

Sharwell *lacked any deference towards adults,* and, much *as he did with children, he begged, borrowed, and stole from any gullible adult* he could use for his purposes. About Sharwell's conscience, the admitting physician wrote, "He has knowledge of major social rules and *knows when he breaks them after the fact because he gets caught and punished.* He acknowledges no inner controls and is subject to *little internal capability for self-supervision."* About Sharwell's *self-concept,* the physician wrote, *"It is poor* with major *delays in the development of object relations.* Despite his superficial bravado and exaggeration, his true self-image is (as he says of himself) as *'bad, dumb, fat, weird, loony, weak, and ugly.'"*

Comment. Sharwell's diagnosis was Borderline Personality Disorder because he met at least six of the criteria of traits listed in DSM-III-R. Thioridazine was used for muting his stormy behavior but it only worked partly to do so.

Somatic and biological studies showed everything to be normal, EEG and CAT scan included, but he had a very mild hearing loss as his only positive finding.

DIAGNOSIS AND DIFFERENTIAL DIAGNOSIS

Since Borderline Personality Disorder involves so many deficits and pathological signs, it is easy to diagnose (and perhaps to overdiagnose) by history and clinical examination. Psychological testing with projective tests is not as useful because the ego fragility is often interpreted as a psychosis, which is not the case in Borderline Personality Disorder; hence, if one is wary of overdiagnosis and discusses this issue with the child psychologist, the testing can be of assistance in the diagnostic process. Neurodiagnostic studies to rule out temporal lobe epilepsy or an Organic Personality Syndrome may be necessary. Such a child needs to be seen more than once in order to diagnose the disorder with assurance.

These are differentiating points:

1. Mania's episodes last longer.
2. Depression's episodes last longer.
3. Schizoaffective disorder has longer episodes of mood alteration along with the A. criteria for Schizophrenia.
4. Organic Mental Disorders show "organicity," Dementia, Delirium, Intoxication, Amnestic Syndrome, etc. (see Chapters 5 and 24).
5. Narcissistic Personality Disorder shows more self-absorption, attention-seeking and, despite lack of empathy, a greater awareness of what other people are really like.
6. Conduct Disorders do not have the severe distortions in mood structure, interpersonal behavior, or self-concept that are seen in Borderline Personality Disorder.
7. Schizoid Personality and Schizotypal Personality Disorders have a separate set of descriptive indices in DSM-III-R.

TREATMENT AND PROGNOSIS

The prognosis is grave without treatment, and guarded before and after rather long-term treatment. The treatment requires a very businesslike therapist, for child and parents, who can empathize with the child's extreme chaos and perplexity but will set rules, give directions and advice, undertake environmental manipulation, and deal matter-of-factly in maneuvers to bring synthesis instead of the enormous "splitting" that Borderline patients are prone to make—a split that does not permit self or other to be a blend of "good and bad," only idealized *or* demeaned. The inordinate rages against the therapist must not be condoned, by saying, for example, "I am sorry I did something to make you angry." Instead, the more effective response is: "I am a doctor wanting to help you pull yourself together so you can be healthier; I know you cannot possibly be angry with me. You have a rage that in your heart of hearts you know is for someone else, not me."

There is a lot of clinical experience showing that the therapist who is accustomed to encouraging inhibited children to express themselves may have trouble setting limits and being as directive as those children with a Borderline Personality Disorder may require. Certainly there is no need to release inhibitions, and "borderlines" do worse when that is the only technique known to the therapist who may unwittingly encourage the child's acting up to get the therapist's attention.

Some Borderline Personality Disorder cases, especially those with separation anxiety, may be helped by imipramine, and also by propranolol if anxiety is intense; and unruly behavior may be curbed with neuroleptic medication, the most used being thioridazine, but chlorpromazine also has calming and sedating effects. The basic modality still, for most people, is relatively long-term hospitalization (6-12 months) for individual psychotherapy, which may continue after discharge from the hospital. Intensive work with the child's odd, occasionally abusive, parents is very much needed.

Dependent Personality Disorder (301.60)

DEFINITION AND CLINICAL DESCRIPTION

The Group for the Advancement of Psychiatry (GAP) Committee on Child Psychiatry in 1966 proposed a category of personality disorder called "Overly Dependent Personality." The children so classified were described as immature for age, passive–dependent, infantilized, chronically clinging, helpless and overdependent, "with difficulties in achieving full autonomy and initiative" (p. 241). Many clinicians liked the GAP scheme of classifying children's disorders (even if "full autonomy and initiative" seemed overdrawn), but DSM-III and DSM-III-R opted for less psychodynamic and more overt behavioral criteria. Dependency is, of course, very much the nature of children, but *overdependency* was the issue for both GAP and DSM-III.

DSM-III-R defines Dependent Personality Disorder in adult terms, but some children could be squeezed into the classification, which is that dependent and submissive behavior are indicated by at least five of the following (bracketed material was added by authors):

1. Prefers others to make most or all of his or her major life decisions [child has little choice].
2. Remains in relationships with people who mistreat him or her, because of fear of being alone [fits most children].
3. Agrees with people even when he or she believes they are wrong, to avoid a disturbance in the relationship.
4. Unable to initiate projects or act on his or her own volition [fits most preschoolers].
5. Offers to do unpleasant or demeaning things in order to curry the favor of other people.
6. Feels powerless or uneasy being alone or goes to great lengths to avoid being alone [sociable child].
7. Feels hopeless and helpless when a close relationship ends [uncomplicated bereavement].
8. Often preoccupied with the fear of being abandoned.
9. Feelings easily hurt by criticism or disapproval [responsive, obedient to adults].

That almost sounds like a docile or obedient normal American child aged five, who is not completely secure in his or her faith that the caretakers love him or her and can be relied upon to meet the child's needs. Still, it is, as the GAP term put it, *overdependent* for an older child of nine or more.

CASE 20-4   After his *father abandoned* him at eight years of age, Chad, whose caretaker had always been his *oversolicitous mother*, did not adapt to his mother's having to go to work outside the home in order to support Chad and herself. The mother, aged 38, was *grieving for the lost marriage* into which she had invested so much before Chad had been born as she worked at a job as an administrative assistant, helping to sustain herself and her husband who was a medical student at the time. Her husband had promised often that he could hardly wait to earn money and let her stay home and care for the baby that they both delayed having until the husband was almost finished with his first year of residency. But, eight years later, liking neither his wife nor child, the father had a relationship established with a divorced woman who was childless and a few years younger than his wife.

When he had been at home with Chad, father was "unmerciful" to Chad, mother said. He criticized Chad's overdependency on grown-ups and called Chad, *"Baby," "sissy,"* and *"lazy,"* urging him to be more macho and self-directing than was appropriate for a child of three-to-seven years. He left home and moved his practice and lover several states away.

Mother, despite *grieving*, found the *job market much less lucrative* than 15 years previously. She could barely make ends meet but had to work, for her husband's promised monthly allotment seldom arrived. Chad made her working a greater strain.

Chad *cried every day when* his *mother left home before him;* so the mother started driving him to school before she went to her job. Chad claimed inability to execute the burglar proof locks on the door. Chad did not want to be a latchkey child or ride the school bus; his mother arranged with an elderly woman in the neighborhood to give *afterschool care* so Chad wouldn't be alone and afraid. Mother liked this grandmotherly afterschool figure but Chad said, "She's *not our family.*"

After he got up in the mornings, Chad *dawdled in dressing* even after his mother had *chosen his preppy wardrobe* for the day. He could *decide little for himself* and burdened his two-job mother with every aspect of homemaking by having *no mind of his own* about food, clothing, straightening up, washing or drying dishes, setting the table, or taking out the garbage. When mother got angry at his helplessness and showed that she needed him with his high IQ (140) *to help her* and *to contribute* to home life, he would *volunteer to scrub the toilet.*

Chad began calling his mother at work to *ask if she was coming home,* and *when* and *if she liked him. "Am I your good boy?"* he would ask repetitively. The mother kept reassuring Chad that she loved him, admired him, was proud of him, because she knew *he was afraid she might leave him.* He seemed *so helpless* and *his feelings were so easily hurt* that she forgave all his enslavement of her. *She would take charge* again, each time after her heart melted, and would go back to *dressing him, spoon-feeding* him when he requested it, and *making every decision* that he called on her for: *what to eat, wear, play, say to his friends.* At age nine and a half, Chad was brought to a psychiatrist.

Comment. Chad had grown accustomed (from birth to age eight) to a greater dependency than normal for a child his age, even before his family was of the mother-only type. But when the father left, Chad became overly dependent and as the months grew to almost two years he developed a Dependent Personality Disorder. The mother-only family has its greatest difficulty in economics and home economics; therefore, if the child(ren) do not help out with housekeeping chores, the overburdened mother often breaks.

DIAGNOSIS AND DIFFERENTIAL DIAGNOSIS

Immaturity, dependency, clinging to adults—those attributes of a child make no sense in the abstract. But when we have a developmental perspective on the age-appropriate behaviors for a child (like Chad, for instance), we see that he was, relative to his agemates and IQ, overly dependent and immature, and would indeed look lazy, sissified, and weak to an unsympathetic observer. Hence, developmental norms and expectations must be invoked in making the diagnosis, for a child, of Dependent Personality Disorder.

The main differential considerations with children are:

1. *Separation Anxiety Disorder,* but the dependent child has no particular focus on avoiding separation and only craves not to be alone. (S)He will seem content when staying with others than familiars.
2. *Passive Aggressive Personality Disorder,* but the overly dependent child's behaviors are not conspicuously stamped with passive resistance or oppositionalism.
3. *Grief,* but the overly dependent child's symptomatic behavior will either predate or be unrelated to a loss, or continue beyond the one-year limit on normal grief.
4. *Depression,* but the overly dependent child does not meet the criteria for Depression and lacks the qualities of an episode of illness. Dependent Personality Disorder is more akin to an unhappy way of life, or a *trait* pathology, not a *state* pathology.

TREATMENT AND PROGNOSIS

The prognosis is for a life of "moving towards others" in helpless dependency (Karen Horney formulation) if no treatment is given. With treatment, which holds prospects of slow reformation and behavior change, the prognosis is not so gloomy. The treatment, for Chad as an example, was mainly by individual psychotherapy, with mother-and-child treatment at the end of each weekly session with the boy and occasional child-and-mother sessions for the entire time. No medications were used. The sessions were devoted to helping Chad learn new things that he could undertake between sessions, giving special attention to his own suggestions and ideas, evaluating his successes, letting him analyze his dreams, and encouraging less clinging whenever possible. Along with psychotherapy Chad joined with others, his agemates (so he was not alone), in scouting and camping endeavors and in karate lessons, which he liked.

The "salvation" of many parent-oriented children is to have an agemate chum and to find comfort in the expanded horizon of peer interaction, for after childhood one does not stand alone, we recall, but in the company of one's peers. Peers help the child to be less clinging and institute more interdependence, give and take.

Obsessive Compulsive Personality Disorder (301.40)

We should note at this point that a "phobic character" such as that of the child with an Avoidant Personality Disorder (Axis II) can, under stress and conflict, move from a personality disorder to a Phobic Disorder and Panic Disorder. For that reason, Avoidant Personality Disorder is discussed in Chapter 17 on "Anxiety, Phobic, and Dissociative Disorders," denoting that it is a *trait disorder* on a continuum with *state disorders,* a personality disorder that turns into a neurosis.

Then why did we not place Obsessive Compulsive Personality Disorder in the chapter with Obsessive Compulsive Disorder (Chapter 17) and present the personality trait disorder as a milder form of the state disorder? Research and clinical experience show that the trait exerts some kind of protective function against developing a full-blown Obsessive Compulsive Disorder. Only rarely does the character disorder become a neurotic disorder, but less rarely do fully treated Obsessive Compulsive *Disorders* turn into Obsessive Compulsive *Personality Disorders.* They have few commonalities despite a prevalent conjecture to the contrary.

DEFINITION AND CLINICAL DESCRIPTION

1) An obsessional (or obsessive compulsive) *character* is one who has an uptight and rigid lifestyle but no stark obsessions and compulsions and not even 2) a personality disorder. An Obsessive Compulsive *Personality Disorder* shows, in

DSM-III-R, "perfectionism and inflexibility" to a degree that creates distress in the affected person and interferes with social or occupational functioning as manifested in five of these nine features:

1. Restricted expression of warm, tender emotions.

2. Stinginess with one's time, money, or gifts whenever no personal gain likely will result.

3. Perfectionism that impedes completion of a task.

4. Preoccupation with details, mechanics, or schedules at the expense of the major point of the activity (this appears to be what Herbert Marcuse called the "overly administered reality principle").

5. Stubborn insistence that others submit to precisely his or her way of doing things.

6. Being a devoted worker to the exclusion of leisure and friendships (going beyond economic necessity).

7. Avoiding, postponing, or extending decision-making, e.g., drawn-out ruminating about priorities.

8. Hoarding, not throwing away, worn-out or useless objects that haven't even sentimental value.

9. Overly conscientious, scrupulous, and inflexible about morality, seeking moral superiority that has no cultural or religious basis.

CASE 20-5   William at age 10 years was brought to a child psychiatrist because of his *"unhappiness, excessive worry and guilt,* and *lack of friends."* Although his schoolwork had always been excellent, he had *ceased to enjoy* it and his *grades were declining* because of his *copying work over* and over, always unsatisfied with what he finally handed in. His parents did not object to his *moralism* and *excessive religiosity* even though they were "lightweight Protestants," they said, but they were annoyed by his *criticism of his parents* for "underpaying" a domestic servant and for "drinking occasional highballs."

With the psychiatrist, William (he rejected any nickname) was always *polite and overly serious* and that persisted for about four weeks of once-a-week psychotherapy sessions. With the psychologist, he remained aloof and "uninvolved" in the testing. It took him a half hour to reproduce the Bender Gestalt figures because of his *slowness, meticulousness,* and *frequent erasures and starting over.* He showed a full-scale *IQ of 117* but did poorly on *timed subtests* because of his perfectionistic *unnaturalness* and *slowness.* Projective testing showed responses replete with *denial, projection, constricted affect,* and *intellectualization.*

William had five younger brothers and sisters who regarded him as *bossy, a nut,* a guy who would never give in and had to have *control* of every interaction: "He won't play with you unless everything goes his way." When William was asked how it made him feel to have so many younger siblings, he said, as stiltedly as a little professor, "Sometimes it is difficult, because *one has the advantage over the younger ones,* and one must remember that." "Clarifying," he explained that he knew he must lead them but not let them know he is in charge.

Eventually William disclosed that he kept thinking from time to time that *there might not be a God.* He regarded that as a hideous thought, he said, but disclaimed any rituals or other outright obsessive or compulsive symptoms.

Comment. William would meet DSM-III-R criteria for Obsessive Compulsive Personality Disorder. He was more than *an obsessive character* because his life was crippled by his personality traits, leaving him *rigid, unfriendly* and *unaffectionate.* But he did not meet diagnostic criteria for an Obsessive Compulsive Disorder.

DIAGNOSIS AND DIFFERENTIAL DIAGNOSIS

This has been covered adequately in the preceding discussion, for an obsessive character has no disorder while the neurosis has symptoms of a true disorder, i.e., obsessions and compulsions, and may assume borderline-psychotic proportions in some cases.

TREATMENT AND PROGNOSIS

Although, as we stated earlier, Obsessive Compulsive Personality Disorder (OCPD) rarely gets structured as a "symptoms neurosis," the child with OCPD can develop other neuroses, notably Phobic Disorder, Dysthymic Disorder, and Anxiety Disorder. Hence, the condition is to be treated and followed up if possible. The easiest outcome is to restore the child to an obsessional character but without OCPD, a character disorder.

Treatment by expressive psychotherapy works best with a therapist who is candid and willing to confront, give advice, make suggestions, stress affects instead of thoughts, talk about affects here and now, avoid vagueness by stressing the need for a concrete example of whatever general thing the child says, and encourage risk-taking and naturalness. Working with dreams can uncover some unvarnished feelings of the child with OCPD. There are obvious combinations of behavioral and cognitive strategies in the expressive or emotive therapy just described. To further the multimodal thought, we can add that such children are usually quite like their parents—they "don't suck a rigid character off their thumbs"—but aren't exact clones of their parents. Thus it is necessary to have the parents also involved.

Psychotropic medications have little relevance currently to OCPD.

Passive Aggressive Personality Disorder (301.84)

DEFINITION AND CLINICAL DESCRIPTION

Children under the sway of parents who demand honor and obedience seem bound to resort to cunning, using Good Soldier Schweik tactics of overcompliance with orders while showing inner opposition and resistance. Some of those children overuse passive defiance to impede their performance when demanded to do things that are not outrageous at all. DSM-III-R gives nine indices, of which at least five are needed to diagnose a condition as Passive Aggressive Personality Disorder:

1. Procrastinates or dawdles so that deadlines remain unmet.
2. Appears to work with deliberate slowness and to do a bad job if does not want to do a task.
3. Unjustifiably protests that others make unreasonable demands on him or her.
4. Avoids duties and responsibilities by claiming "I forgot."
5. Sulks, gets irritable or argues when asked to do a job he or she does not want to do.
6. Overvalues own job performance above others' evaluations of it.
7. Resents cogent suggestions, from others, of ways of being more productive.
8. Blocks the efforts of others by failing to do own share of work.
9. Is unreasonably demeaning or scornful of persons in positions of authority.

Children with Passive Aggressive Personality Disorder are not as openly rebellious as those with an outright Oppositional Defiant Disorder (see Chapter 4). As DSM-III-R presents the former, one can only envision a sneakily obstructionistic factory worker, office worker, or soldier, all adults. Questions of empowerment of workers in ways that would obviate their passive resistance come to mind to us, the authors, but perhaps not to framers of DSM-III-R. Children, fortunately, are not now soldiers or factory or office workers but they are scholars and the school is their workplace. Many children also take up worthwhile chores and tasks at home, so we can hold to DSM-III-R's business-management flavor in describing children who are passive–aggressive to a fault.

CASE 20-6   Zoe, aged 11 years, had a parental reputation for being the *laziest* of their three children. She had an older brother and younger sister who complied readily with the ex-Marine father's demands for work and play. About weekend chores, he'd say, "Let's get this show on the road!" and about games he'd say, "This is fun and everybody has to play—you too, Zoe." He called the children's mother "vice-president in charge of maintenance and social relations" but he oversaw and exercised veto powers over any decision that the mother made on her own. Father was always insisting that "this operation has got to get better organized" and "this family needs to be whipped into shape." Zoe's siblings, by being compliant and uncritical, received the father's favors, but Zoe was *always in hot water,* with him, and sometimes it was *of her own making.*

Zoe stopped whining, because that brought on a physical beating, but she did all assigned chores in a lackluster way and *barely evaded the lash.* She always *delayed,* promising to get to her rotating household chores, but begging *"in a little while."* Often, she *barely got under the wire* in doing chores, hastily doing the job at the very *last minute* and often doing it *inadequately,* just *enough to get by.* If her father insisted on no delays, she worked *perfunctorily and slowly,* with *a hint of distaste* here and there. She compared jobs assigned to her and her sibs and complained that she always *drew the worst jobs,* even though tasks were rotated. She insisted that she *had done the job* well even if her mother or father pointed out egg left on the sloppily washed plate or kitty-cats of lint left under her bed. If she washed the dishes and her brother or sister dried them, she would *go so slowly* that they were held up from meeting friends at appointed times, and so on.

In school, teachers found her to be *passively defiant and antagonistic* to them, too. In Girl Scouts she was always claiming she was *put upon,* objecting that *projects were dumb.* She often *forgot* to bring the materials and records that were required by a certain deadline. Many adults saw her as *sneakily antagonistic* to them. When the entire family learned that the father was having an extramarital affair, a crisis ensued for all; but Zoe's behavior worsened, so the parents brought her for individual and family group therapy. Zoe had even called her father a dictator and a crook.

Comment. The preceding case history illustrates the pervasiveness of the child's resistance and revenge against what were indeed draconian demands by the father. However, the diagnosis of Passive Aggressive Personality Disorder is underscored by the fact that her passive-aggressive attitudes "spilled over" into all areas of her life, including nonconflictual ones such as Girl Scouts and school.

DIAGNOSIS AND DIFFERENTIAL DIAGNOSIS

History, physical exam, mental status examination, and clinical interviews with child and parents (we usually see the parents initially and without the child) will yield the correct diagnosis. Psychological testing may confirm the diagnosis and give leads for therapeutic work by uncovering a new area of problems that the child has.

The differentiation from other disorders is relatively easy. All that is required is a working knowledge of the DSM-III-R descriptive criteria for such conditions as Oppositional, Conduct, Narcissistic Personality, Borderline Personality, and Obsessive Compulsive Personality Disorders.

Schizoid Personality Disorder (301.20)

There are many symptoms of isolating behavior that children can show: egocentric and narcissistic acts, excessive fantasy or shyness or social withdrawal, hoarding or stinginess, inhibition, timidity, avoidance, running away, rejecting or rebuffing others, suspiciousness, delusional behavior, and asceticism. Those symptoms cut across a number of disorders of mood, thinking, and behaving. They are nonspecific but are all effective in reducing interactions with others; in Karen Horney's typology they are like choreographic movements *away from people* towards solitude and social walling off.

DEFINITION AND CLINICAL DESCRIPTION

According to DSM-III-R, the Schizoid Personality Disorder is one that combines *social detachment* with being unfeeling, that is, displaying emotional coarctation and *restricted expression of emotions,* as shown by four of the six unbracketed indicators:

1. Little desire for, or enjoyment of, close relationships, including being part of a family.
2. Nearly always chooses to be alone, solitary activities.
3. Claims never (or rarely) to experience anger or other deep emotions.
[4. Little, if any, desire to have sexual experiences with another (perhaps mainly adults referred to).]
5. Indifferent to, or claims indifference to, others' praise or criticism.
6. No (or only one) friend or confidant other than relatives or members of one's household.
7. Constricted affect—aloof, cold, unsmiling, rarely nodding or reciprocating when spoken to.

The isolating and isolated behaviors are paramount and, since few of such children develop Schizophrenia, the term *schizoid* may be a misnomer. The GAP (1966) classification listed the same index items as DSM-III-R but rejected "schizoid" and labeled these personality disorders *Isolated Personality Disorder.* The disorder is more common in boys but we present here a girl's case.

CASE 20-7   Hester had been weakly attached to and unconcerned about her mother as an infant. By age eight, when she was brought to a child psychiatrist, she had become an isolate and, oddly enough, on a sociogram made by her third-grade peers *she had chosen nobody to be near or interact with.* She had not been chosen by a single child, either. Her mother had a "schizophrenic" male cousin, aged 29, whose illness (it turned out to be a Bipolar Disorder) she compared to Hester's and wanted an answer to: "Is Hester going to be a schizophrenic?"

Hester was evaluated by a resident in child psychiatry whose first comment about her diagnosis was, "Young Hester's diagnosis falls somewhere between *bland* and *blah.*" He noted that she seemed *temperamentally phlegmatic*—"dull, apathetic, cold, unruffled, and indifferent." Someone asked if she was like the "slow to warm up" child (Thomas & Chess, 1977) and the resident, remembering Greek humoral psychology, said, "No, she *never warmed up.* Both her *breadth and depth of emotional expression were feeble.*" He went on to report on these items from his interview with Hester and the history given by Hester's mother:

> She *withdraws from family activities,* fleeing to the *solitude* of her room. She *daydreams a lot* and *reads a lot* but is not made "happy-looking" by these activities. Not only does she *lack any close friend* but also says when being thrown with others, "I'll *go if I have to.*" When asked to describe the maddest (angriest) she'd ever been, she said, "*I've never got angry* about anything." Likewise for joy and happiness, "I *can't think of any times like that.*" When she was asked what sort of person she is and asked how she'd describe herself to a man from Mars, she said, "I *don't see why I'd tell him anything.*" When the resident insisted, "Come on, what would you tell him is your best point, something he'd have to like?" she rejoined rather vapidly, "*I wouldn't care if he liked me or not.*"

Comment. In both her social detachment and her unemotionality, Hester fulfilled the criteria for Schizoid Personality Disorder. "Her Rorschach responses were sparse," the psychologist reported, "and colorless like a child who is so emotionally coarcted she cannot even reveal any conflicts." Her full-scale IQ was 110 on the WISC-R. She showed no thought disorder or psychotic features, and appeared to be "extremely introverted." Surprisingly, on occasion, a child like Hester can blow up or out in wild aggression, a possibility that needs to be borne in mind.

DIAGNOSIS AND DIFFERENTIAL DIAGNOSIS

The child with a Schizoid Personality Disorder is unhappy in his or her socioemotional depletion and needs to be seen three or four times in diagnostic play observation and psychiatric interview and to be probed further for dreams, fantasies, and feelings. Such clinical devices as Sentence Completion, House-Tree-Person, Kinetic Family Drawing, and a detailed survey of what the child likes best and hates most about foods, colors, relatives, other children, songs, and famous persons may give further elucidation to original clinical impressions.

Conditions to be differentiated, and ways to do so, are:

Schizotypal Personality Disorder, but the Schizoid Personality Disorder does not show bizarre, odd symptoms of thought or behavior or feeling shown by the Schizotypal Personality Disorder. (The same is true for Schizophrenia.)

Depression, but the Schizoid Personality Disorder does not show dysphoria, depression, weight loss, sleep disorder, psychomotor retardation, fatigue, and so on.

Mild Mental Retardation, often felt as needing to be ruled out because responsiveness is so bleak, but does not produce the isolated and aloof picture shown by a case of Schizoid Personality Disorder. "Isolated Personality Disorder" would appear to be a more felicitous term for this condition.

TREATMENT AND PROGNOSIS

If minimal socialization can be achieved through treatment, the child with Schizoid Personality Disorder will probably grow up to be less cold and distant but may always remain unobtrusive in social situations, retiring, and introverted. As stated earlier, these children do *not* become schizophrenic, so that is a very remote risk. They may, however, if untreated, be prone to homicidal aggressive outbursts, but rarely.

The treatment is a warming-up methodology, by and large. The targeted features in treatment are the social detachment and emotional restriction, so gently expressive psychotherapy is the treatment of choice, combined with tolerated exposure to peers and nonrelatives. Sometimes small, private schools that do not make introverts miserable are better than the available public schools for such children. They are lucky if they can be exposed to "adults who *follow children, not theories.*"

Schizotypal Personality Disorder (301.22)
GENERAL DISCUSSION

If children have a Schizotypal Personality Disorder, it is probably diagnosed instead as Borderline Personality Disorder, Schizophrenia, or high-functioning Autism. Schizotypal Personality Disorder is a diagnosis rarely made for children. All (Borderline, Schizophrenia, and Autism) are rare disorders, relatively speaking, and difficult to deal with, certainly.

Since Schizotypal Personality Disorder in DSM-III-R is cast in terms of adult experiences, we shall not include further discussion of it here, except to note that it includes bizarreness and deficits in interpersonal relatedness, appearance, speech, behavior, and thinking.

Personality Disorder NOS (301.90)

Anna Freud (1965) wrote, "I warn analysts not to base any of their assessments of children on the degree of *impairment* of *functioning,* notwithstanding the fact that this is one of the most revealing of criteria for the pathology of adults" (p. 123). Furthermore, after pointing to areas of a child's activities that might be used to show impaired functioning—play, freedom of fantasy, school achievement, stability of personal relationships, and social adaptation—she stated,

> Nevertheless, not one of them can qualify as being on a par with the adult's two main vital functions: his capacity to lead a normal love and sex life and his capacity to work. . . . There is only one factor in childhood the impairment of which can be considered of sufficient importance in this respect, namely, the child's capacity to move forward in progressive steps until maturation, development in all areas of the personality, and adaptation to the social community have been completed. Mental upsets can be taken as a matter of course so long as these vital processes are left intact. (p. 123)

A personality or character type may not hinder the child's progression; a personality disorder will, if not treated; a symptom neurosis definitely will; a psychosis or pervasive developmental disorder will interfere most of all.

DSM-III contained a category called Mixed Personality Disorder that became Personality Disorder NOS (not otherwise specified) in DSM-III-R. Our intent here is to introduce the controversial note that Personality Disorder NOS may be the most useful category for children, the one to be employed most often. We say this because children are in a fluid state of being and becoming, because they may settle only briefly on what descriptively is a disorder and soon change, with salutary life events, to a character type, only later forming a Personality Disorder and again heal enough to return to a character type or even to a unique personality.

DSM-III-R defines Personality Disorders as causing significant impairment in social or occupational functioning or subjective distress. Those criteria are also given for neuroses. But those, as Anna Freud indicated, are adult canons: impairments in love and work, with distress about it. Distress, unhappiness, or misery are not even good guides for the most severe disorders of childhood—just witness the child with Autism, mainly devoid of distress.

Children show mixtures of abortive variants of the adult-type disorders more often than they replicate the adults' clinical pictures, especially in Personality Disorders.

CASE 20-8   Casper was eight years old when he was evaluated by a child psychiatrist for his parents' complaints of Casper's *reading and learning difficulties,* his tendencies to be *a loner,* and his *confusion about his sexual role.* Casper proved to have an *IQ of 85* and some *perceptual-motor problems.* His birth was difficult and prolonged, requiring forceps and accompanied by *anoxia.* The parents were warned that he might have difficulties later on. Early in infancy, he was found to have *hyaline membrane disease.*

Casper's parents were high achievers and, hardly knowing what they were doing, *they imposed high expectations* of excellent performance on both Casper and his adopted sister, aged three. Casper reacted by being *a defeatist concerning school* where he was usually *friendless and alone* and identified as having *a reading disability.* At home, however, competing with his little sister, he *tried to act grown-up* and always *played for center-stage.* He attended slavishly to *trying to please and amuse his parents* and, in the process, had *a clobbered self-concept.* In five months of psychotherapy he never reported a single dream, so great was his *guarding and self-concealment.* During long periods of solitude he played at two roles with *single-minded determination,* that of a doctor and a priest. It was as if he *assumed a different identity* when he played. *Such play never seemed to achieve any completion, resulted in no release of tension,* but had *a compulsive, almost frantic quality.* Neither doctor nor priest brought him any relief.

Casper had *confusion about his sex role* identity and at times *imagined that he did not have a penis* and would *dress up as a girl.* This was ultimately understood not to be a gender identity problem but simply some sex role confusion prompted by *castration anxiety* in his Oedipal confusion. During therapy it was revealed with fear and trembling that Casper *felt unloved at home* and also that he had *a very specific phobia of getting onto an elevator.*

Comment. Casper's case was not atypical in its presentation of many symptoms suggesting developmental, neurotic, and personality disorders, but showing a mixed picture that would not easily be written off as only an Adjustment Disorder. With certainty, Casper's case could be diagnosed on Axis II as a Reading Disorder (315.00) and on Axis I as a Simple Phobia (300.29) but his other partly neurotic (anxiety, obsessive compulsive, sex role dysphoria) and character disorder symptoms might be diagnosed, again on Axis II, as a Personality Disorder NOS (301.89).

It does not become disconcerting that we make as many diagnoses as are warranted, and probably in Casper's case we need to make those two diagnoses on Axis II and one on Axis I. Childhood psychopathology is shifting, fluid, and diverse.

Questions for Study and Action

1. Examine their descriptions in DSM-III-R to see if there would be a need for an Oppositional Disorder, listed under the Disruptive Behavior Disorders of children, separate from Passive Aggressive Personality Disorder. Which do you find more severe? What arguments could you summon for keeping both diagnoses? Look at

the case given in this book to illustrate each of the two disorders and note what features of authoritarian parents are present.

2. Why is "causal explanation" so imprecise and tenuous in childhood psychopathology? List five reasons and explain each.

3. Several years ago the Veterans Administration adopted the practice of giving a personality diagnosis as well as a symptom-picture diagnosis on every veteran who was hospitalized. What could you say in favor of such a practice in child psychiatry? What realistic conditions would militate against the practice?

4. Why are the so-called "biological foundations of personality" so important when we are looking for etiology of personality disorders? Would you include congenital anomalies under genetic conditions? under physique? Explain.

5. Which of the Personality Disorders discussed in this chapter show a continuum with neuroses, developmental disorders, and psychoses? Which definitely do not show that continuum, arguing against a spectrum of disorders? How would some Personality Disorders seem to protect a child from developing into a symptom disorder?

6. Which of the Personality Disorders discussed in this chapter would, and which would not, have a better chance of forming a working alliance with a psychotherapist? Make the two lists, explaining your reason for placing the particular item in one list or the other.

7. Would early onset Pervasive Developmental Disorder (PDD) be more likely than a later onset PDD to recover sufficiently to warrant a diagnosis by 12 years of age of Borderline Personality Disorder? Explain. Do you know any research that you can use to aid you in forming an opinion on this matter?

8. Do you agree with the authors' criticism of DSM-III-R's listing of reliance on others, staying with persons who mistreat one because of fear of being alone, agreeing with people just to keep the peace, difficulty in doing things on one's own, doing demeaning things just to curry favor, avoiding being alone, and so on as being the cardinal signs of a disorder, when they so often typify the child's estate? What does a developmental perspective do to alter this odd situation? Is concentrating on *adults only* inconsistent with a developmental perspective? Do adults also have a developing life? Explain.

9. Explain how four different Personality Disorders might result from having been an unwanted child, one who was genuinely hated by the primary caretaker to such an extent that the child concluded, "Something basic is wrong with me and I may have no right to exist." In each case show what symptoms within that Personality

Disorder refer directly or indirectly to being hated. Do parents always refrain from saying to a child that they hate him or her? Is it easier for the child to be told or to have to infer it?

10. Differentiate between the nonverbal behavior of a child with Histrionic Personality Disorder and a child with Obsessive Compulsive Personality Disorder. List at least five distinguishing nonverbal behavioral items and explain each.

For Further Reading

Bemporad, J.R., Smith, H.F., Hanson, G., & Cicchetti, D. Borderline syndromes in childhood: Criteria for diagnosis. *Am. J. Psychiatry,* 139:596–602, 1982.

Bloch, D. *So the Witch Won't Eat Me: Fantasy and the Child's Fear of Infanticide.* Boston: Houghton Mifflin, 1978.

Chapman, A.W. Personality-pattern disturbances. In *Management of Emotional Problems of Children and Adolescents* (2nd ed.). Philadelphia: Lippincott, 1974.

Freud, A. *Normality and Pathology in Childhood.* New York: International Universities Press, 1965.

Frijling-Schreuder, E.C.M. Borderline states in children. *Psychoanal. Study Child,* 24:307–327, 1970.

Group for the Advancement of Psychiatry. *Psychopathological Disorders in Childhood: Theoretical Considerations and a Proposed Classification.* Report No. 62. New York: Brunner/Mazel, 1966.

Horney, K. Neurosis and human growth: The struggle towards self-realization. In *The Collected Works of Karen Horney.* New York: W.W. Norton, 1950.

Mack, J.E., & Ablon, S.I. *The Development and Sustenance of Self-Esteem in Childhood.* New York: International Universities Press, 1983.

Miller, A. *Thou Shalt Not Be Aware: Society's Betrayal of the Child.* (Trans. by H. Hannum & H. Hannum) New York: New American Library, 1986.

Reich, W. *Character-Analysis* (3rd enlarged edition). New York: Farrar, Straus and Giroux, 1971.

Thomas, A., & Chess, S. *Temperament and Development.* New York: Brunner/Mazel, 1977.

21

Attention-Deficit Hyperactivity Disorder

The young subspecialty of child psychiatry has found some of its greatest therapeutic success in treatment of Attention–Deficit Hyperactivity Disorder (314.01)—a success, moreover, that has brought it squarely into the mainstream of medicine by using pharmacological means to reach definable and measurable goals. No longer is expensive and lengthy psychotherapy the only treatment modality; the pharmacotherapy and brief parental guidance used in treatment of ADHD have shown that child psychiatry can offer the same down-to-earth, economical, and accessible service to everyone as can the rest of medicine.

But the dramatic and easily obtainable nature of this pharmacological success has invited shortcuts in diagnosis and treatment of ADHD. These, in turn, have "soured" a number of people, both lay and mental health professionals, on the entire category of ADHD so that the very concept of ADHD, as well as its pharmacological treatment, has been disputed and rejected.

Simple as its definition is, ADHD is not a uniform concept, and requires a thorough understanding for correct diagnosis and treatment. ADHD was previously labeled under several derivations of the word "hyperactive": the "hyperactive child," "hyperactivity syndrome," or "hyperkinetic syndrome or disorder." The seemingly obvious and self-explanatory nature of the word "hyperactive" led to the erroneous belief by many parents that they themselves could diagnose their children—mostly in the negative, by repudiating this diagnosis. Physicians proposed, and parents opposed, the diagnostic label of ADHD.

One previous deviation from the nomenclature based on the word "hyperactive" was the name "minimal brain damage," or "minimal brain dysfunction," or "MBD." While the etiological implications of this term are open to debate (which we shall join presently), MBD offered a less popular, indeed frightening, term. In view of all this, most child psychiatrists have welcomed the introduction of the new term, "Attention–Deficit Hyperactivity Disorder," as being nonthreatening, resistive to "do-it-yourself" diagnosis by the lay person, and descriptively accurate.

DEFINITION

The most basic definition is that ADHD is a syndrome whose core is distractibility and inability to contain stimuli, resulting in excessive and random movements and short attention span. The DSM-III-R defines ADHD as the triad of developmentally inappropriate inattention, impulsivity, and hyperactivity. Built into this definition is the factor of immaturity, as the triad is inappropriate for the child's age. It is indeed fortunate that DSM-III-R cautions that the signs of ADHD may not be observed directly by the examining clinician, and therefore they must be reported by the adults in the child's environment who know the child well, such as parents and teachers. DSM-III-R places ADHD, along with Oppositional Defiant Disorder and Conduct Disorder, under the general category of Disruptive Behavior Disorders.

According to the DSM-III-R definition, ADHD starts before the age of seven years (typically by the age of three years) and has to have been present for at least six months.

CLINICAL DESCRIPTION

The following case illustrates ADHD in its most "classic" form.

CASE 21-1   Jack, aged seven years, was referred because he could *never sit still* ("ants in his pants"), was always *on the go,* and *could not stick* to any one activity. His excessive and totally *random activity* caused problems both at home and at school, where he could *not pay attention, was distracted by every extraneous sight or sound, rushed through* all assignments, but *never finished* them. Even when he ceased his *constant motion,* which happened rarely, he seemed to be daydreaming.

He was *difficult to manage,* not only because he *did not register* whatever was said, but also because he was *impulsive;* he acted without forethought, *on the spur of the moment,* was *easily provoked and angered,* and when angry went into *action* at the "drop of a hat." Consequently, Jack was involved in many *fights* with peers. He made friends easily because he was outgoing and *action-oriented:* he liked to ride his bike with gusto and play various games. However, most of his friends eventually did not want him around because he could *not stick to the rules* of the game, *wait for his turn,* sit still, or delay gratifications.

Jack's mother reported that he had *moved excessively* even in utero. His delivery was complicated by the umbilical cord wrapped around the baby's neck, producing moderate asphyxia, although labor had been quite short, almost precipitous. He was a *difficult baby,* in that he *slept little* and fitfully, with *colic* for the first three months. His motor-development landmarks were *early;* as soon as he could walk, he ran. He was *into everything,* and climbed onto everything. Nothing was safe from him, and he had many visits to the emergency room. He *wore out all his toys,* since he managed to take apart even the sturdiest of them. He could not even settle down in his sleep and would *get up* in the middle of the night and *roam around.*

Although Jack was called "motor mouth" because of his constant talking, he was given to a lot of "fibbing." His verbal accounts of what he did were unreliable, partly due to his inability to stick to one line of thought during his narrative, and partly due to his faulty attention span at the time that the event actually happened.

Family history revealed that his mother considered herself "flighty" and two maternal *uncles* had been in *trouble with the law* in their younger years. On father's side, there was a history of alcoholism. There was no history of suicide or depression.

During the individual interview, Jack at first tried to "put his best foot forward," i.e., he sat in his chair as quietly as possible. But soon he started *fidgeting, shifting* in his chair, then got up, *touching* toys and papers and other paraphernalia on the examiner's desk. Presently, Jack turned the light switch on and off and staged *violent games* with the toys. He *went from one activity* to another in rapid succession. After a while, Jack asked, "What else is there to do?" and indicated that he was *bored* with what was available in the office. He wanted to leave because there was "nothing to do." As soon as he arrived in the waiting room, he started *teasing* his younger sibling and got into a tug of war with his mother, which seemed to *relieve his boredom temporarily.* He *raced* back and forth in the corridor and delighted in making as much *noise* as possible by sideswiping the coat hangers. Mother commented, "As I told you, you always *have to keep two steps ahead* of him." When it was time to leave, Jack lunged towards the door, oblivious to any oncoming traffic.

Comment. This child shows the "organically driven" case of ADHD, with an uninterrupted personal history of all the signs of ADHD and a family history of the syndrome. The diagnosis would be clear without the observable hyperactivity, too.

Out of a veritable cornucopia of symptoms, which we shall organize presently when we discuss diagnosis, we can organize two subtypes: those children who show ADHD under any set of circumstances, and those who show it only in response to an overstimulating environment. It is possible to portray this distinction on a gradient of severity, the most severe ADHD children being unable to stay still and pay attention even in a low-stimulus environment, such as a quiet office, with only the examiner present, and the least distractible being children who become hyperactive and "revved up" only when in a high-stimulus environment, typically a classroom or a school bus.

We discuss the psychological consequences of ADHD separately later in this chapter.

DIAGNOSIS

The diagnosis of ADHD is based primarily on a complete, longitudinal *history*, given by the parent and the schoolteacher—in that order of importance. Secondarily, the diagnosis is based on the clinician's observations, psychiatric examination, and special neurological examination. There still are no laboratory tests of practical use, although a number of neurophysiological and biochemical procedures have been used in research.

The history of ADHD symptoms

In putting the parental history first, we are at variance with a number of other authors who place more trust in the teachers' reports, especially when rating scales are used. It is, nevertheless, our firm contention that the parents (above all the mother if she is the primary caregiver) know the child best and have known him or her longer than any teacher or child psychiatrist. Moreover, without the parents' positive history, the diagnosis is seriously in doubt, and meaningful treatment practically impossible.

When taking the parental history, the clinician need not be unduly concerned with the parents' opinions on whether the child is hyperactive. What matters are the facts: a fair estimate as to the extent of distractibility and attentional deficit can be made on the basis of the parents' description of the child's overall lifestyle and style of reacting, regardless of their disclaimers, such as, "But he is not hyperactive."

Complaints by the teachers are a significant lead to the diagnosis of ADHD and are often the precipitating factor prompting the parents to seek professional help for the child. Rarely will the parents totally negate the teacher's history. When this does happen, it is either because the teacher has prematurely "pushed for" medication, or because the parents simply cannot or will not admit to any imperfection in their child. "False positive" reports of hyperactivity by teachers are rare. "False negative" ones are relatively more frequent, but in general, there is good correspondence between the parents' and the teachers' reports.

Difficulties and apparent inconsistencies arise because teachers, more so than parents, often do not adhere to reporting of their observations only. They add their own views and interpretations of the child's behavior. The use of rating scales eliminates much of this "overlay," yet rating scales are no substitute for clinical inquiry, and clinical acumen cannot find an appropriate container in a questionnaire, however well devised. However, rating scales, especially the Conners' Parents' and Teacher Rating Scales, are an excellent adjuvant for thoroughness, for a written record to remind parents and others of the baseline, and for "tracking" in the course of treatment (see Chapter 1 for specific scales).

The basic syndrome of ADHD consists of three clusters of hyperactivity, short attention span, and impulsivity. Examples of each have been given in the preceding case history. For making the diagnosis, however, the contributory significance or "weight" of each cluster, and of each symptom within the cluster, is not the same.

One symptom that "straddles" two or all three clusters is "organic drivenness" (Kahn & Cohen, 1934). As the name implies, the child gets going and keeps going as if he (most children suffering from this disorder are boys) were driven by an overwrought motor. He is therefore both hyperactive and inattentive, and may, for the same reason, be impulsive. However, even when given such a comprehensive and clear history, the clinician will need to keep in mind that the central diagnostic theme is short attention span equals *distractibility*, and that hyperactivity alone is an unreliable criterion.

Perhaps the most misleading item in both the parental and teacher history is impulsivity. A child who misbehaves for any reason may be suspected of having ADHD by the teacher who hopes for pharmacological relief, and by the parents who scapegoat this particular child. It is here that clinical acumen and comprehensiveness are needed so that behavioral difficulties and hyperactivity that are not part of ADHD can be ruled out.

The duration of symptoms of ADHD varies from "all of the child's life," or "from the word Go" (using the terminology of typical reports by parents), to at least six months, usually beginning with the child's entry into school. The latter point may be an artifact if it was only then that the symptoms started causing trouble.

The following are points to focus on when taking the history:

(a) The attention span is the most central symptom and is worth exploring in detail. In order to be significant, short attention span should occur in almost all situations where sustained mental effort is required. The exception is television—the information that a child can watch television for long periods of time does *not* mean good attention span because the television tube is well-known as the most powerful attention-focusing agent. By the same token, when a child cannot sit still even for television, his attention span is most likely very short.

Short attention span is best inquired into directly, even to the point of asking parents to quantify it. "He cannot sit still for anything" or "He cannot stay with something even for two minutes" are examples of statements that are suggestive, but have to be amplified. Do they apply in all situations? What makes them better, what makes them worse? These questions address the core problem of distractibility, i.e., short attention span is a function of the child's inability to screen out incidental stimuli, both external (sights, sounds) and internal (impulses and "stimulus hunger"). The existence of this stimulus barrier deficit (for details see the section on Etiology and Pathogenesis) can be ascertained by appropriate questions: "Is the child easily distracted by irrelevant stimuli?" "Does he pay equal attention to events that have nothing to do with the task at hand?" "Is his focus constantly shifting?" "Does he never complete tasks?"

Attention span improves for anyone in one-to-one contacts and in quiet surroundings, as well as under circumstances of high motivation. All this holds true in ADHD as well, except that it is virtually impossible to find a task that would fascinate an ADHD child without offering at least some physical activity. Some ADHD children also do surprisingly well on such tasks as building elaborate structures with Lego blocks, which require a relatively small amount of physical activity but make up for little movement with colorful complexity.

(b) Hyperactivity in ADHD is of the erratic, random kind, somehow reminiscent of the Brownian movement of molecules. A high activity level may be suggestive of ADHD, but certainly is not diagnostic. Here occur most of the semantic misunderstandings between parents and clinicians: to the parents, "hyperactive" is a pejorative term, and many of them will say something like, "My child is hyperactive, but not hyperkinetic." High activity level is not tantamount to ADHD. Perhaps another way to refer to the hyperactivity cluster is "excessive and persistent motor responses": the child reacts to all stimuli motorically, i.e., with movement. That is why they are described as "in constant motion."

These children will be described (and will describe themselves) as liking activities that involve speed—racing on bicycles or go-carts, running wild. Some are good at sports; others simply like the commotion, but are poor teammates because of their impulsiveness.

(c) Impulsivity: At its worst, this manifests itself as violence towards siblings, peers, or animals. In these cases we hear statements like, "He constantly hits other children; picks fights; torments and beats up his younger brother or sister;

there is no end to name calling." They "pick on" other children and are, in turn, picked on. Sometimes, these children will tackle adults. The killing of animals (pets are the most accessible) is the most ominous defect in impulse control.

When less severe, impulsiveness is reflected in seemingly thoughtless, "on-the-spur-of-the-moment" actions, such as running out of the house (and into the busy street), daredevil actions on a bicycle, or taking up a new activity just because it has caught the child's fancy—without finishing what was being done previously. Parents complain more about the "messiness" of these children, with things left all over in their wake, "as if a tornado had hit the house."

The classic symptom of impulsivity is a quick temper: these children are easily provoked and often literally fly into enraged action. Another frequent set of symptoms in this category is inability to take "No!" for an answer. Their reactions to frustration, from any source, are always strong, sometimes extreme, and are immediately translated into action—fighting, screaming, cursing, crying, or temper tantrums.

The contributing history

(a) Certain items in the child's developmental history correlate (to a varying degree, and not always significantly) with ADHD. They are not diagnostic in themselves, but are adjuvants in the diagnostic process, helping to "tip the scales" towards ADHD.

The following are useful practically and merit inquiry:

- prematurity
- signs of fetal distress pre- and perinatally, i.e., fetal distress that prompted the obstetrician to hurry the delivery
- precipitated or prolonged labor
- perinatal asphyxia, particularly umbilical cord wrapped around the child's neck, and low Apgar scores
- feeding and sleeping difficulties in the first days, weeks, or months of the child's life, such as day-night inversion ("slept all day and cried all night" or "slept fitfully, if at all"). The most notorious among this group of symptoms has been the "three-month colic," often found to be due to milk allergy.

(b) The family history is of diagnostic value at least equal to the developmental items just listed. The triad of alcoholism, hysteria, and sociopathy in one parent has been shown to correlate significantly with ADHD. A "direct" family history of ADHD is surprisingly common—as a matter of fact, even more common than the triad just mentioned. Specific and straightforward inquiry will often elicit the response: "I was 'hyper' during my childhood"; "My brother could never sit still." A supportive item in the family history is learning disability: "His father never could read"; "His uncle is very bright and can do anything with his hands but his wife has to read him the instructions." This capitalizes on the overlap between developmental learning disorders and ADHD.

Another item capitalizing on yet another overlap, this one between ADHD and Conduct Disorder, is aggressiveness. Violence or trouble with the law (including a history of jail sentences) is suggestive of Conduct Disorder or ADHD in that family member.

The history of brain damage

"When Bobby was eight months old, he fell down the stairs and knocked his head. No, he was not unconscious, but I often wondered...."

This very common vignette from an anxious mother is an example of parental misconceptions about what constitutes brain damage. If the clinician were to inquire into all the questionable head trauma, we would end up with no useful data at all.

What we mean by brain damage is definite injury to the central nervous system, either traumatic or infectious. Although the incidence of ADHD in children with proven brain damage has varied from one author to another (some even claiming that it is no higher than in the general population), a history of brain damage almost ensures the diagnosis of ADHD in the presence of symptomatology in the hyperactivity-attention deficit-impulsivity clusters.

The psychiatric examination

The child psychiatric examination relies heavily on *observation,* as we emphasized in Chapter 1. This is especially true in ADHD, where observation may show the syndrome clearly. The child's verbal communication and play give additional diagnostic clues.

Observation. In typical and sufficiently severe cases of ADHD, observation shows a "driven" youngster who moves quickly from one activity, or from one toy, to another, without giving any one of them enough attention or enough time. As a result, the child does not derive the intended benefit from the toy or activity.

"Drivenness" may be manifested in "perpetual motion," but, as already mentioned in the history section, the excessive movement is not always purposeful and is quite often of an incidental, zigzagging nature. These children are in perpetual motion without a discernible purpose.

There is a certain "tyrannical" aspect to the hyperactivity. The child perseverates either in overall activity or in one or the other aspect. For instance, when a child cannot find a small ball that has rolled under a piece of furniture and become inaccessible, he will make many attempts to retrieve it, repeating the same strategy, with small variations, a dozen times. The examiner who happens to have a playroom equipped with a pool-table had better be prepared to spend the entire session with the child rolling the pool balls over and over again. This perseverative activity is just that—perseveration in the organically "driven" sense, *not* sustained attention span—and the child simply stimulates himself again and again with motor activity, without playing a game of pool.

An associated feature, also related to brain dysfunction and found typically in brain-injured adults and children, is the inability to "change the set," i.e., the child perseverates in one activity and reacts with signs of frustration to a change of activity. The change usually has to be forced upon the child.

To add to the scenario in the examining room, many ADHD children are a source of anxiety to the examiner, because nothing seems safe from their whirlwind activity or their need to touch everything around them. The more objects, especially toys, the room contains, the more the child gets stimulated. Therefore, having only sand, water, or finger paints around is a good idea for the examiner's peace of mind.

Having illustrated the most typical features of hyperactivity and short attention span, we must now state quite clearly that observation may reveal *none* of the signs described so far, and yet the child turns out to be suffering from ADHD. There are two main reasons for this (see also section on Etiology and Pathogenesis): the child's capabilities for inhibition are significant, or the child becomes hyperactive only as a result of overstimulation; the examiner's office is usually a quiet and safe place, quite unlike the classroom or playground.

Therefore, we continue to witness the perennial mistake made by pediatricians and other primary care physicians of diagnosing ADHD according to the presence or absence of observable hypermotility in the office. Again, we urge caution and *not* saying to a mother who complains that her child is or may be hyperactive: "He cannot be hyperactive. He does not show any hyperactivity in my office; he is all boy."

The careful observer can, nevertheless, detect hypermotility even in "quiet" children: their attention span does "deteriorate" after 10-15 minutes, and there are increasingly frequent extraneous movements—shifting legs, poking at objects, and generally getting progressively more restless as the expressions on their faces become progressively more bored. They need sensory input badly, and respond to minor distractions or go in search of distractions. However, the busy primary care practitioner cannot be expected to keep a child under observation for any period from 10–45 minutes; what he or she *can* be expected to do is to listen carefully to the mother's history.

By the same token, not all hyperactivity is ADHD. Even an observation of short attention span, once, does not mean ADHD. It may mean that the child is distraught, unhappy, or anxious. It is the entire, longitudinal picture that justifies the diagnosis of ADHD.

We may mention here Rutter's (1982) division of ADHD children into "pervasive" and "situational." "Pervasive" ADHD cases are more severe and, therefore, are evident even without overstimulation, i.e., even in the quiet one-to-one, office environment. "Situational" ADHD needs the outside trigger of overstimulation to show itself clinically and may be missed in the office examination.

Apart from motility, the examiner will make note of any signs of "stigmata"of immaturity (see Chapter 2). Positive findings are supportive or suggestive, but not diagnostic of ADHD.

Verbal and nonverbal communications. Children with ADHD tend to be superficial and concrete in their thinking, as reflected in how they describe their life and their feelings and in how they play. What they feel and what they express are geared mostly to simple, concrete, "tangible" items. Their fantasies are tied to action, and their interpersonal relationships are simpler than those of the child without ADHD. Although they get angry easily, they get over various psychological traumata faster and possibly with less psychic pain than the average child. This refers to the "normal" type and frequency of mental traumata, such as rejection, negative reactions to the child's actions, or parental disappointment in the child's work. However, since these children cause an above-average amount of negative reactions in their environment, the cumulative effect is considerable and almost always results in their having low self-esteem.

Diagnostic approaches of possible value. Among the less reliable diagnostic approaches are psychological testing, the electroencephalogram, and laboratory tests.

The psychological tests are of some practical diagnostic value, as long as the clinician does *not* rely on them as primary diagnostic tools. Increased scatter on the subtests of the WISC-R or a significant discrepancy (more than 15 points) between the verbal and performance scales suggest perceptual-motor difficulties, which may be related to, and therefore potentially indicative of, ADHD. Positive findings on the Lincoln-Oseretsky test, which measures motor function, may also point to hyperactivity. Abnormal findings on the Bender-Gestalt test are probably the most commonly used, and abused, for helping in the diagnosis of ADHD; we say abused because a useful test is excessively relied on. (The tests referred to here are described in Chapter 1.)

The electroencephalogram often shows nonspecific abnormalities that occur more often among ADHD children than controls, but it should *not* be used for practical diagnostic purposes, as the margin of error is too large.

The biochemical measures of serum neurotransmitters or their enzyme DBH, or measurements of urinary metabolites of neurotransmitters, are chemical quantifications used in research *only*.

Therefore, we may state firmly that at the present stage of our knowledge, there are no laboratory or psychological tests practically diagnostic of ADHD, and that the diagnosis of ADHD continues to depend solely on the clinical evaluation. Finally, there is one clinical procedure that may be viewed as the "ultimate diagnostic test," and that is the response to treatment with stimulant medication. It should not be used in a cavalier fashion, since medicinal treatment of ADHD must be part of a comprehensive approach. We will discuss it in the section on Treatment.

DIFFERENTIAL DIAGNOSIS

The main differential diagnostic issue concerns different etiologies for the same clinical picture. Put differently, when we see a hyperactive child who has difficulty paying attention, we have to determine whether this is due to the disorder of ADHD, or whether it is due to other psychiatric or medical causes.

1. *The first division to be established in the differential-diagnostic process is to rule out medical disorders.* A number of causes can produce symptoms similar to those of ADHD, because children react with hyperactivity, impulsivity, and/or attentional difficulties to a multitude of disturbances, either within themselves or in their environment. Therefore, most physical illnesses may cause symptoms of ADHD. Among the legion of such illnesses, congenital but undetected endocrine disorders, especially hyperthyroidism, should be thought of; among infections, respiratory tract and urinary tract infections. The latter sometimes are associated with congenital abnormalities. Among medical disorders in general, allergies are the most common cause of restlessness, irritability, hyperactivity and hyperreactivity, and poor concentration. In addition, upper respiratory tract allergies produce otitis media that interferes with hearing, further compromising the child's attention span.

2. *The second division is to separate out psychogenic conditions.* There is less pressure to make this differential diagnosis, because time lost is not potentially as irreparable as in organic disorders that call for early treatment. On the other hand, this differential diagnosis is often more difficult to make, partly because of the intertwining of temperamental predisposition in the parents and the child with the psychogenic factors, and partly because emotional conditions produce clinical pictures that are very similar to ADHD, without the availability of differentiating organic signs. One factor that increases the similarity is that psychogenic hyperactivity is often of long duration, just like ADHD.

What helps in the differential diagnosis is a thorough history that rarely shows the long duration or the complete symptomatology of ADHD, but does reveal anxiety in the family and in the child. Paralleling this finding in the history is the finding, in the psychiatric examination, of the presence of anxiety and generally of a richer fantasy life in the child with psychogenic hyperactivity.

3. *Conditioned or lifestyle hyperactivity.* This category refers to syndromes almost identical to ADHD, but which arise out of imitation of a family style of high activity, high reactivity, and volatility. The child either imitates these patterns or, more significantly, becomes conditioned by them. This happens because the child gets rewarded only when he or she attracts attention (positive or negative) through action—the noisier and faster, the better.

There is no specific name for this syndrome, and even the name we have given it does not completely cover all of its aspects; but it does address the most important mechanism. We do not include it among the "psychogenic syndromes" because we would like to separate this "lifestyle" syndrome from the one precipitated by a mentally significant event with resulting anxiety and from Depression, which is absent in the lifestyle hyperactivity.

The diagnosis of "conditioned hyperactivity" is often complex because it may be mixed with mild or moderate ADHD proper. In other words, a highly volatile family may have traits of ADHD that are genetically handed down to the child in addition to the conditioning process. The child may be suffering from an ADHD that is made much worse because impulsivity and action are encouraged. Differential diagnosis is made more difficult because "lifestyle hyperactivity" is also of chronic duration.

We therefore view "conditioned hyperactivity" as occupying a place in between ADHD and psychogenic or reactive hyperactivity. (An example is given in Case 21-5).

The cases presented below illustrate some of these points:

CASE 21-2 Amos was halfway through the third grade when his family started receiving reports from the teacher that Amos was "hyper": he *could not sit* still, he was *fidgeting* all the time, and he seemed to be moving his books and papers to and fro. He was *not paying enough attention* to the work, and his *grades were slipping.* This was *out of character* for him, as he had been a good student and a rather quiet boy up to now. The parents themselves had noted that he had become restless and intolerant of heat—indeed, his skin felt hot and flushed. Amos was found to have *hyperthyroidism.*

CASE 21-3 Malvina was a six-year-old petite girl who had been considered somewhat lively by her parents, but *never* to the point of "getting into everything." Indeed, she was a very cooperative child, who could be relied upon to *stop a certain activity* if her parents thought it was getting out of hand.

As she moved through first grade, however, Malvina displayed progressive *restlessness* at school. There were days when she *could not sit still* and *asked to go to the bathroom* many times—too many for classroom routine and discipline. Her teacher wondered whether she was hyperactive. Malvina also complained about *pain* in her side, especially when she had to *sit still*. Initial examination by the pediatrician was without any findings, but subsequent physical examinations revealed tenderness in the left costovertebral angle; her astute pediatrician included intravenous urography in her workup. This showed ureteral obstruction, which was corrected surgically, and the child's behavior returned to normal.

CASE 21-4   Alex was a seven-year-old second-grader who was referred for psychiatric treatment because he was considered *"hyperactive"* and a "behavior and attention disorder" by his mother and his teacher. Both of them found him hard to deal with: he could *not sit still* when the class was in session or when he was having dinner with his mother and brother, and his *attention span wandered easily away* from school assignments or chores. What mother and teacher were most concerned about, however, was Alex's *irritability*, lack of inner restraints, and *quick temper*. He was *easily provoked* by the smallest friction and simply could *not hold his temper;* he often lashed out at peers, both verbally and physically. He was easily frustrated by any task that did not offer immediate gratification. He was repeatedly apprehended *shoplifting*, and when asked why he took a seemingly meaningless item, he replied simply that he *wanted it at the moment.*

When examined, Alex presented a *confusing picture of restlessness, moving around* the office; *touching everything*, but with a *fleeting flicker* of interest *that quickly petered out;* and then the boy went on to yet another object, to leave that in turn, and so on. His facial expression was one of *apathy*, and he approached the interview and the examiner with a mixture of *disinterest* and *pugnaciousness.*

His attitude changed when the examiner succeeded in sustaining the conversation on the *family scene*. Alex reported that his father had left the family half a year earlier, following years of marital strife between the parents. Of all the children, Alex had always been the *closest* to his father, and his *symptoms had indeed started at the time father left*. As Alex talked about this, he revealed both *sadness* about father's absence and a great deal of anticipatory *anxiety* about the future. He felt *guilty* about what he may have contributed to the parental separation: Had he "sided too much with father"? Had he "told on his father or mother"? and the like. What preoccupied him most, however, was the current *conflict of loyalties*, since he knew that father wanted custody of the children, especially of him, Alex, and he loved both mother and father. He was angry that he was being *put in this situation*, and wished he *could get out of it*. He had thought of running away, but his sense of family loyalty had prevented this. All in all, Alex found himself in a *state of constant conflict* and *anxiety* and *did not know how to deal with it.*

The mother confirmed that Alex's hyperactivity and other problems indeed *started after* father had left home, and that prior to that event, Alex had actually been a rather quiet child, on the sensitive side, and certainly not considered "hyper" by anyone.

Comment. This case highlights, among other features, the *discontinuity* in the history of psychogenic hyperactivity. This discontinuity is not always so abrupt as it was here; however, many cases of psychogenic hyperactivity can be traced to a point of change, often a traumatic event. Change in family circumstances is frequently the precipitating event, but a variety of stresses or traumata can be found here. One such factor is child abuse, of any kind, particularly sexual abuse.

The diagnosis is not only helped by the history, but by the psychiatric examination itself. This reveals an inner life of conflict, with resulting anxiety and depression, behind the symptom picture of hyperactivity.

CASE 21-5   Vito was referred for psychiatric consultation after his first-grade teacher decided he was *too wild* for her classroom. She insisted he be transferred to another class, where the same thing happened, for that teacher also felt that she could not devote most of her time to Vito. When the teachers discussed Vito's problems with his parents, the reaction was one of *incomprehension*—the parents *could not understand* what the teacher was objecting to: Vito was *all boy* and was *smart and a go-getter.* The teachers thought that Vito was "hyper" since he rushed through all his tasks, talked out of turn, went after anything aggressively, —although without malice or intent to hurt. They felt he might have been doing it "for attention."

Comment. This parent's teachers were right. The child was acting for attention, since action was the one known way to get it—it was his family style.

ETIOLOGY AND PATHOGENESIS

The subject of both the causality and the pathophysiology of ADHD has become complex partly because, in the past, we thought we knew more than we actually did. The other factor making for complexity is that older studies lacked precise terminology and comprehensiveness of research design, usually failing to control for interactional factors.

We will summarize the contemporary thinking about etiology and pathogenesis as follows: ADHD is a syndrome arising from any one of several causes, some known, others unknown. There is disagreement on the pathophysiological mechanism that gives rise to the syndrome, there being two contradictory schools of thought.

Understanding of the causes and neurophysiological mechanisms of ADHD is very useful clinically, because it relates clearly to the symptom picture and thus enhances the practitioner's clinical skills, even though the causal reasoning is incomplete and controversial. For purposes of exposition, we are dividing our discussion into that of causes and of mechanisms, but the two are, of course, intertwined.

Causes

Brain damage. This, historically, was the classic cause of ADHD. Careful reasoning has resulted in considerable, although not total, consensus in the scientific community that it indeed *may* result in ADHD, but not predictably so. Demonstrable brain damage, such as arises from head trauma or central nervous system infections, accounts for a small proportion of ADHD children.

Our knowing that gross brain damage does not necessarily produce ADHD has helped to settle some of the controversy surrounding "minimal brain damage" (MBD). The MBD concept arose from the observations by Strauss and Lehtinen in 1947 that known brain damage resulted in hyperactivity, short attention span, and reactions ranging from rage to frustration. If the same syndrome is seen in children without demonstrable brain damage, they reasoned, the syndrome is also due to brain damage, but that damage is "minimal" because it cannot be demonstrated with the relatively crude methods (then) available.

The term "minimal brain damage" has been rejected by most clinicians because it implies an etiology that may not apply in each case. However, this should not be misunderstood: some damage or pathology of the central nervous system may be present in the majority of cases of ADHD. This is borne out by the significantly higher incidence of nonfocal ("soft") neurological signs, associated developmental disabilities, congenital stigmata of immaturity, abnormalities of the electroencephalogram, and biochemical (neurotransmitter) deficiencies. Brain pathology is not supported by a history of prenatal or perinatal trauma, which is found in less than 20% of ADHD children.

Genetic factors. Of all the causes of ADHD, genetic ones are the most frequently encountered (see also section on Diagnosis). ADHD is inherited either directly as the full disorder itself, or as traits, such as impulsivity combined with poor judgment and immaturity (the triad of sociopathy, hysteria, and alcoholism found in parents), or the associated developmental learning disorders. Twin and adoption studies have confirmed the importance of possible genetic or genogenic factors.

"Maturation lag." This is a vague, poorly quantified, but quite cogent term. Almost all children with ADHD act immaturely and have a special, difficult-to-describe, yet nevertheless definite, aura of immaturity about them. In its simplest definition, maturational or developmental lag means that the child's nervous system has not developed to the expected norm; however, this dysmaturation is never global or "across the board" in all areas, but always involves some functions

more than others. For instance, gross motor development is "on time," but fine motor coordination and perception are not. This provides the basis of the "scatter" on intelligence tests and of the abnormalities on tests of perceptual-motor function.

Intrauterine damage. Included here are congenital anomalies on one hand, and on the other the results of various toxic intrauterine influences on the embryo or fetus: factors like subclinical lead poisoning, cigarette smoking, and alcoholism in the mother during pregnancy. These issues await further research, if they are to be more than conjecture.

Allergies and intolerance of dyes and carbohydrates. The assumption that alimentary allergies or hypersensitivity to natural or artificial dyes, causes ADHD is based on anecdotal reports, and has not been confirmed by well-controlled studies. These conditions appear more potent in younger children. The role of carbohydrate (sugar) intolerance is even more speculative; there are single case reports of children becoming overactive on sweets, but there is a shortage of systematic studies on the subject.

Nonorganic causes. The syndrome of "conditioned" or "lifestyle hyperactivity" does not completely fit all the criteria of ADHD. However, it is reasonable to suggest that adverse interactional patterns do produce short attention span, hyperactivity, and impulsivity. The process is one of direct imitation of parental actions and reactions, often combined with a conditioning resulting from the parental reward of certain styles of excessive activity. The learning starts in infancy and early childhood, and is strengthened by unconscious, automatic, parental responses to the child's behavior. As the child grows up, (s)he finds the mature responses of introspection and delayed gratification extinguished by selective inattention, whereas quick action is rewarded and often rendered necessary for emotional survival.

Mechanisms

Anatomically, the proposed mechanisms center in the *reticular activating system* of the brainstem, a structure functioning as the "central switchboard" of all sensory input. There are found both excitatory and inhibitory neurons and, depending on which of these predominate, the reticular activating system may or may not function as an adequate stimulus regulator (Wender's model). Biochemically, inadequacy of function is thought to be associated with deficient quantities of neurotransmitters; there is no unanimity as to which of the known neurotransmitters is most instrumental. The majority of experiments have implicated dopamine.

In the 1950s, Laufer proposed the model of lowered neuronal threshold to stimuli, as measured by the photometrazol test (Laufer, Denhoff, & Solomons, 1957). Because of this lowered threshold in the reticular activating system, there is overstimulation, which translates itself into distractibility and hyperactivity.

A contrasting model subsequently was elaborated by Satterfield and colleagues (1981): there is lowered excitability in the midbrain reticular activating system, therefore the system needs more stimuli. The child seeks stimulation by greater activity—thus, hyperactivity arises because of "stimulus hunger." Other studies have also suggested that ADHD children are "underaroused" or respond with lesser evoked potentials to stimuli, thus creating a need or "hunger" for more stimulation. The result would be random movement and random attention, or distractibility because of the need to follow stimuli.

Both models use response to stimulants as experimental evidence. In Laufer's experiments, amphetamines increased and normalized the sensory threshold, in effect raising the stimulus barrier. Laufer increased synaptic conduction time through the use of amphetamines and explained thereby the paradoxical effect of these agents, since prolongation of conduction time in the midbrain would slow down the excitability of that structure. Most investigators propose that the normal stimulating effects of amphetamines correct the neurotransmitter deficiency and increase the evoked responses, and thereby correct the pathology of underarousal. By stimulating the cortex, psychostimulants also increase cortical control over disorganized brainstem activity, thus improving purposeful behavior and attention span. This view has received added support from the reaction of children with ADHD to phenobarbital, which suppresses cortical activity and, instead of sedating these children, makes them worse, i.e., hyperactive.

TREATMENT

A thorough diagnostic workup of the child with ADHD will provide the clinician with the insights necessary to plan a rational and individualized treatment approach. This self-evident statement bears repeating in the context of ADHD, because the seeming simplicity of the disorder seduces some clinicians into taking therapeutic shortcuts.

As part of our continuing effort to emphasize that interactional and educational measures are just as important and as indispensable as judicious pharmacotherapy, we shall discuss the former first.

Interactional measures

These consist of parental guidance, psychotherapy of the child, and behavioral modification measures.

Parental guidance. This is the linchpin of all treatment of ADHD. Parental guid-ance is a combination of *educational* and *psychotherapeutic* techniques. The former clarify the parents' perceptions of the child and help them to understand the child when they obtain established knowledge about ADHD. The latter explore that part of the parents' psychopathology which is an obstacle to appropriate understanding and management of that particular child. The goal is a better understanding of the child's behavior and of the parents' own reactions, and the gradual building of new skills for handling the child with ADHD.

Counseling of the parents of an ADHD child is a specialized procedure. It is best done by a child psychiatrist as it requires both a thorough grasp of the mechanisms of ADHD and skill in psychodynamics. A parallel to brief psycho-therapy suggests itself since the therapy requires considerable skill in selecting specific issues for work. The clinician working with the parents of an ADHD child needs to work selectively with those sectors of parental psychopathology that interfere with their adaptation to a special problem (the ADHD child), not with their psychobiological functioning, or even parenting in general.

Direct guidance depends on several factors, but the experienced clinician soon finds that giving too much direct advice too early is a distinct pitfall. The basic technique should, instead, be for the parents to acquire a framework of understanding their child and their own reactions, and to absorb the principles of management, and then to apply these principles to their own situations in a learning process spread out over several follow-up sessions.

Nevertheless, there are a few "staples" that most clinicians find useful to impart to parents at one time or another. The first of these is prevention: many parents sense that keeping "a step or two ahead" of their child is a good policy, and the clinician encourages the parents always to think ahead and plan ahead towards situations that will minimize disruption and overstimulation—i.e., intense excite-ment and too many activities in close succession are best avoided. It is very difficult to "bring the child down" from excitement. Activities from which the child learns and uses the knowledge gained should be encouraged. Succeeding in age-appropriate tasks builds self-esteem, an important commodity for any child and especially for the ADHD child, whose self-esteem is usually low.

The screening of peer relationships is yet another area for intervention and prevention. Most parents believe in the value of friendships to the point of being uncritical about the kinds of friends their child associates with. ADHD children are more susceptible to the influence of peers with impulse control difficulties for such children offer them quick stimulation and quick gratification. The parents are the only agents who can select and control these relationships. The child has neither the motivation nor the judgment to do so.

Furthermore, the parents are the intermediaries *par excellence* between the psychiatrist and the school system. All too often, parents displace their frustrations onto the school, and teachers may do the same things to parents. The ADHD child needs structure, and the prerequisite for that is agreement between the adults.

This brings us to one of the basic principles of counseling all of the adults who take care of ADHD children: in order to establish structure, there needs to be consensus among the participants. ADHD children are difficult and provoke a range of feelings and reactions in their caregivers. At times, this amounts to protectiveness; at times, it amounts to a challenge of the adult's self-esteem as a parent or questions the adult's intelligence or personality per se. Disagreements between parents of ADHD children are more frequent than among other parents, the difficult child sometimes becoming the fulcrum on which the parents' marriage breaks up.

Agreement between the parents, and between them and the teacher, is so advisable that it is worth a few compromises. To achieve reasonable consensus among the adults, the clinician uses his/her psychotherapeutic skills.

Reaching consensus is facilitated by the clinician's attitude of not assigning blame, but of seeking solutions. This does not mean that parental reactions and attitudes do not contribute to the child's behavior. It means that the clinician proceeds with sensitivity to the parents' guilt and does not push the parents onto the defensive. "There are no problem children, only problem parents" is still very much with us, in spite of its absurdity, and parents are still made to feel guilty, since they are accused of being causally responsible for their child's ADHD.

Behavior modification. This is based on the principle of operant conditioning. It rewards delay of gratification and self-control. Usually a system of charts is employed, wherefrom children accumulate points, to be traded in for tangibles. Some children can be taught self-monitoring.

These and similar behavioral methods have had mixed success. We believe that success depends on the therapist's skill and on the follow-up: the therapist who has experience with long-term use of behavioral modification will do well, if he/she has regular follow-up appointments with the parents and the child, to reinforce the system and to prevent the mere acquisition of a few basic rewards without subsequent randomization and self-sufficiency.

Psychotherapy. In a broader sense, parent counseling is a form of psychotherapy. What we refer to under this title, however, is individual psychotherapy with the child, specifically that along psychodynamic lines.

In its standard, traditional form, even when fully adapted to the child's age, psychotherapy of the ADHD child has been unsuccessful. The goal of treatment of ADHD is simply too different from what psychodynamic psychotherapy is expected to accomplish, i.e., to restructuring of defense mechanisms.

Individual psychotherapy is, however, useful to treat associated pathology and the mental sequelae of ADHD. Even then, it is usually modified to relate to the concrete, short-term perspectives of the ADHD child. Low self-esteem and inappropriate measures to relieve it are the main indications. An age of at least six or seven years and ability to relate, as well as improved attention span (usually following successful pharmacotherapy), are minimal prerequisites.

What the therapist tries to accomplish are new ways for the child to relate and in which to be successful, based on the child's real abilities. Every child has strengths; these are identified by the therapist, and the child is encouraged to make full use of them. Hard work is supported, praised, and the child is helped to achieve success in school.

Psychotherapy is provided in shorter sessions (half an hour) and at longer intervals (e.g., every two weeks) and always in close cooperation with parental counseling, and any other measures required. (Gardner [1979] advocates using the mother as cotherapist.) It is, however, beneficial to continue psychotherapy over a longer period, i.e., at least several months, to incorporate the normal process of maturation, on one hand, and to prevent relapses, on the other. Psychotherapy of the ADHD case is not for the novice: the therapist should be expert in long-term, psychodynamic psychotherapy, since this seemingly simple psychotherapy of ADHD draws its strength from sound psychodynamic tenets and is then tailored to the special needs of the ADHD child.

To repeat a frequent warning: successful pharmacotherapy should not blind the clinician to the need for psychotherapy. Indeed, when the child has improved with other measures he/she may then show a partial clinical picture of internal conflict (neurosis), which is an indication for psychotherapy.

Educational measures

The coexistence of developmental learning disabilities with ADHD is frequent, and clinicians find themselves prodding the system to bring about or maintain the special diagnostic and remedial measures that only the school system can provide.

In addition, the clinician may be able to offer teacher counseling, or at least attempt to. The counseling is best done along the lines recommended for "parental counseling," as the clinician will find that teachers have as many difficulties and psychological "blind spots" as parents, and will therefore require similar combined therapeutic approaches.

The level of sophistication and open-mindedness varies as much among the teachers as among the parents, and the clinician needs to muster a great deal of evenhandedness and patience. When dealing with teachers, often the clinician will initially encounter simplistic views: pharmacological treatment or nonpharmacological treatment, strict discipline or permissiveness ("understanding"). A learning process will need to take place for the teacher, just as for the parent; therefore, follow-up is more important than trying to have the teacher absorb the information all at once. Both parents and teachers need additional guidance if the child is treated pharmacologically.

Hundreds of parents have reported that a genuinely self-assured teacher who runs a structured classroom does well with the ADHD child. The teacher who is successful with this kind of pupil senses the fine line between making the learning process interesting but not overstimulating to the child. Classroom structure entails predictability and less stimulation (since everyone is rather quiet, too). If the teacher also can motivate the child, the teacher's actions yield practically the same effects as successful treatment with psychostimulant medication.

The psychiatric consultant can discuss various detailed measures with the teacher, always keeping in mind, as with the parents, not to become so specific as to usurp the day-to-day management and education of the child. Teachers may be reminded that the ADHD child needs a more concrete approach and that he/she needs more frequent repetition of the instructions; as a matter of fact, this amounts to the same technique advocated when we suggest that parents divide a longer or more complex task into several segments. Being "two steps ahead" of the ADHD child comes naturally to a talented teacher, but may be taught to many teachers.

Other professionals in the educational system, such as the school psychologist and the school social worker, are very valuable allies since they can afford to view the ADHD child with greater detachment and therefore stay away from the more emotional attitudes taken by some teachers. An ongoing, consultative relationship between the clinician and these professionals provides a platform of interprofessional understanding for the benefit of most ADHD children in a particular school system.

PHARMACOLOGICAL TREATMENT

To borrow from Winston Churchill (himself, in our opinion, probably an ADHD child): "My warnings . . . had been so numerous, so detailed, . . . that no one could gainsay me" (Churchill, 1948, p. 667). We hope to have done nearly as well, by alluding repeatedly to the dangers of treating ADHD exclusively with medication, even if the dramatic effectiveness of psychostimulant drugs tends to preempt all other treatment approaches. The clinician must, therefore, have the self-discipline to treat the ADHD child and his/her parents with all the modalities that a thorough understanding calls for. If pharmacotherapy is administered in combination with the other measures, it is highly beneficial. If it is administered in isolation, it is still beneficial, but may cause other areas to be left unattended when medicating ADHD children.

We shall fully address the two main categories of medications used in ADHD—the stimulants and antidepressants—and discuss the role of the neuroleptics and other medications not in the mainstream of current pharmacotherapy. Finally, we look at the unproven methods of treating ADHD children.

The stimulants

These comprise the standard pharmacological treatment of ADHD. This treatment approach was pioneered by Bradley, who discovered, paradoxically, that benzedrine (rarely used today) calmed children with behavior problems. Among the currently used stimulant medications, methylphenidate (trade name: Ritalin) has become the standard agent. Before prescribing, the physician should ask him/herself: What will the medication accomplish? In this case, the answer is: increased attention span equaling less distractibility and better concentration; a decrease in excessive and random motility, i.e., decreased hyperactivity; and better impulse control. These are behavioral parameters. In most cases, improvement on these parameters will have beneficial effects on the child's school performance. Controversy continues over the question of whether stimulants improve learning performance per se, yet most of the evidence favors the view that the improved learning is solely a consequence of better concentration. The three stimulants in common use now are methylphenidate (Ritalin), dextroamphetamine (Dexedrine), and magnesium pemoline (Cylert).

Methylphenidate (Ritalin). This most commonly used and most frequently studied stimulant drug is popular for the predictability of response to it and, most likely, because it is not an amphetamine and therefore does not bear a "street name." It is also the stimulant with the shortest duration of action (3–5 hours).

Therapeutic dose ranges from 0.3–0.8 mg/kg per dose. Because of its short duration, methylphenidate may have to be given twice or even three times a day. This translates into a range of 5–60 mg per day or of 2.5–20 mg per dose.

The dose quantity obviously depends on age. Nearly all practitioners have found that prescribing stimulants to children below age 5 years is inadvisable in most instances, since the response varies unpredictably, often from one day to another, and confuses and frustrates the child's parents. This erratic effectiveness puts the approach into disrepute prematurely, for most of these parents resist recommendations for pharmacotherapy with stimulants at a later time when the child may really need them.

For ages 5–8 years, the 5 mg tablet of methylphenidate can be used as the basic unit. The dose is then titrated upward as needed to find the lowest effective single dose. The parents are instructed to give the child the medication in the morning only, and then observe him/her (over the weekend) and to ask the teacher to give a report and, if possible, to complete one of the rating scales. The important information to be gathered at this point is whether the child shows improvement, and if so, in what areas and for how long the improvement lasts.

The response to the lowest dose may be very dramatic at first. The observation may be that the child did better the whole day long. Much of this is a mental/symbolic by-product, the "halo" effect: everyone is more optimistic and has positive expectations without putting the burden on the child, and this combines with the immediate and genuine pharmacological effects. Since some of the troubles for the ADHD child are due to a reciprocal action and reaction formula, the beneficial effects of the medication may extend beyond the few hours of its pharmacological effect simply by having interrupted the reciprocal formula for a while.

As time goes on, however, the pharmacological reality takes over and the individual dosage and frequency have to be revised upward. At that point, the clinician may instruct the parents to add half a tablet to the early morning dose (i.e., 2.5 mg) and send a supply to school for noontime administration, following the same gradual escalation pattern. The parents are asked to stop at the lowest dose that gives reasonable results but not to hope for perfection. The lowest effective dose *may* be safer. Still, the main consideration is that higher doses are not markedly more effective, do produce side effects (to be discussed presently), and leave little leeway for later increases which will be mandated by the growth of the child.

There are exceptions, of course, on both sides of the dosage range. Some children cannot tolerate more than 2.5 mg, and a few others require 50 mg per day at age seven years. Psychosocial matters have to be studied carefully in these extremes, especially the "lifestyle hyperactivity" described in the earlier section on the Differential Diagnosis. There appear to exist, however, a few children who metabolize all stimulants so rapidly that a higher dose is needed for normalizing them. A sustained-release form (Ritalin SR 20 mg) exists and is of practical value once that dosage requirement has been demonstrated.

Children 8 years or older may be started with the 10 mg tablet of Ritalin, which can then be titrated in 5 mg increments.

Dextroamphetamine (Dexedrine). The only difference between this agent and methylphenidate is that dextroamphetamine has a slightly longer duration of action. For all practical purposes, including dosage, the two stimulants are very similar in clinical application and actions.

Magnesium pemoline (Cylert). This medication is different from the two just described. Pemoline has a longer duration of action (up to 12 hours) and requires regular administration for up to 6 weeks (or more) to produce solid behavioral effects. Its dosage range is from 18.75–150 mg per day; the usual dose in grade-school children is 37.50–75 mg. The obvious advantage of the longer duration allowing for once-a-day dosage is offset by the "lag time" during which, for weeks, parents and doctor do not know whether the child is responding to the medication.

Side effects of the stimulants. Stimulants as a group (of the three we considered) are safe medications. When pemoline (Cylert) was first introduced over a decade ago, there were reports of mildly elevated liver enzymes; these, however, have proven of no clinical significance and it is not necessary to order routine laboratory tests during long-term use of any of the stimulants, including pemoline.

None of them produces addiction. Tolerance is extremely rare, if it exists at all. The dose increases made for a growing child are predicated on growth, but children often continue on the same dose for a long time, even years, with the same good effect.

The most common adverse effect of psychostimulants is a syndrome of "over-response": the child has responded so well that he/she is too quiet to the point of being described as zombielike by the parents, or wonder if the child is depressed or oversedated—"too down." Another untoward manifestation, not necessarily combined with the first, is paradoxical crying or whining, i.e., with little or no precipitating cause. These side effects are directly related to dosage and will disappear when the dosage is reduced.

There has been a great deal of concern over suppression of growth, either indirectly by suppression of appetite or directly via a hypothalamic-pituitary mechanism. It appears that when controlled follow-up studies are conducted over a long time span (e.g., a decade), growth retardation is not in evidence. In other words, the patients treated with stimulants seem to catch up in late adolescence or young adulthood if there was any earlier growth retardation. Persistent suppression of appetite is rare and the present authors have never been impressed by any change in patients' growth rate. The parents should, nevertheless, be apprised of the essence of the controversy over growth suppression.

The only other major side effect is the emergence of tics or involuntary movements. Several authors have reported the emergence of Tourette's Disorder after the use of a stimulant or antidepressant, presumably because of their action of augmenting active nervous system neurotransmitters. A few children will develop reversible excessive movements, e.g., picking at their skin, which disappears upon discontinuation of the stimulant medication. Parents should be questioned about any prior history of tics, either in the child or among relatives, and the rare possibility of Tourette's Disorder being precipitated (or perhaps more accurately, unmasked) by the stimulant agent, should be discussed with them. Again, this is a rare eventuality. On the other hand, tics may be an expression of the underlying ADHD, and those tics usually improve with stimulant medication. Here, too, a meticulous history and careful follow-up of the response to the medication will usually provide the needed course. Headaches, stomachaches, pallor, or flushing of the face are minor side effects of little clinical consequence that often disappear on their own accord.

It is very useful to remember that, even in the most impressively successful cases, there will be gaps in the pharmacological effects. Such inert drug effects occur usually between times of administration, or because the medication simply "does not do it all." This is where the child and his parents need to be counseled to bridge the gaps by nonpharmacological means, i.e., by their own efforts.

A side effect, which is, rather, the normal response, is interference with sleep, or more usually, with going to sleep. This insomnia often vanishes after the first two or three weeks of medication. It is not possible to predict which child is going to react which way: some will be helped by a bedtime dose of stimulant medication to fall asleep; many others will be indifferent to an afternoon dose of stimulant; some will have trouble falling asleep if the medication is given late in the afternoon. These difficulties may be due to the time gap in pharmacological effectiveness. In all events, the clinician is advised to check his or her own reactions of omnipotence so (s)he does not feel called upon to manage every hour of the child's life. Put differently, there will be periods when the child's problems will have to be handled by the child and his parents, not by the "magic" of pharmacotherapy.

The antidepressants

The heading refers to the tricyclic antidepressants (TCAs) since these and not the monoamine oxidase inhibitors are used with children.

There has been a profound change in adoption of these medications for ADHD in the past few years. Several recent studies have suggested that these agents are as effective in ADHD children as are stimulants. The more traditional view has been that they are the "second line" medications, when the child has entered adolescence and no longer responds as favorably to stimulants.

Recent investigators have been bolder about the dosages prescribed for ADHD by raising the minimum and medium dosages. However, the maximum dose of 5 mg/kg per day of imipramine (Tofranil) continues to hold true. The previous fears of interference with the cardiac conduction system (as reflected in the prolongation of the P-R interval and the lengthening of the duration of the QRS complex on the electrocardiogram) have been somewhat allayed, but we would still recommend being conservative, obtaining an electrocardiogram at dosages above 3 mg/kg or if there is significant rise in pulse rate.

The desired effects and side effects of the whole class of antidepressants are discussed in the section on medications in Chapter 2.

The long-term use of stimulants and antidepressants

When properly used, pharmacotherapy of ADHD with stimulants and antidepressants can make a vital difference in the quality of the child's life, and of his family's, and in the child's prognosis. We affirm the last statement despite some follow-up studies failing to support such a contention; we base our belief on our experience of long-term pharmacotherapy *combined* with the other approaches.

It is true that the results of pharmacotherapy fade as soon as the agent is discontinued. We therefore recommend continuation of pharmacotherapy as long as definable benefits are in evidence. This means periodic (at least once-a-month) rechecks of the child and the parent(s), which really translate into ongoing, supportive, and, where necessary, brief psychodynamic psychotherapy. The child can safely be continued on stimulants until he no longer responds to them with improved attention span, which for many children occurs in pubescence or at puberty. A serious indication for continuing pharmacotherapy as long as it is effective is impulsivity with cruelty to peers or to animals.

Pharmacotherapy can, of course, be discontinued sooner. The criterion is maturation to the point where the child's own motivation (i.e., cortical control) gains control over the disarray of random and excessive excitation in the brainstem, according to Wender's model. Children can easily be restarted on pharmacotherapy if it turns out that our assessment of their self-control was overly sanguine.

The clinician may leave it up to the parents whether to stop pharmacotherapy during summer vacations, but the parents should know that there is no proven need to give "drug holidays." Most parents have no difficulty accepting the physician's reassurance that stimulants and antidepressants are not addictive or habit forming.

The neuroleptics

These agents used to be more widely employed for ADHD before it became clear that better results, with fewer side effects, could be obtained with stimulants and antidepressants. The neuroleptics are now resorted to in those rare instances when stimulants or antidepressants bring about extraneous movements or tics, or in cases where the possible diagnosis of ADHD is overshadowed by severe conduct disorder with serious loss of impulse control. For further details, consult Chapter 2.

Unproven treatment approaches

These have enjoyed such popularity at different times that they need to be addressed. Most of them have focused on exclusionary or elimination diets.

The Feingold diet. The Feingold or San Francisco Kaiser-Permanente (SFKP) Elimination Diet excludes all foods with a natural salicylate radical, tartrazine, and any artificial color or flavor. Controlled studies have not supported the expectation of improvement in most ADHD children, although there are single case reports where it has been successful. The diet is complex and difficult to adhere to.

Low sugar diet. The basis for this is the popular belief that refined sugar is not good for us, and that many children get "revved up" because of eating sugar. Again, controlled studies have not supported this totally, but have conceded the possibility that simple sugars may have some hyperkinetic effect in young children (preschoolers). Many clinicians have been told by mothers that increased sugar intake makes their children "wild." The clinician may take a supportive attitude towards any parental effort to cut down on the consumption of sweets, provided this does not promote an even greater interpersonal problem than originally brought the child to the psychiatrist.

Hypoglycemia. The enthusiasm for this disorder recently has waned considerably. Nevertheless, some parents insist that their child is hyperactive because of hypoglycemia. This belief may stem from parental need to put a more acceptable label on the child and may have been encouraged by a physician's incorrect interpretation of a glucose tolerance test. Hypoglycemia is a rare disorder that requires the presence of observable signs and symptoms concurrent with demonstrated low points in blood glucose levels. The danger with this pseudodiagnosis is that it prompts and abets parental resistance against more effective treatment modalities.

Artificial dyes. The results are the same as with other diets: first, there is no solid evidence that dyes are in fact causally related to ADHD, and second, it is well-nigh impossible to exclude them completely from the diet. The interpersonal difficulties caused by the "cure" are often worse than the disease.

Antivertigo drugs. The use of these drugs is based on Levinson's theory (1980) that ADHD and developmental learning disabilities are mediated by cerebellar-vestibular dysfunction. There are no controlled studies to support this continuation.

Caffeine and similar nonprescription stimulants. Use of these was a very logical idea pioneered by Schnackenberg (1974), and subsequently by one of the authors (Fras, 1974), but eventually found to be ineffective. Caffeine and other stimulants appeared to have the same effects as the standard prescription stimulants but were not concentrated enough; therefore, they were ineffective because the dose was too low.

PSYCHOLOGICAL AND SOCIAL CONSEQUENCES OF ADHD

ADHD is not a psychogenic syndrome per se. It arises presumably from a neurophysiological substrate and is shaped by the reciprocal interaction between the child and his or her social environment. The mental symptoms are secondary, deriving from the conflict between the immature, primitive, and erratic behavior of the ADHD child and the child's interpersonal environment. Conflict with society is a further consequence of ADHD, with ensuing antisocial, even criminal, adaptation being set in motion. When we remind ourselves of the neurophysiological models of ADHD, we can understand the delay with which mental symptoms arise in ADHD children, for these children are distractible and their attention is diverted from grasping the full significance of their interpersonal world and its problems.

But this does not last forever, and the emotional impact of being different, causing animosity in their environment, and being rejected is finally discerned by the child. At that time, the most frequent, almost universal, reaction is low self-esteem. These children find that they cannot measure up to the average peer. The peers, in turn, find that out, too, and this, plus the overreactivity of the ADHD child, makes the ADHD child a ready target for taunts, rejection, and exclusion.

Compensatory measures against low self-esteem and feelings of inadequacy include playing the clown, "buying" friendships (often with money stolen from home), or showing off in reckless or defiant actions. The next phase is for like children to band together and build a group image based on "toughness" and antisocial acts. Thus, the psychological problems become social, moral, and societal ones.

Excessive dependency, especially on their mothers, is still another psychosocial complication of ADHD. This dependency combines elements of hostility, for the mother is used as if a substitute peer, as a source of comfort, and as an outlet for anger. Linked with this is withdrawal from everyday involvement with people outside the family, especially the more average peers, and feeling fear of measuring up to others in any areas, even in those where the ADHD child does well.

Impulsivity, low frustration tolerance, and outbursts of temper not only interfere with interpersonal relationships but ease the emergence of guilt, self-hate and, again, feelings of helplessness, inadequacy, and low self-esteem. Antisocial acts, defiance of authority, and delinquency are social consequences that are multiply determined. Neurophysiologically, these children's low frustration tolerance and immature need for immediate gratification are coupled with immature judgment ("I won't be caught"). Secondarily, the child's prosocial need for visible success and adequacy gets thwarted.

Finally, the need to belong, but to suffer multiple rejection, makes ADHD children easily led, both into gangs and by unscrupulous criminal operators.

Stealing, fighting, truancy, and drug and alcohol abuse are more frequently encountered in ADHD children (and adolescents) than in the average population. In their delinquent gangs, ironically, these children find the structure they need, the acceptance, and the spirit of adventure.

COURSE AND PROGNOSIS

The course of ADHD is highly varied, and depends on several circumstances. The prognosis, too, is closely tied to these several factors. Earlier, child psychiatrists wrote that ADHD is simply outgrown at some time in adolescence. Unfortunately, this is simply not so. One visible change seen in about 80% of adolescents with ADHD is a marked decrease in hypermotility. Most adolescents seem to be able to sit still, but many still show fidgetiness; and a proportion of them (perhaps, again, 20%) will continue to have attentional difficulties, although these are not immediately discernible by casual inspection of their overt behavior.

Many ADHD children retain well into adulthood their traits of immaturity, superficiality, and poor judgment based on concreteness and immediate gratification. Included are residual poor impulse control and a tendency to violence or criminality. Their interpersonal relationships may lack depth, and a larger-than-expected number develop schizophrenia. In their adult lives, ADHD females are more prone to hysteria and males to antisocial personality. Both sexes are at greater risk for alcoholism and drug abuse, especially if not treated effectively during childhood.

The course and prognosis of ADHD depend greatly on the following variables:

(a) *Psychosocial conditions* are probably the most important. The child's family and school, in that order, can make the difference between appropriate structure, support, and encouragement of his/her strength, on one hand, and being lost on a sea of impulsive, random hyperactivity and negative input, on the other.

A cohesive family will be able to instill values which will counteract the penchant for immediate gratification, as will a cohesive larger community. Follow-up studies have shown poorer prognosis in ADHD children from a stormy, disruptive, and impoverished environment.

(b) *Significant overlap with Conduct Disorder*, in particular with physical violence, is a warning that trouble will extend into adolescence and adulthood. Such symptoms as repeated firesetting or cruelty to animals do not augur well for the future. A family history of trouble with the law, especially if repetitive and extensive, is a signal for a possibly serious prognosis.

(c) *Severe developmental learning disorder* associated with ADHD *may* make the course more troublesome and negatively affect the prognosis, but this depends greatly on the quality and duration of remedial help received.

(d) *Treatment.* A review of the literature will result in the impression that several follow-up studies, comparing behavioral or pharmacological treatment of ADHD with no treatment at all, purport to show no significant overall difference between the two groups and that there are actually few studies supporting long-term benefits from treatment. Skepticism is always in order but the reader should take all this information with a great deal of caution, since most studies are methodologically flawed. The latest edition of the *Comprehensive Textbook of Psychiatry* (Kaplan & Sadock, 1985) actually gives more credence to the conclusions of practicing clinicians than to any organized studies.

It is the conclusion of the authors of this book that comprehensive, multimodal treatment of ADHD significantly improves prognosis. Several mechanisms account for this: when the ADHD child behaves and performs better, there is greater intrinsic comfort for the child as well as positive feedback from the environment; the child acquires and eventually internalizes skills at handling feelings; and the entire process of treatment leaves a paradigm of benign and beneficial interaction with adults. The last-mentioned counteracts the tendency of children with ADHD to find support from socially unacceptable subcultures. At the least, treatment bridges the time to later maturation. If such maturation is insufficient in adolescence, prior treatment may provide a positive experience to build on.

(e) No discussion of ADHD's eventual outcome is complete without the encouragement that comes from studying the life histories of successful people. Talent, intelligence, and genius are not denied the ADHD child. Many ADHD children retain their immaturity for the rest of their lives, but may become outstanding for that very reason.

Questions for Study and Action

1. The mother of a seven-year-old second-grader says: "The teacher thinks my son is hyperkinetic, but I don't think so; he is hyperactive all right, but not hyperkinetic." What do you think the mother means by this?

2. The mother of this second-grader eventually agrees with the diagnosis of ADHD, but states that the father, from whom she is now separated and who did not attend any of the sessions with the child psychiatrist, keeps telling her there is nothing wrong with the child, that he is "all boy." How would you proceed from here on?

3. The teacher of a third-grader has told the parents that the child "should be on medicine" because she keeps disrupting the class. You have diagnosed the patient

as ADHD; the parents are opposed to the use of any "unnecessary medications" in childhood. They are, however, willing and able to continue with you in the other modalities of treatment. What will you do?

4. By contrast, you have developed a comprehensive treatment plan with the family of another child with ADHD; this includes the use of stimulant medication. The teacher, however, is opposed to the use of medication. What will be your stance here?

5. An eight-year-old boy has been treated with increasing doses of stimulants, first methylphenidate, then dextroamphetamine, and finally pemoline, and in each case the mother has complained that after initial good response, the child eventually no longer responds to the medicine. She says he is "becoming immune" to the medicine. Suppose you are the child psychiatrist who has been called in for consultation on this case, what are your thoughts about the possible cause or causes of this reported lack of response?

6. The parents of an eight-year-old boy with the full panoply of problems of ADHD say: "What is going to happen in the teens—criminality, drugs, etc?" They fully expect the child to get worse in adolescence. How can you turn this fear to therapeutic advantage? What can these parents do to influence the prognosis?

7. A seven-year-old girl with ADHD uses the excuse, "I can't help it, I am brain-damaged." Should such an excuse always be discouraged? When would you leave it in place?

8. The parents of a hyperactive child are surprised at the treatment plan, and say, "Aren't you going to try to find out what is making the child this way?" What would your reply be?

9. The mother of a nine-year-old girl with ADHD has started parental counseling. The therapist has suggested "toning down" her environment, as she gets easily overstimulated. It soon turns out, however, that the mother is appalled at any thought of cutting down on parties or on the endless parade of visiting friends or relatives. What can the therapist do?

10. The mother of a boy with ADHD complains that the teacher is "stigmatizing" her child by moving him close to her desk, because she cannot control him any other way. The mother insists that "mainstreaming" is the only "fair" way of handling the child in school. What is your opinion?

11. The father of an eight-year-old boy who had been diagnosed as having ADHD as well as Developmental Reading Disorder, objects to his son's being in a special classroom, where there are only 12 students, saying that he does not want his

son to be treated "like a retard." You have never seen this father. What do you think may be going on with the father or with the family?

12. As you finish preparations for pharmacotherapy of a second-grader with ADHD, the mother says that she would rather not tell the teacher about any of the treatment. What do you do at this point? Should you have insisted on teacher input from the very beginning? The child has no developmental disorder (no learning disability) and needs no remedial work at school.

For Further Reading

Barkley, R.A. *Hyperactive Children: A Handbook for Diagnosis and Treatment.* New York: Guilford Press, 1981.

Biederman, J., Gastfriend, D.R., & Jellinek, M.S. Desipramine in the treatment of children with attention deficit disorder. *J. Clin. Psychopharmacol.,* 6:359–362, 1986.

Bradley, C. The behavior of children receiving benzedrine. *Am. J. Psychiatry,* 94:577–585, 1937.

Churchill, W.S. *The Second World War. Vol. 1. The Gathering Storm.* Boston: Houghton Mifflin, 1948.

Connors, C.K. A teacher rating scale for use in. drug studies with children. *Am. J. Psychiatry,* 126:884–888, 1969.

Donnelly, M., Zametkin, A.J., Rapoport, J.L., et al. Treatment of childhood hyperactivity with desipramine: Plasma drug concentration, cardiovascular effects, plasma and urinary catecholamine levels, and clinical response. *Clin. Pharmacol. Ther.,* 39:72–81, 1986.

Fras, I. Alternating coffee and stimulants. *Am. J. Psychiatry,* 131:228–229, 1974.

Gardner, R.A. Psychogenic difficulties secondary to MBD. In J.D. Noshpitz (Ed.), *Basic Handbook of Child Psychiatry, Vol. 3.* New York: Basic Books, 1979, pp. 614–628.

Kahn, E., & Cohen, L.H. Organic drivenness—a brain stem syndrome and an experience—with case reports. *New Eng. J. Med.,* 210:748–756, 1934.

Kaplan, H.I., & Sadock, B.J. (Eds.) *Comprehensive Textbook of Psychiatry* (4th Ed.). Baltimore: Williams & Wilkins, 1985.

Laufer, M.W., Denhoff, E., & Solomons, G. Hyperkinetic impulse disorder in children's behavior problems. *Psychosom. Med.,* 19:38, 1957.

Levinson, H.N. *A Solution to the Riddle Dyslexia.* New York: Springer-Verlag, 1980.

Levy, F., & Hobbes, G. A 30-month follow-up of hyperactive children. *J. Amer. Acad. of Child Psychiatry,* 21:243–246, 1982.

Rutter, M. Syndromes attributed to "Minimal brain dysfunction" in childhood. *Am. J. Psychiatry,* 139:21–33, 1982.

Satterfield, J.H., Satterfield, B., & Cantwell, D. Three-year multimodality treatment study of hyperactive boys. *J. Pediat.,* 98:650–655, 1981.

Schnackenberg, R.C. Caffeine as a substitute for Schedule II. Stimulants in hyperkinetic children. *Am. J. Psychiatry,* 131:228–229, 1974.

Shekim, W.O., Cantwell, D., Kashani, J., Beck, N., Martin, J., & Rosenberg, J. Dimensional and categorical approaches to the diagnosis of attention deficit disorder in children. *J. Amer. Acad. of Child Psychiatry,* 25:653–658, 1986..

Strauss, A.A., & Lehtinen, L. *Psychopathology and Education of the Brain-Injured Child.* New York: Grune & Stratton, 1947.

Wender, P.M. *Minimal Brain Dysfunction in Children.* New York: Wiley-Interscience, 1971.

22

Psychoses and Pervasive Developmental Disorders

The term "Pervasive Developmental Disorder" is a newcomer to the psychiatric nomenclature, introduced in 1980 by DSM-III and retained in DSM-III-R. It replaces a number of terms, such as "early infantile autism," "childhood schizophrenia," "interactional psychotic disorder," "atypical child," and "schizophreniform psychotic disorder." All of these terms cover conditions *without* localizing signs of brain pathology. The reason for the new term is the *absence* of adult-type criteria for schizophrenia, i.e., these conditions may have no formed delusions, hallucinations and loosening of associations, and the striking *presence* of significant, widespread, and severely disruptive deviations in all areas of personality development. Another reason for the omission of the word "psychosis" in DSM-III-R is the questionable relationship of the syndrome to adult psychosis since young children lack a premorbid state, at times, to which their rehabilitation can be oriented.

Although the new terminology has brought a great deal of order and reliability to the diagnosis of Pervasive Developmental Disorder itself, it may have left out some diseases which would qualify for the term "childhood psychosis" because of their psychotic features and their subsequent course. We will, therefore, consider childhood psychosis briefly at the end of this chapter and

357

keep in mind that Pervasive Developmental Disorders are, by and large, the equivalents of some of the functional psychoses of adulthood.

Pervasive Developmental Disorders are subdivided on the basis of their age of onset into autistic and other pervasive developmental disorders. Each of these can be "full syndrome present" or "residual state," the latter usually representing the later stages of the disorder. Making these distinctions is not as important as making the basic diagnosis of a Pervasive Developmental Disorder, which we shall describe by referring to its prototype of "Autistic Disorder." This term is, fortunately, well established and familiar to all professionals, part of the present nomenclature, and now well defined.

Infantile Onset Autistic Disorder (299.00)

DEFINITION

The term "Infantile Autism" was introduced by Leo Kanner in 1943, and the syndrome is now characterized by early onset—before the age of 36 months—and the following three cardinal symptoms, namely, disturbances in:

1. speech and language ("communication impairment")
2. human relationships and feelings (impaired reciprocal social interaction)
3. developmental rate (marked by restricted repertoire of activities, interests, and fantasies)

In addition, disturbance in perception and in mobility are often seen.

CLINICAL DESCRIPTION

CASE 22-1   Jonathan's mother started asking the pediatrician questions when Jonathan was less than a year old, complaining that he was *not responsive:* "When I pick him up, he is like a board—not only does he tense up, but he does not seem to like being held. As a matter of fact, he does not seem to care for me; he is *not affectionate,* he is *not loving,* he is *not cuddly.*" Moreover, the mother asked, "Is it normal for a baby *not to accept* any solid foods except oatmeal and beef, and to reject all others?" The pediatrician tried to *reassure* the mother that the boundaries of normality were broad and that there was nothing to worry about since the baby was physically normal otherwise.

Nevertheless, a few months later the mother had more complaints: Jonathan had started walking on his toes, but showed *no interest in exploring.* He did not play with his older brothers or with his toys, except for a toy airplane whose propeller he would twirl incessantly, literally for hours, and would become extremely *upset* if interrupted. This reaction seemed like either extreme panic or a temper tantrum.

This time the pediatrician attended to the mother's concerns since he himself was impressed by Jonathan's *lack of response to him as a person.* During the examination, the child avoided the doctor's gaze, could not be induced to follow directions, and generally *treated* all the people around him *as if they were inanimate objects—things.*

Referrals to specialists were made, and, at the age of two-and-a-half years, Jonathan was fortunate to be accepted into a *special university-sponsored educational* program. By that time, his symptoms had become more pronounced: he had progressed normally in his gross motor skills but was deficient in fine motor skills. Everything in his environment had to be left unchanged or else a long tantrum would ensue. And, most conspicuously, there was *no communicative* speech: Jonathan frequently babbled incoherently and incomprehensibly, producing poorly enunciated words *devoid of any meaning.* Nor did he respond when talked to—so much so that for a time the parents started wondering if he was *deaf.* However, it could be rather easily ascertained that he was not deaf: he *responded to certain* noises, albeit in a highly *idiosyncratic manner;* if the sounds were grating, he would react with the usual panic/tantrum response; other kinds of noises, even when loud, would produce no response.

Needless to say, Jonathan *did not relate* to other children and had no playmates. He was *socially completely isolated.*

Comment. This vignette illustrates a rather typical case of Infantile Autism. The mother's "gut-level" feeling about her child is of the *greatest diagnostic importance.* It is, perhaps, the earliest "symptom" or indicator of Infantile Autism, and *should never be dismissed* by the physician. It reflects the profound disturbance of human relatedness so characteristic of this disorder. Subsequent preoccupation with *sameness* in the environment, the perseverative preoccupation with certain movements, especially whirling motions, and the extreme and prolonged reactions to change in the environment should confirm the suspicion that something is seriously wrong.

Finally, marked *discrepancies* in the areas of development (e.g., gross versus fine motor functions), *perceptual peculiarities* (tolerating certain tastes, or sounds, and not others) and, above all, *absence of communicative speech,* both expressive and receptive, should suffice to establish the diagnosis.

DIFFERENTIAL DIAGNOSIS

This is of practical importance since some more treatable disorders may show part of the symptomatology of Pervasive Developmental Disorder. A proper diagnostic workup aids us in differentiating an autistic disorder from the others.

We must remember that Pervasive Developmental Disorder may occur in association with organic diseases such as phenylketonuria, congenital rubella, tuberous sclerosis, retrolental fibroplasia, mental retardation from various causes, and brain damage from various causes including, especially, convulsive disorders.

Severe environmental deprivation in infancy resulting in hospitalism or anaclitic depression may have overlapping symptomatology, but can be differentiated on the basis of its special characteristics. The following disorders can cause differential diagnostic difficulties:

Deafness—The deaf child will be *unresponsive* to *all* sounds, with secondary retardation in speech and other areas of development. However, the deaf child is emotionally responsive to affective contact and does not show the highly idiosyncratic catastrophic reactions to change in routine. A similar situation may obtain in some cases of blindness but deafness leads often to confusion with autism, yet can be identified by an audiological consultation.

Mental Retardation—Many children with Pervasive Developmental Disorder also are mentally retarded. Mental retardation *alone* produces fairly *uniform delay* in all areas of development, without the unevenness of developmental delays that occurs in Pervasive Development Disorder. The clinical psychologist's consultation can be helpful in making this differentiation.

Developmental Language Disorder (aphasia), especially the receptive type—As explained in the chapter on developmental disorders, these are specific language disorders, but not disorders of emotional relatedness. They do not, in other words, encompass a broad series of dysfunctions of the entire personality. Children with developmental language disorders try to communicate in nonverbal ways as if to compensate for the aphasia. Although Developmental Language Disorder may give some disturbances in social responsiveness, these are never as severe as in Pervasive Developmental Disorder. Aphasic children are affectively responsive and do not show the other characteristics of autism. The consultation of a neurologist and neuropsychologist, and of a speech pathologist, helps to sort out aphasic from autistic children.

Schizophrenia—This can be differentiated on several characteristics: 1) schizophrenia rarely appears below age 10; 2) schizophrenia often has exacerbations and remissions, i.e., an uneven course, whereas Pervasive Developmental Disorder never has remissions; 3) delusions and hallucinations do not occur in Pervasive Developmental Disorder nor are there loose associations. Those children who eventually develop communicative speech say bizarre things, but although this is so and their thoughts are very concrete, what they say "hangs together" in its own idiosyncratic way. In other words, the classical loosening of associations, the incoherence, and the profound lack of any logic of schizophrenia are not characteristic of Pervasive Developmental Disorder; it is still characteristic only of schizophrenia.

Finally, one senses a more profound impairment in relatedness in Pervasive Developmental Disorder—the warm relatedness never seemed to have been there to begin with, whereas the individuals suffering from schizophrenia have periods when they are trying to reach out to establish human contact, albeit in their own bizarre way. The psychiatrist makes the distinction between autism and childhood schizophrenia by clinical observation, interview and mental status exam, history taking, and psychological testing.

Maternal Deprivation (deprivation of parental care)—This causes developmental retardation and blunting of emotional relatedness commensurate with the severity and duration of the deprivation. Withdrawal, cognitive blunting, and depression can resemble autism; hence, at times, maternal deprivation causes a clinical picture practically indistinguishable from infantile autism. The distinguishing feature of severe deprivation in early childhood is the history, often complemented by physical findings of neglect, or even abuse, and the improvement in the child once a better environment is provided.

CASE 22-2   Wanda was six-and-a-half years old when her parents sought consultation. The child could not function adequately in school because her speech was *rambling* and usually *meaningless*—as a matter of fact, Wanda most often simply *repeated* whatever was said to her—and because she seemed to "*look through*" everybody, treating all *people* as if they were *things*. In addition, she exhibited frequent, repetitive, and stereotyped hand-flapping motions and, although quite restless to the point of hyperactivity, showed little interest in most activities except in rock music, to which she would listen for hours, *swaying and rocking* to the beat and going into prolonged *temper tantrums* when the music was switched off.

The parents reported normal development until age *three-and-a-half* when they thought Wanda was turning *deaf,* since she became *oblivious* and *unresponsive* to people around her. It turned out that she had "tuned people out." Moreover, her *strange motions (hand-flapping and choreoathetoid movements)* were at first suspected to reflect a neurological disease. Initially, the parents had been annoyed by her speech, since they thought her "*aping*" of whatever they said was done intentionally; moreover, the child could *not be taught to use the pronoun "I." They felt hurt* because Wanda seemed to reject them; she often *repulsed them physically,* or she *shrank* away from them, *avoiding looking directly at them.*

Comment. The case vignette is of an example of Pervasive Developmental Disorder, childhood onset. It has practically the same symptomatology as Infantile Autism, except for its onset *after 36 months of age.*

We note echolalia (repeating of words or phrases), motor disturbances (hand-flapping and choreoatheoid movements), meaningless verbiage instead of communicative speech, and inability to use the pronoun "I." None of these symptoms is specific to Pervasive Developmental Disorder, but with the absence of human relatedness and of attempts to establish communication through any channel and Wanda's catastrophic reaction to the interruption of her perseverative activity, they round out the diagnosis.

We further note an absence of neologisms, delusions, and hallucinations (the child gives no indication of a "listening attitude"), which, together with the apparently unremitting course, distinguish it from Schizophrenia. There is no loosening of associations since there is insufficient meaningful speech for any associations to occur in the first place.

Organic Brain Syndrome is partially ruled out through neurological examination (absence of localizing signs). This examination should be repeated at intervals of 6-12 months to establish a longitudinal profile, since we know that a number of neurological diseases mimic Pervasive Developmental Disorder. Although most of the neurological disorders are of the degenerative kind, others are treatable, e.g., temporal lobe tumors or severe seizure disorders.

Finally, a recently recognized syndrome must also be considered in the differential diagnosis: Rett's syndrome, characterized by autism, dementia, microcephaly, loss of purposeful use of the hands, and progressive inexorable organic deterioration, although the latter may extend over many years. Among the neurological manifestations of this deterioration, epilepsy is common. Rett's syndrome can be differentiated from Pervasive Developmental Disorder by the fact that it occurs exclusively in girls, shows loss of previously acquired development, especially of language, and produces characteristic stereotypical movements, especially of the hands. Moreover, these patients eventually lose all ability to walk. The syndrome is now being increasingly diagnosed (Hagberg et al., 1983).

PROGNOSIS

The clinician will be expected to be familiar with the factors affecting the prognosis in Pervasive Developmental Disorder, since one of his or her most important functions in counseling the family of a child with Pervasive Developmental Disorder is the explanation, to the family, of the prognostic significance of the clinical findings.

Pervasive Developmental Disorder of the autistic type is not uniform prognostically. The most important factor in the prognosis is the presence of communicative speech by age five years, making the outlook relatively favorable, i.e., it offers the chance of eventual self-sufficient or nearly self-sufficient functioning.

Tested intelligence (IQ) is a corollary of speech, especially since half of the standardized intelligence tests depend on verbal communication. Because of this aspect and because of the fact that intelligence reflects overall brain development, IQ is a direct prognostic indicator: the lower the IQ, the worse the problems.

Ability to use toys and self-care capabilities, especially toilet training by age three years, are other prognostic indicators. They reflect cognitive motor and social progress.

The foregoing factors are of importance in both subtypes of Autistic Disorder. The childhood-onset subtype usually has a somewhat better prognosis per se than that starting in early infancy.

Seizures and signs of focal neurological impairment augur a poor prognosis since they reflect more severe impairment of brain function. They usually occur in association with significant mental retardation, itself a definite indicator of poor prognosis.

The children with a combination of good prognostic indicators are, unfortunately, few in number. As they grow older, especially when they reach adolescence, their ability to relate to other people improves, although it probably never reaches the "normal" or "average" degree of warmth characteristic of most of us. As adolescents, they are still made anxious by changes in their environment, but much less so. This former characteristic now shows itself mainly as a rather rigid adherence to routine. At this point, these individuals can profit from psychotherapy guided by a specialist. As adults, these fortunate few can expect to obtain jobs commensurate with their skills and interpersonal capabilities, usually performing best in work requiring rigid adherence to routine and not dependent on collaboration with other people. Most of them eventually date, and a small number have actually married.

At the gravest end of the spectrum are the severely autistic children, most of whom are mentally retarded as well. For them the prognosis is definitely poor. They are, and should be expected to continue to be, a severe emotional, and sometimes financial, burden on their families.

Controversy surrounds the prognosis of children who are between these extremes because of the unanswered question of the relationship of Pervasive Developmental Disorder to Schizophrenia. Some of the children with the former disorder do indeed manifest hallucinations and bizarre ideas equivalent to delusions around age nine or 10 years and thereafter. They then have the same prognosis as severe ("process") schizophrenia.

ETIOLOGY AND PATHOGENESIS

There is now consensus that the cause or causes of Pervasive Developmental Disorder are organic but unknown. Therefore, our considerations are actually of possible neuropathological mechanisms after the primary cause has set in. There is one exception: the cause may be genetic with the mode of inheritance being that of an autosomal recessive trait. A number of identical twins have been found to be concordant for Infantile Autism, and those identical twins discordant for the disorder have, nevertheless, shown a high incidence of impairment of cognitive processing. No chromosomal abnormalities have been found so far. This area awaits further research but it already ties in with the main hypothesis of the underlying mechanism, i.e., that Pervasive Developmental Disorder is a disorder of central processing—the processing and modulation of perceptions, symbols, and cognition, the most evident result being impairment of communication at all levels, both verbal and nonverbal. The primary site, if any, may be in the brain stem, but it is important to remember that the disorder is probably the result of multiple, and perhaps quite heterogeneous, causes.

Most experts follow this model and consider Pervasive Developmental Disorder as a disorder of communication and cognition. The old theory of interpersonal factors, such as emotionally cold, "ice-box" parents causing the disorder, is no longer held by any serious investigator or clinician. This theory had actually brought hardship to many parents who were directly or indirectly vilified by professionals, adding insult to the enormous emotional burden brought upon them by having a child so severely disturbed. Some of these parents indeed became reclusive and overcontrolled as a reaction to their children; in the heyday of exclusive emphasis on psychodynamic (interpersonal) factors, this secondary reaction was then misconstrued as being the primary cause of the disorder.

Of course, interplay between organic and environmental factors is a logical and safe approach to the etiology of most psychiatric disorders; however, in the case of Pervasive Developmental Disorder, we are as impressed by the weight of organic or constitutional factors as compared to the relatively negligible effect of *any* specific handling or attitude on the part of parents (environment).

TREATMENT

There is no causal treatment, and, for many patients, there is no effective, symptomatic, or even palliative treatment for this disorder. Nevertheless, it is not a totally hopeless disorder, especially for those children with islands of communicative speech.

The following is a list of treatment methods:

1. *Special psychoeducation*—This consists of structured classroom special teaching and close parental involvement. An example is TEACCH (Treatment and Education of Autistic and Related Communications Handicapped Children). According to its originators, TEACCH is a "highly structured psychoeducational teaching approach," using the parents as co-therapists for their children. This type of comprehensive approach may be the most effective one proposed thus far. Obviously, it is limited by its availability—such programs are still few and far between. Parts of the program can be administered even if the total program has not been set up.

2. *Psychotherapy*—This is a rational approach only in older patients (10 years or older) with communicative language, i.e., in those with the best prognosis. Otherwise, it probably should be considered ineffective to the point of wasting resources better used for other purposes, i.e., psychoeducational measures and parental guidance.

3. *Parental guidance and support*—It is difficult to imagine the suffering of many of these parents. This strain often produces secondary personality changes in them, and their lives become obsessively structured around the one autistic child. The clinician can help inject a note of balance into this situation.

CASE 22-3   Yolanda's parents had been a middle-class, upwardly mobile family six years ago when it became apparent that Yolanda showed symptoms indicative of Pervasive Developmental Disorder. The family faithfully followed the regimen of weekly sessions with a psychiatrist, although the child was still *continuing* with her bizarre symptomatology three years later. By that time, their insurance benefits were *exhausted,* but the parents funded the cost of treatment until they had to face the reality that they could not possibly afford it anymore. Not only the parents' lives but also those of *their other two children were profoundly affected* by the parents' conviction, because they could not face the guilt that they had been somehow responsible for her illness in the first place, that they had to devote extra attention to Yolanda. In addition, the parents asked, "Are we doing everything we can to give her all the chances of improvement?" When they saw another specialist, the *magnitude* of *family disruption* became apparent and was addressed.

Comment. This case is presented here to illustrate the need for flexibility in the treatment; not every disorder should be dogmatically treated with long-term psychotherapy. The clinician must know the expectable natural history and prognosis of the disorder; however, he or she must also impart this knowledge to the parents through a psychotherapeutic process. Sometimes the doctor's rapport with the family is so good that one serious, meaningful session is enough. Often it takes repeated working through of parental guilt to allow the parents' reality testing to assert itself.

4. *Pharmacological treatment*—This is not causal or curative but can go a certain way towards improving the life of the patient as well as that of the family. How much that is will depend on both the nature of the patient's symptomatology and the programs into which the patient can be enrolled. Obviously, pharmacotherapy will be most effective for such "target symptoms" as hyperactivity, destructiveness, excessive amounts of bizarre motions, or excessive—though usually meaningless—verbal productions. Medication will be of little value for the lack of relatedness or absence of meaningful speech.

Recent clinical experience supports the advisability of aggressive pharmacotherapy for suitable target symptoms, *especially* in conjunction with psychoeducational programs and family guidance. At the very least, pharmacotherapy can make the patients more amenable to those programs, although the results may transcend that dimension.

The reader is referred to Chapter 2 for the appropriate details on neuroleptics, which are the first-line medications. In keeping with the trend of the last decade, high-potency-per-milligram medications (e.g., haloperidol, fluphenazine, and thiothixene) are preferred. The risk-to-benefit ratio, particularly respecting tardive dyskinesia, has to be weighed by the clinician familiar with the prognosis of that particular case of Pervasive Developmental Disorder. The physician prescribing medication has to work very closely with the parents and the staff of whatever educational or psychoeducational program the child is in, because sedation not only may interfere directly with the child's ability to learn, but also will exert negative effects on the staff, who will take any sign of sedation as a welcome way to displace their inevitable frustrations when the child does not progress—the lack of progress will indeed occur as part of the natural history of the disorder, but it will then be blamed on the medicine.

Because of the presence of a variable number of neurological "soft signs" and other evidence of brain dysfunction in children with Pervasive Developmental Disorder, attempts have been made to treat these children similarly to those with Attention–Deficit Hyperactivity Disorder. Thus, stimulant medication is a "second-line" approach. The results are variable and neither physicians nor parents should have unrealistically high expectations; however, it is well worth trying since no chance to help these children should be missed.

CONCLUDING REMARKS: PERVASIVE DEVELOPMENTAL DISORDER VERSUS CHILDHOOD SCHIZOPHRENIA

Seemingly, the present psychiatric nomenclature has neatly packaged all childhood functional (i.e., without localizing focal, neurological findings) psychosis into Pervasive Developmental Disorders (PPDs) and subdivided them into Autistic Disorders (of infantile onset before 36 months of age, of childhood onset after 36 months, and age of onset unknown or not otherwise specified) and PDD-NOS (not otherwise specified).

Nevertheless, not all clinicians are entirely happy with this classification. Some are convinced that there is a continuity of morbidity between childhood, adolescence, and adulthood, all representing Schizophrenia. It is indeed a clinical fact that children with some, or most, of the classic features of Schizophrenia are seen in clinical practice. There are no statistics to show how often this happens since the nomenclature has been in flux and disarray until recently. But childhood psychosis appears often enough for the perceptive student to feel comfortable enough to step out of the confines of Pervasive Developmental Disorder and to diagnose "childhood psychosis" or even "childhood schizophrenia." The clinician should do so whenever looseness of associations, incoherence, illogicality, delusions, and hallucinations are encountered, particularly if accompanied by abnormal movements (posturing) and abnormal speech (unusual intonation or monotoning). These abnormalities of thoughts, perceptions, affects, and behavior are similar to those seen in adults. They only need correcting for age and developmental phase in order to be diagnosed.

Questions for Study and Action

1. Describe in detail your diagnostic workup of a four-year-old boy who shows for speech only a bit of echolalia (a soft drink commercial), who twirls a string incessantly, who does not respond to the language of others, and whose motor

coordination is advanced but who cannot reproduce a circle with either right or left hand. Divide your workup into those things that you can do (history taking, observations, etc.) and those that you must ask of others (laboratory studies, consultations).

2. In your diagnostic workup, assume that you asked a psycholinguistics expert to evaluate the four-year-old in Question #1 above. The psycholinguist was cheered to note that, in addition to the reported echolalia, many of the utterances of this little boy, while not intelligible speech, employed the morphemes and phonemes of a pre-English-speaking person. How would you explain and interpret this finding to the parents? Would you advise speech training and therapy for the boy? How would you justify that? Would you advise a "therapeutic nursery or pre-school" for the child? On what grounds? How would you explain the advice to the parents?

3. Add Heller's Disorder to the differential diagnosis listed in this chapter and show how it can be differentiated from deafness, severe deprivation, mental retardation, schizophrenia, and aphasia. (*Note:* Heller's Infantile Dementia, a progressive dementia without other signs of neurological disorder, is a syndrome including diverse cerebral disorders. The onset is from age 1 to 4 years and generally is reported to afflict "pretty" blond children. The child's behavior deteriorates as he/she regresses in both speech and mentation. Look this up in a pediatric text, we suggest.)

4. List five broad areas of habilitation and rehabilitation for a three-year-old boy with Autistic Disorder of Infantile Onset, imagining that he has had no specialized treatment theretofore. Under each general area (e.g., therapeutic work with parents and sibs) specify the various treatment modalities that could be promising.

5. Write out a case vignette describing a five-year-old autistic boy with the most favorable prognosis. Underline each item that denotes better outcome.

6. William Goldfarb differentiated young psychotic children who showed numerous "organic" features from those who showed none or few. The former had parents who appeared to be healthy and intact; the latter had parents who were disturbed or disordered, often having a major mental disorder. Discuss this situation, trying to account for it.

7. Since ADHD is often said to be "organic" and pervasive, list some of the so-called soft neurological signs that appear in children with an Attention–Deficit Hyperactivity Disorder. Explain each. Be certain to include a positive Romberg, dysdiadochokinesis, cerebellar drift, and at least two others.

8. Magda Campbell studied with follow-up a group of psychotic/pervasive-developmental-disordered children and found that those children hospitalized for more

than 40 months were no more improved than those hospitalized for two or three months. How would that affect your thinking about two parents who request that their autistic child be placed in a long-term institution? How would you deal with their request?

9.   Two parents of an autistic child insist that their child has a chemical imbalance that can be corrected by megavitamin therapy, so they take the child from one megavitamin clinic to another, spending megadollars in the process. What would you tell them? How? Why?

10. Describe the disappointment and pain that would be felt if you were a mother with a child diagnosed as autistic at 10 weeks of age. What about the child's relationship with you would be most frustrating and unrewarding? What other features of the clinical picture would upset you?

For Further Reading

Campbell, M. Poor prognosis: The earlier appearing psychosis. Paper presented at the American Academy of Child Psychiatry, Toronto, Ontario, Canada, 1976.

Cantor, S., Evans, J., Pearce, J., & Pezzot-Pearce, T. Childhood schizoprenia: Present but not accounted for. *Am. J. Psychiatry*, 139:758–762, 1982.

Goldfarb, W. *Childhood Schizophrenia.* Cambridge, MA: Harvard University Press, 1961.

Hagberg, B., Aicardi, J., Dias, K., & Ramos, O. A progressive syndrome of autism, dementia, ataxia, and loss of purposeful hand use in girls: Rett's syndrome: report of 35 cases. *Ann. Neurol.*, 14:471–479, 1983.

Kanner, L. Autistic disturbances of affective contact. *Nervous Child*, 2:217–250, 1943.

Menolascino, F.J. Diagnosis of Childhood Psychosis. (Letter to ed.). *Am. J. Psychiatry*, 140:133–134, 1983.

Nelson, W.E., Vaughan, V.C., III, & McKay, R.J. (Eds.) *Textbook of Pediatrics (9th ed.).* Philadelphia: W.B. Saunders, 1969.

Ornitz, E.M., & Ritvo, E.R. The syndrome of autism: A critical review. *Am. J. Psychiatry*, 133:609–621, 1976.

Rett, A. Ueber ein eigenartiges hirnatrophisches syndrom bei hyperammonaemie im kindesalter. (On a peculiar syndrome of cerebral atrophy in childhood, associated with hyperammonemia). *Wien. Med. Wochenschr.*, 116:723–738, 1986.

Ritvo, E.R., Spence, M.A., Freeman, B.J., Mason-Brothers, A., Mo, A., & Marazita, M.L. Evidence for autosomal recessive inheritance in 46 families with multiple incidences of autism. *Am. J. Psychiatry*, 142:187–192, 1985.

Schopler, E., Mesibov, G., & Baker, A. Evaluation of treatment for autistic children and their parents. *J. Amer. Acad. of Child Psychiatry*, 21:262–267, 1982.

23

Delusional (Paranoid) Disorders

DEFINITION

Delusional Disorders, also called Paranoid Disorders, have false beliefs as a central characteristic. Belief systems are seldom *logical* or *empirical,* as scientific statements would be expected to be, so truth and falsity may be hard to evaluate. The disorders pertain to *fausse connaissance,* as the French say, to *false consciousness,* a term used widely by Marxists to depict proletarians who think like the bourgeoisie. The delusion can be held by a single individual, or by two (*folie à deux*) or more (*folie à trois, quatre,* etc.). The worshipfulness of a Nazi or Fascist for his strongman leader may bespeak delusion. Other everyday examples include red-baiters on the radical right or leftists who see a Rockefeller plot behind every Democratic or Republican president or the believers at the Jonestown massacre. Among children, an example other than Jonestown would be the white child who feels that black children are innately inferior. Belief systems always border on delusions when they are zealously held, with fixity and fanaticism. Fortunately, few children are "true believers" in adult causes, both secular and religious, but they can be hoodwinked, brainwashed, and programmed, at times, into blatantly false beliefs.

When a child develops a Delusional (Paranoid) Disorder (297.10), that child at the very least is a) lonely and b) untrusting. The homes, streets, and schools of America are full of lonely and untrusting children, yet not all are suffering from a Delusional Disorder. Some children sustain betrayal and disappointments that may unhinge them only briefly, provoke social withdrawal, and stimulate suspiciousness, but not be ill with a Delusional Disorder.

DSM-III-R specifies that in a true disorder the delusions are not bizarre (for after all, a child could be involved in being poisoned, infected, or followed) and the delusions have lasted more than a month. Further, the child does not have prominent auditory (cf. Schizophrenia) or visual (cf. Delirium) hallucinations; and the rest of the child's behavior apart from the delusional system is not bizarre. Paranoids are quite intact save for their "pockets of insanity."

When a child is induced into a delusional psychosis (297.30) by another person (psychotic parent, hysterical sibling, fanatical cult leader), the induced child is under the sway of a person more assertive and influential than the disordered child. Hence, there are two (or more) cases to be diagnosed, and convention calls the stronger one "the primary case" and the weaker, "the secondary case." Even when a Delusional Disorder is shared between twins, the dominant one is the primary case of a *folie à deux*. The delusions of both have a common theme but the secondary case was *not* psychotic prior to adopting the delusions of the primary case.

We have included Delusional Disorders in this Section on "Thinking and Central Processing Disorders" because of their derangement in thought, a central disturbance in communication and information processing, even if they are not pervasive.

ETIOLOGY AND PATHOGENESIS

The root causes (etiology) of delusion-formation are not as well known as the mechanics of a delusion's emergence and relinquishment. And the mechanics of pathogenesis are better understood for an Induced Psychotic Disorder than for a primary case of Delusional (Paranoid) Disorder. Let us tackle first the still-difficult case of the shared delusion. First, the parent (or other), *the primary case,* becomes psychotic and develops delusions as a part of the illness. The primary case may be suffering from a Delusional (Paranoid) Disorder, but not necessarily, for the primary case may be one of Schizophrenia, paranoid type, or of mania with a dominant affect of suspicion and delusions congruent with that mood, or of Organic Mental Disorder with delusions, or Depression with mood-congruent delusions. The primary case may be hysterical (Conversion Disorder or Dissociative Disorder) with delusion(s), or a religious fanatic, and transmit to the child the delusion(s) attending hysteria or fanaticism. The child, *the secondary case,* does not appear to make strong, "intrapsychic" identifications with the delusional system that (s)he adopts and usually adopts solely the delusions, not the other symptoms. The learning of the other's delusion is copied rather superficially; hence, the learning is by imitation not identification, for when the child is separated from the primary case the delusion will not be retained.

Now, we shall consider the pathogenesis of the child with a primary case of Delusional (Paranoid) Disorder, a rarity, because it is transient in children, seldom fulfilling the criterion of lasting a month or more. Freudian dynamic explanations held, with some validity, that the child's cognitive style was ever close to primitive, primary process thinking and that paranoid developments resulted from overuse of projection and denial, two grossly primitive defensive maneuvers, and anal-stage fixations and regressions (Freud, 1938). Melanie Klein (1958), the child analyst, went further back and postulated a paranoid position that the early infant occupied routinely in life's first two months—her postulation was of not only a pre-oedipal but also a pre-anal, early oral stage phenomenon. Harry Stack Sullivan (1939), a sociobehavioral psychiatrist, stressed the loneliness of the paranoid adult and traced the genesis of paranoid states back to preadolescence, or late childhood, without a close chum. Norman Cameron (1974), a child psychiatrist, described the paranoid's formation of a pseudo-community, i.e., a delusional community in which the paranoid person denies actual loneliness, social incompetence, or isolation or withdrawal by imaginatively inventing a number of important figures who are centering their attention on the paranoid individual.

The fact that the paranoid is generally intact, apart from the compartment of the delusional system, makes many of these speculations (about how the paranoid comes to be sick) doubtful, at best, unless we postulate that the delusions are merely the Achilles' heel of an otherwise functioning person, that little slipped cog that could do the person in at his or her insanity hearing.

CLINICAL DESCRIPTION

CASE 23-1   Solomon, a child who otherwise was intact, had a fixed notion that, despite considerable evidence to the contrary, he was being *infected with toxins* from food additives and environmental toxins and consequently believed he *had "allergies."* His parents *opposed fluoridation* of drinking water but his mother was particularly zealous: she tried to get the school board to *remove fluorescent lighting* from all classrooms last year; she provided Solomon with a highly restricted diet of raw meats, fresh fruits, and vegetables that had been soaked in water overnight, and cereals and breads prepared "from scratch." When Solomon created trouble for her, she *accused him of having eaten junk foods* behind her back. She *no longer ate in restaurants,* but when she used to, she made a "federal case" out of being seated at least five tables away from a smoker. She insisted on leaving Los Angeles to *live in an unpolluted small town* in New England. Her husband acceded to all her demands but had some reservations about their excessiveness.

Solomon, at age eight years, was healthy but found out early that his *mother liked to teach* him and that *she knew a lot about poisons* in food and air. He discussed these with her at length and never ate cafeteria or junk foods at school, only a special lunch packed at home. Halfway through the third grade, Solomon began to *believe that he was sick* from "environmental allergies" for which skin testing, further dietary exclusion, special air filters, and massage were among many things prescribed by a local naturopath. Solomon's *complaints of headaches, burning eyes, and dry throat were not confirmed by abnormal physical findings.* His itching was accompanied by no rash. He had no eosinophilia, no elevated white count, no fever.

Although Solomon was bright and above his grade level on achievement tests, he *began to miss a lot of school.* No classmate felt his absence as a loss. His father insisted that Solomon go to see a pediatrician and, thereafter, a child psychiatrist.

Comment. Solomon was a relatively mild example of a Shared Paranoid Disorder, the same as Induced Psychotic Disorder. When, at age nine and a half, he went to New Zealand for a year with his father (who had been assigned there and had grown unhappy with his marriage), leaving his mother in New England, Solomon lost his allergic illness and his food and air delusions, slowly at first; but by the end of the year, he ate a hot dog without ill effects.

CASE 23-2   When Lynn, an only child, was three years old he heard his maternal grandmother exclaim to his mother, "Why, Lynn is *a girl's name!*" His mother had *dressed him as a girl* all his life and thought of him as a baby without gender. As he had grown older, he developed the *delusion that he was a girl, played almost exclusively with girls,* and had a firmer conviction that his *genitals were not real* and were *not meant to be male.* He did little to adapt to kindergarten and grade-school pressures and found that he *depreciated maleness,* finding it even repulsive to have "those dirty old things" (meaning penis and scrotum with testicles).

Follow-up: By age 21, Lynn had been under psychiatric care for two years. On the psychiatrist's recommendation, he had *received female hormones, surgical castration,* and *plastic reconstruction* of the scrotum into a vagina. As a transsexual he had had all documents indicating his assignment to maleness, such as driver's license, changed to show that Lynn was female. She thanked her mother for giving her a name that could easily be that of a female, since her name did not now have to be changed.

Comment. Cleeta (Case 12-1, p. 175) had a similar delusion but with a different outcome. Also, Miguel (Case 5-1, p. 94) had some persecutory delusional formation that was transient. Moreover, child cases of mysophobia blend easily into paranoid delusions of infection but if they persist less than a month, it is not a Delusional Disorder. Lynn's delusion *began early, became reinforced and fixed,* and ultimately *changed her phenotypic gender identity.*

DIAGNOSIS AND DIFFERENTIAL DIAGNOSIS

When we encounter a child who has a delusional disorder, the first step is to determine whether the child is a primary case or secondary case, as defined in the foregoing. If a secondary case, the next thing would be to ascertain that the child indeed was devoid of psychosis before acquiring the delusion. A third step would be to determine that the delusional behavior does not pervade all of the child's thinking, feeling, and behaving, that the child is not hallucinating, and that nothing is making the child's whole existence deranged or bizarre, for that indicates something other than a Delusional Disorder.

Of help in the diagnostic workup for these three steps is history taking from the child and from collateral informants such as parents, sibs, schoolteacher, grandparents, and neighbors. The physical and mental exams are also good occasions for making added observations for diagnostic enhancement. The history of drugs taken also assists greatly in the diagnostic workup. Psychological testing, to rule out wide scatter on IQ testing, and projective testing, to document the major conflicts, typical defenses, and general style of the child's imaginative productions, are of high value with a delusional child. Laboratory studies of lead, mercury, and other poisons may be helpful, if indicated, and a screen of urine for street drugs could be important. Since the child has a psychosis, although compartmentalized, the EEG and CAT scan might be done.

The major disorders to be differentiated when the child is the primary case are as follows:

Induced Psychotic Disorder, in which the child is the secondary case, not primary;

Organic Mental Disorder, in which the picture of a broader disturbance of cortical functions exists;

Depression, which shows a broader and more deviant mood-picture congruent with the delusional picture;

Mania, in which the mood-picture is altered and congruent with the delusion;

Schizophrenia, in which the mood-incongruent delusions are accompanied by hallucinations, thought disorder, and other maladaptations.

DSM-III-R indicates five types of delusions that need to be specified in the primary case: Persecutory, Jealous (adults), Erotomanic (adults), Somatic, and Grandiose. If none of these fits, the delusion is called "Unspecified." Children have been seen occasionally to develop Persecutory, Somatic, and Grandiose delusions: a child who believes the mother is systematically poisoning his food; a child who has numerous "environmental" allergies; a child who thinks he is turning into a pig; a child who believes he is immortal or invulnerable or omnipotent. Neither of the authors of this book has seen a child with Erotomanic or Jealous delusions.

TREATMENT AND PROGNOSIS

From the clinical cases cited, we see that prognosis may be highly variable: best for the shared delusion because separation from the primary case dislodges the child's secondary case; moderately favorable for the primary case that is treated early; and very grave for untreated cases or cases of such fixity that delusion comes to transform reality. The treatments, as shown, include separation from the primary case and also dynamic individual psychotherapy, peer group therapy, and family group therapy. Cognitive and behavioral therapy have not been reported as treatments with children, to our knowledge. Most efforts by a clinician to "out-argue" or "disprove" the delusion are so futile that even a systematic cognitive therapy would probably not be efficacious. Nor are psychoactive drugs ordinarily useful in treatment.

Questions for Study and Action

1. For a mother and child in a *folie à deux*, outline a treatment plan for each of the pair. Indicate if they are to be seen together or separately, by one or two therapists, and what treatment modalities would be employed for each.

2. Read or reconsider Harry Stack Sullivan's emphasis on the preadolescent chumship as an advantageous step forward in the child's development of self-esteem through sociability. What expanded validation of one's self-worth comes from the love of a close chum?

3. Are there features of childhood, other than proneness to crude, primary-process thinking, that make the child vulnerable to Induced Psychotic Disorder? Explain.

4. Compare and contrast a child with Munchausen-by-Proxy and a child with Induced Psychotic Disorder.

5. Imagine that you were Solomon's (Case 23-1) father and detail what you would have done to help the child when you began to realize that his mother was delusional. Would you have taken the child away for a year?

6. What is your opinion of the psychiatrist who, by condoning it, helped Lynn (Case 23-2) to actualize the delusion by making a transsexual shift? What about the ethics of not condoning or not assisting?

7. Why do male-to-female transsexuals greatly outnumber female-to-male cases? What would androgynous norms do to that incidence pattern? Explain.

8. In what childhood disorders do loneliness and lack of feeling loved figure as an important emotion? List at least eight and explain each choice.

9. Would you "join" a paranoid child in her or his delusions? How so? Would anything be gained by countering the child's delusions? Outline an approach that would combine candor, disbelief, and a desire to help.

10. Would a psychotherapist with a Paranoid Personality Disorder be a good choice as a therapist for Solomon? Explain. Why might psychotherapists in private office practice become prone to paranoid trends? Explain.

For Further Reading

Cameron, N. Paranoid conditions and paranoia. In S. Arieti & E.D. Brody (Eds.), *American Handbook of Psychiatry, Vol. 3* (Revised Ed.). New York: Basic Books, 1974.

Colby, K.M., Weber, S., & Hilf, F. Artificial paranoia (computer simulation). *Artificial Intelligence*, 2:1–25, 1971.

Freud, S. The interpretation of dreams. In A.A. Brill (trans. & ed.), *The Basic Writings of Sigmund Freud*. New York: Modern Library, 1938.

Klein, M. Some theoretical conclusions regarding the emotional life of the infant. In M. Klein, P. Heimann, S. Isaacs, & J. Riviere (Eds.), *Developments in Psychoanalysis*. No. 43 of the International Psychoanalytical Library. London: Hogarth, 1958, pp. 198–236.

Sullivan, H.S. *Conceptions of Modern Psychiatry*. (Originally published, 1939). New York: W.W. Norton & Company, 1953.

24

Organic Mental Disorders

S ince Organic Personality Disorder (310.10) and Intoxications (code depends on the intoxicant substance) were discussed in Chapter 5, they will not be covered here. Our rationale for including those two organic disorders with Disorders of Behavior was that they are typified principally by *behavioral signs*. The remaining Organic Mental Disorders interfere so notably with higher mental functions (doing, feeling, and central processing) that we feel that they belong here with Developmental Disorders, Personality Disorders, and Psychoses. Eight of the Organic Mental Disorders will be reviewed briefly herein. (It should be noted that we made no distinction between "disorder" and "syndrome." For the sake of simplicity, we will use "disorder" throughout this chapter. DSM-III-R regards many organic problems as both syndromes and disorders.)

Delirium (293.00)

CLINICAL DESCRIPTION

A delirious child is one with altered attention and awareness, confusion and disorientation, and possibly memory, sleeping, judgment, handwriting, and speech disturbances. Originally, delirium (*de-lira* = out of the furrow) referred to

Italian farmers of the 16th century who could not plow a straight line when they had delirium associated with malaria. Today, an equivalent phrase, "off their trolley," depicts a similar state by means of a more urban metaphor. The most frequent etiology of childhood Delirium is any condition (chemical, infection, etc.) that can produce hyperpyrexia. Febrile delirium is often seen in infants and toddlers and may precede or follow a febrile convulsion.

A good diagnostic system specifies etiology of its disorders whenever possible. For that reason DSM-III-R makes a sensible commentary about the etiology of Delirium: either there is direct evidence of an organic etiology (demonstrated in the patient's life story or laboratory findings or on physical and neurological exam and recorded on Axis III) or, lacking direct evidence, an organic etiology can be inferred if nonorganic mental disorders have been ruled out.

Delirium develops in a short period of time, varies during each day (worse after dark), is characterized by the following: a clouding of awareness of the child's surroundings and a reduced capability to shift, refocus, and sustain attention to environmental stimuli; by a cognitive disorganization (often shown in incoherent speech content); by perceptual distortions (e.g., tactile and visual hallucinations or illusions); and by two or more of the "cardinal signs of brain disorder." Those cardinal signs are disturbances of orientation, speech, memory, judgment, and handwriting.

CASE 24-1   Clarice was two-and-a-half years old, a bright and verbal little girl who seemed happy and was a source of great pleasure in her parents' eyes. She was prone to suddenly developing fevers of *40° C* with streptococcal infections, during which she became *disoriented, misinterpreted environmental objects,* and yelled out, "Shoot that fly," when *no fly was present.* She was *agitated* and *disoriented, shrinking from her father* and saying, "Go away, bad man!" and *not recognizing familiar surroundings* when her mother carried her, her blanket, and her teddy bear into the living room so that they could be nearer one another. The pediatrician feared she would have a febrile convulsion, so advised the parents how to bathe her in barely tepid water and recommended a pentobarbital rectal suppository whenever her fever had escalated to 39° C.

Comment. Clarice's febrile deliria were transient. They seldom lasted more than two or three hours and were followed by exhaustion and temporary debilitation until antibiotics had overcome her bacterial infections.

Delirium in children is usually acute, not chronic as may be seen often in adults (chronic delirium tremens, etc.). The treatment of the underlying sepsis, hypovitaminosis, or drug reaction will clear up delirium promptly. The best nursing care is to keep on a bright light and simplify the child's surroundings.

This is a good time to clear away mobiles above the child's bed and simplify all verbal communications directed to the child or others.

Dementia (294.10)

CLINICAL DESCRIPTION

In former centuries, cognitive disorders were divided into *amentia* and *dementia,* the former a failure to develop normal reasoning powers, the latter a loss or diminution of intellectual capabilities. For the general psychiatrist, the dementias were early-appearing (dementia praecox, now Schizophrenia), presenile or senile, according to age of onset. Today, a regression from one's former abilities, or a *failure to continue* a mental growth rate that had been established previously, constitute Dementia.

DSM-III-R provides five criteria for the diagnosis of Dementia:

1. Lost intellectual abilities sufficiently severe to interfere with social or occupational functioning
2. Objective evidence of memory impairment
3. At least one of the following four findings:
   (a) impaired judgment
   (b) impaired abstract thinking (concrete interpretation of proverbs, unable to find similarities and differences in word-pairs, difficulty defining words and concepts, and related intellectual tasks)
   (c) aphasia or apraxia or agnosia or constructional difficulty
   (d) change from premorbid personality can be documented
4. Does not meet criteria for Delirium or Intoxication, although these may be superimposed
5. Positive evidence of an organic cause or strong presumptive evidence of intellectual deficit due to organic cause.

CASE 24-2   Cindy was a spunky and curious seven-year-old girl whose *mother had rubella* in the first trimester of her pregnancy with Cindy but declined to be aborted. Hence, Cindy was a planned and eagerly expected child. After an operation in infancy for an *interventricular septal defect,* Cindy had thrived and had reached elementary school with a high level of functioning considering her congenital rubella.

In first grade, she showed *difficulty learning to read* and a *generalized slow-wittedness at home and school.* Fortunately, she was tested in kindergarten by a clinical psychologist who retested her at age seven and found her full-scale *IQ to have declined by 12 points* in the two years. Her *memory* was impaired, some of her *verbal responses were incoherent and off the point,* and she had developed a *staggering* gait by the time she was referred to a pediatric neurologist. She had her first grand mal *seizure* the day before the neurologist's appointment to see Cindy.

She was hospitalized and diagnosed as having progressive rubella panencephalitis (Axis III) after CT scan, EEG, and cerebrospinal fluid studies had been done. A virologist was consulted who confirmed the neurologist's diagnosis. Cindy's dementia progressed rapidly until only her vegetative functions remained intact. *Memory, speech, and handwriting capabilities were lost.*

Comment. When counseling the parents about institutionalization for Cindy, the pediatrician told them it had not really been determined whether Cindy had retained the rubella virus from her intrauterine life which was now producing a viral encephalopathy *or* had acquired a new exposure to rubella which her immune defenses had not been able to control.

Cindy met the criteria for a diagnosis of Dementia in her tragic and precipitous decline in mental functioning, far below her former attainments, due to her experience with rubella *in utero* and again in second grade. Her parents thought they had been doubly (or more) accursed by a virus that ordinarily causes only a mild and transient disorder among school-aged children.

Amnestic Disorder (294.00)

CLINICAL DESCRIPTION

Memory is a great time-binder for a talking animal because it enables *the individual* to store information that can be retrieved whenever it is needed. It is a higher cerebral function that aids individualized adaptation. Some children with eidetic imagery have photographic memories that aid their superior adaptation unless conflict and stress arise to impede their memory. Whenever it has a good memory, any animal needs fewer instincts or phylogenetically preprogrammed behavior.

However, when an insult to the brain occurs, a child may show many brain syndromes but one of the most annoying and embarrassing is a picture of memory loss without Delirium or Dementia. DSM-III-R gives three forthright criteria for making the diagnosis of Amnestic Disorder:

1. Both *short-* and *long*-term memory impairment—the first an inability to learn new matter and the second an inability to remember what was known in the past.
2. No clouded consciousness (as in Delirium and Intoxication) and no general decrement in intellectual capabilities as seen in Dementia.
3. Positive evidence from history, physical exam, or laboratory tests of a causative

organic insult. *Note:* There cannot be merely a presumption of organic insult, only some positive evidence thereof (cf. Delirium and Dementia).

CASE 24-3   Eleven-year-old Doug was enjoying kite flying with his younger brother on the elementary-school playground on a spring Sunday afternoon. The wind changed and quickly carried the kite towards an electrical power line that rimmed the playground. Doug was *knocked to the ground, had a seizure, became unconscious,* but *continued to breathe* after the seizure ended. His little brother ran for help and Doug, seemingly *confused and disoriented,* was taken to a nearby hospital's emergency room.

Doug was hospitalized for 72 hours for observation and laboratory studies. Within five or six hours he had recovered from his Delirium but a dramatic memory defect persisted without any evident Dementia. The EEG was grossly abnormal, but without any localized dysrhythmia, and *remained abnormal* a full year later, although less so. Doug was able, two weeks after the electrical injury to his brain, to *interpret proverbs appropriately* and not concretely; his *visual memory was less deficient* than auditory memory. After two weeks he *could recall playing with the kite* and seemed to accept his parents' view that he got a severe electrical shock through the kite cord. However, he had *amnesia for subsequent events* and was pitiably inefficient in his *spotty processing of new and recent learning. Written reminders* recorded by his mother helped him to cope with his poor memory: "Get up; wash up; eat breakfast; brush your teeth; put on the clothes on the rack at the foot of your bed; at school, go to home room 214," and so on.

By six weeks after his accident, Doug still had *difficulty retelling a brief narrative* after five minutes had elapsed and *seemed puzzled when asked what he did at Eastertime and the previous Christmas.* He *could not remember his camp counselor* whom he liked very much during the preceding summer but when shown Bill's photograph, he smiled and said, "That's him."

Comment. Accidental electrical trauma induced a seizure instantly, with postictal lethargy followed by a few hours of Delirium. When the clouded consciousness cleared, his memory deficit persisted without any serious impairments of judgment, speech, orientation, or handwriting. His Amnestic Disorder had been overcome (largely) by the end of about eight months, although Doug lacked confidence in his memory for the next 18 months. A subjective sense of bad memory could not be corroborated by mental state evaluation or by psychological testing. By ninth grade Doug had resumed being a better-than-average student.

The limbic system subserves memory as well as affects and olfactory sensation. It is impugned in many of the brain disorders that cause Amnestic Organic

Disorder. Memory disorders may dominate the clinical picture after some closed head injuries; amnesia may develop even without loss of consciousness. After herpes simplex encephalitis the Amnesia may be the predominant residual from which a child may not recover. Treatments for amnesia are largely supportive and symptomatic. Acetylcholine, physostigmine, and vasopressin are experimental treatments not generally available or adequately tried out with carefully documented improvements in memory.

Organic Delusional Disorder (293.81)

CLINICAL DESCRIPTION

This is a Delusional Disorder that was not included in Chapter 23 on Delusional (Paranoid) Disorders. Since Organic Delusional Disorder does give evidence of organic causation, it is more sensible to review the syndrome as one of the Organic Mental Disorders, thereby helping us to highlight its differentiation from the rest of the Organic Mental Disorders.

Organic Delusional Disorder is a rare illness among children, even after traumata to the head that produce concussion, fracture, or intracranial bleeding. More often seen are the symptoms of Dementia, Amnestic Disorder, Organic Affective Disorder, and Organic Personality Disorder. The reader may wish to review a transiently delusional picture as shown by Miguel (see Chapter 5, p. 94).

DSM-III-R states as diagnostic criteria:

1. Delusions are the prominent clinical feature
2. No persistent clouding of consciousness (Delirium), nor loss of intellectual capabilities (Dementia), nor prominent hallucinations (Organic Hallucinosis) are present.
3. History, physical examination or laboratory studies show a "specific organic factor" that accounts for the picture seen (no inferences based on global assessment, no presumptions, but real evidence).

CASE 24-4   Martin was eight years old when his father gave him LSD on the belief that "children, too, need to have mind-expanding experiences." The father was an attorney in a poverty law program who used LSD regularly to produce ecstatic (out-of-the-body) enthusiasms (in god) and felt that his vivid visual hallucinations were enriching consolations. Martin, unlike his father, however, became fearful and suspicious after taking the LSD. He then rushed out of their apartment and leapt over eight stairsteps to the mid-floor landing, fracturing his skull in the process. His father wrote it off as a bad trip that went sadly awry and was very attentive to Martin throughout his hospital stay.

When Martin came home from the hospital he had *no conscious recall* of what had happened on the evening of his skull fracture and concussion (i.e., both retrograde and anterograde amnesia that later cleared up). But he became *mistrustful of his father* and developed *the delusion* that his *father wanted to harm him* and perhaps *kill him*. In reality, Martin's father became contrite about his introducing Martin to a hallucinogenic drug. He vowed never to do that again. The father wondered if Martin's "continuing to be so paranoid" was attributable to "minor flashbacks to the bad LSD trip." The astute pediatric neurologist assured the father that Martin was not having flashbacks, but delusions: "no hallucinations, no dementia, and no clouding of consciousness."

Comment. Knowing the father well because he had assisted many of her impoverished clients, the Child Protective Services worker had made an assessment of the father for the agency. As a single parent he had "made a serious mistake in judgment on that single occasion but he is basically a sound parent," she wrote, upon closing the case for her agency. The neurologist did the correct differential diagnosis and had reported the case to Protective Services in a responsible way. The neurologist wished, on referring Martin to a child psychiatrist, that Martin's father could be less zealous about inducting Martin into his own somewhat deviant lifestyle.

The erosion of a child's trust lies in the history of most children with Organic Delusional Disorder but does not adequately explain the symptoms. After a head injury, in trying to fit the pieces together, the child may embark on a fixed delusional course. The delusions are outgrowths of the posttraumatic confusion as well as of the need to give the child's own version of accounting for subjectively perceived changes, risks, and insecurities. It is the organic CNS insult that precipitated delusion making and sustained it.

Organic Hallucinosis (293.82)

CLINICAL DESCRIPTION

A rare organic disorder in childhood, Organic Hallucinosis combines three essential features: 1) a definite history or physical finding or laboratory evidence of organic damage to the brain that plays an etiological role; 2) hallucinations in any sensory modality that constitute the main clinical feature; meaning 3) the disorder is not Delirium (clouded consciousness), not Organic Delusional and not Organic Affective Syndrome or Disorder. Since the exclusionary criteria are rather sweeping, it is not surprising that Organic Hallucinosis is a rare finding even among children with head injuries.

CASE 24-5   Six-year-old Ellie had been *born with difficulty*, since at the last minute the obstetrician had decided to use *forceps* for a vaginal delivery instead of doing a caesarean section. Her *10-minute Apgar score* was low (3) and she had a *mild diplegic spasticity* that was barely noticeable by the time she began *walking at 16 months of age*. She did some *toe walking* from two-to-four-years of age with a *slight tendency to scissors gait*, but that had also stopped by the time she was in kindergarten.

Ellie's kindergarten teacher observed her to *smack her lips, blink her eyes*, and, *"acting like she was in a trance,"* to *tilt her head as though listening* to someone above her and to say, *"Don't say that! It is not nice."* The entire episode lasted less than three minutes but the concerned teacher reported it to Ellie's mother. The father, who was an elementary school teacher, reassured his wife that five-year-olds "just do that. It is probably an imaginary companion."

About 10 weeks later, Ellie had another episode almost identical to the one the teacher had reported, but this time it occurred at the dinner table and was frightening to her parents who arranged the next day for an appointment for Ellie with a pediatric neurologist.

The EEG showed a *left temporal lobe focus* and the CAT scan showed no mass intracranially. Taking diphenylhydantoin, Ellie became thick-tongued but her automatisms and hallucinations became more frequent, more terrifying to her parents, and more upsetting to Ellie. With a *change in medication to carbamazepine, Ellie's Organic Hallucinosis diminished* and her *temporal lobe seizures lessened in frequency*. On the new medication, Ellie became free of hallucinations and was able to be an average student throughout first grade.

Comment. Hallucinations were Ellie's predominant symptoms of an organic psychosis. Finding the right regimen of anticonvulsants for psychomotor seizures and Organic Hallucinosis is often a difficult search. Note that Ellie had some ill effects from phenytoin but a good response from carbamazepine. She met the DSM-III-R criteria for Organic Hallucinosis.

One need not speculate about the etiology of the hallucinations if there are abnormal EEG tracings and a clinical picture of temporal lobe or complex partial seizures. For that matter, a history of a birth injury only reinforces the possibility of organic brain damage and a plausible cause of the epilepsy that leads to the Organic Hallucinosis.

Note: Ellie had cerebral palsy, which is often accompanied by Mental Retardation, but that was not so in Ellie's case. Moreover, toe walking is seen more frequently in Autism than in mild cerebral palsy, despite that not being the situation in this case.

Organic Mood Disorder (293.83)
CLINICAL DESCRIPTION

The varieties of brain insults and injuries are numerous and, although less than with adults, with children, too, the symptoms depend in general on the location, extent, and severity of the injured brain tissue. The only Organic Mood Disorders that the authors have seen are cases that resemble Mania. Yet, DSM-III-R names these three criteria for an Organic Mood Disorder.

1. The predominant disturbance is of mood with at least two of the symptoms for Depression or Mania:
         Mania
   (a) inflated self-esteem
   (b) decreased need of sleep
   (c) more talkative or pressure to talk
   (d) flight of ideas/racing thoughts
   (e) distractibility
   (f) increased activity or restlessness
   (g) overinvolved in risky behavior
         Depression
   (a) sustained depressed mood
   (b) loss of interest or pleasure
   (c) weight change
   (d) sleep changes
   (e) psychomotor changes
   (f) fatigue or anergia
   (g) feeling worthless or guilty
   (h) lowered ability to think or concentrate or decide
   (i) recurrent thoughts of death.
2. Definite evidence from history, physical or lab examinations of a causative organic factor.
3. *Not* Delirium, Dementia, Organic Hallucinosis or Organic Delusional Syndrome.

Note: Depression, if present, should be specified and perhaps ought to include either a depressed mood or anhedonia (symptom (a) or (b) in the listing under "Depression").

Mania, if present, should be specified and documented by any two of the seven symptoms listed above. Again, it is imperative to remember that manics may be dominated by euphoria *or* suspicion *or* anger, so it is important that the dominant affect be specified.

CASE 24-6   Lilith was a pubescent 11-year-old whose mother was taking her for a ride to a fruit-and-berry farm near the city in which they lived. They had seen an ad in one of the papers that read, "Pick your own for half of the price," and had decided it would be fun to try that. On the way there, on a steep-grade railway crossing with only a stationary sign for warning, the automobile stalled in front of an oncoming train. The mother survived but her bilateral head injuries yielded a rather severe Dementia; Lilith survived with Organic Mood Disorder.

Lilith not only talked faster, one month after the accident, but also louder. She told the neurologist who interviewed her, "My *mouth runs fast but nowhere near as fast as my thoughts.*" She *could not sleep until after midnight and awoke at 5 A.M. ". . . feeling great. I don't need any more sleep.*" Her first menstrual period began the third day after her emergence from a week-long coma. Lilith, pleased by menarche, became disinhibited through both her *smutty vocabulary* and her *hypersexuality.* She *masturbated openly* and made indecent *sexual proposals* to any male as tall as she was or taller. Her easy *distractibility,* making her jump from topic to topic in a pressured, high energy style, gave her the appearance of psychosis but she did not have a formal thought disorder. *Neither delusions nor hallucinations* could be elicited.

Given lithium carbonate by the neurologist, Lilith improved for a time but her hypomanic joking and sexual indiscretions soon increased again. A small nightly dose (25 mg) of chlorpromazine was added to the lithium and the combination produced better control of her Mania-like behavior. Her father took small comfort that Lilith's organic disorder was fairly under control but his wife would need constant care and attendance for the remainder of her life.

Comment. With the train-auto wreck, a week of coma, and her clinical picture after she was aroused from coma surely warranted Lilith's diagnosis of Organic Mood Disorder. She met at least six of the criteria for Mania. This "manic release" from mediation and control of speech, thinking, sexual prudence, and overall good judgment is, as we stated, uncommon but not a complete rarity.

Depression, with psychomotor retardation, dysphoria, and vegetative symptoms, has been seen in adults and adolescents. It stands to reason that there are brain-injured children who appear lethargic and dysphoric too. Perhaps Depression is easier to diagnose and treat in the older age groups and Mania, a rarity relatively speaking, more conspicuous in the younger. Whenever Depression occurs in association with an Axis-III diagnosis—such as brain, renal, hepatic, or pulmonary disorders—it is as responsive to antidepressant medication as any other Depression.

Organic Anxiety Disorder (294.80)
CLINICAL DESCRIPTION

Organic Anxiety Disorder, expectably, is a disorder for which an Axis-III diagnosis of organic brain pathology can be given (by history, clinical examination, or lab studies); but it does not fit a diagnosis of Delirium, Dementia, Organic Hallucinosis, or Organic Delusional Disorder. The disorder shows severe anxiety as its predominant disturbance.

The anxiety of this disorder appears in panic attacks (meeting, A, C, and D criteria in DSM-III-R for Panic Disorder or criteria A, B, and C for Overanxious or Generalized Anxiety Disorder). See DSM-III-R for these criteria; they are met in the case we have cited even though our case also has features of Post-traumatic Stress Disorder.

CASE 24-7   Elvis was eight years old when his father killed Elvis's mother by pistol shots, two of which went astray, landing in Elvis's brain. They were removed through neurosurgical intervention. Elvis regained consciousness six hours after surgery. A week elapsed during which time he showed no memory of the murder of his mother. He could not be convinced that she was dead, nor that his father was incarcerated and would not come to see him. Some attending him suspected he was "delusional" or "delirious." A child psychiatry consultant recommended that his favorite aunt spend more time with Elvis, if possible. It was possible, but difficult, since she worked as a clerk in a department store and lost pay when she was absent from work. Still, she made the sacrifices needed in order to be with her deceased sister's little boy.

Elvis cried, confided in his aunt how depressed he was to have nobody who would be his mommy, and seemed reassured that his aunt intended for him to live with her and her own son (aged nine) and daughter (aged six). Child Welfare approved his maternal aunt's caretaking and Elvis was discharged from the hospital in just under three weeks, with arrangements for follow-up visits to neurosurgery and to child psychiatry clinics.

Elvis was soon sound enough on neurological examination to be discharged from neurosurgery, coinciding with the time when he developed *"panic attacks"* that were *unrelated to others' attention,* or lack of focused attention, to Elvis. The *attacks came unexpectedly* but seemed to bear some *relation to times of transition—* when he was getting ready to go to church with his aunt, when he was leaving church, when it was time to go out playing with his cousins, when he stopped vigorous activity to "calm down and watch TV." Some of these changing situations seemed to bring on separation panic. Some of the panic episodes, that is, were times of separation but not all; yet all times of panic were times of change or anticipated change.

Elvis first of all—during a panic attack—*clutched at his anterior chest wall,* saying his *heart hurt,* then quickly became *dyspneic* and *"croupy-sounding."* He *sweated, trembled,* and *felt dizzy, fearing he was going to die.* Within a week after his first experience of panic, he had had a total of six such attacks that really worried his aunt. She noted that he was *easily frightened,* quite apart from the times of panic, and sadly forecast that he was fated to be a "nervous" orphaned boy. He had *nightmares* two or three times a week—dreams of his father either beating up Elvis or Elvis's mother or trying to shoot both of them. He would *jump* and *look terror-stricken* if a door was slammed or a car backfired. He would *leave the room* in anxious *trembling if a television story depicted guns and violence*—and many did.

Comment. Elvis began having pathological symptoms as a captive witness of his father's wife abuse. He was acutely psychotic (Delirium) postoperatively, became grief-stricken thereafter, and then, when at home with his aunt and cousins, he developed an Organic Anxiety Disorder that showed features of Separation Anxiety Disorder, Panic Disorder, Post-traumatic Stress Disorder, and Over-anxious or Generalized Anxiety Disorder. That he was basically conservative, clinging perseveratively to his present security and resisting any change, is characteristic of brain-injured children. They want their worlds and their sched-ules to be simple and devoid of novelty or abrupt changes. The treatment modalities helpful to Elvis were expressive (insight-producing) psychotherapy and a tricyclic antidepressant for relief of his severe anxiety symptoms.

Organic Mental Disorder NOS (294.80)

This residual category is saved for combinations that may not meet criteria for any of the seven subtypes presented in this chapter or in Chapter 5 concerning Organic Personality Disorder; for behavioral disturbances associated with epi-lepsy; or for "other." Developing young persons may often fall in this *NOS* category, according to the authors' experience. Such children require a multi-modal therapeutic approach and as much diagnostic acumen as possible, but an acumen that is seasoned with an understanding that the given child may present a mixed and shifting clinical picture. We have chosen this point to discuss epilepsy and the psychopathology that attends its course. See also Ellie, Case 5, who had temporal lobe epilepsy and Organic Hallucinosis.

CLINICAL DESCRIPTION

The child with epilepsy provokes great anxiety in many parents and also in the affected child because the child feels "seized" by conditions beyond his or her control. Pre- and postictal phenomena qualify for consideration as illusions, hallucinations, delusions, twilight states, trancelike phenomena—all being or-ganically driven symptoms. It is the interphase to which we shall give concentrat-ed attention, the period between seizures. There is no evidence for a hard-and-fast "epileptic personality" but there are some general patterns that merit the clinician's attention when dealing with a child with "major motor generalized tonic-clonic seizures," a child with grand mal, the most frequently encountered form of childhood epilepsy.

The etiology may not be easy to identify since neuropathological, genetic, chemical, toxic, infectious, and unknown causes may prompt epilepsy. Idiopathic (grand mal) epilepsy is the most frequently seen form of seizures, probably having two or three times the incidence of seizures of known or presumed causation. Grand mal seizures are much more common than other types, such as focal, petit mal, psychomotor, gelastic, running, mixtures, and others. No child who has grand mal and undergoes the diagnostic-etiological-localizing studies usually undertaken can feel anything but the center of others' attention, preoccupation, and puzzlement—and hence become self-concerned and egoistic into the bargain. Many children with seizures do become "narcissistic" and self-absorbed but with external locus of control.

CASE 24-8   Harry, now 10, was five years old when he had his first generalized major motor seizure: he experienced *aura* and *lost consciousness;* his *arms and legs stiffened* and then *jerked rhythmically;* he *became incontinent, ground his teeth, and bit his tongue.* When he "came to," he seemed *dopey, sleepy,* and *disoriented;* he *complained of headache.* Since he had two such generalized seizures, he was considered to have a *seizure disorder* and had taken phenytoin and phenobarbital since he was six years old, with only three seizures subsequent to being originally medicated. The parents did not consider that good control, so they changed neurologists, but to no avail for he had two seizures after seeing the second neurologist.

Harry changed *from being happy and upbeat,* though *at times demanding and irritable* prior to having seizures, into a child who *felt inferior, inadequate, and different.* He became a *shy and retiring* boy, but for a half-day prior to a seizure he would be *belligerent* and *verbally abusive.* Then after the seizure he would *act* in a *guilty* manner and return to being *withdrawn.* He showed *no intellectual deterioration* as would be expected when idiopathic grand mal is under fair control.

Comment. The parents were alarmed by their anxiety and guilt that his epilepsy might be hereditary. The boy responded both to the seizures and to the way others regarded them. He certainly had a brain disorder before and during, as well as immediately after, seizures (postictal), and showed altered behavior and personality between seizures. Children with seizures often benefit from personal and family counseling.

GENERAL COMMENTARY

The Organic Mental Disorders can be thought of as psychophysiological or psychobiological disorders for they integrate in their etiologies and courses a number of psychical, social, economic, and organic factors. A society in which accidental poisonings and injuries are so frequent has a part to play, or one in which children are subjected to being victims of so much violence, or one in which health care is needed and so often unavailable. Familial and interpersonal chaos or conflict almost always worsen the course of the organic mental disorders. The children themselves are problem children at home and at school, suffering from low self-esteem and lacking in feelings of security, as well as having particular cognitive, emotional, and behavioral symptoms.

The development of classification for these disorders reveals some interesting changes: in DSM-I and DSM-II they were classified mainly by etiology, a perfectly sound way to classify but with little utility to the clinician. DSM-III and DSM-III-R have remedied that by including etiology in the diagnostic scheme but giving first rank to the clinical symptom picture. Hence, Doug (Case 24-3) would have been classified in DSM-II with other physical injuries to the brain and not according to his amnestic syndrome; Elvis (Case 24-7) would have been diagnosed according to his weapon wounds and his anxiety would not have been emphasized; Cindy (Case 24-2) would have been diagnosed as "Organic Brain Syndrome associated with infection" but her Dementia would have gone unhighlighted. For both clinical and research purposes, predominant symptoms make more sense to be underlined in our nosology, as has been done by DSM-III and DSM-III-R.

Oddly, DSM-III-R conforms to the older format of specifying the etiological agent only with substance use disorders. DSM-III-R codes those disorders in a way that overemphasizes the specific substance that is misused. Either way would be helpful for statistical compilation and health planning, but health services planning is not a top priority at the national political level today.

Questions for Study and Action

1. Explain why a child with epilepsy often shows a perception of "external locus of control." Why would a child whose father has died be likely to show the same imputation of sources of control? Why might young children in general be persons who perceive the motors of influence on their lives as being outside of themselves?

2. How would Clarice's (Case 24-1) diagnosis have altered if there had been a criterion of two weeks' duration? Explain.

3. In the case of Cindy (Case 24-2), would anything have been gained if she had received the DSM-II diagnosis of Organic Brain Syndrome associated with viral

infection (rubella)"? What are some advantages in our diagnostic label, following DSM-III-R?

4. Doug (Case 24-3) underwent a transient Delirium followed by Organic Amnestic Disorder. Were there signs of a persistent Delirium as well as of memory loss in Doug's case? Explain.

5. In Martin's (Case 24-4) Organic Delusional Disorder, what work would be needed to help the boy and his "avant-garde" father? List three modalities that may be helpful and explain each.

6. For Ellie's (Case 24-5) Organic Hallucinosis, involving a seizure disorder's manifestations, outline a sensible diagnostic workup that includes more than CAT and EEG studies. Specify the kind of EEG, too.

7. In Lilith's case (24-6), specify the features of her symptoms and course in responding to treatment that substantiate the diagnosis of Organic Mood Disorder (Mania). What was the predominant affect in her Mania—suspicion, euphoria, or anger?

8. For Elvis (Case 24-7) outline the elements in a comprehensive treatment program, other than environmental change, educational placement appropriate to his needs, and pharmacotherapy. What other sectors of his life needed therapeutic care and attention? Should he, under optimal conditions, have been taken to his mother's funeral? Explain.

9. What is there about children that makes so often for combination and NOS diagnoses? Should Harry (Case 24-8) be in the NOS category or in one of the other organic mental disorders?

10. How many types of brain injury to children can you list? After you have made your list, consult the list in the International Classification of Diseases–9.

For Further Reading

Laufer, M.W., & Shetty, T. Acute and chronic brain syndromes. In J.N. Noshpitz (Ed.), *Basic Handbook of Child Psychiatry, Vol. III, Disturbances of Development.* New York: Basic Books, 1979, pp. 381–402.

Prugh, D.G., Wagonfeld, S., Metcalf, D., & Jones, K. A clinical study of delirium in children and adolescents. *Psychosom. Med.,* 42:177–195, 1980.

25

Specific Developmental Disorders

LANGUAGE AND SPEECH DISORDERS

These disorders encompass "central" communicative disorders, i.e., the *language* disorders; "peripheral" speech or communicative disorders, e.g., Developmental Articulation Disorder and the other *speech* disorders; and one purely psychogenic communication disorder, Elective Mutism. Note the distinction between speech and language in the communication disorders.

LANGUAGE DISORDERS

Language disorders can arise at any point in the child's life. *Congenital* or developmental or specific language disorders are present from birth. *Acquired* language disorders arise whenever the etiological noxious agent affects the central nervous system. The acquired language disorders are the domain of the neurologist. We will address the developmental or congenital language disorders here.

OVERALL DEFINITION

The disorder is defined as delayed language acquisition not explainable by general mental retardation, hearing impairment, emotional trauma, or other

391

disease. In DSM-III-R, there are two subtypes: *expressive,* involving impairment in encoding and production of language, and *receptive,* for which *both* the understanding and production of language are impaired. *Receptive* developmental language disorder is the more severe of the two. The DSM-III-R code is the same for both subtypes but the specific subtype of disorder is recorded.

EPIDEMIOLOGY

Estimates of the prevalence of Developmental Expressive Language Disorder range from 0.2% to 13% (Baker & Cantwell, 1985). Most estimates, however, cluster around 6% (National Institute of Neurological Diseases and Strokes, 1972).

ETIOLOGY AND PATHOGENESIS

This is unknown, but an organic etiology—either "brain damage" such as "birth trauma" or developmental lag—is thought to underlie most language disorders. Most investigators are of the opinion that they are related to other learning disorders (genetic factors) and that they all share in a perceptual dysfunction, especially an impairment in auditory discrimination. Variations on this latter theme are deficiencies in auditory memory span, deficit in storage of speech, slow processing of speech, and inability to recognize sounds in their linguistic context. In actuality, the causes of most cases are *unknown.*

The following are the descriptions of the subtypes:

Developmental Expressive Language Disorder (315.31)
DEFINITION

The Expressive type of Developmental Language Disorder is defined in DSM-III-R by the developmental inability to acquire vocal expression, or encoding, of language, even though the comprehension, or decoding, of language has developed intact or relatively intact. Another way to put this is that the child has normal or near-normal inner language, or processing and understanding of what is heard or seen, but cannot express or say it. As a result, the child's vocabulary is restricted, and grammar is poor.

CLINICAL DESCRIPTION

CASE 25-1   Mark was seen at age eight because of significant *emotional difficulties,* poor relationships with peers because of reacting to any frustration by either *temper outbursts* or *withdrawal,* and poor relationships with adults (both parents and teachers) by being stubborn and disobedient.

Past history showed that Mark had walked at about one year, but had *not developed speech* until he was close to two years old. Even then, he was able to say *only the simplest words* ("ma-ma," "da-da"), while *simple sentences* were not mastered until well *after this third* birthday. Nevertheless, he was always in *good contact* with his environment, *understood* what was said to him and *expressed himself* by gestures and simple words.

When seen by the physician, the eight-year-old talked with *a simple vocabulary*, but was in excellent contact with reality and seemed naturally bright. His fund of knowledge was hard to determine because of his relatively limited vocabulary, but his school records indicated that he *read at grade level*, without, however, being able to express or reproduce the information thus gained. His grades were, therefore, not the best.

Comment. Mark's case is an example of Developmental Expressive Language Disorder, with retarded development of expressive language, but with normal hearing, intelligence, and inner language. Psychological testing for IQ and cognitive skills would have been helpful.

Developmental Receptive Language Disorder (315.31)

DEFINITION

The Receptive type of Developmental Language Disorder is defined in DSM-III-R as the developmental failure to acquire comprehension (decoding) *and* vocal expression (encoding) of language, i.e., the developmental absence of both inner and expressive language. Deficits occur in sensory perception (recognition of symbols), integration (or awareness of relationships between symbols), storage recall (reproducing the symbols) and "sequencing" (recognizing or reproducing sequences of symbols). Since effective decoding of others' messages is absent, this gives a very severe language disorder.

Associated features are common and prominently include symptoms and signs of developmental delay in motor-perceptual areas. The most important associated features, however, are reading and writing disorders, which, according to DSM-III-R, are invariably present.

CLINICAL DESCRIPTION

CASE 25-2   Henrietta was six years old when she was brought to the child psychiatrist because of *"excessive shyness"* and "withdrawal." When the *complete* history was taken, it became clear that the girl had only *seemed* withdrawn because she *spoke very little*, in short sentences, with *poor pronunciation and enunciation* of sounds, and sometimes *"did not make sense."* This was noticed by the kindergarten teacher, who had also reported that Henrietta had had occasional difficulties with the use of toys and play materials—it looked as if she sometimes *did not know* either the proper function or the relationship of one toy to another, such as the recognition that chalk was used on the chalkboard and not on paper. On the other hand, Henrietta learned all the essentials of her kindergarten program except that she printed letters "atrociously." She was ahead of the class in simple arithmetic. The school system finally decided that Henrietta was "too immature" to be promoted to first grade, especially since her attention span was thought to be quite short. Thus, at the time of her psychiatric examination she was repeating kindergarten.

When in the playroom, Henrietta was a very active child who *related well* to the examiner, was often clumsy, and appeared at her best with stuffed animals, in play activities that reflected *interpersonal skills and warmth,* but she did poorly with a house and furniture. She had a vocabulary of a few dozen basic words but was difficult to understand because she omitted most of the final consonants and could not pronounce "L." She was, however, eager to communicate, and used gestures and little dramatizations to get her messages across. According to her parents, she had started to talk after her second birthday.

Comment. This child was in danger of being misdiagnosed in the direction of psychiatric disorder (withdrawal), although her interpersonal skills were essentially normal. She showed, however, immature speech and delayed and poorly developed language in all spheres, without other features suggesting mental retardation (since she learned all the tasks of kindergarten). Also noted were associated features of clumsiness, difficulties writing or printing letters, and short attention span.

DIFFERENTIAL DIAGNOSIS (BOTH SUBTYPES)

This is important. Hearing disorders, Mental Retardation, Pervasive Developmental Disorder (psychosis) and Developmental Articulation Disorder can all be ruled out on the basis of absence of other, specific symptoms of those disorders. What then remains, in the exclusionary diagnostic process, is strictly a disorder in language, with the child's response shaped by that impediment. For instance, the mentally retarded child responds to sound predictably within his/her mental capacities, whereas the language-disordered child responds discrepantly—i.e., his or her behavior in general indicates a much higher level of functioning than the child's response to auditory verbal input would indicate. Similarly, the psychotic child will show abnormal responses and behavior in many areas outside the response to strictly auditory verbal cues. The child with a Language Disorder is in full emotional contact with his/her environment.

In Developmental Articulation Disorder, the language is intact, but the production of the sounds of speech is obviously impaired.

TREATMENT (BOTH SUBTYPES)

This is not within the expertise of the average physician. After complete psychological testing has been done, speech pathology is the discipline most likely to offer some help, and the psychiatrist is often needed to deal with the secondary emotional problems. Parental counseling helps parents to avoid the extremes of unrealistic expectations and demands on one hand, and overprotectiveness on the other.

COURSE AND PROGNOSIS

Outcome depends on the severity of the disorder. Prognosis is best in simple Developmental Expressive Language Disorder, and worst in severe cases of the Receptive subtype that show serious auditory perceptual difficulties.

SPEECH DISORDERS

Developmental Articulation Disorder (Dyslalia, Dysarthria) (315.39)

This disorder of mispronunciation is the most frequent speech disorder, occurring in approximately 6% of male and 3% of female schoolchildren, and at an even higher rate in preschool children. It is more frequent in males, nonfirstborn, and working class or poor children (Baker & Cantwell, 1985). DSM-III-R classifies this disorder among the Specific Developmental Disorders, together with Language Disorders.

DEFINITION

The disorder is defined in DSM-III-R as the frequent and recurrent misarticulation of one or more sounds when compared to the majority of speakers of the same language and dialect who are of the same age. Developmental Articulation Disorder is the developmental failure to articulate specific, later-acquired, parts of speech, i.e., sounds of phonemes. Instead, the child omits those sounds and/or substitutes other sounds. If the sound misarticulated is *l* or *n*, it is also referred to as "lalling"; if the "fricatives" such as *s, z, sh,* or *ch* are involved, it is called "lisping." Other sounds involved are *th* and *f*.

Vocabulary, grammatical structure, and all the neurological aspects of language reception (comprehension and expression) are normal.

ETIOLOGY

Most experts now agree that a developmental lag that never catches up or a delay that may be compensated underlies Developmental Articulation Disorder. A contributing factor may be a large family size and linguistic understimulation of the child. The child's pronunciation is not up to age level.

CLINICAL DESCRIPTION

The clinician should bear in mind that Developmental Articulation Disorder rarely comes in pure form. It is usually associated with other developmental delays. Attention–Deficit Hyperactivity Disorder and Developmental Reading Disorder are frequently found to coexist with Developmental Articulation Disorder. Delayed landmarks of speech development and enuresis are other often-associated findings.

The symptomatology of this disorder is based on the misarticulation or mispronunciation of certain sounds in words, not of entire words or syllables. These abnormalities are mainly of two types: first, substitutions of an incorrect sound, such as substituting th for the s and z sounds (lisping), saying do instead of go, or w for r (as in the famous "Bugs Bunny" cartoon, where the hunter pronounces "wabbit" instead of "rabbit"). The second type is the omission of sounds, such as "ow" for "house," or "coo" for "school." A third type, less frequently encountered, is distortion, in which the speaker mispronounces a sound in a way that approximates the correct sound ("Apistopal" for "Episcopal").

It is not necessary for a doctor to memorize the ages by which certain consonant sounds should be mastered. Suffice it to say that by the age of five or six, most children will master the articulation of all the consonants and th in English. More than half the sounds are attained by age three, and the rest by age five, with s, the and z being the last.

CASE 25-3   Todd was six years old when he was referred for psychiatric consultation because of a string of difficulties, chief among them being hyper-activity, reading difficulties, impulsivity with aggressiveness, and bedwetting. He was the second to youngest of a sibship of seven, and his parents had a hard time taking care of the family, both economically and emotionally.

Examination showed Todd in constant motion, both motorically and verbally. He heard and understood the examiner and communicated readily, but at first was hard to understand because he mispronounced several phonemes, espe-cially s and z, and omitted r. He further showed a number of neurological soft signs, including poorly developed laterality.

One of the reasons Todd's family had always experienced economic difficulties was that Todd's father had never been able to go beyond 10th grade in school because of a severe reading difficulty for which no compensatory education was furnished. Todd himself had been enrolled in remedial reading even though he was only in first grade, as his communication disability was quite severe. Psychological testing showed no severe deficits except in his speech.

Todd's hearing and comprehension of the examiner's speech were normal, and he related well emotionally. Once sense was made out of his mispronounced speech, it became obvious that his grammar and syntax were normal for his socioeconomic level.

Comment. Developmental Articulation Disorder rarely occurs by itself, and the above case demonstrates the context of other developmental delays: Developmental Reading Disorder, Attention–Deficit Hyperactivity Disorder with soft neurological signs, general immaturity, and a family history of verbal nonfluency and reading disability. Moreover, Developmental Articulation Disorder occurs more often among children of large sibships, possibly reflecting lessened individual attention (including verbal attention), rare correction and guidance when the child misarticulates (guidance lacking for most children), and fewer opportunities for modeling correct pronunciation.

DIFFERENTIAL DIAGNOSIS

Although Developmental Articulation Disorder is sometimes called "dysarthria," that is incorrect. Dysarthria is, in reality, an impairment of enunciation of entire syllables and words, due to organic lesions located at any point from the cerebral cortex to the "end apparatus," i.e., in the muscles of speech articulation. Pervasive Developmental Disorder (Infantile Autism), Developmental Language Disorder and Mental Retardation show difficulties in language and poor articulation, but can be distinguished easily by a comprehensive history and examination. To recapitulate, Developmental Articulation Disorder has normal receptive and expressive language, hearing, and intelligence, but deviates only in pronunciation or enunciation.

TREATMENT AND PROGNOSIS

Whether to institute treatment depends on the child's age and the severity of the disorder, as well as the extent and severity of associated difficulties. Among the latter, psychosocial and sometimes psychiatric sequelae must be considered. In other words, a Developmental Articulation Disorder may at times produce ostracism or ridicule by peers and lead to withdrawal, various Anxiety Disorders, or Depression.

An experienced speech pathologist or specialist in "communicative disorders" can determine whether the articulation disorder needs treatment considering the child's age, but it is the duty of the expert in child mental health to assess the overall status of the child and recommend treatment.

Speech therapy is the specifically appropriate treatment; however, adjunctive treatment measures may be indicated. Involvement of the family (usually the parents) is always necessary, as with all remedial measures, such as speech therapy, that involve training by repetition. Speech therapy itself is a specialized procedure administered by specialists.

Prognosis, given treatment, is generally good, at least before age eight. Speech therapy is an effective treatment approach, especially when supported by the adjunctive treatment modalities.

Stuttering (307.00)

DEFINITION

Stuttering is defined in DSM-III-R as a disturbance of both rhythm and fluency of speech through the mechanisms of blocking, hesitation, repetition or, rarely, prolongation, involving single sounds, syllables, or entire words. Stuttering is, therefore, a dysrhythmia and a dysfluency of speech. Unfortunately for the child afflicted with this disorder, Stuttering is most severe when there is pressure to communicate, and often the most important words are the ones with which the child has the greatest difficulty.

Characteristically, Stuttering is often absent during oral reading, singing, and when talking to inanimate objects or pets—when the child is amused, curses, or says obscenities.

Conceptually, we can thus view Stuttering as placed in between Developmental Articulation Disorder, where motivation and psychological factors play virtually no role, and Elective Mutism, in which motivation is the main determinant.

Stuttering is frequently accompanied by associated movements in specific groups of muscles of the head: periorbital tics, tremors, or jerking of the lips or jaw or the entire head. Accessory hand movements may be made and the anal sphincter is typically tightened during Stuttering.

ETIOLOGY

The plenitude of theories about the etiology of Stuttering shows that nobody really knows what causes Stuttering. From the plethora of theories we will pick out a few samples to help the clinician get a better understanding of the disorder.

The easiest theory to follow is the psychodynamic one—so easy, in fact, that it is suspect: the psychoanalyst Fenichel considers Stuttering an anal-sadistic sexualization of speech; underlying this, in turn, is the primitive belief in magic: "words can kill." The hesitations of Stuttering are thought to represent aggressive acts against the impatient listener.

A more recent, and perhaps credible, theory is the organic "brain function" theory. Based on such experimental neurological findings as bilateral representation of speech in the cerebral hemispheres (i.e., both hemispheres have speech centers) and different rates of blood flow to Broca's speech areas (speech center) in one versus the other hemisphere, depending on whether the subject was stuttering, this theory has considerable appeal to many.

These theories can then be linked with the genetic theories, viz., that Stuttering is inherited. The resultant theory is the "breakdown theory," which holds that inherited constitutional characteristics produce a temporary incoordination in speech, which becomes Stuttering (Silver, 1985).

Another explanation for the occurrence of Stuttering, with or without the postulate of inherited factors, is that the stutterer anticipates difficulty with speech (Bloodstein, 1969). Parental reactions are seen as the instrumental condition: the child experiments with speech, and his or her normal repetitions of syllables or words are criticized and focused on by the parents, and prematurely termed Stuttering. Finally, learning theories have been applied to Stuttering. All of them seem to have had difficulties explaining what maintains Stuttering, i.e., what could possibly reward a socially maladaptive behavior such as Stuttering? Reduction of anxiety *after* the anticipatory struggle to speak has been viewed as the main reinforcer.

Except for the organic theories (e.g., bilateral speech representation), none of the theories has been based on experimental evidence. Therefore, the organic theories are now thought to be the most credible. Surprisingly, however, all nonorganic theories have had at least partially successful treatment applications.

CLINICAL DESCRIPTION

Stuttering usually has a sequential, protracted history. In a typical case, it starts somewhere between ages two and nine (there are peaks at ages two to three and five to seven), and develops through four phases. The fourth phase is in late adolescence and/or adulthood and represents the completed and chronic clinical picture, with significant anxiety and defense mechanisms elaborated against it. This is an area for adult psychiatry.

Phase 1 is the initial, episodic phase, where the normal repetition of sounds in the acquisition of speech becomes invested with what appears to be an extra intensity. This phase occurs in preschool children, i.e., during the age of acquisition of speech. Since it appears to be an extension of a normal process, it is hard to determine when actual Stuttering begins. Almost one out of every two of these children recovers, i.e., they never become true stutterers.

If the problem continues, the intervals between these repetitions become shorter, the tendency to stutter under pressure (either general excitement or intense need to say something) becomes more pronounced, and Phase 2 sets in. By this time the child has reached kindergarten or the first grade in school. Different from Phase 1, the child now considers himself (most are boys) a stutterer, but surprisingly shows little concern. There is usually an increase in stuttering with pressure of speech.

Phase 3 is in late childhood (age eight or older), and stuttering in response to particular situations is more pronounced: oral reports in the classroom, speaking on the telephone, addressing a stranger, and the like. "By-pass" mechanisms make their appearance: the child substitutes words for which he has more fluency in place of those with less fluency, and he "talks around" words or phrases that he has come to remember as obstacles. Nobody values perfect fluency as much as a stutterer, it is said.

CASE 25-4   Xavier was eight years old when he was seen by the child psychia-trist to "rule out" emotional factors in his stuttering. The parents had difficulty remembering exactly when it all began. They did recall that Xavier repeated consonants at the *beginning* of *new words,* and of words whose usage he was *learning,* such as "He took it f-f-from m-m-me." However, this *ceased* and he was fine until his younger sibling was born, which coincided with Xavier's beginning school. At that point, Xavier seemed to take forever to get certain words out, especially more complex ones: he would *take deep breaths, grimace,* and try endlessly to get the word completed. When Xavier had to *answer a question during classroom* discussion, he stuttered a great deal.

His parents and his teachers tried not to make too much of Xavier's stuttering, but this *benign neglect did not seem to influence* the stuttering in any way. The *parents* were *ambitious, upwardly mobile* people, who had read up on stuttering and finally concluded that something must be done. They thought that perhaps the birth of the sibling had been a traumatic event, and generally looked for psychological explanations, especially as they had had a number of marital difficulties. Father eventually recalled that he had stuttered when he was in kindergarten.

When seen by the doctor, Xavier was stuttering severely at first. This improved slightly when Xavier became more familiar and comfortable in the interview. He reported that he had difficulties making *new friends,* but that classmates and *longtime* neighborhood friends went along with his stuttering and *"did not make too much of it,"* since he proudly reported that he was *good* at sports and at electronic games where talking was not at a premium. However, he felt he was *different* from the others in oral presentations, from which many teachers had excused him. Perhaps because everything depended on his written work, he had become *anxious* and *compulsive* about it.

Comment: The case history illustrates the insidious beginning, fluctuating, and then chronic course of stuttering. This child's subsequent adjustment remained good, although he became anxious, with threat to his self-esteem because of his differentness in school. His parents hoped for a psychological cause, but probably that is not a hope to be fulfilled in Xavier's case.

DIFFERENTIAL DIAGNOSIS

Few other conditions are likely to be mistaken for Stuttering. Developmental Articulation Disorder, when severe, may be mistaken for Stuttering at first glance, because words may be cut down by omission to simple sounds, and similar sounds may be mistaken for repetition. However, the child's breathing and pausing between sounds and words is normal in Developmental Articulation Disorder, and there is no anticipatory anxiety. Cluttering, a disorder in linguistic organization, can be distinguished by its blanking out, extreme efforts at word finding, faulty sequencing, repetitions of entire syllables and words, but all devoid of anxiety. Clutterers are unaware of their troubles with language.

Most differential-diagnostic difficulties arise in the young child when it is impossible to distinguish between normal hesitancy during the acquisition of speech and future stuttering. Unfortunately, there is no reliable way to tell which way the speech is going to develop and, therefore, most clinicians prefer to err on the side of reassurance so as to minimize the element of the parent's perfectionistic tension that might aggravate a child's stuttering.

TREATMENT AND PROGNOSIS

"The trouble with treatments for stuttering is that almost all of them work for a while at least." This, according to Van Riper (1973, p. 144), summarizes the state of the art.

Psychotherapy of various denominations probably has been the least effective, for it results only in some lessening of the stutterer's anxiety and improvement of his or her overall functioning and reactions to the stuttering, without, apparently, lasting benefits.

Specialized forms of behavior therapy are now the mainstay of treatment: desensitization is aimed at reducing the anticipatory blocks, and a variety of positive responses are substituted for the stuttering. Variations on this theme include the use of electromyographic feedback and special "airflow" techniques (to relieve vocal cord tension).

Obviously, the treatment should be conducted by qualified specialists, usually from among speech pathologists. Most children will be older (10 years or more) by the time treatment is decided on. The mental health professional has a constructive "standby" role, to attend to the secondary emotional reactions.

Prognosis is good for long-term adjustment and even control of stuttering *provided* the child and the parents are motivated to continue with treatment for a long time.

Cluttering (307.00)

Cluttering is a rapid speech that moves by fits and starts but the child is not self-conscious about these gaps in talking punctuated by repeating of syllables or words. There are times when a child appears to blank out and to be hunting for the right word, indeed, for any word. The child's reading comprehension too is usually patchy; the written language of such a child is also fitful, skimpy, and poorly organized. Clusters of words are thrown onto a page but they do not fit the semantical, grammatical, or syntactical patterns of the language in which one is trying to communicate. On rereading them, the child himself may or may not know what message was intended.

Cluttering is very rare and may have a more basic neural impairment (than stuttering) as its underlying cause. Cluttering shows global linguistic processing difficulties. Its differential diagnosis was considered under that of Stuttering in the preceding subsection.

Elective Mutism (313.23)

DEFINITION

Children suffering from Elective Mutism have "normal speech equipment," i.e., they can comprehend and speak, but they choose not to speak as an important part of their social lives. Elective Mutism is, therefore, defined as continous refusal to speak in almost all social situations, especially school, despite normal language ability, i.e., normal receptive and expressive language (see DSM-III-R).

ETIOLOGY

Elective Mutism is a psychologically patterned disorder and is not caused by organic factors. When there is a definite precipitating, traumatic event, the resulting mutism is called traumatic mutism. This is *not* equivalent to Elective Mutism.

Elective Mutism appears to be caused by a variety of psychological factors—early emotional trauma, such as hospitalization early in life, or early rejecting or ambivalent parental (especially maternal) attitudes. However, there are more clinical descriptions of ongoing emotional conditions that appear to cause Elective Mutism, and therefore such ongoing, chronic, or pervasive emotional difficulties generate a more convincing hypothesis of causality. The most frequent scenario is one of "taking sides": the family is split into warring factions, the child siding with one parent and "punishing" the other, or "punishing" the outside world. Why the child chooses speech as the weapon may be explained on the psychodynamic ground of persistence of magical thinking ("words can kill"). Fixation at the anal stage is another way of explaining the symptom choice—the younger the child, or his/her mentality, the more magical that thought will persist. Moreover, children with Elective Mutism are "anal" in their character: controlling, stubborn, oppositional.

In summary, a combination of family pathology and intrapsychic conflict is the most common psychodynamic blueprint. Hayden (1980) considers "symbiotic" Elective Mutism the most common, reflecting excessive siding with mother in the context of severe family pathology, with the child assuming a powerful, controlling and often manipulative role through the selective withholding of speech. "Passive aggressive" Elective Mutism follows somewhat similar lines, whereas "speech phobic" Elective Mutism occurs in children with higher levels of anxiety which are displaced onto the function of speech.

CLINICAL DESCRIPTION

CASE 25-5   Marybeth, aged five-and-a-half years, was referred to a child guidance clinic by her kindergarten teacher because she still would *not talk to anyone six months* after beginning school. The teacher stated that she had seen other children be shy and reticent when starting school, but their refusing to speak never went on for so long nor was it done so *completely and consistently* as by Marybeth.

The *mother* reported that the child *spoke freely* with her and the *eight-year-old brother.* At school Marybeth *comprehended* what was said to her and *responded nonverbally to verbal* communications, although there was "a *stubborn streak* in her."

When examined, the child would not speak to the psychiatrist, but had been *overheard to talk to her mother in the waiting room.* When she was subsequently seen jointly with mother, she *whispered* to her mother when the examiner kept engaging both of them in conversation.

Past history showed that the child had *spoken very little to persons outside her family,* although she managed to maintain several "lukewarm" relationships with peers in the neighborhood. With these, she communicated by gestures and occasional short utterances.

Mother further reported that Marybeth was often *difficult to manage* due to her *frequent temper tantrums and stubbornness* and that, seemingly as a result of obstinacy, the child was often *encopretic*. The father had tried to discipline the child, whereas the mother had felt overwhelmed by her and usually gave in. Marybeth was reported occasionally to "punish" father for his disciplinary measures by not speaking to him.

Comment. All the salient characteristics of *primary,* that is idiopathic, elective mutism are shown by this child, as well as most of the associated features: stubbornness, difficult temper, encopresis, shyness, and reticence in most social situations. No precipitating events can be found. The obvious voluntary control of this syndrome has been reflected in the previous name of the disorder: voluntary aphasia or *aphasia voluntaria* (the term was coined by Kussmaul in 1877, according to von Misch, 1952). The child thus withholds speech in certain (actually most) social situations, most commonly and typically at the most important of all social functions of childhood—in school.

DIFFERENTIAL DIAGNOSIS

The cornerstone of all differential diagnosis concerning speech and language is the presence of speech in Elective Mutism. Once this is established, the rest is relatively easy. Slight difficulty in the differential diagnosis may arise because Elective Mutism may be associated with *delayed language development* or with Developmental Language or Articulation Disorder. The salient point is the observation of such difficulties in *all* situations with the other disorders but only in *specified* situations with Elective Mutism.

Mental Retardation and childhood psychosis (Pervasive Developmental Disorder—childhood Autism) are further examples of observable difficulties in speech and communication; but again, the overall, relatively unselected scope of their language difficulty is the feature differentiating them from Elective Mutism.

Another area requiring differential diagnosis is in interpersonal functioning. Children with Elective Mutism are often shy and oppositional as well. By the same token, depressed children, or those suffering from Avoidant Personality Disorder or Social Phobia, may be tongue-tied in many situations, especially when seen for a psychiatric examination. The point of differentiation is the persistence and long duration of Elective Mutism, and, on detailed examination, the domination or predominance of the refusal to speak over all other symptoms in Elective Mutism.

Finally, undetected deafness will result in speech and communication difficulties that may mimic Elective Mutism. Hysterical aphonia is the loss of voice as a conversion symptom but it then occurs in all contexts of the child's life.

TREATMENT AND PROGNOSIS

Our elaboration of etiological hypotheses was intended to give the clinician a framework for selecting and focusing treatment.

Obviously, the treatment should be selected on the basis of the particular relevant psychodynamics. Since family pathology usually is present, most therapeutic approaches should include work with the family and, since individual psychotherapy is almost always indicated, most treatment interventions become multimodal. Some authors have a preference for psychiatric hospitalization of the child as the most effective treatment, others prefer behavior modification in an outpatient setting. Over the longer term, almost all approaches are successful and Elective Mutism, per se, has a good prognosis.

Questions for Study and Action

1. Outline how you would proceed in a diagnostic workup of a child with an articulation problem. What would you ask for from (a) laboratories, (b) consultant clinicians?

2. Why does Cluttering appear to be a language problem while Stuttering seems to be a speech problem?

3. What truth is there in the quip that nobody reveres fluency as much as a stutterer? Explain.

4. In what ways could a specialist in communicative disorders work on a child psychiatry health team? List at least half a dozen ways in which his/her skills would be valuable for a team effort.

5. Why would Elective Mutism be a possible manifestation of:
    (a) passive-aggressive noncooperation with someone who physically punished the child?
    (b) sexual abuse by grandfather?
    (c) phobia about associating with ethnically different persons?
    (d) mild Mental Retardation?
    (e) harsh interparental predivorce conflict?

For Further Reading

Baker, L., & Cantwell, D.P. Developmental language disorder. In H.I. Kaplan & B.J. Sadock (Eds.), *Comprehensive Textbook of Psychiatry,* (4th Ed.). Baltimore: Williams & Wilkins, 1985.

Bloodstein, O. *A Handbook of Stuttering.* Chicago: National Easter Seal Society, 1969.

Eisenson, J. *Aphasia in Children.* New York: Harper & Row, 1972.

Fenichel, O. *The Psychoanalytic Theory of Neurosis.* New York: W.W. Norton, 1945.

Gualtieri, C.T., Koriath, U., Van Bourgondien, M., & Saleeby, N. Language disorders in children referred for psychiatric services. *J. Amer. Acad. of Child Psychiatry,* 22:165–171, 1983.

Hayden, T.L. Classification of elective mutism. *J. Amer. Acad. of Child Psychiatry,* 19:118, 1980.

Human Communication and Its Disorders: An Overview. Monograph No. 10. National Institute of Neurological Diseases and Strokes. Bethesda, Maryland: Department of Health, Education and Welfare, 1972.

Shapiro, T. *Clinical Psycholinguistics.* New York: Plenum, 1979.

Silver, L.B. Speech disorders. In H.I. Kaplan & B.J. Sadock, (Eds.), *Comprehensive Textbook of Psychiatry* (4th Ed.). Baltimore: Williams & Wilkins, 1985.

Van Riper, C. *The Treatment of Stuttering.* Englewood Cliffs, NJ: Prentice-Hall, 1973.

Von Misch, A. Elektiver Mutismus im Kindesalter. *Zeitschrift für Kinderpsychiatrie,* 19:49–87, 1952.

Weiss, C.E., & Lillywhite, H.S. *Communicative Disorders: Prevention and Early Intervention.* St. Louis, MO: C.V. Mosby, 1981.

ACADEMIC SKILLS DISORDERS (LEARNING DISABILITIES)

These are disorders of specific areas of academic development not due to another disorder. (They are coded on Axis II in DSM-III-R.) The specific areas of development are subdivided into those of reading, spelling, arithmetic, and writing but the clinician should remember that the impairment is broader than the particular category implies. Thus, Developmental Reading Disorder, for instance, affects thought processes in various subtle and sometimes less subtle ways; comprehension, composition, ability to glean the essence or the nuances from communications or interactions are variously impaired.

The clinician is careful to remember that although Developmental Reading Disorder is the most notorious and the most frequently diagnosed, the other developmental disorders of academic skills can cause important impairment too, but are easily missed because of the diagnostic focus being primarily or exclusively set on reading disorder.

The older term—"specific learning disorder" or simply "L.D."—therefore has some advantage, but the confusion with a psychogenic learning disorder probably cancels out its usefulness. The Academic Skills Disorder may be in reading, writing, or arithmetic or combinations of those "three Rs."

Developmental Reading Disorder (315.00)

DEFINITION

A brief definition is that this is an Academic Skills Disorder presenting with impaired reading ability not due to inadequate intelligence or faulty schooling, poor eyesight or emotional problems. A more detailed definition is that Reading Disorder is a developmentally determined significant impairment in the rate and quality of acquisition of reading skills. It is due to constitutional and genetic factors, and not due to any other handicap. "Significant" impairment is defined as a one-to-two-year discrepancy in reading skill for ages 8 to 13; below that, there is no fixed definition for "significant impairment."

Synonyms sometimes used have been "dyslexia," sometimes "alexia," "specific learning (reading) disability," "word blindness," and "constitutional aphasia."

EPIDEMIOLOGY

Estimates of the incidence of Developmental Reading Disorder among American school children vary between 1% and 15% (depending on the strictness of diagnostic criteria [Jansky, 1985]). The prevalence is higher among juvenile delinquents and the socially disadvantaged. The male to female ratio is 2 to 4:1. The incidence of Developmental Reading Disorder is thought to be lower in oriental cultures using writing that goes from top to bottom rather than from one side to another and where the characters are symmetrical from right to left. Children with Developmental Reading Disorder are a heterogeneous biosocial group, with admixtures of verbal, perceptual, and other problems.

ETIOLOGY AND PATHOGENESIS

The etiology is unknown, but the following hypotheses have been advanced: lesions in various parts of the brain, such as left occipital lobe or left posterior temporal-parietal region; a high incidence of prenatal and perinatal difficulties; and a high incidence of neurological disorders. The main current theory is one of dysfunction of the left hemisphere of the brain, perhaps combined with a skewed dominance of the right hemisphere. There is an interesting historical corroborative aspect to this theory: many famous painters and sculptors had learning disabilities—their right hemisphere is thought to have "overwhelmed" the function of the left hemisphere with the strength of spatial relations and three-dimensional activity. Examples are Leonardo da Vinci and Auguste Rodin. The hypothesis really remains unconfirmed.

The true cause or causes for this disorder are unknown; the most commonly accepted hypothesis is developmental or maturational lag.

CLINICAL DESCRIPTION

CASE 25-6   Frankie's parents had noticed even before school began that he had great *difficulty following directions.* Although seemingly bright and quite verbal, his descriptions of even the most interesting (to him) events were often somewhat "fuzzy" and confused. He did *not* develop *any grasp of the alphabet* in kindergarten, although practically all of his classmates in that kindergarten class did by being able to write their first names. In first grade, he managed to identify letters, but kept *being confused* by the lower case *d*'s and *b*'s and *p*'s and *q*'s. Invariably he would write "dab" or "bab" for "dad." By the end of first grade, very few syllables "clicked" in his mind: he would name the letters but simply could *not synthesize them into a meaningful whole.* His second grade teacher noted that he was much *better in arithmetic* than in reading and could do arithmetical operations at least at *grade level.* He did them all in his head, though, since *writing* down anything seemed *an ordeal* to him: he *labored over writing* and his letters looked atrocious. Many of his letters were *turned around in a mirror image* way; others were simply illegible. In the course of second grade, the diagnosis of reading disability was made and Frankie was enrolled in a remedial reading class, having been examined by the school psychologist, *who ruled out mental retardation and speech disorder,* and by the school nurse and his pediatrician, who ruled out *visual and hearing difficulties* as well as gross *neurological abnormalities* (in view of the reported *clumsiness, mixed laterality* and *difficulty finding his way* around the school).

In third grade, Frankie finally started putting together some *syllables,* but frequently *reversed them:* "was" was "saw," "pool" was "loop" and "no" was "on." Other words or parts of words appeared to be *seen by Frankie differently* than what was written: "bag" was "day," "dog" was "boy."

In spite of intensive work in the remedial class, Frankie was by now *about a year-and-a-half behind his classmates* in reading and writing, and he was starting to express *feelings of being different.* His peers started to drift away from him, as he was quite unable to follow their social development, which involved sharing more complicated games with *more elaborate rules.* Frankie, in turn, drifted towards *younger children* whose games were more at his level and in whose company he could still *feel successful.*

Frankie's parents had gone through a bewildering sequence of reactions: first, they were perplexed, but then they recalled their latent *fears* that their son would have *inherited father's learning difficulties. Father* had had a *very hard time in school,* but had advanced to a supervisory position in industry by dint of considerable *skills unrelated to formal reading and writing.* Moreover, the parents vacillated between *guilt* about their genetic contribution and resulting *overprotection* of Frankie and bursts of *expectation* that their son would do better than father in formal educational accomplishments. When it became apparent that his formal progress in school was below average, they *projected* much of their anger *onto the* school: "Why wasn't something done before second grade?" "Why had the kindergarten or first grade teacher not diagnosed his problems?" These *parental attitudes* only *aggravated Frankie's* very real problems.

Comment. This case is typical of Developmental Reading (and Expressive Writing) Disorder. First, there is the important family history; then, there are early signs of clumsiness and difficulty in comprehension and spatial orientation, and finally specific difficulties recognizing letters and putting them into syllables, such as reversals and misperceptions. As a result, the child was one-and-a-half years behind the average in educational achievements, in spite of normal intelligence and absence of primary physical (e.g., visual) and emotional handicaps.

What happens then in the older child?

CASE 25-7   Wilfred was a *charming, popular* 11-year-old who developed a number of phobias. Careful psychiatric evaluation brought to light undiagnosed learning disability: the patient had *never liked reading,* but somehow always *got by* because of superior intelligence and the talent of *"getting around" problem areas,* either by having others do his tasks for him or by *picking up information via the spoken word* (auditory input) and *remembering* practically everything.

By the beginning *of fifth grade, his disability had "caught up"* with him: there were assignments which he was supposed to *read* (not everything was read or explained in class anymore) and there were *written instructions* on tests. His work *started to suffer* and *his anxiety* increased. He became defensive and *angry,* but underneath he was *questioning his ability* to do anything and became *scared of failure.* For a while he talked his parents into believing *that his teacher* was *mean and incompetent.*

Fortunately for him, his natural social and athletic *skills* helped balance out some of these negative consequences. Nevertheless, it took all of fifth grade for him to overcome the *phobias and other secondary defensive measures,* while at the same time he was enrolled in an intensive course of *remedial reading.*

Comment. In children with graceful social and motor skills, a reading disorder can go undiagnosed until the auditory input becomes inadequate. Psychiatric consequences because of defense mechanisms against low self-esteem may be the symptoms leading to eventual diagnosis of the Developmental Reading Disorder.

DIAGNOSIS

Finding a case of Developmental Reading Disorder depends first and foremost on clinical alertness. A careful *history* is a must. Points to remember are:

• Family history of learning disorder.
• Early observations of a "feeling" by parents that the child is clumsy, has trouble

orienting himself or herself in space (time concepts are developed later), and subtle trouble understanding and communicating.

- Difficulties understanding directions or rules in kindergarten or first grade.
- Persistence of difficulties recognizing, sounding, and writing letters into second grade.
- Typical letter and syllable reversals persisting into second grade and beyond.
- Difficulty synthesizing letters into syllables, syllables into words, and words into meaningful sentences and messages. This naturally leads to inadequate comprehension.
- A frequent finding of poorly developed or mixed laterality.
- Attention–Deficit Hyperactivity Disorder is often associated with Developmental Reading Disorder.

In addition to the history, the clinician has a few simple methods of examination at his/her disposal:

- Ask the child to read an age-appropriate text of the clinician's choosing, or administer the Gray Oral Reading Paragraphs Test, which is a series of grade-level paragraphs, 1st grade through 12th grade (Gray, 1955).
- Ask the child to write (or print) simple words and short sentences (depending on grade level) and look for the typical signs: reversals, confusions, omissions, substitutions, both of letters and of syllables, even words.

The special neurological examination is of adjuvant value, as is the use of the designs of the Bender Visual Motor Gestalt Test (both are described in Chapter 1).

DIFFERENTIAL DIAGNOSIS

Mental Retardation can be ruled out by the overall, across-the-board delay. Retardation shows all mental functions affected and neuromuscular development often visibly delayed. Psychometric testing clinches the diagnosis. Problems of visual acuity manifest themselves in areas other than reading and are, of course, screened out by simple optometry. The same is true of hearing difficulties, which in their milder forms may at first be elusive.

Reading difficulties with emotional causes usually have a different course in that the child often did well at first and subsequently showed a growing decrement in his academic performance. Inquiry will often uncover a precipitating event or set of traumatic circumstances (e.g., divorce) in such a case but not in cases of children subjugated to chronic psychosocial stresses.

In other words, the history of psychogenic learning disability is likely to be discontinuous, whereas developmental disorder presents a continuous history.

Other symptoms are often present in pychogenic learning disorder: generalized anxiety, phobias, and psychosomatic symptoms. Psychological testing is of help here, too, because it can document specific perceptual and cognitive difficulties in Developmental Reading Disorders. Special educational testing shows, with a psychogenic case, none of the specific reading disabilities.

Socioeconomic deprivation often results in a broad spectrum of linguistic, conceptual, cultural, and academic impairment. This category is perhaps the most "mixed" because developmental disorders abound in this group *and* are combined with lack of cultural input or environmental stimulation and an oversupply of hostile attitudes towards "book learning." Again, careful comprehensive history taking is the most helpful diagnostic tool for the clinician, supplemented afterwards by psychometric and educational testing.

The key to the diagnosis and differential diagnosis is in the detective work done by an alert clinician. He or she is not obliged to establish the definitive diagnosis of any Developmental Learning Disorder, since that is a combined educational-pedagogic-developmental diagnosis confirmed by the educational psychologist.

The physician or mental health clinician is, however, often the first, or the only one, who raises an informed question about the existence of a developmental disorder. The clinician does this on the basis of a sensitive, comprehensive (all-around) assessment of the child and the child's environment.

TREATMENT

What has been said about the role of the clinician in making the definitive diagnosis can be said even more strongly about his or her role in treatment. The direct "hands-on" part of treatment of these disorders is not in the physician's area of expertise. The direct treatment is educational—remedial—and is usually administered by the school system to smaller groups or classes of pupils by specially trained teachers. The functional basis of remediation is (a) the systematic reduction of the reading process into the basic, primary "building blocks" and their assimilation by the child through repetition; and (b) the use of alternative channels of perceptual input to support the learning process in general and the assimilation of the above-mentioned "building blocks" (sometimes referred to as "graphemes" or "phonemes" by the educational specialists). Hearing, touch, and position sense are such alternative channels.

However, the physician's role outside the direct treatment is crucial, since the medical practitioner is often the only one to integrate the interplaying constitutional, emotional, and environmental conditions that affect the reading-disabled child.

The most obvious ancillary treatment is the treatment of the Attention–Deficit Hyperactivity Disorder that frequently coexists with developmental disorders. This treatment will enable the child to pay attention to the learning, thereby supporting the remediation process.

The child's emotional reactions to his disability are another area for the physician's intervention. Anger, regression, anxiety disorder, and depression are only some of the potential secondary psychiatric problems. These must be diagnosed, treated or referred to the specialist. Perhaps the most important role for the physician is the management of the parental reactions. When faced with the enigma and the frustrations of a learning-disabled child, the parents may experience a variety of untoward psychological reactions. Some parents undergo a sequence of emotions akin to grief: denial, protest (this includes the projection of blame onto the school system or individual teachers), and finally despair—giving up all hope and all efforts to help the child. The other type of reaction is overprotectiveness, which encourages dependency and an attitude of invalidism on the child's part. Neither type of parental reaction helps the child.

The clinician can be helpful in several ways: first, as an interpreter or translator of a confusing concept (developmental disorder). Abstruse concepts and jargon should be translated into intelligible language. With the correct understanding of the disorder, a realistic prognosis will be espoused by the parents, and realistic hope based on support and remediation will make many of the pathological defense mechanisms unnecessary. Second, the clinician can be an authoritative mediator with the school system. This does not mean joining the parents' pathological defense mechanisms of blaming the school system, but rather ensuring that the child gets his or her due in terms of real remediation (a right guaranteed by federal law—Public Law 94-142). Furthermore, the physician is a protector against fads (e.g., "sugar-free diet" or orthoptic training), which divert attention and effort away from needed educational measures—remediation.

In summary, the clinician's role is in comprehensively diagnosing not only the Developmental Learning Disorder but its ramifications and consequences as well. This means attending to the child as well as the parents and mediating between them. Because the practice of medicine is based both on the scientific and humanistic approach, the physician is the ideal coordinator of all the treatment approaches.

PROGNOSIS

By way of introduction, let us remember that there have been famous people who had very clear developmental learning disorders. Nelson Rockefeller and Winston Churchill are cases in point (Levinson, 1980; Major, personal communication, 1987). There are physicians who can hardly put a few words on paper and have to dictate all their progress notes. Unfortunately, for each one of these stellar cases there exist hundreds of poor outcomes. The prognosis has probably brightened considerably in recent years and is likely to continue to do so because of the great increase in remedial educational programs in public schools. Although the quality of these programs varies greatly, many of them appear to be at least of some help, so that the person is subsequently not completely "word blind."

The prognosis, therefore, depends on the same factors already mentioned in the discussion of the treatment: correct remediation, perseverance in it, treatment of associated problems, adequate economic resources, and support by the family. In addition, the prognosis is improved by the creative use of the patient's strengths in other areas. For instance, many of these patients have abilities in art, music, architecture, or skills in various crafts.

Prognosis, in summary, is always highly individualized and multidetermined, and the clinician is warned against generalized, sweeping statements.

Developmental Expressive Writing Disorder (315.80)

DEFINITION

Developmental Expressive Writing Disorder is defined in DSM-III-R as a level of skills, both in the technique of writing and of composing a written text, significantly below the child's intellectual and academic level. Composing a written text includes the choice, spelling, and writing of correct words, correct grammar, and appropriately clear communicative style. To qualify for this diagnosis, the disorder should be continuous and permanent, not merely a transient occurrence, such as "neurotic writer's block," and it should not be an integral part of another developmental disorder (e.g., Pervasive Developmental or Language Disorder).

Considerable differences of opinion exist among different authors on this subject. For one, there is no overall agreement about what should be included here, since Writing Disorder overlaps with Reading Disorder to a certain extent, but not completely. For purposes of clarity, Writing Disorders may be viewed as including the following two categories.

> *Specific Writing Disorder*—the child has acquired knowledge, can utilize it, can talk about it, but has severe difficulty writing, both "peripherally" (i.e., the very act of writing is difficult) and "centrally" (i.e., there seems to exist a block or inability to transmit information into writing). These children sometimes suffer academic failure in the higher elementary grades, because many tests are written at that stage. They do better on multiple choice examinations and oral tests.

> *Spelling Disorder*—this disorder may be part of the preceding category, may coexist with Reading Disorder, or may present in its own right. Recent research by Frith (1983) has shown that spelling problems, when they are manifested by themselves, last longer than Reading Disorder, and that Spelling Disorder should therefore be considered a cognitive deficit rather than only a reflection of maturational delay. It is, however, conceivable that the longer duration of Spelling Disorder may be due to the fact that more effort is spent on the remediation of Reading Disorder.

What the clinician may wish to focus on in a confusing field of writing and spelling difficulties is the amount of difficulty resulting for the child in terms of communication and academic success or failure. The doctor urges the educational system to accept the fact that some children spell either differently (e.g., phonetically), or not at all, or cannot process words into intelligently written symbols, and that this is a disorder that warrants serious attention.

TREATMENT

Since nomenclature and concepts are not standardized yet, there is no settled body of knowledge on how to pursue remediation for writing disorders, but inventive and intuitive teachers are still a valuable help.

Developmental Arithmetic Disorder (315.10)

For the physician, by far the most important aspect of this disorder is the fact that it exists and that Developmental Reading Disorder (dyslexia) is *not* the *only* developmental learning disorder.

DEFINITION

Developmental Arithmetic Disorder is defined in DSM-III-R similarly to its reading disorder equivalent—i.e., a serious impairment of the development of arithmetic skills that cannot be explained by mental age and mental retardation, inadequate schooling, or primary emotional factors.

EPIDEMIOLOGY

Because no single test of mathematical ability has the universal application and acceptance of many of the tests for Developmental Reading Disorder, the incidence and prevalence are unknown. Girls, as a general rule, have higher verbal than arithmetic skills (Vm), and boys the reverse (vM).

ETIOLOGY AND PATHOGENESIS

Not only are there no specific, definite causes known, but also just as in Developmental Reading Disorder, there is indeed a feeling of greater uncertainty and multiplicity of factors even among the hypotheses. Spatial ability, verbal ability, verbal abstracting ability, approach to problem solving and, perhaps most frequently, an almost indefinable "genetic predisposition," or lack of it, may contribute to mathematical abilities.

CLINICAL DESCRIPTION

CASE 25-8   By the time Zelda had reached the third grade, she had accumulated a *history* of *impulsivity, clumsiness,* and *right-left confusion* as a preschooler and great difficulties in *"getting" her numbers* in kindergarten and first grade. In second grade, she could *barely count.* Towards the end of second grade, she improved by the use of *rote memory,* but had *no understanding* of any *mathematical operations.* The concepts of *"plus"* or *"minus," "tens"* and *"ones,"* for instance, were meaningless to her. Zelda had *not* learned how to *tell time,* either. On the other hand, she *read* quite well for her age and *by and large* grasped *the meaning* of what she read, although often in a very *broad and superficial sense only.*

Comment. The preceding description is of a severe case of Developmental Arithmetic Disorder with a *total* deficit in math skills. Obviously, many milder forms exist more often.

DIFFERENTIAL DIAGNOSIS

Anxiety as a "block" to the learning of arithmetic may play a more significant role than in Developmental Reading Disorder, as do poor or inappropriate teaching methods. Therefore, Developmental Arithmetic Disorders are more difficult to tease apart in the diagnostic process, which is not usually done by the physician. The psychologist's evaluation is almost indispensable.

TREATMENT

This is highly specialized and beyond the reach of the primary care physician. The effect of this disorder on the child's overall functioning and self-esteem is less devastating than that of Developmental Reading Disorder. As in Developmental Reading Disorder, the physician's most important role is that of an advocate for the child's interests.

Developmental Coordination Disorder (315.40)

Following the lead of the ninth revision of the International Classification of Diseases, DSM-III-R now gives Coordination Disorder separate status, thus formalizing what practitioners and lay people have known for years, namely, that some children are immaturely clumsy and that this clumsiness need not always be associated with other developmental disorders, although it often is.

DEFINITION

Developmental Coordination Disorder is defined as a developmental level of motor coordination, in performing daily activities, that is notably *below* what one would expect considering the child's age and IQ. An incoordination problem may be manifested by marked deficits in achieving motor milestones, by dropping things or clumsiness, by poor performance in sports, or by poor handwriting. The coordination deficit is not due to a known physical disorder or a more severe developmental disorder such as Mental Retardation or Autism. Developmental Coordination Disorder is coded on Axis II of DSM-III-R, since it is regarded as a Specific Developmental Disorder.

ETIOLOGY AND PATHOGENESIS

Likely to be multifactorial, this disorder is assigned some putative causal factors that may not be specific for this disorder. Developmental decrement in perceptual-motor function may be genetically determined and relatively fixed. Organic contributing factors may be prenatal and perinatal complications, malnutrition during the early weeks or months, or toxic influences.

CLINICAL DESCRIPTION AND DIAGNOSIS

Diagnosis is based on the history and examination of the child. The history shows impairment and significant delays in motor skills. Milestones are definitely late, and the child has difficulties with such basic tasks as tying knots (shoelaces), buttoning clothing, putting puzzles together, building with blocks—especially the "Lego" type—and, in grade school, building models.

Since coordination difficulties include clumsiness and inability to participate gracefully in various games and sports, the presenting complaints, when the child is brought to a mental health specialist, may be social difficulties, especially with peers. The child may have developed feelings of frustration and low self-esteem, and manifest behavior problems, withdrawal, or depression.

The examination shows a child with gross and fine coordination problems as well as associated movements such as choreoathetoid movements of the fingers and mirror movements. These signs are picked up easily on the special neurological examination (examination for "soft" or nonfocal neurological signs), as described in Chapter 1. Specialized psychological tests, such as the Lincoln-Oseretsky Test of Motor Development, may also be used.

Since Developmental Coordination Disorder is a developmental *motor* disorder, it is not surprising that a speech articulation disorder is fairly frequently associated with it. In addition, it may occur in tandem with a Developmental Reading

Disorder and Attention–Deficit Hyperactivity Disorder; all of these associations help in the diagnosis and point to common pathogenetic mechanisms.

DIFFERENTIAL DIAGNOSIS

The first task in the differential diagnosis is to rule out organic medical and neurological disease. This is done by careful history and neurological examinations. The history will almost always show an onset at a definite time in the child's life, rather than being continuous from birth forward. The neurological examination will identify a child's muscle strength or weakness, persistent abnormal movements, atrophies or hypertrophies, and changes in sensory function; it can be supplemented by specific tests, such as electromyography, and medical tests (e.g., when rheumatic fever is suspected). Another group of disorders to be differentiated are the Stereotyped Movement Disorders, with which there may be overlap because of the Developmental Coordination Disorder's episodic choreoathetoid movements. However, stereotyped movement disorders and the movements of Habit Disorder occur spontaneously and, in the long run, arise uncontrollably from a resting state, whereas Developmental Coordination Disorder needs movement to show itself.

Similarly, Attention–Deficit Hyperactivity Disorder (ADHD) may have motor manifestations of excessive, sudden movements; the child may have overlapping Developmental Coordination Disorder as well. In this case, ADHD can be diagnosed in its own right as a second disorder. Pervasive Developmental Disorder and Childhood-Onset Schizophrenia may exhibit abnormal movements and posturing; these are more severe, and more patently abnormal, than what is seen in Developmental Coordination Disorder; in addition, the mental status examination will reveal specific abnormalities. Finally, Mental Retardation (MR) is accompanied by poor neuromuscular development reminiscent of Coordination Disorder. The diagnosis of MR is, of course, made on the basis of deficient global development, especially decrements of cognition and of adaptive functioning.

TREATMENT AND PROGNOSIS

Specialized perceptual-motor exercises are moderately effective in improving coordination. These and possibly general coordination training (modified active physical therapy) are the only specific treatments for this disorder.

Because of the secondary mental problems, psychotherapy and parent counseling may be indicated when the child is awkward and clumsy. Associated Attention–Deficit Hyperactivity Disorder, Developmental Speech Disorder or other Academic Skills Disorders will, of course, call for appropriate treatment and remediation. Thus, in most instances, treatment will be multimodal and interdisciplinary if it is to help.

Prognosis for Developmental Coordination Disorder per se is probably more favorable than for other Academic Skills Disorders. As the child grows older, some of the Developmental Coordination Disorder is attenuated by maturation; the main resolution, however, comes from focusing on other areas of success, especially academic and interpersonal skills. It is here that compassionate, focused psychotherapy can play a significant part.

Questions for Study and Action

1. A 10-year-old white boy who could not read told the child psychiatrist, tearfully, "If you can't read, you ain't shit." What measures could be taken to enhance his self-esteem and to improve his reading? Outline your (a) diagnostic workup, (b) treatment plan.

2. Discuss the differential diagnosis of a child's Spelling Disorder, showing how to rule in and rule out the various disorders that you want to differentiate from Spelling Disorder.

3. Trace the various normal neurological pathways needed for a child to write normally in his mother tongue, i.e., *not* to have an Expressive Writing Disorder. Include specifically the interacting hand-eye-mouth-larynx-and-brain in your discussion.

4. For a Developmental Arithmetic Disorder in a 10-year-old girl show how sex-role stereotyping made a contribution to its genesis.

5. How would children's games such as hopscotch, horseshoes, ringtoss, and Tiddly-winks be of help for a child with Developmental Coordination Disorder? What would the risks or hazards be?

For Further Reading

Aiken, L.R. Language factors in learning mathematics. *Rev. Educ. Res.*, 42:359, 1972.

Arnheim, D.D., & Sinclair, W.A. *The Clumsy Child.* St. Louis: C.V. Mosby, 1975.

Benton, A., & Pearl, D. *Dyslexia: An Appraisal of Current Knowledge.* New York: Oxford University Press, 1978.

Doehring, D., Trites, R., Patel, P., & Fiedorowicz, C. *Reading Disabilities.* New York: Academic Press, 1981.

Eisenson, J., & Ogilvie, M. *Communicative Disorders in Children.* New York: Macmillan, 1983.

Fritch, V. The similarities and differences between reading and spelling problems. In M. Rutter (Ed.), *Developmental Neuropsychiatry.* New York: Guilford Press, 1983.

Gray, W.S. *Gray Standardized Oral Reading Paragraphs.* Indianapolis: Bobbs-Merrill, 1955.

Jansky, J.J. Developmental Reading Disorder (Alexia and Dyslexia). In H.I. Kaplan & B.J. Sadock (Eds.), *Comprehensive Textbook of Psychiatry (4th Ed.).* Baltimore: Williams & Wilkins, 1985.

Johnson, D., & Myklebust, H. *Learning Disabilities: Educational Principles and Practices.* New York: Grune & Stratton, 1967.

Levinson, H.N. *A Solution to the Riddle Dyslexia.* New York: Springer-Verlag, 1980.

Margalit, M., & Heiman, T. Family climate and anxiety in families with learning disabled boys. *J. Amer. Acad. of Child Psychiatry,* 25:841–846, 1986.

Slade, P.D., & Russell, G.F. Developmental dyscalculia: A brief report on four cases. *Psychol. Med.,* I:292, 1971.

26

Mental Retardation

I n this chapter we will present a focused view of the psychiatric aspects of
mental retardation. As a consequence of this approach, no attempt will be
made to furnish a comprehensive dissertation on the various known disorders
causing Mental Retardation, nor will we go into detail about the special education and care of the mentally retarded. Therefore, this chapter could be called
"some psychiatric aspects of mentally retarded children." In DSM-III-R Mental
Retardation is listed with Developmental Disorders, all of which are recorded on
Axis II.

DEFINITION

In few other areas of child psychiatry is definition as important as in Mental
Retardation. The reason for emphasizing the correct definition is that a large
portion of the public and, unfortunately, a certain number of health professionals,
too, have erroneously equated mental retardation with low IQ.

Mental Retardation is defined similarly by DSM-III-R and the American
Association on Mental Deficiency (AAMD): the child has to function on a
retarded level both intellectually *and* in terms of adaptive behavior. Therefore,

the definition comprises two parts: significantly subaverage general intellectual functioning *and* concurrent impairment in adaptive behavior (Szymanski & Crocker, 1985).

"Significantly subaverage intellectual functioning" refers to an intelligence quotient (ratio of mental age to chronological age), or IQ, of 70 or below on an individually administered IQ test (IQ = Mental Age/Chronological Age × 100).

"Adaptive behavior" is the effectiveness with which an individual meets the standards of personal independence and social responsibility expected of his/her age and cultural group. The importance of this definition is that it is based on two parameters: intelligence *and* adaptive behavior. This means that, within reasonable limits, relatively good social and emotional adaptation can make up for lower intelligence. The student should note the word "*relatively* good"; some impairment of adaptation is expected in all instances in order to diagnose mental retardation. Axis V should specify the highest level of adaptive functioning in the past year and, if it is good relative to IQ, that could erase or qualify a diagnosis of Mental Retardation. DSM-III-R explicitly states that good adaptive functioning may be present in individuals whose IQ is near but below 70, and thus these individuals do not really meet the criteria for mental retardation. Although DSM-III-R consigns it only to a V-code, there is a Borderline Intellectual Functioning category in general, informal use, with an IQ of 70–85 or even higher.

This "gray area" underscores the fact that mental retardation is a syndrome which is defined by behavior. Otherwise it would only represent the natural variation (distribution curve) of the development of the central nervous system, starting with two standard deviations below the mean. As we shall see presently, not only do mentally retarded children have behavioral symptoms because they have expectable difficulties adapting, but also these difficulties are often augmented by mental illness.

When dealing with agencies and special educators, the student will encounter subdivisions and technical terms which need defining:

Mild Mental Retardation (= educable: IQ levels 50–70) (317.00)

Fortunately, some 80% of mentally retarded children fall into this mild group. These are the slow learners, but most of them, as a group, can master the basic communicative skills for near-independence in our society, i.e., a grade-school vocabulary, and ability to read and write to the extent that they can read signs, labels, and simple directions. Arithmetic is learned to the extent that they can go shopping and perform measurements. They often play with children of average intelligence.

Moderate Mental Retardation (= trainable: IQ 35-49) (318.00)

They learn to take care of all their physical needs, to communicate simply, and to follow simple instructions. They are behind their average peers in the understanding and assimilation of social conventions and therefore rarely play with them consistently.

Severe Mental Retardation (IQ 20-34) (318.10)

As preschoolers, these children are limited in motor as well as communicative skills. They learn to talk in later childhood, but have a very limited vocabulary. They need constant supervision.

Profound Mental Retardation (IQ below 20) (318.20)

These children are so limited in their development that they require not only constant supervision, but constant care and attendance if their survival is to be sustained.

As a general rule, since the communicative, social, and motor skills decline with declining IQ measurements, the gross neurological abnormalities will increase. In severe and profound mental retardation, there is a high incidence of severe neurological disease, especially seizures, and defects in vision or hearing.

ETIOLOGY AND PATHOGENESIS

The foregoing educational and pragmatic subdivisions are useful in discussing the various etiologies of mental retardation.

The mildly retarded group has the least circumscribed etiology. In other words, this is the group for whom the concept of variation of the normal distribution curve of intelligence applies. Genetic factors are often in evidence, and the term "familial" is often used to refer to this etiology. In addition, environmental conditions (sociocultural deprivation, economic and physical suffering, lack of stimulation, etc.) play an equivalent part in the etiology of mild mental retardation so that separation of sociocultural and familial etiologies is extremely difficult.

Moderate mental retardation may also be familial, or may be caused by some of the definable etiologies: internal (e.g., metabolic disease, chromosomal abnormalities) or external (e.g., injury to the central nervous system, trauma, infection).

As we proceed to *severe* and *profound* mental retardation, definable and gross central nervous system abnormalities are the rule, summarized as follows. External or extrinsic causes are represented by congenital cytomegalic inclusion body disease, congenital rubella, congenital syphilis, toxoplasmosis, and various traumata. Intrinsic or endogenous causes include such disorders of metabolism as the histiocytoses, the lipoidoses, phenylketonuria (PKU), hepatolenticular degeneration, porphyria, or galactosemia. Another set of endogenous factors are the malformations (e.g., microcephaly, macroencephaly, porencephaly, craniostenosis) and the various chromosomal (e.g., Down's syndrome) anomalies seen in inherited or congenital diseases.

The student is referred to standard textbooks of pediatrics and psychiatry for the descriptions of these many syndromes.

CLINICAL DESCRIPTION AND DIAGNOSIS

The clinical health professional makes the presumptive diagnosis of Mental Retardation, but only the psychologist–psychometrist can establish the definitive diagnosis by means of standardized tests of intelligence.

The clinical picture with which the health professional is going to be confronted, for purposes of making a diagnosis, will depend on the severity of the Mental Retardation.

Mild Mental Retardation

The most difficult to diagnose are children with Mild Mental Retardation, since there are no specific signs or symptoms. The preschool child shows delays in developmental landmarks, for instance, speaking in sentences or taking care of him/herself. Many mildly retarded children, however, are not diagnosed as such until they are in school; that is where their adaptive functions start to fall short. They cannot meet academic demands, and further problems, including psychiatric difficulties, may ensue.

CASE 26-1   Orville was seven-and-a-half years old when seen by the child psychiatrist. The reason for referral was that he could *not get along in school,* neither with peers nor teachers. His parents had entered him one year late in kindergarten because of his *"immaturity."* Nevertheless, he had had a rough year of it, and *first grade,* where he was now, was *even worse.* Orville was *inattentive, restless,* and *easily provoked.* He seemed especially set on resisting the teacher's requirements for *academic work;* he either pretended *not to hear the teacher's instructions* or else "raised a ruckus" while she was giving assignments. At home, by contrast, he was reasonably well behaved; he was a very *active* child but willing to do the *simple chores* that his parents required of him.

Examination showed a boy who became *defensive* when the doctor discussed school with him; the defensiveness turned out to be a reaction to cover up feelings of *inadequacy* and *low self-esteem*. He wished he did not have to go to school and do all those assignments.

Orville also showed a tendency to be quite literal and *concrete* in his thinking and simple in vocabulary, not imaginative; he also showed several neurological *"soft signs."*

On careful questioning, the parents reported that, compared to his older brother, Orville's developmental landmarks were *slightly slower:* he walked at 13 months, talked in sentences at "2+ years," and was generally clumsy and uncoordinated (he could not tie his shoes until recently).

He was referred for psychometric testing and obtained a full-scale IQ of 62 on the WISC-R, without much variation among the performance and verbal subtests.

Comment. Mild mental retardation was not noticed until the demands made by school resulted in Orville's behavioral difficulties. This is sometimes referred to as the "six-hour syndrome" (the time that the child spends in school).

Moderate Mental Retardation

Unlike the previous group, children with Moderate Mental Retardation usually are detected *before* they start school. Their developmental landmarks are definitely delayed, and they are late in taking care of their bodily needs.

CASE 26-2   Ryan was seven years old when he was seen by the psychiatrist for severe *temper tantrums* when *demands* were made on him to do simple tasks *involving self-sufficiency in personal hygiene* and *simple chores.*

He was described as *hyperactive* ("getting into everything, pulling things off dressers, accident-prone"). In addition, he had developed *separation anxiety* in regard to both parents, especially mother. Ryan had already been diagnosed as suffering from the "fragile X syndrome," and his full-scale IQ was tested at 42 on the WISC-R. His Vineland Social Maturity score (mother as informant) was just under a mental age of four years.

Examination showed a boy of short stature and disproportionately large head, including large ears. It took a great deal of patience to deal with him, as he appeared to be in *constant motion.* He showed difficulties *buttoning and unbuttoning his winter coat,* as well as other difficulties suggestive of *dyspraxia.* Whenever he had trouble performing a task, he became quickly frustrated, stamped his feet, and insisted that the examiner or the parents *help* him immediately. Because of *separation anxiety,* he was seen together with his parents, and it was obvious that he was quite *dependent* on them.

His vocabulary was *limited* to simple words and phrases and he tended to be *clumsy* and careless with the toys. In general, he was *not self-sufficient* in play, but looked to those around him to amuse him and direct his activities.

Comment. There was no difficulty diagnosing this boy as mentally retarded; indeed this had been done prior to his entry into school, since the delay in attaining motor landmarks had been perceptible.

His psychiatric difficulties were typical of Attention–Deficit Hyperactivity Disorder as well as Anxiety Disorder (Separation Anxiety Disorder); the former responded to the standard treatment with stimulant medication. The Anxiety Disorder appeared to have grown out of the child's dependency as well as the parents' overprotective attitudes towards him. Their overprotection was partly a result of considerable ambivalence about having a mentally retarded child.

Severe and profound mental retardation

These usually present no diagnostic difficulty in the preschool child: the diagnosis is made by both history and evidence of delayed developmental landmarks. Severely delayed or never-reached ability of the child to take age-appropriate care of himself or herself will be apparent. Since most of these children show physical signs depending on the specific etiology, physical examination is useful in deriving the diagnosis. Again, the reader is referred to standard textbooks of pediatrics for appropriate study of these rarer forms of Mental Retardation.

ETIOLOGY, PATHOGENESIS, AND CLINICAL CHARACTERISTICS OF MENTAL DISORDERS IN THE MENTALLY RETARDED

The foregoing case examples will introduce the reader to the fact that mental illness in the retarded child is no different from mental disorders in the child with normal intelligence. In DSM-III-R all mental disorders attending Mental Retardation would be listed on Axis I, with the Mental Retardation itself recorded on Axis II.

As a group, mentally retarded children have a higher incidence of psychiatric pathology. There are two schools of thought concerning the etiology and pathogenesis of psychopathology in the mentally retarded: on the one hand, the "organicists" contend that most, if not all, of the psychiatric symptomatology arises from the same substrate as the Mental Retardation itself.

The other line of reasoning is that psychopathology arises through the same processes as in a person of normal intelligence. Special consideration is given to such interactional factors as the greater dependence and differentness of the retarded person, and such constitutional–temperamental factors as individual basic adaptability, or lack thereof, or overreactivity. This second school of thought probably represents the majority view.

Any description of psychiatric illness in the mentally retarded child really consists of two sets of psychopathology: that of the parents and that of the child.

Parental psychopathology

This may not be immediately discernible since normally intelligent parents of mentally retarded children have sectors of their lives in which they function without direct reference to these children. However, in their relationships with the mentally retarded children, they are often suffering from anger towards the child, compensated for by overprotectiveness, guilt for having brought a defective child into the world, low self-esteem for the same reason, and compensatory mechanisms to deal with those feelings. It is these compensatory mechanisms that precipitate many of the behavioral difficulties in the retarded children.

When looking at parental psychological defense mechanisms what we encounter first is *denial:* the parents claim that their child simply is not retarded ("Look at all the things he/she can do!"). After the initial shock and disbelief, there may be a period of mourning and depression, because of the loss of the hoped-for normal child. This is frequently associated with projection of blame: first, the diagnosis is doubted (the school psychologist "did not know what he was doing"); then, the cause may be attributed to somebody else's wrongdoing ("the obstetrician was late"). The final stage should be one of realistic acceptance of, and adaptation to, the child's limitations, and the seeking out and support of the child's strengths.

The psychopathology of the child

As we have already stated, mentally retarded children will have the same spectrum of psychopathology as their average counterparts. Thus we encounter psychotic disorders with or without demonstrable thought disturbances and severe Depression, as well as Organic Brain Syndromes, at one end of the spectrum of severity, and Conduct Disorder, Attention–Deficit Hyperactivity Disorder, Anxiety Disorders, and so forth towards the less severe end.

In our experience, the most frequent psychiatric disorder among mentally retarded children is *Attention–Deficit Hyperactivity Disorder* (ADHD). In many of these children, the physical cause of their mental retardation is probably the cause of the ADHD as well. In other children, environmental factors, such as parental permissiveness as a compensatory mechanism for their own difficulties, may be the major causative factor. ADHD in the mentally retarded child can be diagnosed easily by history and observation; ADHD responds well to pharmacotherapy with stimulants and the setting up of a more structured environment.

Affective Disorder, chiefly Depression, is also frequent among mildly and moderately retarded children. They perceive their lack of ability to hold their own against average children. Their self-esteem is low because the average standards are too high for them to reach. Without appropriate support, they feel helpless and hopeless.

Diagnosis of Depression in the mentally retarded child may be difficult because mentally retarded children have less vocabulary at their disposal; this is especially true of putting feelings into words. Therefore the clinician will have to observe very carefully and infer Depression from nonverbal clues and general attitudes. Treatment is similar to that of other Depression in childhood, with the provision that the therapist work closely with special educational services and agencies that provide opportunities for the mentally retarded to develop skills and mastery that will enhance their self-esteem.

The entire range of Adjustment Disorders can also be seen in this group, especially in the mildly and moderately retarded.

Stereotyped Movement and Habit Disorders are seen mostly in severely and profoundly retarded children. These rocking, head banging, hand flapping, and repetitively self-stimulating activities are more in evidence when the environment is barren and insufficiently stimulating, i.e., when these children are left alone without minimal attention and supervision. Sometimes the self-stimulating activities extend to self-mutilation. These movement disorders and self-mutilating behaviors are a direct result of the brain damage underlying the Severe or Profound Mental Retardation. Related to these habit disorders is Pica, which in this context may be viewed as another primitive habit and self-stimulating disorder.

A special issue is Infantile Autism (Pervasive Developmental Disorder—Autism). Almost 70–80% of autistic children are in the mentally retarded range when tested for intelligence. The two conditions therefore overlap to an extensive degree, with Infantile Autism contributing more to Mental Retardation than vice versa. However, there are several organic disorders which produce both Mental Retardation and Autism: the highest incidence of Autism is found in congenital rubella; other organic disorders causing Autism in a limited number of children are phenylketonuria, tuberous sclerosis, congenital syphilis, and congenital hydrocephalus. The differential diagnosis of Mental Retardation and Infantile Autism will be discussed below.

Finally, pathological personality traits develop in a large number of mentally retarded children, especially traits of dependency in excess of their actual helplessness.

DIFFERENTIAL DIAGNOSIS

The longer mental retardation has lasted, i.e., the older the child, the clearer the diagnostic picture becomes—and vice versa. Thus, differential diagnosis is most difficult, yet most crucial in the early stages, as correct diagnosis of treatable disorders makes a lifelong difference.

The most important category to be differentiated, then, is obviously the group of organic disorders that produce delayed developmental landmarks and, ultimately, mental retardation if not diagnosed and treated. These are metabolic disorders, such as phenylketonuria or hypothyroidism, cerebral malformations or neoplasms resulting in hydrocephalus, and sensory deficits such as blindness and especially deafness. Diagnosis depends on a high index of clinical suspicion and medical knowledge.

Another set of disorders mimicking Mental Retardation at first, and then actually developing into Mental Retardation, are the deprivation syndromes: reactive attachment disorders of infancy and early childhood, hospitalism, or anaclitic depression.

Finally, mental retardation has to be distinguished from the other Developmental Disorders. If Developmental Language Disorder, either expressive or receptive, is so severe that the child is aphasic, differentiation from Mental Retardation may be difficult. Likewise, severe Developmental Reading Disorder may cause the child to be suspected of mental retardation. In rare instances, the reverse situation may obtain: one developmental *ability* is unusually developed, whereas all the others are retarded; this is the "idiot savant."

The most severe developmental disorder—Pervasive Developmental Disorder, Infantile Autism—has, as already mentioned, a large area of overlap with Mental Retardation. The differentiating characteristics for Infantile Autism are the uneven developmental landmarks (they are mostly delayed, but unevenly so) and the lack of emotional relatedness to the caretakers. The mentally retarded child, by contrast, is evenly retarded in development and, within his or her capabilities, relates emotionally in ways appropriate to the environment.

One last general caveat: appearances are deceiving and this works both ways, for better or for worse. A child with cerebral palsy or hydrocephalus may look retarded but may be of normal or even bright-normal intelligence. By contrast, many mildly or moderately mentally retarded children have no physical characteristics whatsoever to distinguish them from their peers with average intelligence.

TREATMENT AND PROGNOSIS

If it is true that mental disorders arise in retarded children for the correspondingly equivalent and similar reasons as in children with average intelligence, then it follows that treatment is similar, too. This is indeed so, with the understanding that psychotherapy has to be simplified to address the cognitive level (i.e., mental age) of the child. In other words, the therapist should not go by the chronological age or size or appearance of the child.

Psychotherapy is appropriate for the mentally retarded child, as is pharmacotherapy. Most of the indications for both modalities are the same as for children with average intelligence.

Prognosis does not depend solely on intelligence. Adaptability, flexibility, and pleasant personality positively influence prognosis. A case in point is Down's syndrome: experience with children with this syndrome has indeed confirmed the traditional view that they are more gentle and less aggressive than average, and they have, as a group, done very well in both personal achievements and public acceptance. This has certainly been helped in no small measure by the concerted efforts of their loyal parents, another example of what can be achieved by successful and creative resolution of defensiveness in the parents.

Finally, we come to the important question of whether to treat the mentally retarded child at home or in a specialized school, i.e., institution. The trend now is to keep and treat as many mentally retarded children as possible in their homes, since the level of emotional and cognitive stimulation and enrichment is usually higher within the family than in any specialized institution. However, there are indications for institutionalization: Profound Mental Retardation overtaxing the emotional and practical capabilities of the family; intolerable aggressiveness, especially associated with definite signs of brain pathology unresponsive to outpatient treatment; and inappropriate expression of sexuality unresponsive to intervention. Certainly, in many instances, the deciding factor will be parental abilities. In severe cases, parental ability may be realistically inadequate to keep the child at home, yet unresolved guilt in the parents prevents referral to a residential center. These and similar situations call for our counseling with the parents, which is an *indispensable* ingredient in all treatment of the mentally retarded child.

Questions for Study and Action

1. You may have heard the statement "Once mentally retarded, always mentally retarded." How do you feel about it? If you do not agree with it, give examples to disprove it.

2. What is meant by "mainstreaming"? Which group among the mentally retarded has done especially well with this approach? Is the term used only with the mentally retarded?

3. One of the stereotypes about mentally retarded children is that they are impulsive, potentially dangerous, and that "normal" children should not be allowed to play with them. Discuss your views about this fallacy.

4. One of the rationalizations for institutionalizing mentally retarded children is that the mentally retarded are happiest among their own kind. Discuss the fallacy of

this view and ways to counteract it. What resources are available in your community to help its mentally retarded children?

5. The staff physician at a residential school for the mentally retarded has prescribed a neuroleptic for a severely retarded and behaviorally difficult child. The parents have questions about their child's being all "doped up." Discuss the pros and cons of pharmacotherapy in this case.

6. A child psychiatrist proposes to prescribe a stimulant for a mildly retarded, hyperactive child. The parents question the rationale for this approach: "Will it help our child to learn or is this done solely for the convenience of the teachers, so that they do not have to work so hard with him?" How would you work with the parents on this matter?

7. A parents' group would like to discuss the issue of behavior modification at the residential treatment center. Some parents feel this "robotizes" their children. What do you think? Have you ever dealt with a parent group like this? How would you approach them?

8. What is meant by *Propfschizophrenia*? How would it be treated?

9. Why is mild sociocultural Mental Retardation, said to be the most frequent type in the U.S., not found in Norway? Explain.

10. Why is the incidence of Mental Retardation among American children said to be from 3%-5% and, among American adults, to be 1%. Give three reasons for this shift in prevalence in the two populations.

For Further Reading

Featherstone, H. *A Difference in the Family: Life with a Disabled Child.* New York: Basic Books, 1980.

Hulse, J.A., et al. Growth, development and reassessment of hypothyroid infants diagnosed by screening. *Brit. Med. J.,* 284:1435-1437, 1982.

Menolascino, F.J. (Ed.). *Psychiatric Approaches to Mental Retardation.* New York: Basic Books, 1970.

Szymanski, L.S., & Crocker, A.C. Mental retardation. In H.I. Kaplan & B.J. Sadock (Eds.), *Comprehensive Textbook of Psychiatry* (4th Ed.). Baltimore: Williams & Wilkins, 1985, pp. 1635-1671.

Szymanski, L.S., & Tanguay, P.E. (Eds.). *Emotional Disorders of Mentally Retarded Persons.* Baltimore: University Park Press, 1980.

SECTION D

BEING VICTIMIZED

Forensic child psychiatry, aided by its link to the biobehavioral sciences, brings to the legal profession a large body of meaningful theory and research findings that are translated into practical, legally relevant applications. "Forensic" originally referred to a forum or a public discussion but now denotes the ways in which scientific work done in other fields can be applied primarily to criminal law but secondarily to civil law as well. Hence, lawyers may call upon pathologists, psychiatrists, toxicologists, and other physicians to bring their forensic expertise to bear in disputes before judges. Operating where two professions meet, the forensic child psychiatrist is called upon to be sufficiently knowing of the law to "translate" child psychiatry into legal terms and thereby be of service to the legal profession.

Forensic child psychiatry may be involved whenever children commit crimes (psychiatric criminology), or are victimized by the crimes of others (psychiatric victimology), or are involved in civil suits. Forensic child psychiatry attempts to understand and explain both *the child*—as participant, criminal, or victim—*and the situation* in which the legal transgressions occurred. The goal is not to blame but to account for behavior. The most frequent activities of forensic child psychiatrists pertain to child custody disputes, divorcing parents, delinquent behavior, emancipation of minors, terminating parental rights, competency determinations, automobile-accident injuries, and involuntary commitments to mental hospitals. Forensic child psychiatrists also are concerned with a number of rights of children, encompassing their rights to special protection (from abuse or neglect), special services (e.g., the right to education or treatment), and rights to greater freedom of action as they grow older and more competent.

This Section focuses mainly on child psychiatric victimology—particularly on children's neglect and abuse by their parents or parent surrogates. Forensic child psychiatry affords the practitioner an opportunity to speak out as a scientific healer and citizen advocate on behalf of children's needs, capabilities, interests, and rights, helping the court to understand the child's behavior. The student of victimology soon realizes that children are an almost universally oppressed group, not only in families but also in schools, courts, mental hospitals, welfare agencies, group homes, correctional facilities, and medical and psychiatric clinics. Hence, it has been said that children need protection against their protectors who are often the *perpetrators* of child abuse and neglect. In particular, parents can become effective advocates *against* the nonfamily professional child caretakers.

At the end of this Section there is a chapter on the role of the child psychiatrist in the courtroom.

27

Neglect

Children rely on their parents both for the refinements of respectful, loving care and for survival itself. Some parents, often because of their own unmet needs for nurturance and support, come to parenthood unready to meet their children's wants, wishes, and needs. As a result, these parents envision their parenthood as an ordeal, a drain, and may never capture the slightest notion that parenthood is a time of life for joyful fulfillment, for being reliable or dependable. Children by nature are dependent on adults and benefit greatly when they have dependable parents as caretakers; if they are fortunate, the odds increase that the children will grow to live out lives of satisfaction in expanding networks of relatedness and, when in their turn they become parents, they will *be* parents and dependable. Many young parents realize that growing autonomy does not have to lead to loneliness and self-absorption but growing up does produce amortization of infantile dependency through achieving adult dependability. But healthy human beings are always related to and loving others.

DEFINITION

Child neglect is a sign of caretaker failure. In religious terms, child neglect consists of "sins of omission" and the root Latin work *neglegere* means "not to pick

433

up." Neglect always occurs (according to common morality) when adequate or appropriate care and attention are not given to someone who has proper claim on that care and attention: a child, an invalid, a friend, or a neighbor. Neglect is a psychosocial stressor (Axis IV) contributing or leading to diagnoses on Axes I, II, and III of DSM-III-R.

ETIOLOGY AND PATHOPHYSIOLOGY

Numerous conditions have been adduced to explain child neglect by caretakers. Some examples are: failure in infantile attachment or bonding, unwanted pregnancy, depression or other mental disorder in the caretaker, conflicts between parents and focus on their marital interaction, ignorance of parenting skills, parental reactions to child's handicap or unusual temperament, infanticidal impulses. Clearly, parents who neglect children have themselves been neglected— by parents in early childhood and by a larger community when they grew older.

Neglect becomes manifest in varied clinical syndromes of children (marasmus, anaclitic depression, failure to thrive, Psychosocial Dwarfism, Depression, Conduct Disorders, Attention–Deficit Hyperactivity Disorder, Learning Disorders, Anxiety Disorders, and others) through mechanisms that are known to be complex at times but poorly explicated at present.

The diagnostic workup with neglected children consists of the following: a sensitive physical examination to ferret out anomalies and deficits; astute observation of the child's behavior in the clinic, at home, and at school; comprehensive laboratory studies to rule out anemia, parasitic infestation, infections, or liver, kidney, or lung malfunctioning; obtaining a full social and family history; and utilizing appropriate consultants. The latter include a clinical psychologist almost certainly (intellectual level and potential, child's self-concept, child's view of her or his place in the family, special strengths or gifts, typical coping or defending strategies) and, as warranted, opthalmological, audiological, neurological, genetic, or endocrinological consultation.

CLINICAL DESCRIPTION

As an antichild (or not pro-child) phenomenon, neglect bears affinity with all forms of child abuse and with child murder. It may be the prodrome or *forme fruste* of abuse or murder for some young parents. Neglect, especially with an infant, can be life-threatening.

CASE 27-1   Ulrich was an accident-prone four-year-old who obtained medical care through the emergency room of a charity hospital run by a medical school. He was Caucasian, *born out of wedlock,* and the eldest of three children who lived with their *mother only.* Although deserted by Ulrich's father during her first pregnancy at age 18 years, Ulrich's mother declined to pledge the unborn child to be adopted near the time of birth. In fact, she roomed in with the baby and breastfed him. She refused to apply for welfare because she wanted to be "independent" and retain her self-respect. She became a live-in maid and was able to look after Ulrich during his infancy while she performed domestic chores for her employers.

Ulrich *thrived* until his *next sib* was born out of wedlock and the *mother lost* her job as a domestic servant. She wanted to marry the second baby's father, whom she had met at a bar on one of her nights off. But he disclosed that he was married already and would not rearrange his life to marry her. She lived briefly with her own mother (and *her* boyfriend, 12 years junior to Ulrich's maternal grandmother) before she began to receive welfare payments from Aid to Families with Dependent Children (AFDC), food stamps, and a subsidized rental apartment in a seedy housing project. At this point, Ulrich's mother began to feel *hopeless, overburdened* by the added demands of Ulrich and the new baby, *bereft of adult companionship,* and *oppressed by her overload* of child care, homemaking, and duties. She felt that she had to get out of the mess, and a vocational rehabilitation agency backed her in obtaining a beautician's training. While at the Beauty College she *left her two children with a neighbor* who had two children of her own to care for and charged very little to baby-sit. She formed a friendship with a self-proclaimed "gay" fellow student, but he turned out to be bisexual; he, too, declined marriage but she became pregnant again, delivering the third baby when Ulrich was three-and-a-half years old.

Ulrich had been hit by a car when crossing the street *en route* to a neighborhood convenience store to buy potato chips for his mother. Brought to the Emergency Room, he was found to be unscathed except for a large bruise on his left thigh and abrasions on his right elbow and hand. *Numerous healed scars* were evident; he was observed to be wiry but muscular and his medical chart had recorded on it *over 40 earlier visits for accidents,* cut, poisons, and *20 bouts of otitis media.* His navel, axillary, and pudendal skin folds were *grimy* and his clothes were *filthy.* He was *unkempt* and had "the appearance of a street urchin," according to the pediatric note. He gazed attentively at the TV in the waiting room, while his mother talked to his doctor.

Comment. Ulrich's case illustrates many features of neglect and high risk for pathology in children who are neglected: threats to the mother-only family's economic survival; the relative isolation of the impoverished family from medical care or other community's resources; the mother's early pregnancy; her determined but unsuccessful efforts to be independent and a reliable provider; her lack of contraception and family planning; her vulnerability to sexual exploitation and abandonment by men; her disadvantages in the labor market; her "creeping neglect" of the children; her tendency towards role reversal in sending her son to fetch snacks from a convenience mart; her overwhelming loneliness, deprivation, and overload of work and responsibility; Ulrich's receipt of inept childcare; his "accident proneness," untidiness, frequent bouts of otitis, and musculoskeletal precocity and agility. Please note that the mother-infant bonding during Ulrich's infancy had been better than with either of the two other offspring. In a sense, Ulrich got a headstart over both of his sibs; by comparison to them he will be, and will seem to be, lucky—relatively advantaged.

DIFFERENTIAL DIAGNOSIS

To be differentiated in cases of obvious neglect are mildly mentally retarded children, who may be as depleted and vacuous in demeanor as some neglected children; conduct-disordered children, who may be as action-oriented, taut, and vigilant; children with Attention–Deficit Hyperactivity Disorder, who may appear equally tense and distractible as are some neglected children; and depressed children, who may also appear gloomy and needy. Neglect may coexist with any other childhood disorder, in fact, and parceling out neglect from the other concurrent conditions may be the physician's task, not merely ruling out other conditions. Abuse (physical, mental, or sexual) may also be present when neglect occurs; both abuse and neglect must be reported to child protective services by the physician who is a child's advocate.

TREATMENT

A comprehensive plan of treatment must include:

1. The child's well-being
    - reporting neglect to child protective services
    - crisis care (e.g., by providing homemaker services to the family, giving parents respite from child care)
    - individual psychotherapy if the damages and traumata have been internalized
    - treatment of coexistent disorders, related or unrelated to neglect
    - appropriate academic placement and progression
2. Helping parent(s) to succeed in parenting
    - effectiveness training/group therapy focused on child care
    - family casework and counseling
3. Helping the family group
    - family group therapy/casework
    - assistance in obtaining services from health, welfare, and educational agencies

- budgeting, meal planning, marketing advice, and assistance
- encouraging family participation in neighborhood and community activities

PROGNOSIS

Neglected children do not have happy outcomes as a group. They are at risk of succumbing to an array of social, medical, and psychical pathology. Many grow up to be only mercenary and ungenerous, self-seeking, criminally deviant, untrusting, and suspicious. They are particularly vulnerable to failure in parenting when they bear children; their own parenting will be rife with distortions such as splitting, role reversal, projective identification, narcissistic identification, and identification with aggressors; they are likely to be abusive and neglectful parents.

Questions for Study and Action

1. Can you find out from child welfare or child protective services how many children were reported to be neglected last year in your city or county? Did you call them or write them for these statistics? Which is more effective, generally, when a physician is dealing with agents of public bureaucracies?

2. Assuming that Ulrich would show an Attention–Deficit Hyperactivity Disorder by the time he reached first grade, how would you evaluate his concentrated watching of TV in the Emergency waiting room at the time he was hit by a car? Why is TV called "the great American babysitter"?

3. List five indices of neglect in Ulrich's case.

4. List five markers of Ulrich's mother's being neglected by her community's helping agencies.

5. Why was Ulrich actually advantaged by comparison with his two younger sibs? Explain, showing how dependency in his earlier years may be transformed gracefully into dependability when he becomes a parent.

6. What kind of treatment plan would you devise to aid Ulrich's healthy growth in future? Be very specific in your planned items for Ulrich, those primarily for his mother, and those for the entire mother-only family.

7. What plausible hypotheses can you formulate to cover this situation? In many communities, reported cases of child neglect were outnumbered during the 1980s by reported cases of sexual abuse.

8. How might it devolve that radical feminist groups energetically oppose child pornography but remain rather silent about child neglect? Be detailed and sensible.

9. What sorts of medical facilities might be preferable to a charity-university hospital's Emergency Room for Ulrich's family? Sketch out the ideal health/welfare/education agency to serve him and his family best.

10. Can you advise an impoverished mother about budgeting/shopping/nutrition for a family of one adult and three children? Find out about welfare payments, public housing, available markets, and the essentials of good nutritional foodstuffs for two poor families known to you professionally.

For Further Reading

Katz, S.N. *When Parents Fail: The Law's Response to Family Breakdown.* Boston: Beacon, 1971.

Oates, K. *Child Abuse and Neglect: What Happens Eventually?* New York: Brunner/Mazel, 1986.

28

Sexual Abuse

Sexual abuse of children is not a child mental disorder per se, but the consequences of being sexually abused may result in a mental disorder for a child. Particularly when there are abrupt personality changes—for example, in the preschool child who suddenly becomes hypersexual or sexually aggressive or who shows a gross panic disorder, or the school-aged child who quickly becomes isolated or withdrawn from peers, or the adolescent female who runs away from home or becomes wildly promiscuous—all these may be disorders that arise to give evidence of sexual victimization. In such cases, sexual abuse may be seen as the precipitant of true disorders, a trauma that triggered the mental disorder of the child. The difficulty is that parents and physicians, much less teachers, do not think to ask children simply if someone has touched them in the area covered by a swimsuit or done anything sexually abusive. Whenever otherwise inexplicable aberrant behavior occurs, *the first big diagnostic accomplishment is to inquire whether sexual molestation has taken place.* If we do not ask, we cannot say, "The history is negative for sex abuse."

DEFINITION OF SEXUAL ABUSE AND CHILDREN'S RIGHTS

Definitions of sexual abuse of children vary with the times. The sexual abuse of children has become an issue whenever and wherever children have been

439

accorded a semblance of rights to protection from adults' rape, sodomization, genital fondling, rubbing (frottage), and being seduced into performing orogenital, anogenital, genitogenital, or manual-genital or other sexual acts with adults. Sexual abuse of children is unthinkable (or not "conceptualizable") in eras and places that disallow children a separate existence, or do not concede that children's mental and bodily integrity is their right; it becomes an issue only when there is a set of values that gives meaning and importance to children's rights to "proper" care, consideration, and autonomy. If a father has ownership and control of children, there cannot be abuse, regardless of what the father did, since the father has all the rights and the child has no rights. Thus it is that abuse reflects at least a minimal societal consensus about rights of children.

The rights of children fall into two groups: rights to *liberties* and rights to *protection*. At times, children have had relatively greater claim to protection than to freedom of choice, but one set of rights does not have to be at odds with the other. For example, some legal scholars contend that children have a right to sexual enlightenment and freedom with their agemates at the very same time that they have a right to be protected against adult sexual abuse ("molestation"). One right releases the child from control, while the other protects the child as a minor who is not equal to any adult. Perhaps another way to state the point is: While rights to freedom stress the child's full humanity, rights to protection emphasize the child's dependency or "minority" status—although the child will be expected to grow up and not require forever his or her special services and supplies that must derive from others. Rights to a guardian's care and protection always have as their endpoint the full competency of the one under guardianship.

Many ideas from earlier epochs persist to strengthen the notion that a child has no rights, or few. "Honor thy father and mother that thy days may be long on the earth" conveys a literal reminder that disobedient children have been murdered with impunity in bygone days. Moreover, incestuous fathers (and their defense attorneys) speak fervently, even today, about a father's prerogatives or the sanctity of the family against external interference, using terms that hark back to a patriarchal society quite unlike ours of the present time. Today, children's rights are being enunciated increasingly in both law and public policy and are framed as *rights to both liberation and protection*. Children's sexual abuse is sometimes seen as the last frontier to call for reform and as the cutting edge for gaining children's rights.

ETIOLOGY AND PATHOPHYSIOLOGY

Sexual abuse has its necessary and sufficient causes in the helpless dependency and trust of a child, in the antichild (or other) motives of an adult, and in the specific milieu in which the adult turns to a child for gratifying a mixture of power and sexual intentions. The child victim is usually abused sexually by a familiar adult; in fact, the victim is generally a young girl and the perpetrator of the crime the girl's father, stepfather, other close relative, or the partner of a single parent.

Four classes of sex offenders against children are the sadistic, the pedophiliac, the carnal-narcissistic and, rarely, the person with episodic dyscontrol.

1. The *sadistic* perpetrator of child sexual abuse is more suffused with cruelty than with libido. Hence, sadism is considered a perversion. That sexuality is involved at all seems almost accidental; rather sexuality seems to be selected only for its misapplication to possibilities for inflicting pain, achieving conquest and dominance, or symbolizing the brutal enslavement of an inferior. A child's body usually is not of the size that permits easy entry by an adult's genitals or finger, so the size differential requires the adult male to desire to seduce, overpower, and inflict pain on the child who is made a sexual victim. Such a child molester has an ideology of carnality straight from the Marquis de Sade, insisting that a child screams and weeps only from enjoyment of sexual excitement; in reality, a child feels the pain as pain and the adult enjoys inflicting that pain. The antichild sadist is likely to be a sadist in other ways too; e.g., he likes to rape adult women (and/or men, too), he prefers "buggery" in his homosexual encounters, and he enjoys being the enslaving master in sadomasochistic games. The sadistic child molester employs a *macho* rhetoric, extols the rough and tough, enjoys being hated by mistreated subordinates at work, praises another man for being imperiously insistent or bossy, and so on. The sexual patterns only mirror the character patterns.

At times, "normal" parents delight in violent battling with their children only because they are certain to win, to conquer, to break the child's will, and to feel masterful. Zealous teachers also fall easily into sadistic relationships with children, obtaining "moral superiority" over the young, and sometimes becoming sexually aroused while administering corporal punishment to a child. On the spectrum of child victimization, brutal sodomy or rape stands only a few steps beyond brainwashing and inflicting bodily pain.

2. *Pedophilia* is a sexual perversion in which, rather than a person of one's own age, a young child is the preferred "sexual object," heterosexual or homosexual. It is not uncommon for an incestuous father to claim he has no pedophiliac leanings when first discovered, but subsequent data disclose a history of numerous sexual assaults on children from his adolescence onward. Moreover, in the polygraphic or psychophysiological laboratory such individuals demonstrate greater alertness and sexual arousal when shown photos of nude children than when exposed to nude photographs of women or men. As with any of the perversions, in pedophilia the man (usually) undergoes arousal and buildup of excitement and guilt as he plans and prepares either to seduce or to force a child victim into compliance with whatever he prefers to lead to his orgasm. Some

pedophiles proclaim their "straightness" and rationalize what they did by asserting that they behaved very gently and gave the child a lot of kind reassurance; they insist that if anal or vaginal penetration was not accomplished, no conceivable harm was done. They refer to their seduction as "nonassaultive," meaning there were no sadistic bodily injuries inflicted on the child. The child, however, often feels frightened and exploited by the perceived cruelty of the self-labeled "nonassaultive pedophile."

3. The *carnal-narcissistic* perpetrator of child sexual abuse is not exclusively focused on children for his "kicks" but may be what earlier psychoanalysts called "polymorphously perverse," or simply childish and immature, or chaotic. With adult males or females, male or female children, groups of people, animals, pornography, masturbation—such a person is sexually tuned up and turned on by a large array of "objects." He discriminates little as he acts out a diversity of sexual interests and fantasies. Knowing little of love, such a person does not relate to others, only to the diminished self. His satyric spirit leads him to seek sexual thrills and to experiment in numerous ways, including with young children. He damages the child when he seduces or rapes her (or him). The carnal narcissist's rationalizing statements often sound like sexual revolution jargon; "screwing everything that moves" is justified as being of *no harm*. He questions that there could possibly be anything wrong with whatever leads to adult orgasm and release. Apologies for sexual immorality are not new. Earlier examples were ancient Rome (Petronius), ancient Sodom and Gomorrah (The Bible), and—closer to our current sensate age—19th century Europe when both carnality (promiscuity, rape, sexual experimentation) and childism or child oppression (infanticide, abandonment, sodomy, child labor, brainwashing) were rampant. Children are harmed if victimized by these insistently sexually preoccupied adults. Just as the goal of sadism is to dominate, to control another's behavior, the goal of narcissistic carnality is to have "kicks" and obtain orgasms.

4. The *dyscontrol* perpetrator of sexual abuse is rare but merits mention. He loses control of his behavior and becomes antisocial; he claims to "go out of his mind" and becomes unable to curb either lust or actions. Usually, he ascribes his disorder of self-control to *alcohol or other drugs* and insists that he has no basic character flaw that would lead him to sexual abuse of a child. His reasoning is defensive, but criminals need to be defensive when charged and tried, we have to recall. One other, seldom seen cause of sexual abuse from episodic dyscontrol is *brain disorder:* psychosis, mental retardation, temporal lobe or psychomotor epilepsy, and pathological intoxication from small amounts of alcohol. Knowing this, the doctor who is asked by the defense attorney (of an accused child molester) to do a diagnostic workup should remember to obtain an EEG, preferably after depriving the accused of a night of sleep. The sleep-deprived subject will fall asleep during the tracing and only then may temporal lobe spikes appear on the EEG.

DIAGNOSIS

A. The *diagnostic workup* for a *reputed child molester* would include:

1. history, physical, and mental examination
2. complete battery of psychological testing
3. drug screening
4. neurological evaluation, including sleep-deprived EEG
5. full clinical psychiatric evaluation

If the perpetrator of child sexual abuse agrees to it, studies can be made in a *polygraphic laboratory,* usually by agreement of the prosecuting attorney and the defense attorney. Since a child's accusations are so well-founded, perpetrators will ask that the child first submit to polygraphic studies; then they will abscond or refuse to live up to their part of the agreement, claiming their constitutional rights not to submit to such studies—after the fact. Timing is important when polygraphy is agreed on; the putative molester should be required to go first. Perhaps a brief explanation will aid the beginner in child psychiatry to understand why legalistic documentation and caution are needed in cases of child sexual abuse: the typical pattern of the molester is first of all to deny any such allegations, then (if the charges are incontrovertible) to engage in a convoluted rhetoric of self-justification, and finally to stick with a defensive stance or else to come clean, even apologize to the child and to his other family members and embark on a program of remediation or treatment.

The incestuous father or stepfather, a paradigm for child sexual abuse in many ways, reacts *immediately* to a child's accusation by claiming that the child is lying, that the child does not separate fact from fantasy, or that the child has been coached to lie by her mother. Projective identification ("the child is a devil, not I"), role reversal ("she was supposed to love me and support me, not blow the whistle"), identification with the aggressor (a father should be in control of what his children do or say—many sex-abusing men have themselves been sexually abused during their own childhood), simple conning, self-deception, narcissism, and claiming loss of control with amnesia are among the numerous defense mechanisms that come into play at the point of the initial allegation.

The pattern continues in the second stage of self-justifying rhetoric: the father may claim that what he did was not harmful, particularly if no vaginal intercourse was completed or no lacerations and contusions are evident. Or he may blame his wife for being "frigid," excuse himself because he lacks potency with adults but must have sex with someone nonthreatening, or try to excuse what he did by contending that he was simply giving sex education to the child or that it was only his way of showing love for the child. Towards his wife, especially, the incestuous father takes an adversarial stand, accusing her of being unloving, of working through the daughter to get him in trouble, or of labeling her as a wife who is not subservient as the Scriptures require. Patriarchal ideology flows freely from the child sexual abuser: a man has rights; a father is like the deity's representative on earth and cannot do wrong; the family with a father is sacred and effective, but without a father there can be no family; and so on.

In the third defensive stage the incestuous father will begin negotiating to get a suspended sentence or to obtain a pretrial diversion to "treatment" or to sue his wife for divorce and try to make the sexual abuse a part of the domestic court proceedings—anything to decriminalize his criminal behavior.

B. What sort of *diagnostic workup* is required for the child who has been sexually molested? First of all, the health professional should obtain the best possible evidence or data, since he or she may be called on to testify in court. Retrievable and accurate recording is necessary, for which a *videotape* is superior; next best after the videotaped interview and physical exam come the medical chart and audio recordings. If the videotaped segment can be done with a police officer present, so much the better. "Polaroid" shots of the victim may also help in documentation of findings. Second, anogenital, anovenereal, and pharyngeal smears for the presence of sperms and bacterial cultures should be done. Third, the interview with the child should be conducted as effectively as possible: talking with the child alone (neither parent present) if the child is verbal, i.e., roughly more than two years of age; using realistic dolls with genitals obvious on the dolls in order to get on tape the story in the child's own words; employing only those terms that the child uses; and doing everything conceivable to minimize the amount of questioning to which the child will be subjected. To that end, a *videotaped interview with doctor and police* using anatomically accurate, naked dolls is superior since it may obviate any excuse for further quizzing by court, police, health, and welfare personnel.

Sexually abused children often have been interviewed on more than 100 occasions from the time of abuse until the court has tried and closed the case. Considering that these interviews are often hostile and adversarial to the child's interests and occasionally framed as, "You lied about what your father did to you, didn't you?" it is not surprising that sexually abused children might seek respite more than truth.

CHILDREN'S ALLEGATIONS AND RETRACTIONS

Although children *can* be coached to fabricate a story of sexual abuse, it is not difficult for a knowledgeable psychiatrist to discern when the allegations are false. In brief, whenever the allegations are made up, the child does not use a child's vocabulary; does not show a child's mode of understanding; makes the charges too easily and with descriptive details that show adult formulation more than a child's; makes unabashed charges in the presence of the "accused" only when the "plaintiff" parent is present but seems comfortable when the accuser is absent and accused is present. Moreover, there is some evident pathology, such as depression or vindictiveness, within the accusing parent. Nobody knows better than such a child how "dirty" the fighting can get between two angry and estranged parents.

It means "doubtful" to the legal system, but "more credible" to the behavioral scientist when a child who alleges incest by the divorced father, as an example, manifests the following picture: disclosure was rather hesitantly articulated and told; at least a retraction or two have been done and undone; the child talks in a pained fashion, in a child's vocabulary, and with a fearful and apologetic air if the accused is present; the child also has some of the pathological stress responses that are appropriate for the age group to which the child belongs.

A child who knows that telling lies is not moral is competent to testify whenever (s)he promises to tell the truth; but an astute defense attorney tries (if allowed to do so) to undermine or demean the child's cognitive grasp of the actual situation. Most judges permit queries to be set forth in adult language and wording that presupposes adult logic and explanation. A child can tell the truth by age two or more years; in fact, it is nearly impossible for a child to dissimulate or fabricate a sexual attack. The laws of cognitive development make it unlikely that a child under 11 years of age will "invent" or "fantasy" sexual behavior that the child has not actually experienced. Even in the rare custody battle where a parent has coached a child to concoct a lie of being molested, the child uses terms and explanations that are transparently "adultish," not the child's own. The sensorimotor stage lies too close at hand for a child to dream up sexual abuse out of the blue. The prelogical child does not fabricate sexual experiences; also, that child does not reason by the same logical patterns that adults may reason; hence it is important to get the *child's* story—even if in unrelated fragments—and *not try* to squeeze it into an adult-style causal narrative.

In a victim-blaming era, it is not surprising that charges of false allegations of sexual abuse will be leveled routinely against children, principally by defense attorneys for alleged perpetrators. Alas, at times certain views held by psychiatrists also serve to undermine or impugn reports given by victims of sexual abuse, e.g., the view that children, uncoached and unrehearsed, may have incestuous longings for the parent of the opposite gender and that these longings and fantasies may impede a child's reality sense. Cop-outs are sought on all sides in order to demean and minimize the reports and testimony of children. Hence, we need to devote a brief section to false allegations, admitted even by antichild zealots to be a minority of cases, but an issue much heralded by defense lawyers and others.

There are some five situations in which a child's report of sexual abuse might alert the professional to possibly false allegations. These five include coaching by an irate parent, molester displacement or transposition, shared delusional thinking, vindictive fabrication, and (possibly, though rare before adolescence) fabrication based on incestuous fantasies by the child. We consider each of these five in turn.

During an angry postdivorce battle between a child's mother and father, children are easily formed into pawns of their conflict. Easy divorce, no-fault divorce, and joint custody have been sought by married adults; when those easy divorce conditions have materialized, as we have noted, all ferocious litigation is delayed and displaced to the postdivorce phase of intemperately "dirty" fighting between the divorced parents of a child. Mothers of young girls might prompt their daughters of heterosexual fathers, or sons of homosexual fathers, to claim falsely that the father has sexually molested the child during times of visitations; the father likewise with the child who has visited the divorced mother from whom the father wishes to wrest custody or visitation "rights." Children who have been coached to tell lies regarding the other parent tell their lies in a rather mechanically rehearsed fashion, are easily thrown by simple questions about the alleged incident, and seem to have very shallow comprehension of the behavior that they are alleging. In the presence of the alleged perpetrator, the child recites the same lines, often with little congruent affect displayed.

Another situation in which false allegations may emerge would be, for example, a small girl who hates her stepfather and who might accuse him of sexual molestation when in reality she had been molested by a friend or relative of the stepfather. This situation would probably arise with great rarity, and then only with children who were 9–12 years old or, more likely, older adolescents. Most younger children lack the vindictiveness or sophisticated cunning required to transfer blame from a true perpetrator to a patsy.

The principles of cognitive development must be borne in mind whenever we undertake to play detective or adversary against a child who alleges sexual abuse. For instance, transposition of witnessed details of a pornographic film to a falsely accused molester would become increasingly likely with advancing age, but an account showing both internal and external consistency would almost certainly not be fabricated out of the whole cloth by a child under 11 years of age. That would also be the age at which some guilt and remorse that attend cognitive-moral development would also have been established as a curbing influence on the child's lying. Also, we should recall that before 8–10 years of age, a child does not have the power to sequence events precisely as they would have occurred to adults and would have been stored by adults; temporal veridicality is weak in children who have not attained the Piagetian level of formal operations. Experienced time can be altered from a conventional pattern even in normal adults and adolescents, or adults with fever, head injury, and possibly schizophrenia; so incorrect temporal sequencing does not negate a child's truth telling. A child's cognitive schemata, into which all experiences are incorporated and assimilated, are not as highly differentiated as are the schemata of adulthood. Hence, a child can, step by step, be duped into collaboration with an adult molester, only belatedly reaching a threshold beyond which the molestation will be processed and reschematized by the child as traumatic sexualization/betrayal/stigmatization/victimized powerlessness (Finkelhor & Browne, 1985). For processing new experiences that are unfolded gradually, the child both adapts the new to old schemata and moves into new ways of categorizing and schematizing experiences.

Shared Delusional Disorder was discussed in Chapter 23, but not in the explicit context of false ideas about child sexual abuse. A mother who was sexually abused herself might, finding her own sexuality, parenting, and mental health adversely affected, come to hold the false belief that, just as her own father molested her, so her husband probably will have molested their daughter. If she involves the daughter in her deluded thought, the daughter may present false charges against her father. It must be evident that such a child needs help; this is often overlooked in the literature on false allegations. Such lying in a child is not indicative of merely a Conduct Disorder.

Vindictive fabrication has been seen but twice in the combined experiences of the two authors, and in both cases they were concocted by 15-year-old females who had reason to be spiteful towards their respective father and father's brother. In both cases, the young women had temporal lobe epilepsy and after treatment recanted on their earlier stories; in one case the accused father, also, had temporal lobe dysrhythmia. We have not seen cases in any younger females or males, but must note that many writers with an antifemale and antichild bias always mention the possibility of vindictive fabrication. Such writers also bear down heavily on the next situation, entailing fantasies borne of incestuous longing and converted into lies of actual incest.

Fabrication by the child of incestuous molestation when all the child wanted was to have incest with the father is taken very seriously by many followers of Freud who followed him into a certain casuistry when he decided to discredit and discount his patients' reports of childhood sex abuse, preferring to attribute the patients' accounts to their longings to have incest. That shift of onus from adult male to female child has been addressed over and over by feminists and other child advocates and antiFreudians. As a theory, it seems to have a special allure to male psychoanalysts, and from our perspective it is an unproven tenet of Freudian doctrines.

Hence, only the first three of the five possible situations for children's lying about sex abuse are tenable, in our opinion, and those three occur only on extremely rare occasions. Perhaps as easy divorce becomes institutionalized and ramified, more instances of the first situation will appear in the future. In all events, the children who bring false allegations of sex abuse are in need of psychiatric attention.

Psychological testing is helpful in the diagnostic workup of a sexually abused child. The psychological consultant is asked to advise the physician about:

1. The child's IQ: to see if there is anxiety-bred decrement or scatter in the verbal or performance IQ.

2. The child's cognitive stage: to determine if the child's cognitive style is age-appropriate.

3. The child's self-picture: self-assurance or doubt, sense of autonomy or powerlessness, ability to cope under stress, ego strengths.

4. The child's image of her (or his) family; if the child is angrily antimolester, is either parent trusted for support and protection?

5. The child's gender identity, sexual knowledge, and sexual imagery as revealed in the testing situation; sexual preoccupations or fears.

6. The indications of psychic trauma and Post-traumatic Stress Disorder, of depression, of generalized fear or anxiety, of dissociative or conversion-hysteria tendencies.

When integrated with the physician's own diagnostic data, the psychologist's consultation can be highly useful to the team of physicians, other health and mental health specialists, social workers, and police and court officers. The team, through conference and collaboration, is the main vehicle for both diagnosis and treatment of sexually abused children.

CLINICAL DESCRIPTION

The outward and inner phenomena of psychopathology vary according to the age of the molested child. Overt phenomenology is manifested in the global stress responses of a very young preschool child, the abrupt changes in social interaction (or sociability) of the school-aged child and the runaway or even promiscuous behavior of the older child. Eroticization of behavior may be present in children of all three age groups. Looking at the child's inner life and attitudes, one is impressed that any age shows narcissistic wounds and psychic traumatization, with feelings of disloyalty, resentment, fear, and betrayal. The child's greater feelings of self-worth and autonomy, coupled with some angry blaming of the molester, seem to protect in particular the older child who has been sexually abused. Otherwise, if the mother and siblings do not rally round and help the child to extrude and reject the perpetrator and transcend by undoing repression of the experience, the child himself/herself feels guilty, perplexed, confused, and responsible for the entire family's welfare—a huge burden for an already-victimized young person.

CASE 28-1   Julie was two years old when she was brought by her mother to the emergency service of a charity university hospital with a foul-smelling *vaginal discharge, vaginal and anal lacerations, edema* in the pudendum, and rubor and turgor of the *external genitalia*. Culture proved that she had *gonorrheal vaginitis and proctitis*. The case was reported to Protective Services, who determined that the *mother's live-in boyfriend* had been sexually molesting her since he had moved into the household four months earlier. When the gonorrhea had been treated, Julie manifested condylomata acuminata, which did not respond fully to treatment with podophyllin and were eventually removed surgically.

Julie's *mother disclaimed* any knowledge of her boyfriend's sexual molestation of both Julie and her four-year-old brother. The *brother* had to be treated for anal lacerations and fissures, which the child said had been induced by a table knife being repetitively inserted by the mother's boyfriend; then later he was also treated for condylomata. When the boyfriend was accused, he *claimed that it was an outright, bold lie* that had been fabricated by the children. Later, he plea bargained and was given a prison term of five years; he was paroled after one-and-a-half years. He *neither admitted* what had actually occurred, nor *was tried for* that; in addition, he offered no apologies to either child or to their mother.

One year after the sexual abuse, Julie appeared *shy and withdrawn*. Her paternal grandmother had been awarded custody of the children. Julie experienced *scary dreams* and occasional *temper tantrums* and did not seem happy, so her grandmother requested that she be seen by a child psychiatrist.

CASE 28-2   When Alan, who lived in a small western town, was nine years and four months old, he was surrounded and *overpowered* by three *older* boys, two aged 13 and one aged 14. These three grabbed him by the arms and took him off into the woods adjacent to the school playground. There, two of them held knives against his neck and chest while the third undressed him from the waist down and forced him to suck on the older boy's penis until he ejaculated into Alan's mouth. In less than an hour Alan had been forced to fellate all three of the older lads before he was released to go home but *instructed that they would kill him* if he ever told anyone about the events.

When Alan got home he brushed his teeth a couple of times and used mouthwash, *behind the closed bathroom door*. He was *afraid* he would be killed if he told his mother, with whom he and his three siblings lived, but he *felt "bad"* and thought he ought to tell someone: his divorced father who lived in a nearby town and had visitation there with the four children one weekend each month. The father was irate, told Alan he would kill those three "little perverts," and blamed Alan's mother for not protecting her oldest son from such a shameful and stressful experience. The father took most of the initiative in reporting the case to Protective Services, who replied that they would "take care of it" and advised the father not to speak to the boys who had perpetrated the offense, nor to their parents.

The three "juveniles" were brought before a judge who castigated them for being such bullies and warned them to stay away from Alan. The boys were *not* adjudicated further and Alan continued to feel uneasy when he was around all older (teenage) males, especially the three perpetrators of his oral-sex rape. Seen soon thereafter by a child psychiatrist, Alan reported *bad dreams* of being captured and beaten by gangs of older boys. He did not dream of their forcing him to engage in fellatio; it was only a *physical endangerment* that he felt in his frequent anxiety dreams. He also had *flashbacks* accompanied by feelings of *fright and near-panic* during his waking hours, often when nobody male and older was near him. He became *more concerned about sexual matters* after his rape experience but his concerns were mainly about parental sexuality; his father had a live-in girlfriend and his mother a live-in boyfriend, but Alan said he thought grown-ups ought to get married if they were going to live together.

The case that follows, although not of a child, is included because it shows the frequent sexual problems of older youths who were sexually abused and not supported by the nonperpetrator parent.

CASE 28-3   Edna was 12 years old when referred to a child psychiatry center for evaluation and treatment. At that time she had not attended school for more than a year, having seen a general physician who determined that she was depressed, homosexual, and given to running away from home. For the past several months, Edna had identified herself as homosexual because she had developed an eroticized "mother–daughter" kind of attachment to an older woman in her local town. In referring to her relationship to the older woman whom she loved, she persistently contrasted the good relationship she had with her older friend and the bad relationship she had with her mother. The child psychiatrist pointed this out to Edna and her story of sexual abuse by her stepfather two years earlier unfolded.

Edna's mother had immediately repudiated Edna's story, called her a liar, asked if she had been trying to make passes at the stepfather, and accused her of being seductive. Edna said she felt disillusioned with both her mother and stepfather and began running away from home, being truant from school, and not knowing where to turn for support; her older "homosexual" friend had been her only confidante and supporter. Edna had developed ulcer symptoms, which had responded poorly to a bland diet over the past two years. She became irritable, uncommunicative, and spent a lot of time at home in solitude; she would run away at times that her mother thought were totally unpredictable and unprovoked, only to be apprehended and returned by the state police after a few days—once after almost two months. She had never had a date, claiming she did not like males.

DIFFERENTIAL DIAGNOSIS

Once it has been suspected and established that a child was sexually abused and now shows signs of a mental disorder, the differentiation to be done on the psychiatric consequences includes:

1. *Adjustment Disorder* with probable healthy response eventually (dependent on treatment provided, however).
2. *Anxiety Disorder*—generalized or situational.
3. *Avoidant Disorder*—many sexually abused children will actively avoid any adult, especially male.
4. *Post-traumatic Stress Disorder*—delayed or immediate.
5. *Dissociative Disorder*—although we do not know how often sexually abused children develop multiple personality, we do know that most contemporary cases of multiple personality were sexually abused in childhood.
6. *Depressive or Dysthymic Disorder*—most likely if the child has been habitually molested and not been believed when she or he "squealed," or has been threatened and persuaded not to reveal the sexual abuse.
7. *Eroticized behavior, premature pseudoadult sexuality, and seductiveness and provocativeness*—"Cinderella complex," although an antichild concept, is a possibility.

As stated earlier, when these psychiatric conditions appear, the astute clinician will inquire about sexual abuse, since these disorders may give us the first alerting signs of sexual abuse.

TREATMENT

Treatment planning is geared to the child's needs in: 1) the initial crisis phase (six to eight weeks after the incident has occurred); 2) the six-week period following the crisis of disclosure; and 3) the more prolonged phase of reclamation, reorientation, and reconstitution of both the child and the family without the perpetrator. Phases 1 and 2 together should, optimally, take no more than three months, the period during which (ideally) the criminal case should have been tried and decided. Ideally, respecting the child's welfare, the first and second phases would occur simultaneously in six-to-eight weeks, but often there is a lag between occurrence and disclosure and again between disclosure and prosecution.

In the initial crisis phase, when the child shows changes in thinking, feeling, and behavior, no explicit revelation of the crime may occur. Or perhaps we should say that the crime, going undetected, may continue to imperil the child, because the childcaring persons in the abused child's life are negligent (parents, teachers, social workers, physicians). The most appropriate treatment during this initial crisis is for the parent(s) and all adults who are responsible for the child to be able to read the behavioral signs and help the child to articulate the sexual abuse that took place, to discern that the change in the overall mood state and behavior of the child may signify sexual abuse of the child, and to move for a speedy end of the abuse in order to save the child from further harm. Interestingly, in all 50 states' laws, the physician is required to report suspected sexual abuse of a child.

What the child does before detection has occurred, especially if he or she has been threatened, should (s)he report the abuse, depends on age. The *preschooler,* devoid of abstract thinking, shows mainly biological changes in eating and sleeping, and bedwetting, and starts displaying gross signs of cruelty—all these signs could alert a sensitive and vigilant parent, teacher, or doctor. The school-aged child's alerting signals for the careful adult observer include sudden changes in school work, the appearance of sexual preoccupations, discomfort or fear when around the perpetrator or others who are "like" the perpetrator, withdrawal from play and companionship, and sadness. The older child victim typically starts running away or engaging in delinquency. If the mother in particular can surround the child with a protective mantle of support and safety, that is the most appropriate treatment; it will allow the child to divulge the full details as the child experienced and comprehended them. If handled properly by the adult caretakers, the period of initial crisis quickly becomes the crisis of disclosure. Then the caretakers can stop guessing about the "hidden signs" of child sexual abuse.

In the period following the crisis of disclosure, the child's needs for a firm bonding with the nonperpetrator parent (the mother, in nine out of 10 cases), for prompt medical care (including psychiatric crisis care), and for protection against further abuse by the perpetrator lead the child protection agency (usually a division of the local or state department of social services) to remove the perpetrator from the home, report the crime to both police and child welfare agencies, offer crisis help to the mother-headed residual family, and remind the prosecution that, while we acknowledge that a heinous crime occurred, we also acknowledge that after a trial is completed the outcome of psychiatric or endocrine therapy for some types of molester may be more efficacious than imprisonment alone.

It is contraindicated to bring the incestuous father or stepfather or mother's friend back into the family—thereby "reconstituting" the family—until after the legal case has been tried and, if the abuser is found guilty, the sentence imposed, suspended, or probated. The few child abuser treatment programs that have attained any success in treating an early-reconstituted family have always required that the treatment be imposed by and conducted through the authority of a court of law after sentencing. This generalization covers broad experiences with family-based child sexual abuse in Canada, the U.S., and Great Britain: Pretrial "diversions" by courts into "treatment" of the reconstituted incestuous family have had poorer and vaguer results because such families drop out or move away, coalesce to keep their secrets, intensify their pathologies, and otherwise resist or refuse treatment. Hence, while on faith some propose *only* a family-group therapy (including the molester), a more judicious practice would be to cooperate with law enforcement in order to protect and "save" the child, hoping for a quick resolution of the legal case so that a humane approach can *then* be taken to the entire family.

In the third phase of longer term healing and reclamation, help for the child consists of a strengthening of the mother-child bond, finding extrafamilial, community supports and aids for the mother-only family, facilitating further ego-strengthening within the child through a period of accelerated learning that she or he is a child and a victim—galvanizing her or his identity as a child with rights, and a victim with rights. This rapid learning may necessitate a temporary period of disenchantment with adults in place of an earlier, more naive view that adults are benign and friendly, as well as a quick training period in realizing that she or he is a victim but can identify with victims rather than aggressors and forge some practical devices for ensuring against further victimization. Group membership with other mothers and children who have been sexually abused is helpful to the incest victim for increasing awareness and establishing a supportive network. A young child can learn that she (or he) has exclusive say-so about being touched by anyone in the areas of their bodies that are covered by a swimsuit. A young child can learn that (s)he may refuse to do anything with another's body parts; the young child also can learn how to get help if his or her rights are denied.

In summary, the psychotherapy for the child may be conceived as multimodal, individual psychotherapy, behavioral modification, and group therapy, as well as judicious pharmacological treatment.

PROGNOSIS WITHOUT TREATMENT

The treatment of the sexually abused child in the crisis period and thereafter is imperative so that grave psychopathology and dysphoria do not ensue. Chief among the disorders to appear (at once or later) in untreated or mistreated cases of children sexually abused by adults are the following:

1. *Sexual disorders and deviations*—Sexual unrest, promiscuity, manhating prostitution in girls, disorders in arousal and orgasm (impotence, frigidity, inhibition), and perversions (especially sadomasochism and practicing child molestation when the child becomes adult).

2. *Mental disorders*—Chronic fear, Depression, Dissociation, Anxiety and Panic Disorders, Stress Disorders, and Schizophrenia, because, even if the disorder that emerges has a high familial incidence, sexual abuse triggers its phenotypic appearance.

3. *Distortions in parenting*—Role reversal, cruelty, projective indentification, identification with the aggressor, narcissistic identification, suspicion or mistrust of one's male spouse as a prospective child molester, gross failures in empathy for children, and generalized demoralization about marriage and child care.

Questions for Study and Action

1. Describe the elements of a suitable diagnostic workup for Julie (Case 28-1) after she had had surgery for the condylomata and recovered but was brought to a child psychiatrist. List each item of the diagnostic workup, along with its justification and rationale.

2. Realizing that Julie's mother had absconded when the heat of her boyfriend's crime was on him, but returned to claim visitation rights after his plea bargaining and sentence, draft a letter to the court making your recommendations about when and how the mother's visits to Julie would occur, whether with or without supervision, where, and for how long. Consider primarily what the child needs in her traumatized state.

3. Make a case for the treatment of Julie's Post-traumatic Stress Disorder to be carried mainly by supportive work with the grandmother, environmental manipulation, training in parental effectiveness, ascertainment of day care, and so on. What arguments can you muster to justify a focus on the grandmother primarily with relatively little direct contact with Julie at age two years?

4. Assuming that Alan (Case 28-2) met the major criteria for a Post-traumatic Stress Disorder, discuss other conditions that need ruling in or out as a part of a diagnostic differentiation. Discuss three other childhood mental disorders that need to be included in such differential diagnosis.

5. If children do need parenting from any or all sources available, what is there about Alan's receipt of parenting that may need shoring up and expansion? What would you advise his custodial parent, the mother, about ways to give Alan more security at this time in his life? Be detailed and specific.

6. Alan as a sexually abused preadolescent is now placed at risk for psychosocial problems that may in themselves lead to further psychopathology in adolescence and young adulthood. First, list some of the difficulties that he may be expected to encounter (especially if he becomes lonely and phobically withdrawn from peers and from a loving chumship with an agemate); second, list some of his strengths or assets as a bright male that could help him be "immunized" from subsequent stressors.

7. Discuss the statement that follows: The outcome for a sexually abused child is less pathological if the child has a strong ego and sense of self and can rely on the advocacy of some important adult. Make a list of at least six concrete indices of a "strong ego" that would benefit a sex abuse victim in childhood.

8. Outline the details of a treatment program for a residual mother-only family after incest occurred. Classify your program constituents according to those directed towards the child individually, those directed towards the mother, those towards the siblings, and those towards the family as a whole.

9. If Edna met all the criteria of DSM-III-R for a Major Depressive Disorder, how would you treat her? Review the earlier chapter (Chapter 15) on mood disorders and their treatment. What dosage would you begin with, if you chose to use a tricyclic, and how would you know whether she is absorbing the right amount of the medication? What would you expect the TCA to do for her peptic ulcer symptoms? for her idea that she is homosexually inclined? for her runaway behavior?

10. Do you see some aspects of Edna's behavior suggesting that she needs the support and protection of a mothering person? Could the therapist provide that or should some other measures be suggested? Would you as a child psychiatrist want to include Edna's mother in the psychotherapy? What about including the older woman friend?

For Further Reading

Adams, P.L., & Roddey, G.J. Language patterns of opponents to a child protection program. *Child Psychiatry & Human Development*, 11:133–157, 1981. Also appears in S. Chess & A. Thomas (Eds.), *Annual Progress in Child Psychiatry and Child Development*. New York: Brunner/Mazel, 1982, pp. 667–688.

Burgess, A.W., Groth, A.N., Holmstrom, L.L. et al. *Sexual Assault on Children and Adolescents.* Lexington, MA: Heath, 1978.

Finkelhor, D., & Browne, A. The traumatic impact of child sexual abuse: A conceptualization. *Am. J. Orthopsychiatry,* 55:530–541, 1985.

Journal of American Academy of Child Psychiatry, 25:449–492, 1986. (Articles on sexual abuse by A.H. Green, L. Claman et al.; L.C. Terr, B. Nurcombe, A.A. Rosenfeld et al.; P.J. Racusin, J.K. Felsman, & D.H. Schetky).

Stuart, I.R., & Greer, J. (Eds.). *Victims of Sexual Aggression.* New York: Van Nostrand Reinhold, 1984.

29

Physical Abuse

Unless physical abuse is disapproved generally, its definition is problematic. A nation whose Supreme Court upheld the rights of schools to administer corporal punishment to children is a nation for which the demarcation of physical abuse to children is difficult. The U.S. is such a nation. If corporal punishment in schools is justified by the doctrine that while the child is at school, the school stands *in loco parentis* (in the status of a parent), then obviously parents' physical punishment of children is assumed to be correct and can be transferred to school authorities and others. The child psychiatrist as a citizen, and also a scientific healer, generally understands that an angry parent may occasionally box his obnoxious child's ears but may or may not concede that such parental behavior, especially if apologized for by the parent, gives schools and other institutions a right to administer physical pain to children. Again, the reader is reminded that awareness of physical abuse is only possible when the child is seen as having rights (as with neglect, sexual abuse, and mental abuse). Without rights being defined, no victim can be defined. For many child psychiatrists as citizens, the whole matter is one of numerous ethical and pragmatic dilemmas. The dilemma of physical punishment that slips over into physical abuse or battering has a history that will be briefly noted now.

Members of the three influential religious groups of Judaism, Christianity,

457

and Islam, basing their reasoning on a mistranslation from the Jewish King Sol-omon, have made parents responsible for rebuking and beating their children. They equate the Bible's "Bring up a child in the way he should go and when old he will not depart from it" with the secular rule of "Spare the rod and spoil the child." In reality, the Solomon wisdom may be more aptly translated as, "Bring up a child in that child's own way, then when old he or she will not depart from it." Even today, many parents see their mission as one closely akin to an animal trainer, requiring much grit and violence on the part of the parent. The law traditionally has held that a minor son or daughter is the property of the father—or of the child's parents—and may be beaten with impunity. As a result, children have been lashed freely (usually in the zone of the buttocks), physically restrained, deprived of food, warmth, clothing and companionship, and so on. Only in 1871 did a New York statute protect children from such abuse by including them under an earlier statute protecting horses and other animals (Radbill, 1974).

Although a pediatric radiologist first described in 1946 a "syndrome" of multiple fractures of the long bones along with subdural hematomas in a number of children (Caffey, 1946), there was no explicit suggestion that such injuries may have been inflicted by the parents; it was not until the 1960s in the U.S. that *the battered child syndrome* came to public awareness. Since that time, there has been a relative decline in the reported incidence of physical abuse of children. Some experts regard physical abuse as a default or renunciation of parenting second only to sexual abuse, although, today, sexual abuse and neglect have grown more common than physical abuse. Physical abuse is aimed at murdering the child and is seen to occur mostly with infants or very young children and children who have special needs because of their mental or physical handicaps. Accurate incidence figures are not easy to obtain but the best estimate is that in 1983 there were one million physically abused children in the U.S. and about three thousand of them died as a result of physical abuse.

DIAGNOSTIC WORKUP FOR PARENT(S) AND CHILD

The most effective detection can be done by a professional who suspects inflicted abuse when children sustain repeated injuries or poisonings that are said to be accidental or when children show the bodily scars of multiple traumata—from cigarette burns, choking or throttling, puncture and laceration wounds, bruises, welts, lumps on the head, scalding, or fractures. *Neglect* may be a precursor of such abuse, so the height and weight measures of the child as well as a full developmental evaluation need to be done to determine if there is a developmental delay. Review Chapter 10 on Eating Disorders. Signs of undernutrition and fluid deprivation should be noted, as well as "ground-in" dirt under the nails and in the umbilicus, diaper rash, and so on. The clinician should be duly suspicious if a child with positive signs is brought in by a standoffish parent who seems disinterested in the child's condition. The parents may give very feeble explanations of the way the injury was sustained, show a history of repeatedly moving from one county to another, have little involvement with neighbors or social agencies, proclaim a belief in violence as the way to modify a child's behavior (e.g., spanking a month-old infant to stop its crying), and give a history of having been abused and neglected when they were children. Questioned separately, as they should be, the two give conflicting stories. A child over age two years should be interviewed separately from either parent; the child's independent story is important even if the parents have vigorously coached the child ahead of time.

Distortions are rampant, if these parents are interviewed at some length. They show projective identification ("the child is a devil, wicked, malignant"), role reversal ("no matter what I do for her, she won't sleep and let me get any rest"), identification with the aggressor ("my parents beat me, even broke both my legs one time, but it was good for me"), narcissistic identification ("she made me sick and ashamed of her deformity"), crude denial, and so on. When such parents cooperate with psychological testing (Wechsler Adult Intelligence Scale, Thematic Apperception Test, Rorschach Ink Blots, Draw-a-Figure, and Sentence Completion, for example), they show a shortage of personal resources and a primitive nature in their defending and coping strategies, making them unable to supply nurture and protection to young children.

The child, too, may enter into rapid complicity with all the foregoing parental distortions, not disclosing the abuse, not complaining, and not contradicting the parents' instructing the child what to say. Indeed, the most abusive parent is often the one to whom the child clings with a guilty demeanor, believing the parental version of physical abuse and feeling responsible for increasing his or her parent's happiness.

There are certain traits in the *child* that make him or her more vulnerable to abuse, although not blameworthy. Chief among these are developmental, constitutional/temperamental, and organic disorders that produce symptoms of difficult adjustment, overactivity or overreactivity, impulsivity, and attention deficit.

CLINICAL DESCRIPTION

Implicit in the foregoing discussion of diagnosis or detection of physical abuse is a clinical picture that is exemplified in this vignette. *Italicized* are risk factors for physical abuse.

CASE 29-1   Marie was *three years old* when she sustained a skull fracture and showed roentgenographic findings of multiple rib and long bone fractures in varying stages of healing. She had been *born prematurely,* weighing four-and-a-half pounds, to an *unwed, adolescent* woman who was 15 years of age. Her mother did *not complete high school* and had *not held a job.* She derived her own and the child's sustenance from Aid to Families with Dependent Children, which *amounted to about two hundred dollars per month* in her state of residence. Since Marie was kept in the hospital for two weeks after her birth, the mother felt *little attachment* to the young baby and decided to *bottle-feed* because that *would not tie the mother down* to the helpless child. Marie was an easy, docile baby who progressed well except for a *febrile convulsion* when she was eighteen months old and numerous myringotomies for *otitis media,* chronic and recurrent. The mother "developed a liking for her" when she was a healthy and responsive infant but *became enraged* by Marie's *toddler negativism and resistiveness* and began to inflict more and more severe *corporal punishment* when the *child would not obey* the mother's commands regarding toilet training, walking, picking up her toys, and eating what was put on her plate. The mother had herself been *physically and sexually abused* as a child, when she lived in her maternal grandmother's home after her *mother had abandoned her* to move to *seek employment.* After Marie was placed in foster care, her mother obtained help from an antipoverty program lawyer in fighting to regain custody of Marie. She was not immediately successful in getting Marie back but she did win the *fight not to have her parental rights terminated.* Consequently, she kept occasional and critical contact with Marie and the foster mother; the latter, she claimed, was ruining Marie *by spoiling her.*

DIFFERENTIAL DIAGNOSIS

The physical and roentgenologic signs of child abuse must be differentiated from organic disease (blood dyscrasias, neoplasms, etc.), on the one hand, and from accidental processes due to developmental or central nervous system pathology (e.g., convulsive disorder) on the other.

DIFFERENCES BETWEEN PHYSICAL AND SEXUAL ABUSE OF CHILDREN

Sexual abuse was regarded as criminal behavior long before physical abuse. Even today, lawyers do not show much interest in physical abuse, leaving it to welfare departments and to professionals who take a soft approach—encouraging parent education, family group therapy, peer group work through Parents Anonymous and similar groups, setting up respite care centers for assaulted children, and making efforts to socialize the parents more fully and to give them a supportive community network. Physical abusers are poorer economically and more often women than is the case with sexual abusers. Also, physical abuse is a readily visible part of an overall family pattern of violence, while sexual abuse may not leave so many telltale physical signs and may on rare occasions be committed by persons outside the family. If any paraphilia or perversion is involved in the genesis of battering, it is sadism, but that appears to be rarely remarked in the literature; in general, child molesters do get orgastic gratifications that child batterers do not obtain. Because of these differences in epidemiology and pathogenesis, the sexual abuse paradigm will not fit for physical abuse, nor vice versa.

TREATMENT

Physical abuse, also a reportable crime, is inextricably imbedded into societal values and strenuously tests the preventive and treatment thinking of the physician. When young families are needy but neglected, it is difficult to prevent child abuse and neglect. When children are viewed as unwelcome and draining consumers—mouths to be fed—infanticide hovers in the social air. If family planning and parent education are not provided to people, unwanted and problematic children will be numerous and will be victimized. Treatment planning in its medical and psychiatric particulars comprises those interventions aimed at the child victim, those aimed at the parent-perpetrator, those aimed at the pair of parents if one is not a perpetrator, and those aimed at the family unit within the larger community.

For the child a sensible treatment plan is as follows: early detection and crisis care of the injured child in a safe milieu; possible placement in foster care to include adoption; crisis psychotherapy to support the child's opposition to the violent parent(s) and to relieve guilt and separation problems; longer-term psychotherapy for Post-traumatic Stress Disorder if present; and every step possible to see that the child can have some experience of a childhood surrounded by adults who delight in taking care of children—empathic and truly mature grown-ups. Simultaneously, the strengthening of community structures to end violence as a reflex act should be sought.

For the parental perpetrator, invoking the authority of a court of law seems to be both responsible behavior and conducive to a more structured, businesslike psychotherapy. Yet psychotherapy yields little as long as the economic wants, the strains and humiliations of poverty, the absence of adequate health care, and the institutionalized violence of our domestic lives remain unaddressed.

For the parental pair, a review of their own childhood experiences in their families of origin helps to clarify their attitudes about parents and children, even if distorted; a review of their conjugal relationship from the time of meeting to the present is also educative and helpful, as is a survey of their roles as parents of children. If this kind of exploration, accompanied by an orientation to make changes, is carried out within a context of helping the parents to visit their children's schools and day care centers, churches, neighborhood organizations and to learn what to do when they can foresee violent blowups brewing, the treatment plan will be more rational.

Questions for Study and Action

1. It has been said that deviant parental behavior can be brought under most effective social control when it has been either "criminalized" or "medicalized." Read on the history of child battering (as in "For Further Reading," at the end of this section, items #1 and 5), then discuss how child battering became medicalized first and criminalized later, in contrast to sexual abuse which was criminalized before it was medicalized. All told, what does this say about the influences of physicians and attorneys in consciousness-raising and public-opinion-shaping?

2. List 10 conditions that augment a child's risk of being battered by nonempathic parents. Looking over the list, does this say that the child is to blame in some way?

3. List five community-related characteristics of families in which violence is most likely to occur.

4. Discuss how each of the following would tend to augment or reduce physical abuse of children:
   (a) a policy of physical restraint and punishment for hospitalized children
   (b) Supreme Court approval of corporal punishment in schools
   (c) having a father who is a wife-beater
   (d) having a mother who does not use contraception
   (e) having a father and mother who do not condone divorce as a way out of an impossibly unsatisfying marriage
   (f) having two parents who pay more heed to their own physical pleasures than to parenting
   (g) having a priest who advised surrender and obedience to a violent parent
   (h) having a pediatrician who believes that childhood is a carefree, happy era, or who says the child will "grow out" of a problem
   (i) having a radiologist who suspects a bone disease when he sees multiple fractures on a child's X-rays
   (j) having a teacher who zealously believes in brainwashing and indoctrination
   (k) attending a school in which self-government by the students is policy

(l) working with a psychiatrist who wants to see things from a child's standpoint

(m) living in a community where children are informed about protective services for abused children

(n) being a child patient who is present at staffing conferences in the child psychiatry hospital

5. Knowing what you do about "hatred and anal-eroticism," give a plausible explanation of why adults who administer corporal punishment to children prefer to strike blows behind the child in the "bad and hidden" area of the buttocks. Don't refrain from speculation and conjecture about unconscious determinants as you draw up a "dynamic formulation" of such child-spanking.

For Further Reading

Bakan, D. *Slaughter of the Innocents.* Boston: Beacon Press Paperbacks, 1971.

Caffey, J. Multiple fractures in the long bones of infants suffering from chronic subdural hematoma. *Am. J. Roentgenol.,* 56(2):163–173, 1946.

Green, A.H. *Child Maltreatment: A Handbook for Mental Health and Child Care Professionals.* New York: Jason Aronson, 1980.

de Mause, L. The evolution of childhood. In L. de Mause (Ed.), *The History of Childhood.* New York: Harper Torchbooks, 1975.

Newberger, E.H., & Bourne, R. (Eds.). *Unhappy Families: Clinical and Research Perspectives on Family Violence.* Littleton, MA: PSG Publishing, 1985.

Radbill, S.X. A history of child abuse and infanticide. In R.E. Helfer & C.H. Kempe (Eds.), *The Battered Child* (2nd ed.). Chicago: University of Chicago Press, 1974.

30

Emotional Abuse

DEFINITION

This, as defined, is perhaps the most common form of abuse but since it has to do with brainwashing, demeaning, bossing, overcontrolling, indifference to the child's needs, condemning and humiliating the child, emotional abuse is difficult to detect, and incidence and prevalence figures are not accurate. The outward signs of the damages are subtle but may be devastating to the child's feeling human or "okay." Emotional abuse may be defined as anything an adult does that destroys self-esteem and sets the child on a course of forever fearfully, and not lovingly, trying to please the parent(s) or other emotionally abusing adults or older children, while feeling he or she has a basic fault. Emotional abuse is another form of denying human rights to children—by rejecting, isolating, terrorizing, ignoring, or corrupting children (Garbarino, Guttman, & Seeley, 1986).

ETIOLOGY AND PATHOGENESIS

Although emotional abuse of a child is not coded as a disorder in DSM-III-R, it can be coded as a stressor which can precipitate coded disorders. If the adult perceives the child as satanic through projective identification, the parent robs both self and child of genuine self-acceptance and lives in an illusion of perfect parent and wicked child. If the parent parades the child about like a trained show animal, the child feels like a narcissistic extension of the parent, not a separate person. Children of narcissistic parents may feel incomplete, act browbeaten, and overstrive to please the parent. The same kinds of distortions of parenting as those described more fully in Chapter 35 provide the parental substrate for emotionally abusing a child: emotional rejection, neglect, scapegoating, incomprehension of a child's needs.

Not only parents but also teachers, doctors, older children, judges, police officers, pediatricians, psychologists, social workers, child psychiatrists, guidance counselors, shopkeepers, park attendants, and camp counselors can instill an infanticidal terror in children, producing emotional abuse. Disrespect for young people and a zealous determination to control their minds and bodies are ubiquitous. So are betrayal, refusing to apologize, deception, and conning. Introducing children to addicting drugs, while producing an Organic Mental Disorder, is adult abuse of children. Emotional abuse looms as an effect of antichild ideology and behavior. Being so pervasive, the charge of emotional abuse of children carries no punch and it is almost impossible to amass any evidence that will hold up in courts of law, "manned" as they so often are by male adults.

To deprive a parent of his or her ownership rights in a child is virtually unheard of. All the legal empowerment is for adults. Even the child born out of wedlock must submit to a father who neglected mother and child until the child reached elementary school age, with no visits, no presents, no phone calls, until suddenly he wishes to be Dad to the child. To support his claims to a formerly unclaimed child, the men on the Supreme Court gave a decision in the 1970s, in almost poetic language, holding that if such a father at any time "shows a flicker of interest" in his offspring, his parental rights are then guaranteed. Hence, the etiology of emotional abuse of children is societal in both attitude and behavior. For the individual adult, his or her own emotional abuse during childhood reappears in adult life, seeming to be appropriate for children to undergo and for adults to inflict. That is, parents identify with their childhood aggressors and not with the child's status as a victim. If one's own parents were brutal, one feels morally correct if one refrains from abusing a child physically and sexually but does inflict neglect, itself a mode of emotional abuse. Adams (1979) has remarked that emotional abuse shows sublimated infanticide.

CASE 30-1   Zora, who had lived in a mother-only family since birth, acquired a new father when she was five years old. The new father was so kindly attentive to Zora initially that some neighbors believed him to be "too good to be true." He talked with her, played with her, fed her, entertained her, read to her, and put her to bed. Indeed, putting her to bed was when he discovered that she stroked her labia and clitoris as she fell asleep. Both her behavior and his own excited interest in her behavior alarmed him. He told Zora that she must *never* do that, but she persisted and he always found her out, it seemed. He rebuked her as a bad and dirty girl, warned her of hellfire and brimstone, and began tying her hands together behind her back. At that point Zora substituted leg movements with her pillow and toy animals, and her new father's zeal grew faster. He tied her knees together and made her wear a chastity belt. He spanked her once on her bare buttocks, but apologized soon after, pleading that he only wanted her to be pure and wholesome and not grow up feeling ashamed of herself for her bad sexual behavior and for being illegitimate. Zora, sobbing, told him she did not know what "illegitimate" meant. He told her how shameful it is to have no father and no name. She seemed puzzled but mostly fearful and disvalued, wanting to please him but being unable to comply with his requests. She was a tyrannized child, conflicted because her bodily comfort and enjoyment were considered to be grave sins. She was a victim of a stepfather's "religious" zeal to modify her behavior and to bring her under the control of his ideas and attitudes. Because he believed she had been possessed by the devil, he had her stand in the corner with a paper bag over her head.

Comment. Zora's stepfather could not have been convicted for the physical abuse of imposing restraints on her limbs, nor for sexual abuse contained implicitly in his preoccupation with her sexuality, but he assuredly abused her emotionally. Yet no conviction was obtained. Zora's mother felt very dependent on her new husband, wanted to be subservient to him, and opted "to stay out of it when he tried to correct Zora about playing with her privates." The court's opinion was that the mother was not culpable and that her only wrongdoing was her bad judgment in selecting her husband. Zora received no treatment.

DIAGNOSIS

As we stated, emotional abuse may be severe but remain imperceptible and undetectable if one's observations are superficial and stereotyped. Only an index of suspicion alerts the more thorough observer. There may be signs of neglect (Chapter 27), physical abuse (Chapter 29), or sexual abuse (Chapter 28) as concomitants and indices of emotional abuse. In frequent clinical contacts with parent and child, the observer notes a deficit in parental empathy and a high level of parental authoritarianism. The child may wince if the parent makes a sudden move; that is eloquent nonverbal testimony that the child is gun-shy. Children who will not respond to a doctor's innocuous questions without first checking it out with a parent are possibly emotional abuse cases. Children who ward off any simple inquiry about their families with the warning, "I don't want you to ask me anything about family secrets," may also be vulnerable. Emotional abuse is seen in parental failure to show helpful empathy to the child.

Projective testing that employs the Rorschach, Thematic Apperception Test, or Children's Apperception Test can be helpful in raising needed suspicions and giving indirect corroboration of our clinically discerned signs of emotional abuse. Overly compliant children when in an interview room with parents may go to the playroom without parents and vigorously beat up on child dolls with parent dolls—not necessarily signifying physical abuse but certainly connoting some failure in the child's received parenting or consumed security.

TREATMENT AND PROGNOSIS

If the abuse is severe enough to cause symptoms of a disorder, even a personality disorder, the treatment of the disorder by expressive therapy is facilitated if adequate parenting, whether by new or accustomed parents, can be brought to bear. Foster home placement, educational help, and any sources of healthy-adult help will make a difference.

The prognosis is brightened if restorative parenting of the child is offered and taken and if the child learns to cope without expecting very much from the original parents. The most dire outcome may be the difficulty that the child, grown up, will have in establishing trust and intimacy with agemates, in marrying and being a reliable and empathic caregiver for children.

Questions for Study and Action

1. Does the indefiniteness of emotional abuse mean, as some lawyers claim, that it should be removed from the statutes that permit the government to intervene in family privacy? Argue each side of the case, and note which side takes the child's welfare into greatest consideration.

2. Should it be easier for an adult to empathize with a child than for a child to empathize with an adult? Explain, using your best vocabulary from child development theory. What do we call the process in which parents demand children to have understanding of the parents' needs?

3. What does it mean to a child if his or her most natural and "soft-fuzzy" comforts are pronounced as wickedly subhuman? Distinguish, for Zora's case, between a stepfa-

ther who showed empathy and one who did not. What specifically would an empathic stepfather say and do? What could Zora's mother have done if she had been more empathic towards the child?

4. Why has it been said that emotional abuse is hard to pin down in a country that allows corporal punishment of school children and the death penalty for certain criminals? Explain the general frame of mental attitudes that are broadcast by both corporal punishment and the death penalty.

5. If you were Zora's parent, male or female, what would your reaction be to her question, "All the kids, even some of my friends, ganged up on me and teased me today. They said I am a bastard. What does that mean? Why don't they like a bastard anyway?" Be very thorough in your reasoning it out.

6. What kind of cultural and emotional climate would lead a 12-year-old child to assert that in his entire life no adult had ever said "I am sorry" to him. Be specific and complete.

7. How hard or soft would be the evidence adduced through projective testing in a court of law? Explain ways that a psychologist's testimony might highlight the greater value of projective testing to ferret out covert attitudes and experiences.

8. Write down what you can imagine Zora's attitudes and fantasies would be at the time her stepfather contrived a chastity belt for her to wear day and night. Don't be afraid to guess and imagine, for that may be a good way to enhance your empathy for a child like Zora.

9. What diagnostic possibilities come to mind when a boy of seven years, fearful and shy, goes into your consulting room after asking you, "You don't think I am a bad boy, do you?" List five outright disorders that such a child might have.

10. What is there about nebulous emotional abuse that may lead to dissociative disorders in childhood as well as adulthood?

For Further Reading

Adams, P.L. The legacy of child murder. In J.L. Carleton & U.R. Mahlendof (Eds.), *Dimensions of Social Psychiatry*. Princeton: Science Press, 1979, pp. 113–121.

Armstrong, L. *Kiss Daddy Goodnight: A Speak-Out on Incest*. New York: Hawthorn, 1978.

Bettelheim, B., *Surviving and Other Essays*. New York: Alfred A. Knopf, 1979.

Garbarino, J., Guttman, E., & Seeley, J.W. *The Psychologically Battered Child.* San Francisco: Jossey-Bass, 1986.

Green A.H. *Child Maltreatment: A Handbook for Mental Health and Child Care Professionals.* New York: Jason Aronson, 1980.

Journal of the American Academy of Child Psychiatry, 24:515–589. (Special section devoted to Children of Divorce.)

Miller, A. *Thou Shalt Not Be Aware: Society's Betrayal of the Child.* New York: New American Library, 1986.

Rush, F. *The Best-Kept Secret: Sexual Abuse of Children.* Englewood Cliffs, NJ: Prentice-Hall, 1980.

Schatzman, M. *Soul Murder: Persecution in the Family.* New York: Random House, 1973.

Stenger, R.L. The Supreme Court and illegitimacy: 1968–1977. *Family Law Quarterly,* VI:365–405, 1978.

31

Child and Doctor in Court

P eople who operate our courts are usually attorneys; they are as adult-oriented as are most laws. For testimony regarding children, these attorneys turn, for more expert information and attitudes, to those who understand child development and children's feelings, thinking, and behavior. Thereupon, the child psychiatrist is invoked for practical advice ("opinion") and for theoretical and hypothetical answers to questions about children. Such testimony by child psychiatrists might help the attorneys to advance the child's welfare, limited, of course, to the degree that a child's well-being pertains to courts and legal matters. In this chapter we shall consider briefly some of the practical clinical issues that involve child psychiatry in these matters.

The major call for a child psychiatrist comes in legal situations such as neglect, various forms of child abuse, custody battles between parents, postdivorce disputation about custody and visitation, infractions of the law (whether status offenses or delinquent acts), privacy and confidentiality, involuntary commitment to mental hospitals, personal injuries to children, emancipation of minors, and termination of parental rights. Each of these will be considered, in this chapter, in an elementary form. There are good texts, listed in "For Further Reading" at the end of this chapter, for the reader who finds forensic child psychiatry to be deserving of a greater depth of understanding.

470

WHAT MAKES FOR FORENSIC EXPERTISE?

Many child psychiatrists feel estranged, even to the point of derealization, during the first few times that they are called to testify in court. Many training programs give child psychiatrists too little preparation for testifying as a partisan child advocate, or as an expert who is presumed to be neutral and fair, or as an identified expert joining in the adversarial system. The expert witness is appointed as such to aid the judge to make a just decision; the adversarial witness has been engaged by one of the adversaries in a litigation—although the uncorrupted child psychiatrist might testify to a truth as (s)he understands the truth, thereby not pleasing at all the adversary who requested the testimony.

What is the point of the adversarial system—a system in which there is a plaintiff ("the people" legally represented by a district attorney, for example, in a criminal charge, or, as another example, the father, postdivorce, who seeks to wrest custody of a child from his mother) and also a defendant? The two sides undertake to contest and demolish the evidence brought by the other side; the accused faces the accuser and cross-examines opposing witnesses. Then, out of the contesting views and evidence a judge makes a decision that accords with the law. If we choose to deprecate the adversarial system, we must be prepared to state whether the inquisitorial system is preferable to the adversarial system. Most people who ponder the only alternative (inquisitional approach) will agree that the system of having adversaries confronting, questioning, and even confounding one another may be better than undercover inquiries, unnamed accusers, and dossiers compiled to be read by the "authorities" who govern. Children, too, in all likelihood benefit most from legal procedures that employ more adversarial than inquisitorial methods. Acceptance of the adversarial, stylized-rhetorical process makes sense generally to the expert medical witness, even if the expert has been appointed by the court and agreed to by both adversaries. Knowing the rules of adversarial proof will help the medical expert to make a better forensic contribution, and not to take too personally the animosities and attacks of lawyers and judges.

Knowing the relevant laws will enhance further expertness. The goal is not to be an attorney but to understand, as an enlightened child expert and citizen must, the general intent and effect of statutes that govern the case about which one will testify. The child psychiatrist knows the general and specific tenor of all the laws that pertain to child victims of abuse and neglect: whether the physician must report suspected cases, what liability the doctor entails in reporting, and so on. Knowing what rules of evidence govern the termination of parental rights, what the law considers to be the age of "accountability" for heinous crimes, what the law holds as the child's rights in courts or mental hospitals or schools, all these are imperatives that rest on the medical specialist who cares for children. This "homework" in knowing the law must be taken up in addition to the duty of long-continuing medical education of the child psychiatrist. One forensic exercise that helps us to learn about relevant law is to have a pretrial conference with the attorneys for one or both sides and to ask them to define or describe the legal issues.

Knowing the jurisdictional domain of the specific court to which one has been called to appear also enhances expertness and know-how of the child psychiatrist. Do matters about children go to a family court or domestic relations court? to a special juvenile court? or to a regular circuit court? In the last mentioned, the "suffering" is shared equally—through a rotation system—by the respective judges, few of whom ordinarily delight in hearing cases concerning children and families. Children and women remain the softest of constituencies for political figures the world over; still, a few attorneys genuinely like to specialize in work with children, serving as advocates or counselors to them, guardians *ad litem* for them and in other ways.

Thorough understanding of the case at hand, from both a psychiatric and legal perspective, is the best preparation for expert testimony. Diagnosis originally meant just that, thorough understanding, so that the case at hand truly can be distinguished from others. Even if one side in a custody battle has subpoenaed the child psychiatrist, the doctor may wish to see the involved persons on the other side too. Even if they refuse, as is their right, some stab at the needed homework has been made. Home visitation, school visitation, adequate diagnostic studies, observations in a variety of settings, conferring prior to trial with the attorneys, all of these will augment expertness and make the testimony more telling.

The last enhancer of expertise to be discussed here in brief outline is the psychiatric report to the court. This should contain little unexplained jargon, should strive to be plain and direct, giving documentation by dates and examples, and be obedient to the rules of grammatical, expository, and effectively rhetorical writing. Otherwise, generalizations that seem impressionistic, prejudicial, and unwarranted will be written down but not inform or persuade the reader and not help the child.

CUSTODY FIGHTS

These fights, legally based on parental ownership of children (remotely by fathers, lately by mothers, more recently by jointly divided ownership), may occur as part of the divorce proceedings or after the divorce has been granted. Many states permit *no-fault divorce* but provide forums for viciously adversarial squabbling about the rights of one or both of the parents to have "possessory conservatorship" or legally mandated proprietorship or joint custody or split or sole custody. It seems doubtful that either no-fault divorce or joint custody will ever be chosen primarily on the basis of the child's best interests; they seem to have been forged in the interests of adults. What children need is the freedom to love *both* parents and to have some emotional access to both parents, without being tossed from pillar to post as may be done when joint custody is defined as 50% of each week with each parent. A child up to the age of puberty and full conscience (usually by 14 years if IQ is normal or above) needs to have a sense of residential and custodial stability, to have a home, to be surrounded by familiar objects and persons, and to be dealt with empathically by responsible adults— not as their extensions, chattels, or projection screens.

The child psychiatrist may be involved in a variety of ways regarding child custody but all of these are in the service of doing the best job possible for the child. Some of the variety of functions is indicated in the following list: encouraging the respective parents to enter into an agreed judgment (Solow & Adams, 1977) about custody for the child's welfare; reporting on the special circumstances of the child's age, gender, and preferences as these affect custody; outlining the needs of the child (or the wants and values) even when these are contradictory and inconsistent among themselves (after all, what most children want respecting parental divorce may be for the parents to be reunited, a wish that does not jibe with reality); tying social/cognitive/emotional/behavioral developmental principles into the observed life situation of the child; speaking out about the primacy for most children of the tie to the mother, and so on. In all these ways, the child psychiatrist does not aim to be adversarial but enters into the adversarial framework and speaks up for the child's interests and rights. Some courts welcome such testimony.

LEGAL INFRACTIONS BY CHILDREN

Children can be rule-breakers and lawbreakers, and when so accused they wind up in court. The two major categories of offenses charged to children are status offenses and delinquent acts. A status offense is a violation of a law governing only children (persons in their minority status, i.e., not having reached their majority). Examples include sexual promiscuity of the female teenager, truancy from school, running away from home, disobeying teachers and parents, or consuming alcoholic beverages. These antisocial acts are not crimes, but they indicate that a young person is at risk and in need of at least an offer of special services and programs.

Juvenile crimes are alleged and tried and, if proven guilty, the young person is adjudicated as delinquent and placed under the direct care of the court. Although psychiatric care and other human services may be mandated or strongly urged on the minor and parents, the corner has been turned for the child as soon as delinquency adjudication occurs. For a record of delinquency (capable of being expunged in later years in some states) is set up, and the spotlight of the criminal system, not the sociopsychiatric one, is turned decisively onto the youngster so adjudicated. Technically, the court has been interposed between the child and the parent(s) *and* between the child and the psychiatrist. The correctional system is ever close at hand for the court, and placement in a correctional facility remains the ultimate threat that courts can impose on children. It deserves emphasis that the courts and correctional agencies show a higher rate of recidivism for delinquent and criminal acts than do the clinics and hospitals of the mental health system. The crude metric of repeating crimes indicates, therefore, that court diversion into a mental health clinic would be more salutary than a quick and easy adjudication of delinquency.

While child psychiatry and child guidance clinics failed on their promise of solving juvenile delinquency in the U.S. between 1920 and the present, their greater efficacy (compared to that of the courts) for normalizing many delinquents has been well demonstrated. Approaches taken by the FBI, the Law Enforcement Assistance Administration, and even the juvenile courts have been far less effective, if the truth be told.

When the child psychiatrist is at court with a child who has been adjudicated delinquent or, as seems to be increasingly popular with some jurisdictions, with a "minor who has been certified to be tried as an adult," the child psychiatrist again speaks out as a developmentalist who has appraised a minor against a backdrop of developmental norms and principles, as a medical expert who knows both the external behavior and the inner world of significances and fantasies of the youth in question, and as a friend of the court whose special focus is on the interests and rights of the young person who stands before the bar of justice.

The child psychiatrist cannot be unmindful of the fact that ethnic minorities are overrepresented among youths hauled into court, sentenced to corrections, given probation, and seldom referred for psychiatric help; the child psychiatrist knows that poor people's young offspring are also vulnerable to earlier and more frequent arrest and conviction than are the offspring of the affluent. Several child psychiatrists known to the authors have been very assertive in their advocacy on behalf of young delinquents and criminals, and this advocacy has been displayed in child psychiatrists' court appearances, prehearing and presentence psychiatric evaluation and reporting, and willingness to serve as friendly counselor or informal probationer for the young person. Such work is very costly for any child psychiatrist—in time, energy, frustration, and income.

CHILD ABUSE AND NEGLECT

These involvements of child psychiatry have already been considered (Chapters 27–30) and will not be repeated here. The reader might review the earlier chapters.

INVOLUNTARY COMMITMENT TO MENTAL HOSPITALS

So few are the statutes concerning the rights of children, and so new are the judicial decisions in the main, that there is little uniformity across the U.S. in mental health laws governing minors. In some states, because of advocacy on their behalf by concerned "special interests," the laws are more eloquently explicit about retarded youths than about any other subgroup of mentally disordered youngsters. The basic question is whether children are persons or nonpersons, and if nonpersons do they have as much right to liberty and protection as that legal fiction of a person, a profit-making corporation, has?

If the child *is* a person, the constitutional lawyer may assert that a child has a right to be protected under the Fourteenth Amendment to the Constitution of the United States, which holds that no state may "deprive any person of life, liberty or property, without due process of law. . . ." Due process for a child about to be committed (against her or his will) to a mental hospital is held increasingly to involve the following: proof that the youth 1) is deranged by a mental disorder 2) that promises to be amenable to treatment in a mental hospital and 3) not in any less restrictive environment, besides 4) the dangerousness of the youth to self or others; a hearing at the time of commitment with rehearings regularly scheduled, providing legal aid to the youth whenever requested; the child's disorder being thoroughly studied in its history, its probable genesis and etiology, its course under alternative treatment regimens, and the like. It is precisely in all these fact-finding efforts that the child psychiatrist can make a forceful and valuable contribution, for it is fact seeking that reduces both legal and medical error and serves the child best in the long run. The child's mental incompetency must be demonstrated in court before the child can be involuntarily committed to a mental hospital. And incompetency itself is a relative concept. Incompetency varies in degree and over time within the same individual.

COMPETENCY DETERMINATIONS

The law has adopted some rough and ready guides for ascertaining competency and criminal responsibility of young people. Full competency assumes that a person is possessed of a full complement of wits that render one able to distinguish between right and wrong. If a person is substantially deranged by a mental disorder, including mental retardation, the person is not competent. Other forms of handicap or incompetence before the law include: minority status (i.e., simply being young and not at an age to make adult judgments); having a guardian appointed to act on one's behalf; being under the influence of mind-altering drugs when a criminal act was committed; not understanding what one did that was wrong; and not being able to mount an adequate defense of oneself against legal charges or to cooperate with one's attorney. Obviously, the metric for competency is both crude and open to different opinions and conclusions in the specific case, but in law that is not a problem, for the specific case needs a fresh appraisal each time one arises. Law and medicine show similarities here, for in medicine, too, the case of a disorder may not always be a classic case but simply an individualized variant that meets diagnostic criteria only in a general way; the treatment has to be individualized more than the diagnosis does.

The safest course for a psychiatrist when making competency determinations is to do a full evaluation, including psychological testing and neurological workup, as well as the mental examination and an examination of competency per se, both at the present and at the time that the alleged crime was committed. A developmental assessment along social, biological, emotional or affective, cognitive, and behavioral dimensions will be most effective.

CASE 31-1   A 12-year-old Hispanic male named José, accused of having attempted to rape a Hispanic woman of middle age and apprehended by a policeman, was roughed up by the officer arresting him. Thereupon, José attacked the police officer with his fists. Because of the serious charges against him, the state's attorney asked that José be certified to be tried as an adult. The certification followed promptly. The child psychiatrist who evaluated José for his defense attorney (a public defender, since José was impoverished) questioned if the lad would be competent to stand trial as an adult because intellectually his IQ showed him functioning at the level of a normal nine-year-old; his academic achievement was at the fourth-grade level; his cognitive stage according to the Piagetian model was at the level of a ten-year-old; his moral development was that of a five-year-old; his psychosexual adaptation was at the level of a six- or seven-year-old; and his general social skills for the activities of daily life were those of an eight-year-old.

Since José lived on the edge of the Bible Belt, his attorney pleaded that he had not achieved moral "accountability" for his behavior and should not have been certified initially as ready to be tried as an adult. If José were *not* found competent to be tried as an adult, he could—if found guilty—be remanded to a juvenile correctional program for three years; if he were deemed competent and tried as an adult, he ran a good chance of being set free (in an adult probation program) without any form of treatment being provided him. He was "found competent to be tried as an adult," declared guilty, given a suspended sentence, and hospitalized for six months.

CONSENT AND ASSENT TO TREATMENT AND RESEARCH

If a child is not competent to stand trial, that child is probably not capable to give competent consent to treatment or to research participation, but he or she may be—it depends on specific conditions and times. The courts ask repeatedly what criteria can be used to determine a youth's capacity to give assent and consent to medical programs; most hospitals have special committees or boards set up to scrutinize consent and assent (Human Studies, Human Subjects Board, Institutional Review Group, etc.) by minors and adults. Ratios are devised to determine whether risks outweigh benefits; standards are drawn up to determine if the human subject has had a detailed description provided for, and moreover has comprehended, the ordinary ill effects of such a procedure. Even so, at times the agreements and comprehensions actually attained fall far short of true understanding because persons have been presumed to have understood and then consented when, in reality, they only consented without genuine understanding.

If a youth is found not competent to give assent or consent, the parent(s) may do so in their role as guardian(s). If the parents—usually lower-class or belonging to a "nonstandard" religious sect—fail to consent to "necessary" treatment (blood transfusions, antitoxins, antivenoms, vaccinations, and the like), the court (i.e., a judge) may intervene, utilizing the doctrine *parens patriae,* and order that the treatment be provided against the will of the parents. *Parens patriae* originally meant that the king could act as guardian to anyone who was unable to act on his or her own behalf; later it came to mean that the more democratic state was like a parent to all. Invoking this doctrine, governmental authorities have intervened in families where parents as well as children were thought to be acting incompetently. Children's protective services have been based on this doctrine.

TERMINATION OF PARENTAL RIGHTS

Final legal dissolution of a parent-child relationship is rare but some abridgments of the parent-child relationship are not rare whenever parents fail to parent or are not needed by a child. Almost all such "intrusions" into the property rights of parents have been fought fiercely and remain on the top of the list of many rights attorneys who seek to protect parents from any incursions by the state or its agencies. State incursions, however, may include the following: a parent's own petition that the child is uncontrollable; temporary foster care placement of children; adoptive placement of children; legal emancipation of children; and termination of parental rights because of neglect and abuse.

An incorrigible or uncontrollable child *(a status offender)* is made a ward of the court by parental default and petitioning in line with their default. The parents in such situations abdicate some of the legal aspects of their parenting and give their former rights over to the court. Likewise, when parents disappear and children are left abandoned, the governmental agency (such as Children's Protective Services) takes up temporary custody and guardianship of the child(ren) and may require an accounting before custody is returned to the parents. The same situation of relinquishing parental rights occurs when parents are found guilty of heinous neglect or abuse of their children.

Foster care has grown as a way of caring for children who have been abandoned, neglected, abused, or declared uncontrollable by their original parents. It is estimated that over three hundred thousand children are fostered each year in the U.S.; for half of these the fostering is long-term, not brief. Many foster children are not freed up to be adopted and the biological parents are given great advantage over foster parents in most jurisdictions. Foster parents, poorly paid and unsung, can be turned into vigorous advocates for children and their rights, as well as for children's mental health, through what the child psychiatrist Paul Fine has called "networking"—building support groups of foster parents.

Minors can take steps to be *legally emancipated*. It is a legal device to give them adult status. To qualify for emancipated minor status, a child usually is self-supporting (from working for or inheriting funds, usually in fairly large amounts), is competent to manage his own funds or to oversee the distribution of an inherited trust and, in general, can meet the requirements of a fully accountable adult in social skills and judgment. Occasionally, a working class youth of 15 or so can establish himself as an emancipated minor when he can prove that he does not need further guardianship. The child psychiatrist can help greatly in the developmental assessment of youths who wish to be emancipated.

PERSONAL INJURIES TO CHILDREN

A big destroyer of youth in the U.S. is the automobile. Children are killed, maimed, and crippled in automobile accidents. Child psychiatrists (along with orthopedists, neurosurgeons, and physiatrists) may be asked to go to court on such personal injury cases; parents or guardians seek some monetary recompense for injuries resulting to a child from reckless and drunken drivers, truck drivers who fall asleep and crash into family cars, and so on. The ideal would be to have a valid evaluation of the child before the injury—IQ, mental status, presence of psychopathology—so that these could be compared with functioning after the injury. But that ideal may not be possible and inferences about pre-injury functioning must be based on "softer" psychosocial data that can be amassed, such as school records and reports from religious instructors, neighbors, and the like. Then, often aided by experts in vocational rehabilitation, the physician can give an estimated sum as the probable monetary shortage incurred by the injury and aid the court and jury in their award of money for the damages incurred.

PRIVACY AND CONFIDENTIALITY

Since a few children have grown up to to sue their parents for violations of privacy during childhood—as when parents gave permission for an autistic child to be videotaped for medical educational purposes—the issues of confidentiality and respect for privacy are important and practical matters. The child psychiatrist has to know what the age levels are that the law actually uses in granting protections and rights to children, even if some child advocates would choose to extend the age downward from what the law permits.

Parents do have a right to know about the treatment regimen in which their children are involved; often this is not a problem because child and parents come together to the child psychiatrist. Our own ways of dealing with confidentiality are to see the parents first, getting the story of their personal histories and their marriage, as well as developmental history on the child. Only later do we see the child both alone and in the parents' presence. But once we have seen the child alone, we have no further separate contact with the parents, only seeing them or communicating with them in the presence of the child. Parents sometimes regard this as a rather strict and unwelcome way of proceeding, but the children like it and most parents do eventually. The only exception is to notify the parents that there is some danger of serious harm being done. Even on such occasions, the child psychiatrist alerts the child and gives the child an opportunity to out-argue the psychiatrist.

Certainly no written communications to courts, schools, or other agencies should be undertaken without prior knowledge on the part of the child and a general right of the child to veto what is written. Even when the child has agreed, parents may need to be consulted, for they may have substantial objections to the written report. Many children seem to benefit from that spirit of respect shown to them by an adult.

In all of these operations on behalf of children before courts, the child psychiatrist is a biomedical and biosocial expert on human development and on mental state who makes developmental science available to lawyers and judges, thereby advocating for what is best for the involved child.

Questions for Study and Action

1. Distinguish between the legal doctrines of *patria potestas* and *parens patriae*. In what kind of family or social fabric did these doctrines originate?

2. Argue for parents as time-limited *guardians* of their children, as opposed to owners and arbiters. What differences would it make if parents were legally defined as temporary guardians for their children, whose guardianship would terminate as soon as the "defect" of the child disappears?

3. Explain, as if to a newcomer to the U.S. from an Asian country, the differences between the adversarial and inquisitorial systems of adducing legal evidence.

4. Outline for a surgical colleague, who has been called to court to testify about a brain-injured child, what steps he can take to give more effective expert testimony. His original contact was in the emergency room, with the comatose child, the mother who was driving and died the next day, and the mail carrier who had only minor abrasions and contusions and kept pleading how guilty he felt to have lost control of his truck and hit the mother and child head-on. Advise your colleague fully about what he can do to upgrade his forensic expertise and give more meaningful testimony.

5. You have been invited to join a panel presentation before a social work group on the topic of "Mothers Are Best for Preschool Children." On the panel with you are:
    (a) a male psychologist, spokesman for Father Power, a group contending that fathers should have more rights to custody of preschoolers;
    (b) a lesbian social worker who, despite her husband's muckraking and denunciations, obtained custody of her four-year-old son;
    (c) a civil liberties lawyer known to be an advocate for gender-neutral legislation and who says, on statistical grounds, too many women are awarded custody of young children.
    Outline your approach so you could counter their various arguments and take a decisive stand of your own.

For Further Reading

Adams, P.L., Berg, L., Berger, N., Duane, M., Neill, A.S., & Ollendorff, R.H.V. *Children's Rights.* New York: Praeger, 1971.

Block, J.E. Beyond parenthood: Toward a guardianship model for parenting. *Social Policy,* pp. 41–46, March/April, 1980.

Caffey, J. Multiple fractures in the long bones of infants suffering from chronic subdural hematoma. *Am. J. Roentgenol.,* 52(20):163–173, 1946.

Chesler, P. *Mothers on Trial: The Battle for Children and Custody.* New York: McGraw-Hill, 1986.

Giarretta, H., Giarretta, A., & Sgroi, S.M. Coordinated community treatment of incest. In A.W. Burgess et al. (Eds.), *Sexual Assault of Children and Adolescents.* Lexington, MA: Heath, 1968.

Radbill, S.X. A history of child abuse and infanticide. In R.E. Helfer & C.H. Kempe (Eds.), *The Battered Child* (2nd ed.). Chicago: University of Chicago Press, 1974.

Schetky, D.H., & Benedek, E.P. (Eds.). *Child Psychiatry and the Law.* New York: Brunner/Mazel, 1980.

Schetky, D.H., & Benedek, E.P. *Emerging Issues in Child Psychiatry and the Law.* New York: Brunner/Mazel, 1985.

Solow, R., & Adams, P.L. Custody by agreement: The child psychiatrist as child advocate in custody determination. *J. of Psychiatry and Law*, 5(10):77–100, 1977.

Wallerstein, J.S., & Kelly, J.D. *Surviving the Breakup: How Children and Parents Cope with Divorce.* New York: Basic Books, 1980.

West, D.J. *Delinquency: Its Roots, Careers and Prospects.* Cambridge, MA: Harvard University Press, 1982.

III

CHILD AS
FAMILY MEMBER

In Part III we consider more systematically the family context of the child. Most of a child's life, even survival, depends on the functioning of his or her family. There are some irreducible patterns, functions, and structures that will aid a child, while others will be heavily pathogenic, and we believe the beginner in child psychiatry should be challenged to work with a sick child's siblings and parents.

Families are heterogeneous and diverse and have a host of ways of responding to stresses and crises. Chapter 32 takes a look at the phenomenon of divorce—or, better stated, the phenomena of divorce—in its impact on a child. Divorce and remarriage, adoption and de-adoption are fraught with psychiatric significances for children. Chapter 33 reconsiders the family that the child leaves whenever the child has to be hospitalized, as well as the meaning of the separation and of the hospital to a child. Chapter 34 examines the snags and pitfalls besetting parents and children who are easily the gravest victims of parental distortions. In Chapter 35 we venture to sketch the outline of what a wholesome family can do for children.

32

Divorce, Adoption, and De-Adoption

DIVORCE

There is now little doubt that the effect of divorce on children is deleterious. The incidence of psychiatric problems in these children is higher than in those children from intact families, and the long-term and second-generation effects have only just begun to be realized.

The student should bear in mind that the older professional literature tended to take a much too optimistic view of the potentially harmful effects of parental separation and divorce. Such complacent attitudes are no longer justified in the face of the better scientific methodology of the new studies. The effects of divorce constitute a clinical problem.

ETIOLOGY AND PSYCHOPATHOLOGY

The impact of divorce on children is predicated on the disruption that divorce conflict brings to the developmental process. Predivorce adjustment is of lesser significance than the process of divorce and its effects on parenting. The handling of the divorce by the parents and collateral caretakers, such as relatives and teachers, and the reconstructive work done by all concerned adults significantly influence subsequent development. The central psychopathological features are regression, grief that sometimes develops into depression, anger, guilt, lowered self-esteem, and yearning for the absent or noncustodial parent. Psychosexual and moral identifications suffer, perhaps especially in male children.

CLINICAL DESCRIPTION

This depends partly on the child's age (i.e., developmental stage) when the divorce occurs.

Preschool children (up to 5 years of age)

Regression, especially in the most recently acquired developmental achievements, is the hallmark of the reaction in the preschool age group.

CASE 32-1   Olga, age 3½, had just begun attending nursery school when her father moved out. Although a shy girl, she had mastered an initial moderate separation anxiety about leaving her mother and joining the nursery school class. Following the parents' separation, Olga *clung* to her mother and *cried inconsolably* when her mother brought her to school. With great difficulty, she was persuaded to stay, but then *hung onto the teacher* and *barely participated* in the activities. At home, she reverted to *"baby talk"* at times and had "accidents" of *wetting* the bed at night and *soiling her underwear* during the day. She had great *difficulty going to bed* and *would not fall asleep* for hours, frequently coming out of the bedroom and checking whether her mother was still there. On these occasions, she expressed the *fear that she would be left* as soon as she fell asleep.

Early school-age group (5–8 years)

Open grieving and deterioration of school performance are typical.

CASE 32-2   Bruce was 7½ years old when his parents separated. Previously well-adjusted, he became *listless,* responded with *crying spells* to frustrations that he previously took in stride, *lost much of his ambition* in Little League baseball (where he had been one of the better players), and was *in turn querulous and aggressive with* or *withdrawn from peers.* His teacher complained that Bruce *did not pay attention,* seemed to *daydream* a lot, and *did poor schoolwork,* which was unlike him, as he had been a good student.

Older school-age children (9–12 years)

The characteristic response is anger, in addition to the responses described for the younger group.

CASE 32-3   Andrea had just turned 11 when her parents' marital difficulties culminated in a separation, closely followed by divorce. Although her relationship with her father had had a number of ups and downs, she now felt he was the "good guy," being booted out by the mother "witch." She turned all her *anger* toward her mother and *yearned* for her father's rather irregular visits. She started *associating with "the wrong crowd,"* a peer group who *tested* the outer limits of their parents' discipline, of which there was not a lot to begin with. Whenever Andrea's mother tried to intervene, Andrea became very *angry, accusing* her mother of "*not caring for my needs.*" Her *behavior at school and academic performance* took a nose dive and, at the same time, she started spending a great deal of time in the school nurse's office. She had a seemingly *insatiable need* to talk with the nurse and showed the same *clinging behavior* with some of her teachers, while she presented severe discipline problems to others.

DIFFERENTIAL DIAGNOSIS

This is obviously no problem when the onset of the child's reaction is clearly related to the marital breakup, but may present difficulties when the child's symptomatology is of long duration. Here, careful inquiry may reveal a long history of impending divorce. At times, however, Conduct Disorders and Attention–Deficit Hyperactivity Disorder may coexist or the child's anger, depression, and scholastic difficulties are very similar to those diagnostic entities. Referral to a specialist is then necessary.

TREATMENT

Treatment is almost entirely psychotherapeutic and always multidimensional; that is, it must address all parties and problems appropriately:

1. *Psychotherapy* of the child gives support and reassurance (whenever that is appropriate and realistic) that he or she will be cared for in spite of the parental split. Insight-oriented psychotherapy may be required to deal with the child's guilt that (s)he brought about the divorce.

2. *Parental counseling* offers support and guidance to the parents so that the divorce does not result in too drastic a decrease in parenting. Some disruption of the parenting function is to be expected, and the usual diminution can be handled by short-term counseling. If, however, depression in a parent seriously interferes with parenting, appropriate psychiatric treatment for that parent is urgently indicated.

3. *Family therapy* is very helpful. It is best, of course, if both parents are willing to participate. Even if one parent, usually the noncustodial one, refuses, it has value in being both economical and effective unless the individual psychopathology (usually the parent's) is more than can be handled by this approach.

4. *Psychopharmacology* with antidepressants may be indicated if the child's grief reaction has turned into clinically substantiated depression. This should be decided by the specialist.

PROGNOSIS

Separation and divorce are *always* very stressful to the children. This is the case even where there had been a great deal of marital strife and even abuse. How the child will come out of this crisis will depend to a great extent on how the loss of the intact family is dealt with and, to some extent, on the quality of new relationships. We should remember that even under the best of circumstances, a loss will be sustained.

The following factors promote good prognosis:

1. The strengths the child brought to the crisis.
2. A continuing good relationship between the child and both parents.
3. A reasonable degree of understanding and absence of fighting between the parents.
4. The willingness of each parent, regardless of custodial arrangements, to take responsibility for all aspects of the child's development and coordinate it with the other parent. Reliability, continuity, and good quality of the visitations by the noncustodial parent are necessary facets of this factor.
5. The availability of a supportive network outside the family—teachers, school counselors and, of course, relatives.

By the same token, a *poor* prognosis will result from continued strife between the parents, rejection and neglect by one of the parents, lack of resolution of previous difficulties (especially abuse) by the divorce, and continued psycho-pathology (usually depression) in a parent, especially the custodial parent.

Some of the negative *consequences* of divorce are chronic depression (in both mother and child), difficulties in sexual role identification and, especially in boys, a possibly higher rate of delinquency. When parents divorce, if the children are left with the mother (which may be warranted emotionally), the family will often be plunged into poverty, which does not help their morale.

QUESTIONS FREQUENTLY ASKED BY PARENTS

Q. Isn't joint custody the ideal way to settle custody disputes?
A. On the surface, perhaps so, but in most instances there are considerable practical difficulties. Many authors have, by now, rejected this solution except in highly individualized instances. The children often complain that, far from giving them two homes, it gives them no home. Joint custody appears a popular idea with noncustodial parents (usually the father) and many lay-men argue its merits more for their personal needs than for the best interest of the child.

Q.   Is it not better for the parents to divorce than for the child to be exposed to their unhappiness or strife?

A.   This used to be a popular notion, and one wonders how many adults have used it as a rationalization to pursue their whims and gratify their own needs. It appears, though, that children will put up with a lot of parental difficulties for the sake of the security of being cared for by both parents. It is the *parenting, not* the *general* or sexual or occupational functioning of the parent, that is important to the child. Moreover, the relationship between the parents does not end with divorce: fighting, arguing, even assault, do not end with divorce. With "no-fault" divorce, custody has become the last domain to be gained or lost, and many parents, especially the fathers, now make it a personal competitive issue to win or lose custody, regardless of their long-term ability to care for the child—that is, regardless of the interests of the child.

Q.   Should a parent remarry as soon as feasible in order to give the child a two-parent family?

A.   No matter how problematic the relationship with the biological parents, that relationship is not given up by the child. Therefore, haste on the single parent's part is inadvisable, not only for obvious adult reasons, but even in the face of the child's pleadings "for a daddy" (or "mommy," as the case may be). Leaving a residence and moving into a new one and change in school systems are other considerations. The interrelationship of stepparent and child and stepparent and parent can produce a number of outcomes, depending on the child's personality, the new stepparent, and the "hidden agenda" of the biological parents. The situation can be further complicated by stepsiblings. The physician's role should be one of a cautious, empathic participant observer without preconceived notions or theories.

Q.   How do I explain the divorce to my child?

A.   Every child deserves an explanation. The timing and content, however, should be appropriate to the child's age. That is, a preschooler should not be told explicit details nor far in advance. A 12-year-old boy, by contrast, will appreciate some of the background issues and should have some advance notice. It is difficult for the parent to keep his/her anger and vindictiveness out of the explanation, but a definite effort should be made in that direction. The advice is cogent, that a parent should apologize for the conflict and disruption brought onto the child by the divorce and then say, "You have a right to love both parents as much as you wish to. I don't love the other parent any longer but you have a right to love both and have access to both."

ADOPTION

We address here not only the parents' and children's reactions to adoption but also the thorny issues of incidence and types of pathology manifested by adopted children. Adoption is one way for people to rear children without giving birth to them. Adoptions have kept down the numbers of American children who have no parental force in their lives to around one million children, most of whom are in "children's institutions."

Any consideration of the psychiatric aspects of adoption has to begin with the current socioeconomic and demographic situation. Nowadays, more couples are seeking to adopt, adoption often occurs at later ages for both the parents and the children, transcultural and transracial adoptions are becoming more common in this country, and the adoption of children with a variety of handicaps is no longer a rarity. All of this provides a much larger arena for a broad range of problems to develop. Recent laws allowing adoptive children access to their biological parents have added a forensic complexity to an already intricate situation.

PARENTAL REACTIONS

A range of emotions and defense mechanisms occurs in the parents of adopted children.

Preadoption reactions—These have become more varied since the advent of transracial adoptions and the adopting of children at a later age of both the parents and the child. The classic reaction of parents was to their infertility, still a common problem, but its incidence has been modified downward by the present trend to adopt children in addition to one's own, biological children. Another preadoption inclination is to desire the adoption of the children from a new spouse's previous marriage.

However, the main preadoption issues are still the inability to have children, and the feelings of inadequacy and low self-esteem on the part of the infertile parent; the other parent often feels angry. The couple may have feelings of loss and depression because of the absence of any children. Adopting is a reminder that people want to care for children for many different reasons.

Reactions to adoption—These reactions are usually the final common pathway of a welter of cultural, social, and personal preconceived notions, biases, prejudices, and misconceptions. Morality enters the scene, too—the adopted child was illegitimate, therefore conceived in sin according to Puritan logic—and finally, pseudoscience makes its appearance, claiming that all adopted children are of inferior biological endowment (Adams, Milner, & Schrepf, 1984; Hersov, 1985).

Other psychopathological features in the adoptive parents at the stage of adoption are increased anxiety, self-doubt, and, above all, overprotection.

Postadoption reactions—Successful raising of an adopted child requires reasonable resolution of the psychopathology just mentioned. This is sometimes interfered with by the child him/herself when the child's psychogenic or biological difficulties appear to confirm the parents' worst fears. Dire prophecies seem to be fulfilled—in the worst way—when the child's behavior does not conform to expectations; normal variations of experimentation, aggressiveness, and assertion of independence are misinterpreted and magnified to the point of becoming self-fulfilling prophecies. As we shall see presently, the *potential* harm that this array of parental psychopathology represents is converted into *real* harm by the contributions of the adopted children's very *real* problems.

THE REACTIONS OF THE ADOPTED CHILD

The child's reactions, viewed chronologically, show as the first and most complex reaction that of the infant to the interrupted bonding process with her or his natural mother. The effects of this intervention are almost impossible to delineate with any certainty, given the deficient state of the art of clinical mental evaluations of infants.

The next emotional hurdle for the child to overcome is the acquisition, processing, and integration of the fact that (s)he is adopted. *When* to tell a child about being adopted has been a longstanding matter of dispute. No longer is the seemingly easy and straightforward rule of telling the child almost immediately universally accepted. It has been realized that telling a child, "You have been chosen," may have different, not always benign, meanings. Most important, a young child does not understand the full meaning of such general statements until after starting first or second grade (around age 7).

Therefore, many authors now recommend that adoptive children be told at a later stage about adoption, in terms that are less likely to induce a feeling of insecurity and exert less pressure to perform or to conform to the parents' expectations. Such terms omit the theme of being "chosen" in favor of a more honest and realistic, yet nonetheless positive, explanation of the adoption.

This is all the more important since adopted children fantasize that their natural parents rejected or did not want them, perhaps because the latter were "bad" or unworthy of them.

Beyond the question of when and how to impart the knowledge of adoption, this knowledge causes a feeling of unwelcome differentness and difficulties in forming a comfortable and stable identity. Moreover, it constitutes one of the issues in the psychopathology of adopted children.

PSYCHIATRIC ILLNESS IN ADOPTED CHILDREN

This is the most controversial and emotional topic of the entire subject of adoption. A great deal of psychiatric literature has tried to maintain that there is no difference in the biological parameters between adopted and natural children. This position was particularly popular and suitable to the state of the art prevailing in child psychiatry in the two decades following World War II, when nurture (i.e., environment) was deemed paramount, to the near exclusion of hereditary nature (i.e., innate biological factors). The following is an attempt to present a balanced overview of the "common ground" of psychopathology in adopted children.

First, there is a substantial body of literature, in addition to a great deal of clinical experience and anecdotal reports, that adoptive children have a disproportionately high incidence of emotional disorders and psychiatric disorders in general. The specifics are as follows:

The most frequently reported difficulties having a higher incidence among adoptive children are those involving poor impulse control. In the younger child (through the primary grades), this impulse dyscontrol involves primarily aggression; in the prepubescent and pubescent child, it also involves sexual impulses. Associated with these impulse control disorders are antisocial behaviors and runaway episodes.

Ten-year follow-up studies on adoptive children in Sweden likewise have uncovered a significantly higher rate of maladjustment in school, with poor attention span, hyperactivity, and interpersonal problems with peers (Bohman, 1972). Other studies, both here (Offord, Aponte, & Cross, 1969) and in Britain (Humphrey & Ounsted, 1963), have emphasized the differences between children adopted within the first six months of life and those adopted after six months of age. The latter had more psychiatric difficulties as well as more disruptive behavior, stealing, and destructiveness. These results were, however, influenced by the quality of care in the adoptive homes.

Although we cannot be certain, we can offer some plausible speculations about the causes of the difficulties mentioned for adopted children. Many adopted children have young (teenage) mothers; these mothers are often exposed to a lot of stress, and the infants themselves have a high rate of pre- and perinatal difficulties, such as low birth weight (Crellin et al., 1971).

Moreover, genetic selection is another factor. Parents who have to give up their children for adoption are often immature, impulsive, and have histories of developmental disabilities (learning disorders); and, almost as often in the case of men, they have delinquency or criminality and trouble in general with authority (Hersov, 1985; Seglow et al., 1972). The difficulty in drawing direct conclusions from the latter considerations (antisociality) lies in the finding that most adoptive children also have problems other than delinquency. However, the first part of the "equation" holds true in many instances: many adoptive children have developmental delays, manifested in Attention–Deficit Hyperactivity Disorder and/or Developmental Learning Disorders, with their symptomatic ramifications.

Another set of possible etiologies are the interactional disharmonies between the adoptive parents and the child, i.e., the reactions to adoption by parents and children that we described earlier in this section. To illustrate the complexity of factors operating when an adoptive parent and child have drifted apart, we present the following case vignette.

CASE 32-4   Norice was 11 years old when she was seen in psychiatric consultation designed to assist the department of social services. *Norice's mother* had requested social services to find a *foster home* or residential treatment facility for Norice, because the two of them just *could not get along* with each other anymore.

Norice was *adopted* at age five years, but had been raised by her adoptive parents since the age of three months as their *foster child*. When she was three years old, the foster father died, and her foster mother never remarried.

When Norice was interviewed, all of her *complaints centered on mother*. She was angry at always having her older siblings (mother's natural children) *held up as sterling examples*. The three older siblings, now all out of the home, had been good students and were supposed to have been *"perfect."* But Norice knew that one of her sisters had to get married because she was pregnant. Every time Norice was friendly to a boy, mother would *"predict"* that she, Norice, would *wind up in the same trouble* as her sister.

Norice stated that she was convinced her mother had not adopted her out of love, as she had been told, but in order to please her husband and cement a crumbling marriage, i.e., the patient attributed *ulterior motives* to the adoption. She felt mother was *racially prejudiced* against her (Norice was part oriental and her foster mother was white).

The report by the mother and caseworker indicated that Norice was doing poorly in school because she had a short attention span and seemed to be more involved in constant interaction with peers (lately mainly boys), instead of paying attention to her teachers. She had been described by most of her teachers as having *a problem with authority* and her relationship with *peers* had always been *"turbulent"—possessiveness* towards friends, followed by *animosity* when friends did not devote as much attention to her as Norice thought they should. Most recently she was described as "willing *to do almost* anything in order to be *popular with boys.*"

Norice herself stated that she *"hated" her adoptive mother* and did *not consider her as her mother* at all; she told the examiner that her biological mother, whom she had never seen and knew nothing about, was and "would always be" her *"real and only"* mother.

Nevertheless, when it came to discussing the notion of foster home or similar placement, Norice showed *little enthusiasm for living anywhere except* with her adoptive mother. She expressed anger as well as anxiety over what she termed her biological mother's wish to get rid of her. As a matter of fact, Norice had made several abortive *suicide* attempts when she was *overwhelmed* by loneliness and feelings of rejection, worthlessness, and not belonging anywhere.

Comment. Norice showed problems specific to being an adopted child in that she could reject the "bad mother" (adoptive mother) and keep the idealized "good mother" (the natural mother), thus splitting her image of her mother long past the age when both images should have been fused. As a result, her sense of identity and feelings of belonging and of security were poorly developed; her suicide attempts, at a relatively early age, reflected this lack of a secure "base." On the other hand, we can guess about the genetics of her attention deficits and poor impulse control without even starting to take a look at the adoptive mother, who may, after all, be the major factor in making this child's life so problematic. The point we want to make is to approach this, and other cases, without preconceived notions of etiology or pathogenesis.

The same statement can be applied to treatment: It is more helpful when embarked on with an open mind.

TREATMENT AND PROGNOSIS

Treatment has to be highly individualized; the clinician's view of the adoptive child patient should be broadly comprehensive. Some adoptive children will present with disorders for which a positive family history would be expected, e.g., Developmental Learning Disorders, Attention–Deficit Hyperactivity Disorder, or Conduct Disorders. Without a real family history to relate to, the way is open to fantasies of exaggerated proportions. On the other hand, the problem may be predominantly based on the parents' reactions, or even their psychopathology. The fact that the child is adopted, together with the knowledge of that fact, often provide first the parents and then the child with a convenient scapegoat and resistance to getting at the underlying interpersonal problems. In other words, adoption is blamed for all the troubles. It is the therapist's task to see through this and to seek out all the underlying etiological factors, including (but not limited to) the facts and fantasies of adoption.

Once this has been done, therapy can proceed along whatever lines are indicated, again *including but not limited to* working through the contributions of adoption to the clinical problems at hand.

Prognosis should be viewed both as short-term and long-term. Short-term prognosis (i.e., symptomatic improvement) is more directly a function of treatment than long-term prognosis, which is less influenced by treatment and more so by constitutional/genetic factors in the child and the psychological "profile" of the adoptive parents, *and* the "fit" between the two.

By and large, the long-term prognosis for adoptive children is good, and, at the very least, better than if these children had been left in their original circumstances. No such general statement can be made about short-term prognosis, which is individually determined.

DE-ADOPTION

In our experience, this has become a clinical entity, pathogenic but fortunately still quite rare.

As the name spells it out, de-adoption refers to the undoing of a previously consummated adoption. Although this can occur at any age, it appears that most cases have been observed when an older child was adopted. This age group can also be expected to be most directly hurt by de-adoption.

CASE 32-5   Oscar was *seven years old* when he was *adopted* by a couple who had been his foster parents for a few months.

Oscar's own history consisted of a series of foster home placements after removal, at age three years, from his biological mother's home because of neglect. Prior to the most recent placement, Oscar was known as *hyperactive* and *difficult to manage;* he was enrolled in remedial classes in school for a *Developmental Reading Disorder.*

The adoptive parents were in their *early thirties, upwardly mobile, childless,* and this was their first experience with having a foster child. They decided to adopt Oscar soon after his arrival at their home, for they concluded that Oscar needed a sense of belonging and the assurance that he would stay in one environment and have predictability and love. They were convinced that this would help his hyperactivity, too.

Five months after the adoption had occurred, the parents sought psychiatric help, because they found it increasingly difficult to cope with Oscar and because their own relationship (their marriage) was imperiled. They complained how Oscar repeatedly managed to mobilize one parent's protective instincts for the child against the other parent. In spite of weekly psychotherapeutic sessions, the parents felt that these difficulties were insoluble. Their initial enthusiasm to *"save this child"* turned to despair and an attitude of complete *nihilism.* They felt there was *only one* solution—de-adoption—in spite of psychotherapeutic, pharmacological, and educational help then being given to Oscar.

The de-adoption took place eight months after the adoption. The child reacted with obvious sadness. Fortunately, he had entered treatment together with his adoptive parents, and was being treated both individually and in family therapy until his family ceased.

Oscar had initially been found to have difficulties in communicating verbally in psychotherapy. Following de-adoption, these difficulties escalated to the point of near mutism. There was a change of therapist and the new therapist encouraged Oscar to communicate through drawings. This turned out to be a very productive medium, and Oscar communicated both his pain and sadness and his willingness to try new relationships, after all. His subsequent improvement took everybody by surprise: the therapist, the school, and his new foster parents. Five months later, Oscar communicated well and was content in the new foster home. He expressed relief that he was in his present foster home, which he considered "normal," as compared to the adoptive home, which he called "too pushy" and "hard to understand what they wanted." Whatever it was, to Oscar it was too much. Oscar was also helped by "post-de-adoption" intervention, i.e., by family sessions with his former adoptive parents so that all three of them might work through their feelings.

Nevertheless, the process of de-adoption was viewed as *terrible punishment* for having done something *bad.* Oscar felt *guilty* because he *did not meet* whatever *expectations* his adoptive parents had of him; he thought it was *his fault* and because he could not measure up, he was *worthless* and *unlovable* and *deserved to lose the adoptive parents.* He later came to see the de-adoption more realistically and became less self-lacerating.

Comment. Oscar's case had a relatively good ending. Probably due to the lack of "fit" between adoptive parents and child, an incompatibility of such proportions developed that the return to what the child knew as a "normal" foster home environment was perceived as a great relief. The environmental change was accompanied by psychotherapy before and after the de-adoption. The pain of such a blow to the child's self-esteem was typical and severe. The case presented also illustrated the expected scenario: adoption late in the child's life; unrealistic "rescue fantasies" on the part of the adoptive parents usually caused by previously unnoticed psychopathology; and contributing difficulties intrinsic to the child, such as Attention–Deficit Hyperactivity Disorder or Conduct Disorder.

There is as yet no secure body of knowledge about de-adoption, and the clinician should follow his or her clinical skills and knowledge of child psychiatry in general, as applied to adoption and subsequent "object loss," viewing de-adoption as the loss of a relationship very important to the child. The parental reasons for de-adoption most often cluster around personality disorders or unresolved neurotic conflicts affecting *their* self-esteem. A tenuous marriage, no matter how good it looks on the outside, is the hinge for the revolving adoption–de-adoption door, be it to save that marriage or as a consequence of a breakup of their marriage, for which adoption of a difficult child was the "last straw."

Questions for Study and Action

1. A white, middle-class, childless couple in their late thirties ask your advice about adopting as a means to bolster their sagging marriage. What are your thoughts, especially when we add that this couple may have to wait several years for a white, healthy infant but may be offered sooner a transracial adoption of an older, or handicapped, child?

2. You are working with a couple in marital counseling. It seems to be nothing but a chronic agony. Somebody suggests that you should recommend divorce and make "successful divorce" a goal of your treatment. What is your thinking about the

appropriateness, propriety, and clinical aspects of this approach? Should you remain neutral? or should you try to "save the marriage"?

3. What is meant by "divorce counseling"? Is it the same as the suggestion in Question #2? What postdivorce counseling may be called for?

4. Discuss your own thoughts about the old theme, "We stay together because of the children." Is it possible to take a stance either for or against this line, i.e., is it possible to be absolutist about this issue? Why?

5. You are asked to help save the marriage of a couple, knowing that the husband has abused both children and is still considered dangerous in that respect. What kind of treatment contract will you make? What will be the goal of what treatment?

6. A white single woman would like to adopt a black child. There is a body of opinion that opposes transracial adoption on the grounds that this black child will be accepted neither by the white community of the adoptive parent nor by the black community of his biological parents. Articulate the arguments for and against such a proposed adoption.

7. A 10-year-old adopted child tells her adoptive parents that she wants to meet her biological mother. Formulate a plan to evaluate the causes for this request and how to help the parents and the child. Should they become locked in a struggle over this issue? How would you proceed?

8. You have evaluated an eight-year-old child as part of a custody fight. The child, not surprisingly, wants the parents back together; however, this is also the earnest wish of one of the parents. How will you proceed?

9. Discuss the statement, "No-fault divorce has moved the conflagration *from* between adults *to* among child(ren) and parents."

10. From the child's interests, what are some disadvantages of joint custody? Do the advantages outweigh the deficits?

For Further Reading

Adams, P.L., Milner, J.R., & Schrepf, N.A. *Fatherless Children.* New York: Wiley Interscience, 1984.

Bohman, M. A study of adopted children, their background, environment, and adjustment. *Acta Paediatr. Scand.,* 61:90–98, 1972.

Crellin, E., Pringle, M.L., Kellmer, D., & West, P. *Born Illegitimate: Social and Educational Implications.* Windsor, England: National Foundation for Educational Research, 1971.

Hersov, L. Adoption and fostering. In M. Rutter & L. Hersov (Eds.), *Child and Adolescent Psychiatry. Modern Approaches.* Oxford, England: Blackwell Scientific Publications, 1985.

Humphrey, M.E., & Ounsted, D. Adoptive families referred for psychiatric advice. I. The children. *Brit. J. Psychiatry,* 109:599–608, 1963.

Offord, D.R., Aponte, J.F., & Cross, L.A. Presenting symptomatology of adopted children. *Arch. Gen. Psychiatry,* 20:110–116, 1969.

Seglow, J., Pringle, M.L., Kellmer, D., & Wedge, P. *Growing Up Adopted.* Windsor, England: National Foundation for Educational Research, 1972.

Sorosky, A.D., Baran, A., & Pannor, R. *The Adoption Triangle: The Effects of the Sealed Record on Adoptees, Birth Parents, and Adoptive Parents.* New York: Anchor/Doubleday, 1978.

Wallerstein, J. The impact of divorce on children, *Psychiat. Clin. N. Amer.,* 3:455–463, December 1980.

33

In the Hospital

GENERAL CONSIDERATIONS

We shall introduce first of all the basic reactions to hospitalization by both the child and the parents, and the factors influencing their reactions. Next, we shall illustrate some of them more closely, with descriptions of the child with congenital heart disease. That particular diagnostic category was chosen as the paradigm because of its great technological complexity today, as well as its realistically life-threatening seriousness, calling for all the technical and psychiatric skills of all involved health care providers.

The most important psychic reaction of both child and parents—the common denominator—is to the separation that occurs when the child is hospitalized. The form and consequences of this reaction will depend on several circumstances:

IN THE CHILD

1. *Age*—The most vulnerable age is from one to four years of age; under the age of one year, the effects of separation depend on the quality of substitute care. For children over four years of age, the effects of separation are influenced more heavily by the nature of the specific illness.
2. *The nature of hospitalization*—Hospitalization may include procedures that bring

499

sensory deprivation, considerable pain, possible embarrassment (especially in older children) and immobilization. These are stressful for the child.

3. *The basic personal characteristics of the child*—More active, perhaps more oppositional, children seem to fare better, even though they are more troublesome to the staff. Children with preexisting anxiety will usually do worse.

IN THE PARENT

The most troublesome factor here is a constellation of insecurities, or needs to control, or guilt of whatever origin, resulting in conflict with the hospital staff. Such parents may be unable to let hospital staff take over when that is appropriate and may displace or even project their own anger onto the staff. This may go so far as signing the child out against medical advice, or result in continued strife which increases the child's anxiety.

Other noxious factors in the parents are reaction formations resulting in staying away from the hospital, and, in the worst case, using the child's hospitalization as a welcome opportunity to "take a vacation" from "the burden of child rearing."

THE HOSPITAL

These are mainly matters of hospital policy. Most hospitals are now quite aware of the importance of allowing parental (especially maternal) attendance; nevertheless, the level of sophistication among hospital staff, especially those with less training than the registered nurses, varies. Poorly trained and poorly motivated ancillary staff can wreak havoc, even where the official hospital policy is enlightened.

THE LENGTH OF HOSPITALIZATION

Hospitalization is no longer considered to produce inevitably all of Bowlby's stages of complete separation from parents (protest-despair-detachment) (Bowlby, 1951; Bowlby et al., 1956). Children make adjustments to the hospitalization, some positive, some negative (regressive).

THE REACTIONS TO HOSPITALIZATION

Having discussed the contributing factors, we will now address the reactions themselves. We may again point to a common denominator: regression. Not all children regress perceptibly, but many show signs such as whining, thumbsucking, wanting to be fed, or wetting the bed, even though they had mastered those tasks prior to hospitalization. Behavioral difficulties, such as agitation or hyperactivity, are also encountered and are often precipitated by circumstances of partial sensory deprivation, confinement, or immobilization.

PREVENTION AND PROGNOSIS

When hospitalization is planned, the child can be prepared by age-appropriate explanation of what to expect, including the pain and discomfort attendant upon the procedures to be performed. It is very helpful to involve the parents in this process since they, and especially the mother, are potentially the most effective therapists.

Preparation is, of course, impossible when the hospital admission has been an emergency; nevertheless, preventive work can be started upon admission, especially with and through the parents.

Preparation/prevention improves prognosis, especially for short-term hospitalization. Good prognosis in long-term hospitalization requires regular parental support and affective input on one hand, and "mainstreaming" (i.e., near-normal activities and tasks, especially schooling), on the other hand. Depression, various anxieties (e.g., equivalents of castration anxiety or fears of death) call for appropriate psychotherapy and, in the case of depression, pharmacotherapy, both usually fairly short-term.

THE CHILD WITH CONGENITAL HEART DISEASE AS A PARADIGM

Some children have unsettling experiences, maddening home lives, crippling accidents, and are born with congenital defects, inborn errors of metabolism, and temperamental styles that may make parenting of them difficult. Or, they may acquire serious diseases and injuries that soon usher in an attendant mental disorder. Our point is not to argue for a chronology that puts trauma or injury ahead of the mental disorder but simply to introduce the notion that serious mental disorder sometimes interacts with a physical impairment—the "reactive disorders." The child with a congenital heart defect is the subject of this section and will exemplify this interaction. One place to locate this problem in DSM-III-R is in Psychological Factors Affecting Physical Condition (316.00).

Three problems can be delineated for easier overview: first, the effects of the congenital heart disease itself on the child's functioning and development; second, the impact on the parents of the child with heart disease and the resulting special interactions that parents enter into with these children; and finally, the effects of the modern hospital's diagnostic and operative procedures on both child and parents.

CLINICAL DESCRIPTION

The effects on the child

These depend on the particular congenital cardiac anomaly but can be broadly divided into the acyanotic and cyanotic group. Cyanosis produces greater developmental delays and greater overall incapacitation. Since it often demands multiple operations, the cyanotic group demands more psychiatric attention.

CASE 33-1   By the time he was eight years old, Ben had had five operations to correct his Fallot's tetralogy. He was a *thin* youngster, the *smallest* child in his class. His parents were concerned about his *nightmares,* his *persistent worries,* and his *recurrent complaint, "Why me?"*—i.e., why was he the one to have to suffer all these difficulties? When a *sibling* had been born two years earlier, Ben fully *expected* her to have the same difficulties and was sorely perplexed to find that she was *healthy.*

Ben was a *daydreamer* in school and could make up the most *fantastic stories* at the drop of a hat. Yet he never directly expressed his anger in words, although he was showing progressively more tantrums and destructive rages. His mother came to the conclusion that she had contributed to this by *granting his every wish* in the past, especially before operations. But, she added, it was so difficult to see him scared and suffering, particularly when he had *repeated operations.* When hospitalized, he clung to the parents and perceived their leaving him as *rejection* and as punishment; indeed, he viewed the operations as *punishment,* too.

Comment. Ben's reactions underscore the child's perceptions of what modern cardiac procedures are all about; *we* know that they are lifesaving, but the child interprets them in the only way he can at his age: as a hostile intervention. And since every effect has its cause, it must be parents' anger that has resulted in punishment.

The effects on the parents

The parents' trials and tribulations start with the diagnosis of congenital heart disease and usually affect the mother much more than the father. As the diagnosis is often made soon after the birth, while the mother and infant are still in the hospital, mother is then caught in a highly vulnerable state, especially if the delivery was exhausting for her. Guilt and inability to deal with the anger over such a misfortune are almost universal reactions. Reaction formation is one defense mechanism used; denial is another; displacement onto the medical staff yet another. The most frequent attitude towards the child is overprotectiveness. However, withdrawal from the child can also occur.

CASE 33-2 Erica's mother was *told* about her daughter's transposition of blood vessels on the third day following delivery by an *alarmed* (and alarmist) nurse. The message was that Erica was seriously ill and would have to be transferred to another medical center for specialized surgery. This was followed by a more considerate explanation by the cardiologist, who nevertheless told mother that the transfer was *urgently* necessary.

Mother vividly remembered this episode and developed an attitude of *expecting danger* for her daughter at all times. She would not *let the child* out of her sight. Mother admitted that she thought Erica's heart condition was really her—the mother's—*fault* and *retribution* for her *not wanting* to have yet another (the third) child at that stage in her life.

Mother's *overprotectiveness broke down* when Erica faced her third hospitalization. She had insisted on a "rooming in" arrangement but subsequently *could not face Erica's crying* and *refused to visit* her except rarely. Fortunately, the *father* was a sensitive and supportive man who sat with Erica and made up for mother's absence to a significant degree.

Comment. Although early lifesaving intervention is necessary in a number of cases of congenital heart disease, the way in which the diagnosis and treatment plan are presented to the mother carry additional noxious potential. Guilt, self-blame, and regressed, infantile thinking characterize many a mother's reaction to being confronted with information that her newborn child, an extension of herself, has a life-threatening "deformity."

Highly ambivalent feelings in Erica's mother resulted in denial, reaction-formation (overprotectiveness), and, finally, overt rejection.

The interaction between parent (usually mother) and child is colored by both the parents' and the child's reactions to the illness and to the procedures. There is really nothing specific to either set of responses. The heart is imaged by many people as *the* most vulnerable organ. Therefore, most responses are more intense than would otherwise be the case.

The younger the child, the more the child will reflect parental reactions with fears of abandonment or rejection; that seems to be the special perspective that the child brings to the interaction. Rage is an almost universal reaction of children—they mirror the parents' rage. In the child, the rage is often overt; in the parents, it is repressed. The postoperative depression so often seen in grade-schoolers may represent further rage turned against themselves, or may be a defensive posture against further injury (as is sometimes seen in nonhuman animals). In addition, depression arises from the pain and incapacitation of the operation, the separation from the parents, and the sense of helplessness in the face of an extensive surgical procedure; the latter brings in its wake severe restriction of activity. Both the child's rage and depression present the parents with affects that they may not be able to deal with: controlling the child's rage may seem inadvisable ("if he cannot let his anger out, it will make his heart strain . . . and kill him . . ."), yet the more permissive the parents are, the worse the expressions of rage seem to become.

Relationships with peers are often interrupted because cardiology checkups do not allow the child to participate in all activities, and the identification with peers and the spreading of emotions to peers is thus interfered with. The drives continue to be largely focused on the parents, for whom this is an added burden.

The effects of the hospital procedures

Modern corrective surgery not only involves the usual fear and pain of any operative procedure but also surrounds the child with a confusing array of high technology. Although the medical centers specializing in these procedures have considerable psychiatric sophistication, there is still often a considerable gap between the children's and parents' emotional needs and what is provided.

CASE 33-3   Georgina was six when she was scheduled for her third corrective surgery. She was an outgoing child, and there existed excellent communication between her and her equally outgoing parents. She was *prepared* for her surgery with the help of the *therapeutic playroom,* where she delighted in trying out the various pieces of equipment. She tolerated the procedure well. However, it turned out she would have to be *operated on again two weeks later because the procedure* could not be done in one session. Although this had been entertained as a possibility, the social worker who was taking care of the family counseling felt that the *preparation* should be done "one step at a time." The parents, too, stated that they "did not have the heart" to tell Georgina of the possibility of the fourth surgery. When this operation was undertaken, the child reacted with *depression: crying, poor appetite, irritability, lack of interest,* and above all, *poor cooperation* with the medical and nursing staff. The child accused the parents of lying to her; she developed separation anxiety and vacillated between *solicitous anxiety* and *truculent oppositionalism* to both parents and doctors.

Comment. Repeated operations represent a dilemma to the parents. They have "their hands full" with the operation at hand; the child wants an optimistic assurance that "this will be it." The decision about whether to forewarn and prepare the child for multiple operations is a highly individual one and depends on:

- *The child's age*—The younger the child, the more advisable it is to prepare *only* for the immediate future, i.e., *one* operation;

- *The parents' tolerances*—If the parents are guilt-ridden and anxious and have put up overdetermined (i.e., multiply determined) defenses against this guilt and anxiety, they (the parents) may be unable to prepare the child for multiple interventions;
- *The child's adaptive capacities*—Children with Developmental Learning Disorders, Attention–Deficit Hyperactivity Disorder, or similar maturational difficulties are less suited for multiple operations. By contrast, children who are verbal and used to communication can better absorb multiple operations.

TREATMENT

This consists of two entities: prevention and the treatment itself.

In terms of prevention, dynamic verbal counseling should be (and usually is) undertaken both pre- and postoperatively. Preoperative counseling should start simultaneously with the diagnosis (i.e., as soon as the diagnosis has been made) and should be initiated and initially carried out by the cardiologist; subsequently, it should be done by the surgeon. The attending medical specialist's involvement in the counseling for the child and the parents cannot be overemphasized: the parents as well as the older child (late preschool, but certainly school-age children) understand the central role of the physician and need to hear explanations and plans directly from him or her. Communication between the physician and the parents is of paramount importance. The cardiologist or cardiac surgeon is not expected to become a psychiatrist; however, it is his duty to explain the diagnosis and procedures patiently, and as clearly as possible, to the patient's parents. This can go a long way towards defusing their guilt, fear, and shame. If he or she can, the medical specialist should try to gain some knowledge of children's perceptions, so that the procedures can be explained to the child in terms of intelligible *gains,* thus defusing the child's fantasies of pain and punishment.

The foregoing are minimal skills expected of the medical specialist. Certainly, the more he/she can counsel the patient and family, the better he/she will be as an all-round doctor in the real sense of the word, and the better will be the results of the surgical procedures.

The physician-specialist is no longer alone, however. Most centers have a "child development specialist" at hand to help in the preventive work. This is usually a specially trained social worker or nurse. Teamwork is the leitmotif in the psychosocial management as it is in the surgical procedures. Teamwork does not mean "passing the buck" when it comes to facing distraught parents or difficult children; it means directly facing as many questions as possible and referring to the other discipline those situations where one staff member feels additional work is necessary.

The use of special toys has become fashionable to the extent that they are used as a "shortcut" or easy way for some staff to avoid the more time-consuming traditional give-and-take of appropriate play interaction and dialogue.

CASE 33-4   Purnell, who was seven at the time, was given a special doll with representation of the heart and large vessels to play with and was asked to show the specialist what *he* imagined was going to be done. This was done the day after the hospitalization at the medical center where the operation was to be performed. Purnell *refused* to do anything with the doll and actually appeared to be *scared* of it. However, he established a *good relationship* with the resident physician assigned to him. This young woman addressed his fears and questions during her *rounds*, listened and talked to his parents, and, when it was time for the operation, Purnell was prepared.

Comment. No "stage prop" can take the place of human interaction. Moreover, a child cannot absorb all the information at once. Children, as well as their parents, need more than one session to grasp the essence of the operation *emotionally.* People do not entrust their lives to a knife-wielding surgeon primarily out of intellectual understanding; they do so out of trust. This trust exists as faith in an institution (the prestigious medical center), but this is often barely enough to get the patient through the door. For the patient really to turn his or her body and soul over to the doctor, there must exist a *relationship* of personal trust based on considerations more primitive, and more compelling, than mere intellectual grasp. Such a relationship must be established through personal contact, both verbal and (especially) nonverbal.

Adults regress when in the hospital, i.e., go back to less mature, more primitive, modes of mental functioning, when immersed in the specialty-focused atmosphere of the medical center. In the case of the parents, transference reactions take place—they endow the institution and staff with parental, magical qualities and powers. A similar reaction occurs in the child, who, in turn, has a limited repertoire of coping devices, the chief ones being reliance on helpful adults and mastery through repetitive play, so that being passively victimized is turned into active mastery. This is the basis for "playing doctor."

The skillful staff makes constructive use of these attitudes. The staff must always be supportive. The parents must be kept from excessive expectations of magic or miracles (excessive positive transference) without destroying their positive expectations of help.

At this juncture, we will offer a word of reassurance to all members of the cardiac team: parents and children bring varying degrees of preexisting psychopathology to the present cardiac situation. The child's congenital heart disease in the first place, and the subsequent stress around its diagnosis and treatment, exacerbate and intensify previous psychopathology. The regression just referred to brings transference reactions that are both positive and negative. The latter may be expressed as accusations that the staff had not communicated clearly or sufficiently or not shown enough empathy and sensitivity. The staff may have tried very hard but, because of excessive psychopathology, cannot succeed. This is where the psychiatric consultant *must* be called in: the regular team can be expected to take care of average and expected reactions but cannot undertake the kind of crisis intervention that only an experienced psychiatrist can provide.

PROGNOSIS

This will logically depend on the underlying heart disease, the child's constitutional/temperamental endowment, and the parents' adaptability and the extent of their psychopathology. By and large, the prognosis for the acute reaction is good. Overprotection and similar reaction formations by the parents may result in chronic neurotic disorders and personality disorders. The handling of anger and the self-image and, subsequently, self-esteem in these children often reflect their special status in both the family and school. A significant factor in the prognosis is the overall treatment given.

Questions for Study and Action

1. In the case of Ben (33-1), outline an intervention involving work exclusively with his parents. What would you ask them first of all? What suggestions would you offer them?

2. How would you proceed to help Erica's mother (Case 33-2) if your time with her had to be limited to three one-hour sessions? List the agenda items you'd want to cover as you plan the three sessions.

3. What helpful psychiatric suggestions would you make to the pediatric surgeon working with Georgina (Case 33-3) in order to prevent and treat her reactive mental disorder?

4. Many infants born with congenital anomalies or defects find their parents in a grief reaction. Describe four major elements of such a grief response in the parents, trying to explain their grief in more depth than the realistic situation provides. Specifically, include in your discussion concepts of parental bonding, the husband-wife relationship, parental narcissism, and parental empathy for a helpless infant.

5. Viewing congenital heart disease (CHD) as one precipitant of a reactive disorder in the infant's mother, contrast the maternal symptom picture when a child is born profoundly mentally retarded to that when the child has CHD.

6. Try to imagine the situation of an expectant father who would prefer a healthy boy baby but delivery brings him a girl with severe cerebral palsy. List 10 of the pathological symptoms that the father may display.

7. Handicapped children are at risk of reactive attachment disorder. Why? Review a) the symptoms of the disorder, b) the relevant psychosocial stressors (ordinarily Axis IV), and c) argue for the symptoms being direct resultants of the stresses.

8. DSM-III-R permits us to make some imputations of etiology—both genetic and psychosocial. The psychosocial stressors are in the forefront for Reactive Attachment Disorder and Post-traumatic Stress Disorder. What are some psychosocial stressors associated with:
    (a) Attention–Deficit Hyperactivity Disorder in a six-year-old?
    (b) Simple dog Phobia in a four-year-old?
    (c) Adjustment Disorder with depression in an eight-year-old whose parents divorced?
    (d) separation anxiety in a five-year-old entering kindergarten?
    (e) Obsessive-Compulsive Disorder in an 11-year-old following masturbation to orgasm?

9. Name four disorders for which genogenesis ("genetic causation") seems important. Next, list 10 disorders for which sociogenesis ("psychosocial causation") seems weighty. What did a famous psychiatrist mean when he stated, "People drive people mad; people make people sane"?

10. Discuss preventive intervention, preoperatively, with a two-year-old and a five-year-old boy who must have his right leg amputated. What are the cognitive differences between the two? body image differences? verbal communication differences? differences in play skills? differences in "castration anxiety"? What difference would there be in preoperative intervention?

For Further Reading

Apley, J., Barbour, R.F., & Westmacott, J. Impact of congenital heart disease on the family. *Brit. Med. J.*, 1:103–105, 1967.

Bowlby, J. *Maternal Care and Mental Health*. Geneva: World Health Organization, 1951.

Bowlby, J., Ainsworth, M., Boxton, M., & Rosenbluth, D. The effects of mother-child separation: A follow-up study. *Brit. J. Med. Psychol.*, 29:211–247, 1956.

Cassell, S., & Paul, M.H. The role of puppet therapy on the emotional responses of children hospitalized for cardiac catheterization. *J. Pediat.*, 71:233–239, 1967.

Douglas, J.W.B. Early hospital admissions and later disturbances of behavior and learning. *Develop. Med. Child Neurol.*, 17:456–480, 1975.

Ferguson, B.F. Preparing young children for hospitalization: A comparison of two methods. *Pediatrics*, 64:656–664, 1979.

Prugh, D.G., Staub, E.M., Sands, H.H., Kirschbaum, R.M., & Lenihan, E.A. A study of emotional reactions of children and families to illness and hospitalization. *Am. J. Orthopsychiatry*, 23:78–82, 1953.

Quinton, D., & Rutter, M. Early hospital admissions and later disturbances of behavior: An attempted replication of Douglas' findings. *Develop. Med. Child Neurol.*, 18:447–459, 1976.

Vernon, D.T.A., Foley, J.M., Sipowicz, R.R., & Schulman, J.L. *The Psychological Responses of Children to Hospitalizations and Illness.* Springfield, IL: Charles C Thomas, 1965.

34

Distortions of Parenting

Parenting presupposes our learning of basic attitudes, information, and skills that we are never taught. Since parental behavior is not instinctive—phylogenetically preprogrammed—we are left for the most part unprepared and ignorant of how to be effective parents, or else to catch bits and pieces through an idiosyncratic ontogenetic learning and development. Most of our childhood training for parenthood results from imitation and identification with our own parent or parents. But that may be slipshod and incomplete, leaving us to learn for the most part on the job, by trial and error, when we are adults and thrown into parenting. Playing by ear is not an ideal way to learn it, for the resultant role playing is based on unconscious determinations of identification, transferences, and repetition compulsion, and so is prone to distortion, lack of full awareness, and comes to us *faute de mieux,* with a lack of informed choices. Perhaps, with such a universal shortage of training for parenthood, the surprise is that so few parents kill, ignore, neglect, and abuse their children. Some do all of those things, as we saw in Chapters 27–30. Now in this chapter, we focus on the mechanisms played out within parents as they copulate, bring children into their lives, and move towards either sharing an existence with their children or not. It is far easier to become a parent than to *be* one.

INDIFFERENCE TO THE CHILD

If a parent is committed to life as usual, not even wanting to take a leave of absence from work when the baby is born and avoiding contact and attachment to the baby, that mother or father is probably an indifferent parent. Fathers, because of societal structuring of the male adult role, more easily than mothers find ways to exempt themselves from any meaningful child care. Workaholic leanings conveniently take a parent away from children.

Also, the ease with which some fathers can leave marriages with children is an index of how little those fathers feel involved in parenting. When they do claim custody, on the other hand, the balance is tipped to the father's advantage, for then the mother is put "on trial" (Chesler, 1986). Finally, a stark example of parental unconcern for children is seen in the unwed fathers who never take up a committed relationship with either the baby or the baby's mother. By 1982, this became a situation of epidemic proportions when 56.6% of the black babies born in the United States were born out of wedlock (*Statistical Abstract,* 1986) and, therefore, usually each baby became the sole responsibility of the single female parent. Married or not married, fathers display widespread indifference to their offspring, often taking comfort from the social ideology that child care is women's work.

Sometimes a young couple who have had little occasion for adolescent sexual opportunity and expression (they may even have repudiated a certain "promiscuity") exult in the permitted sexuality within marriage. As if making up for their late start, they become so enamored of conjugal relations that they are an embarrassment to old friends and relatives. Their lives become overly domesticated as they withdraw their conjugal pair from wider social contacts and, behind the closed doors of monogamy, they "discover" the joys of lust old and new, plain and fancy.

Aided by contraceptive technology, a young couple may develop sexuality as a form of recreation (not for procreation) and may decide together that each will, in imagination, be a baby to the other. They keep their relationship sexually focused and seldom consider the option of bearing a child or children. The Satyricon spirit will prompt them to "open marriage" or group sex more readily than to childbearing. They do not want to be parents but to revel in eroticism that, on health grounds, they would have done better to start earlier, for then they might have been ready to move on before they got to be 30. Since they do not want children they may remain barren.

If such a hypothetical couple do have a baby, they arrange to keep their former roles paramount and thereby develop a family with a strictly conjugal emphasis, in which family a baby is an interloper made to adjust to the parents' wants. That sort of family is made for role reversal: "The baby can just accept our terms and adjust to our lifestyle." That attitude entails an abdication of parenting that falls short of outright neglect and abuse: "Let the baby cry, for (s)he has to learn some time; why not now?"

Hired child care is sought and if it is of high quality, the child certainly is luckier than when abandoned or put in a foundling home (as a lot of parents all over the world still do with unwanted offspring). Not all day care is beneficial to children because some programs lack a focus on the children. Yet we acknowledge that day care now, at the end of the 20th century, is essential because maternal employment is a necessity for financial reasons. Perhaps the marketplace breeds and reinforces indifference to children. Surely, since 1980, hundreds of thousands of women and children have joined the poverty class in the U.S. Our nation is the only "advanced" country in which most of its children live in poverty.

Indifference to a child emerges not only from the conditions mentioned up to now (the baby was unwanted, the parents are centered on their own sexual relationship, the parents demand that the baby serve their wants and meet their expectations, the child is abandoned, the child is eagerly turned over to *anybody* else for child care), but also from certain unavoidable situations that make the parents unavailable to the child. The child, needing parental care for his/her very survival, experiences parental unavailability *for any reasons* as if it were indifference and rejection. A mother who grieves for a dead parent is not available to her infant; a father in prison or in a mental hospital is not available; a poverty-class mother works and is not available; a parent who gets attention diverted to another child who happens to be sick is not available to the baby; a parent who can be "present" for a helpless baby may not be "with" the walking and talking child to such an emotionally involved extent. In all those examples, the child may *feel* abandoned and rejected and that the parents are indifferent, while in reality the parents are devoted, but human, playing other social roles simultaneously with being caretakers for an infant. It would be an egregious mistake to hold the parents totally responsible for all the frustrations and disappointments that come to infant and parent.

TOLERATION OF THE CHILD

Certain parents want to have children because they feel that a good marriage is only a prelude to a good family. They may do what others expect, however, and not what they profoundly desire. Then, when the wife becomes pregnant—perhaps mainly because she has been scripted to obey the motherhood mandate—and then the baby is born, little joy attends the child's presence with the adult couple. Or joy may be outweighed by sorrow. A detachment—a drawing back from parental empathic engagement—occurs, and in its place is a spirit of cool toleration. That toleration maneuver does not make for a happy child. Indifferent to the child and to the child's wants, such parents set up a cold war coexistence with the child, never wanting to give in (or give out) much more than they have to.

The child may be well fed, protected from gross harm, well regulated, and allowed a home life like that of a cooperative boarding house in which the child plays a nonpaying boarder's role. The child perceives it as a nonloving arrangement, as (s)he puts in time growing up without expecting warmth and caring from others. The child is seen but not heard. An unwanted child is rejected, and feels it, even if the parents practice coexistence.

Obviously, the child who is merely provided for and merely tolerated will be lucky to find a loving grandparent, teacher, or adult family friend who is truly interested in children and has warmth to share with that child. While still young, a preschooler, the child may be love-hungry and, when older than five or six years, may despair of getting any love from adults and rely for acceptance on agemates, peers. The tolerated child is probably better off than the child with highly intrusive parents, much as a cold-war reign of terror internationally is better than nuclear holocaust.

TAKING OVER THE CHILD

Certain parents are like animal tamers, trainers, zealous pedagogues, wanting to lead the child and follow theories and notions, not children. They find a child's wildness and strong will to be an embarrassing reflection on their competency, so they take over control of the child's behavior and total existence.

In 1858, the widely read German pediatrician, Daniel G.M. Schreber, wrote in favor of this attitude in his *The Book on Educating Body and Soul,* describing how the child, *one year old,* should be brainwashed:

> Our entire effect on the direction of the child's will at this time will consist in accustoming it to absolute obedience. . . . The thought should never even occur to the child that his will could be in control; rather should the habit of subordinating his will to the will of his parents or teachers be immutably implanted in him. . . . There is then joined to the feeling of law a feeling of impossibility of struggling against the law; a child's obedience, the basic condition of all further education, is thus solidly founded for the time to come. (cited in Schatzman, 1973, pp. 21–22)

Schreber was that type of parent in dealing with his two sons. He devised restraints to prohibit touching of genitals, instituted a regimen of punishment to keep them ambidextrous and using alternate hands in motor activities, and imposed a domestic war against children's natural learning proclivities. He effectively brought his two offspring under his domination. One son committed suicide in adolescence; the other became the famous paranoid judge of Freud's

"Schreber case," whose delusions centered on being robbed of his mind and of his soul being murdered. The delusions reflected one by one his actual child rearing, causing some reviewers to question whether madness originated in son or father (Schatzman, 1973).

Contemporary examples of what Wilhelm Reich (1945) called "emotional plague" and others, such as Alice Miller (1981), called "poisonous pedagogy" are to be found in parents who provoke their children to wrath and oppositionalism, only in order to overcome the rebellious child by brute force. Scenes of this kind of provocation are daily occurrences on public transportation, in supermarkets, and on playgrounds. The final appeal is to the child's guilt that (s)he has her or his own mind, own will, own attitudes, and own feelings. The guilty child, abjectly defeated, conquered, gets started on the path of forever pleasing parents or feeling bad. Happiness is equated with hierarchy: the parents are rulers and children are their subjects. Living in this kind of family gives the child training in irrational authority, an authority based on unshared power, rank, and privilege: "Do as I say." *Why?* "Because I can force you to do things my way."

When the taken-over child grows up and has children, the child-become-parent identifies not with victimized children but with aggressors and again imposes irrational authority on the next generation. The cycle of guilty subservience does not end.

If the taken-over child becomes a psychotherapist when grown up, the likely preference will be for directive, intrusive approaches. Behavioral therapy that seeks only to modify the child's behavior according to values that are the parents' and not the child's may illustrate this. In expressive therapy that disbelieves the child's feeling unloved or persecuted, the secret agenda may always be to get the child to acquiesce to the parents. In family group therapy, the now-adult therapist who was subjugated to parents as a child will ask, "Who's in charge in this family?" and will endeavor to "join with the family," meaning the parents, doing whatever possible to enshrine the parents (or one of them) and to bring the family under the effectively reigning Fourth Commandment: *Honor your father and mother so you won't be killed by them but can live a long life.*

AGGRESSING AGAINST THE CHILD

Oftentimes, parents who were abused in their own childhood will identify with the active aggressor and not with the person who was victimized. They "convert" passive victimization into active aggression against children. Identification with the aggressor gives them a mindset to justify almost any form of violence against children, ranging from infanticide to child battering to justification of corporal punishment. "Spare the rod and spoil the child," they say. Or, having become co-conspirators with their oppressors, they proclaim, "My parents gave me many a shellacking (or whipping or beating) and it didn't harm me," or "It was for your own good."

Infanticide reached a peak in the 19th century in Europe. It is still widely practiced in India, Japan, and other countries. Female infants in particular are regarded as dispensable. Today, in the U.S., many children's deaths are actually infanticide but are written off as sudden deaths, crib deaths, or accidental smothering, falling or drowning. The taboo against infanticide in the 20th century does not always hold strong.

At the international level, the U.S. ranges between placing 10th and 17th in lowering its infant mortality rates; other nations with fewer resources have lower rates that are reported to the World Health Organization. Although higher infant mortality rates do not mean infanticide automatically, those rates are indicative of a low valuation on the survival of young children—a kind of moral extension of the infanticidal spirit into public policy, it would seem. Another way to view these high infant mortality rates is that they are institutionalized infanticide, impersonal but reflective of social arrangements within a given nation.

Physical abuse and punishment of children also seem to be partial materializations of this same infanticidal spirit (see Chapter 29). Parents who would not kill or batter their children may justify stringent corporal punishment of children. And many parents, even if they exercise restraint and seldom thrash the child, see it as an expected thing that children may be beaten, are often beaten, and will always be beaten. "A child is being beaten" is an accurate statement about reality, not an odd fantasy, in our times.

Young children often have the idea that as they grow, their parents will diminish in size and power. They plan a revenge, identifying with the aggression that they have suffered: "When I am grown up, I shall beat my parents." Many do grow up to beat their parents, according to numerous observers of maltreated elderly parents.

Parents of child psychiatry patients frequently report that their offspring remind them of one of their own parents. They say that to highlight their animosity, not love, towards the grandparent-equals-child. Hence, it is not a compliment to the child but a criticism. It is a distortion of who the grandparent is, who the parent is, and who the child is. It is a distortion that has been called "life negating."

RELATING TO THE CHILD THROUGH SPLITTING AND PROJECTION

The mechanisms of splitting, overidealizing and debasing, and projection (described as operative in childhood personality disorders in Chapter 20) are also used by parents, in distortions of parenting. All that is evil within the parent is denied, through splitting into an idealized good self and a derogated bad self. The bad self is then projected onto the child and made to take over the child. The child is no longer perceived as a separate being but as a projected extension of the parent, needed as an emblem of Satan, close to the parent because it is a projected part of the parent, but also distanced from the parent because the child has been converted into an alien persecutor.

Some clinical examples of splitting and projective identification are the following: an incestuous father who believes that if his daughter had not been seductive he would not have molested her; the single mother who believes that her two-year-old son is a hyperactive and incorrigible sociopath; the father in a mental health profession who believes his child is innately bad, originally sinful, and sees "clear indications" of innate sin or aggression in his child; the mother who looked into her daughter's eyes and saw the Devil there so vividly that the mother shuddered and drew back.

The child who is the repository of parental projections feels an obligation, first of all, to be as bad as (s)he is regarded by the parent to be. The child senses the distortion, but does not know quite what it calls for. The child truly has an identity problem under those conditions: "If I am only a projection screen for my parent(s), then who am I? How can I discern and be my real self when I am so inundated by my parents' projections?"

The child who is aggressed against—whether sexually as in fondling and molestation accompanied by brainwashing or by being exploited through kiddie pornography or prostitution, or physically or mentally—is a child on whom are heaped inner distortions by the parents: role reversal, identification with the aggressor, splitting and projective identification, as well as a number of less crude distortions in everyday family life.

NARCISSISTIC MERGING WITH THE CHILD

The parent who relates to the child with narcissistic identification lacks even the capability for separation and individuation shown by the projecting parent. Such a narcissistic parent cannot know normal admiration and empathy for another person, so the other person (the child) is perceived as a part of the parental self, an appendage, a pseudopod that can be let out and retracted but the child is not permitted to exist as a separate being. The parental self or Ego is amoeboid and the engulfed child is not a distinct Thou. The basis of parental narcissism is usually said to lie in a defective self-concept, elaborated when the parent was an infant, under 30 months of age, and reflective of an ambivalent, inadequate attachment from which the infant (now our parent) was unable to differentiate and become imbued with an adequate sense of autonomy.

Otto Rank (1930) described how a parent finds in the child-offspring the embodiment of the parent's idealized Self and the parent's vehicle for biological immortality, but the child struggles against that narcissistic engulfment by the parent. Many writers describe difficulties in individuation in children but few describe it from the parent's angle. Rank was an exception to that trend. Harry Stack Sullivan was another. Sullivan, while not believing that the Oedipal triangle was universal, pointed out that the father (or mother) would presume that the same-sex child was "easily understood" merely because the parent could recall a same-sex childhood. So the parent would deal in stereotyping and, by a kind of narcissistic merger, would never talk with the same-sex child about feelings, motives, and experiences. Presuming everything, the same-sex parent tended to question nothing and, hence, to live in an illusory relationship with the same-sex child; the child sensed the lack of empathy and turned to the opposite-sex parent for comfort and genuine acceptance, according to Sullivan (1953).

Some narcissistic parents, narcissistically identified with their child, do not gloss over what the child is really like and turn away, having become unavailable emotionally. Instead, they bedeck the child, through compulsive overintrusion, with clothes, skills, and belongings. Child and parent become mirrors of each other and the parent tries to ward off any shame by pushing the child to excel, look good, and not reflect badly on the parent. That leads to overmonitoring the child for fear that the superadequate façade will break down. Ballet, music, sports, math, karate—the "enrichment" is unending. Such children are miserable with their overly administered lives and resultant deficits in spontaneity and self-esteem. Alice Miller (1981), in her *Drama of the Gifted Child,* wrote:

> The parents have found in their child's false self the confirmation they were looking for, a substitute for their own missing structures; the child, who has been unable to build up his own structures is . . . dependent on his parents. He cannot rely on his own emotions, has gained no experience in trial and error with them, has no sense of his own real needs, and is alienated from himself to the highest degree. Under these circumstances he cannot separate from his parents, and even as an adult he is still dependent on affirmation from his partner, from groups, or especially from his own children. (p. 14)

Over and over, because the primary self is formed by age 30 months, we see how distorted parenting is transmuted from generation to generation. That first 30 months, as we have stated earlier, is not only formative of all our attitudes of self-regard but also of our parenting skills—the gut-level, willy-nilly reactions that one day we shall replicate with our own offspring.

Parents under the influence of narcissistic identification with a child may be overprotective, guarding against any breach of infantile symbiosis. David M. Levy (1943), the child psychiatrist who brought the Rorschach test to America, studied "maternal overprotection" closely. Levy concluded that the earmarks were "excessive contact, infantilization, and prevention of independent behavior" (p. 37). Beside those three, he named a fourth marker, "lack or excess of maternal control" (p. 38), referring to a biomodal distribution among his overprotecting mothers, with one group being "dominating" and the other being rather like "indulgent" lackeys to their overbearing children. Today, we would have to remark the perpetuation of an infantile symbiosis in overprotective parents, their predilection for the helpless child who admits of only mirroring and merger in a narcissistic undifferentiated membrane of parent-child.

Many parents feel best with young infants and, if they have more than one child, will "dread the day when the baby can stand on his own and say no." If they are narcissistic parents, they will finds ways to delay separation and individuation between themselves and the infant. The last statement would be objected to by Heinz Kohut who disagreed with Sigmund Freud's view that narcissism is a regression from object relations or that narcissism is normal for infants but pathological for adults. Kohut did not see narcissism as fading out, with object relations taking over. Kohut thought narcissism develops along its own lines, and relatedness to others develops along a separate pathway, a Kohutian formulation directly echoing the early formulations of Otto Rank. By that token, parental narcissism only develops and changes consonant with the changing of the growing child's own narcissism. And, the child's narcissism *and* relatedness do mature, again along separate developmental lines.

CONCEPT OF THE GOOD-ENOUGH PARENT

As a gesture of compassion towards often-maligned parents, some people in the mental health professions cite (perhaps wrongly) the late Donald W. Winnicott, British pediatrician and child analyst, in a lowering of ideal standards for parents when they espouse the doctrine of "good-enough" (if not optimally good) parenting. The rationale of some writers about parenting is that children can forgive some parental blunders—indeed they can, particularly if the parent apologizes to the child—and so parents need not feel called (employing a metaphor from Roman Catholic dogma) to live by counsels of perfection, only by the counsels of everyday moral living that apply to an ordinarily moral and empathic human being (in the Roman Catholic tradition).

The parent who is good-enough, in the figurative language of the Gospels, would be one who obeyed the law, the Ten Commandments, but the one who did better than that would "get rid of worldly goods, give them to the poor, and follow me," striving for something above a bare minimum of good parenting. The gap between good-enough and good can be quite wide. And, unfortunately, what seems good enough to the parent may not be good enough in the eyes of the child. We shall return to optimal parenting in the next chapter, "A Family for Children," and show there what is good for the child, from the child's perspective.

Suffice it to say now that an almost slavish servitude by an adult is all that will be good enough for the infant. Winnicott (1953) defined the good-enough mother as one who "starts off with an almost complete adaptation to her infant's needs and as time proceeds she adapts less and less completely, gradually, according to the infant's growing ability to deal with her failure."

A mother, because of her depression, may not be good enough to attend to her growing child, in empathic commitment. A delusional parent, as we saw in Chapter 23, may move to inculcate her delusions into the child. That is not good enough. A father more eager to succeed in business (even the business of a medical practice) than in child care may be of zero worth in the eyes of a child, however rapidly his "net worth" in property may be augmented. A parent with detached study habits, coldly observing the child's behavior while withholding "libidinized interaction," may not ever abandon detachment and adopt a posture of loving empathy. That seems not good enough.

DISTORTIONS OF EVERYDAY LIFE

We want parents to tell us of their own "baby families," their position in the sibling group, and the nature of their parents' interactions with them. It is a good tactic to ask both mother and father, if both are available, about her and his life situation when they were the age of the child whom we are to see. We also ask parents who this child we are to see reminds them of, in order to see what "identifications of everyday life" they may be imposing on the child.

The little girl whose mother blurs together the little girl and a hated younger sister (the girl's maternal aunt) finds it difficult to retain her true self when her mother keeps distorting who she is. The little boy whose father unconsciously equates him with an alcoholic older brother (the boy's paternal uncle) finds it difficult to assume his true selfhood, for his father's expectations induce him to be other than the boy is. We have seen sensitive, imaginative children who took to heart a parent's contempt when the parent said, "You eat like a pig," or "You had better stop wetting the bed so you can set a good example for the new puppy." In a flash, both children in our examples felt dehumanized and cast into subhuman roles by what the parents said. Those everyday-life indentifications by parents came as concrete derogation to the children. These equations, like parables, were very short sermonettes to express disapproval of the involved child's behavior and to admonish the child to behave better. But, to the child, the infanticidal glance stuck, the demeaning metaphor clung, as an invitation to lower the child's self-esteem.

These equations, of course, "do not go the full nine yards," but do carry overtones of splitting, projection, role reversal, aggression, and narcissism. They are risky figures of speech to be used when addressing a preoperational child or a child employing concrete operations; they are too incisively belittling. Consequently, we prefer to ask with what or whom the parent "identifies" the child when parents are seen *before we see their child.*

Our intention is not to be too idealistic but to impress upon the reader that what may seem harmless to a parent may seem harmful to a child. Parental distortions are to be changed, not condoned, if parenting is to improve—a benefit to parent(s) as well as to child(ren).

Questions for Study and Action

1. One interpretation of Winnicott's usage of the term "good-enough mother" is that he referred to a mother whose performance was sufficient for a child to enjoy the symbiotic tie to mother, then to differentiate, separate, and have a proper start on the child's life cycle. Explain the difference between this interpretation and one that would require less of the parent.

2. Explain Lloyd de Mause's assertion that the shift to and fro between role reversal and projective identification in the parent "produces a double image that is responsible for much of the bizarre quality of childhood in the past."

3. Although unconcern about child care has lessened since the Middle Ages, there are residuals of unconcern and abandonment even today. List six markers showing us that empathic service to children has not won the day, and explain how these markers are present today.

4. Explain how the gifted child is an especially easy mark for the parent who tends towards narcissistic identification with the child.

5. What criticism would you be able to mount against the concept of *identification with the aggressor* as the sole motive or defense absorbing the child who has been physically abused by a parent? What else is needed to account for the child's fascination with cruelty forever afterward?

6. How do you account for the fact that many psychoanalysts, whether followers of Melanie Klein or Anna Freud, impute projective identification, identification with the aggressor, splitting, onmipotence fantasies, etc., not to adults but to children? Explain.

7. What options are there for young people who do not want to bear children or rear

children when they grow up? Discuss at least three alternatives that they might choose.

8. Is it a blessing for children that so many females in our society have been programmed and indoctrinated to become mothers? Name several disadvantages of this "reproduction of mothering."

9. How is it possible for a person to be creative, generative, and committed to serving the young of their species without bearing children? Name three types of persons who can do this.

10. Explain how parenthood can be distorted by the parents' transferences and repetition compulsions.

For Further Reading

Chesler, P. *Mothers on Trial: The Battle for Children and Custody.* New York: McGraw-Hill, 1986.

Cohen, R.S., Cohler, B.J., & Weissman, S.H. *Parenthood: A Psychodynamic Perspective.* New York: Guilford Press, 1984.

Levy, D.M. *Maternal Overprotection.* New York: Columbia University Press, 1943.

Miller, A. *The Drama of the Gifted Child.* (Earlier Title, *Prisoners of Childhood*) New York: Basic Books, 1981.

Miller, A. *Thou Shalt Not Be Aware: Society's Betrayal of the Child.* New York: New American Library, 1986.

Rank, O. *Psychology and the Soul.* (Trans. by Turner, W.D.) Philadelphia: University of Pennsylvania, 1954. (Originally published 1930.)

Reich, W. *Listen, Little Man.* (Drawings by William Steig.) New York: Noonday, 1971. (Originally published 1945.)

Schatzman, M. *Soul Murder: Persecution in the Family.* New York: Random House, 1973.

Statistical Abstract of the United States (106th Ed.). Washington, DC: U.S. Government Printing Office, 1986, pp. 59, 62.

Sullivan, H.S. *The Interpersonal Theory of Psychiatry* (pp. 218–219). (Edited by H.S. Perry and M.L. Gawel) New York: Norton, 1953.

Winnicott, D.W. Transitional objects and transitional phenomena. *Int. J. Psychoanal.*, 34:89–97, 1953.

35

A Family for Children

In this chapter we attempt to articulate some of the family's structural and functional characteristics when that family is adequate to the needs of children. There are numerous examples of families that we know to function well. Our instances are drawn from literature and from professional–clinical and personal-nonclinical experiences of the two authors. In carrying out a search for family features that permit children to grow up as healthy and natural persons, we shall range over the structures, developments, and functions that are particularly salient to children's welfare in families. Thereafter, we turn to some plausible and empirically based definitions of "good" parents and "good" children, closing with a series of generalizations made from a viewpoint that looks to society as well as family for adequate services to children.

STRUCTURES

The basic requirement of a family *for* children is that it be a family *with* children. Two generations at the very least are present within such a household. One of them is a generation of parents (producers) and the other a generation of children (consumers). Traditionally, the family consisted of father, mother, and child(ren), but today one-fourth of U.S. children are living in one-parent households

—mostly with the mother only (U.S. Dept. of Commerce, 1982). The statistical norms have already shifted away from a traditional family. Hence, we must recast our notions of what is normal in the way of family structure, leading us to observe that one caretaking adult and one child, at least, now constitute the irreducible family for children. Although traditionally the mother did not work outside the household, today most young children live in families with both parents working (U.S. Dept. of Commerce, 1982). Economic necessity and other societal forces have brought about that current situation; the economic supports to families that would be required to alter the present scheme of parental employment would be prohibitively enormous, hence it seems certain that the working mother is bound to persist as a basic role of women in families, necessitating nonparental child care of ever-mounting proportions. That is an inescapable fact of life late in the 20th century, so policy problems are raised concerning day care being made available that is fit for children, an issue that we leave for later. Child, family, and society are inextricably intermeshed.

The basic personnel of the family for children is at least a dyad, one child with a parental caretaker. Some find it difficult to concede that a family can exist with but one parent. The mother-only family is a structure (with realistic and fantasy problems, it is granted) but that it is viable is unquestionable. Since it is working, it is not broken. It works for some 12.5 million children in the U.S. The poverty of this structure creates far more of its difficulties than the absence of an adult male within the household (see Adams et al., 1984). Other types of family structures include the father-only family, a rarity, but one usually not afflicted by so much poverty; the two-parent family; the three-generational family with grandparents (or surrogates) in residence in the household; and rare forms such as those seen, for example, when two women or two men head a household with children or when children grow up in a communal form of living.

Family pluralism reigns today. It is wise for us to recall that over half of the black babies being born in the U.S. are born out of wedlock and will grow up in mother-only or mother-grandmother families. So we must not be too idealistic, but can realistically conclude that with one of every two marriages ending in divorce, the family may not match our personal values concerning what family life should be—either before or after the breakup. Health professionals them-selves form rather rigid views about an ideal family during their childhood, but such stereotypes and prejudices disserve us *and* the families we seek to serve when we have become professionals. It is best to address each particular family structure afresh and anew, so that we do not try to impose our conceptions or values on the one family coming to us for help.

A family is a small group of persons related by marriage or blood kinship, but we know a family also may be formed through one or two parents' adopting a child. The structures of families are so fluid and variable that almost any imaginable configuration can be expected to be seen in urbanized America today. Family systems theory was formulated with an eye on the traditional patriarchal two-parent family in which only the father worked outside of the home, so it often gets faulted because its theory shows pro-male biases, yet it would be foolish to discard family systems theory entirely.

What is there in family theory that we can use? For one thing, the idea of an interactive, mutually dependent system of roles and relationships: the notion of subsystems. Family subsystems erect and energize boundaries between internal subsystems and around the family system in its entirety. Those boundaries, once in place, give definition and delimitation to the family as a unit, demarcation from other families and other groupings in which family members may participate.

Internally, boundaries surround sexual activities, confining them to those of the married pair, the conjugal pair who constitute a conjugal subsystem. Sexual relations of that pair are not only permitted and positively sanctioned, but children and others in the family are excluded from the sexual intimacies of the marital pair. Naturally, housing level can alter the parents' sexual and erotic boundaries, so that parents may wish to protect their children from witnessing parental intercourse and its foreplay and afterplay, but in the presence of overcrowding the goal may be impossible to achieve. Once again, economic circumstances set limits on family functioning even in so "private" a matter as adult sexuality, for parents in crowded quarters will not always make certain that the children are out of the room, or actually asleep, during lovemaking. In most of the world, this situation may not do irreparable harm to children, although it fires their imaginations and sometimes leads them to mistaken notions of what adult sexual love truly is. Perhaps the moral is that partitioning boundaries are preferable for all concerned.

Other subsystems within the family show similar boundaries. The parental or parenting subsystem, centered on parents' relationships to the child(ren), is strengthened by the incest taboo, which is really two taboos or negative sanctions wrapped up in one: an imperative not to have sex with a child and an imperative not to have sex with a close blood relative. Those negative sanctions serve as subsystem boundary reinforcers, and when they are operative, the parenting subsystem is protected, limited, and defined to the benefit of the family as a whole. Of note is that a child may be *parented* by a sibling or relative who is not actually the child's parent.

The sibling subsystem, when it is present (more than one child in the family), is also a strengthener of differentiations and boundaries internal to the family and its functions. Siblings share their common fate as children, as dependent minors, and as people for whom parents serve as guardians as long as the siblings are dependent and deficient in their minority status.

Children can coalesce, too, drawing first one parent and then the other into their coalitions, until they have effectively eroded the boundary around the conjugal pair and brought one or both parents down to being in collusion with the children against the other parent. When there are two parents and two or more children, family boundaries are enhanced, it would seem, because both conjugal and sibling subsystems are potentiated, giving the entire life of the family greater effectiveness. When there is only one parent, by definition there is no conjugal subsystem, yet the sibling subsystem often rallies, marking off its space from the residual parent's, and helping to make the family function, at times, more effectively and more democratically than it ever had done when both parents lived there.

Any institution takes its character from the customary roles that activate it. The family contains interacting roles of husband-wife (conjugal subsystem), father-mother (parenting), son-daughter (bigenerational), brother-sister (sibling). In the preceding sentence the related roles, when combined into family subsystems, are shown in parentheses. If a father and mother did not consistently show the behavior that they expect of each other and that their children expect of both of them, there could be no nuclear family. Families are dependable and expectable ranges of "appropriate" activities by the family members. Without living up to a certain proportion of expectations, the family evaporates as an institution.

Family theorists assert these system and subsystem principles, using somewhat different words, as they attempt to describe a workable, healthy, and functional family along the following eight structural/functional parameters:

1. stability, i.e., not disorganized or undependable
2. clear roles (not ill defined or conflicted)
3. reciprocal roles (not unrelated or too overlapping or conflicted)
4. clear generation *boundaries* (not diffuse or abrogated)
5. clear perceptions candidly expressed (not vague or concealed or distorted)
6. flexibility, not rigidity
7. individuation, not enmeshment
8. mutuality, not isolation or pretense of mutuality

A family meeting the eight criteria just specified would be a family that possessed the requisite basic structure for serving the needs and wants of children of different ages. Static criteria of family structure or function will not work because the family is a dynamic system that must be capable of changing over time.

DEVELOPMENTS

The changing family makes adjustive and adaptive changes both to the larger world of which it is a part and to the new demands of its individual members. For that reason, a *dynamic* family system is required, one that will develop and change and retain its serviceability as long as its services are needed by its members. Every family lives through a series of developmental crises, although not all of them are really deeply upsetting. The nodal points for family coping with changes are multiple, but the ones that we cover in this chapter are sexuality, gender role, intimacy, wanting a child or children, increasing empathy, growing autonomy in children, discipline, acceptance of grandparents, growth of parents in synchrony with the growth of the children, need of outer resources and supports, and finally how the family will empty the nest of its fledglings.

Sexuality is how the family began. Conjugal relations had to be established before the advent of children and had to have persisted when the children were present, so the family life of adults is very much permeated with lust and sexual activity. Nevertheless, parents are not preoccupied with their sexual arousal and opportunities, so that their focus on conjugal relations is not to the exclusion of concern for the children and they will be able to carry out their effective functioning to serve children. Instead, the parents do a small amount of sublimation, scheduling around the children's needs and seizing opportunities that are presented to them for sexual activities. Flexibility and innovation help them in maintaining a wholesome conjugal relationship while devoting major energies to child care during the first five or six years of each child's life.

Children, too, are sexy creatures, because they are zesty, alive, and need to be in intimate dealings with others. Parents who function well and show a varied repertoire of coping skills can accept the lusty expressions of young children, without promoting the child's eroticism or exploiting the child's libidinal expressions. As children get older they may become genitally active with agemates. That, of course, may be regarded by parents as something shockingly new, but sooner or later the parents must concede, and perhaps celebrate, the sexual maturation of their offspring. Ordinarily, parents do not admit of childhood genitality except for masturbation, "playing doctor," and other such activities. But when the child has reached or passed puberty, the entire family begins to admit of, or assent to, the legitimate sexual interests and appetites of the horny youth. At that time, depending on their real values (much more than on their professed values), the parents will find ways to welcome their offspring into adulthood, including adult sexuality. Few parents are eager to give information or guidance about the details of sexuality to their child or adolescent offspring, but even when they are willing to be consultants to their offspring, it is usually the offspring who reject it out of hand. Young people seem to sense that their sexuality is their own and out of the domain of parental guidance or intrusion. Hence, as a part of the younger generation's growing up and individuating from the family, sexuality is not shared with one's original family but brought under the sway—entirely—of the young person's individuality. Some parents may find this difficult to accept and may prefer not to relinquish such a heavy matter to the discretion of young people, but in time it works out for parents to accept their offspring's privacy and individuality.

In consequence of all the considerations that we have detailed, the family, while not ordinarily a hotbed of incestuous longings, *is* a kind of erotic double hotbed, because both the generations (on either side of the boundaries needed to preserve family living) are sexually attuned, ready, and able. The way a family copes with all these sexual desires and behaviors is an acid test of family effectiveness.

Gender-role definitions and assignments are not rigidly elaborated in the healthiest of families. Since the adults, in their conjugal pairing, can imagine and take on the attributes of one another, most openly communicative families move willy-nilly to a more androgynous format. An adult male who has been absorbed in child care for an entire day finds it awkward to adopt a Tarzan-versus-Jane division of labor and, as an alternative, comes to derive comfort from his feminine as well as his masculine trends and leanings. An adult woman who has rushed a croupy child to a hospital, managing all details of traffic and hospital bureaucracy very well, finds it a bit silly to reject her more competent tendencies and interests just to appear feminine/subservient or to feed the hungry male ego of her spouse or lover.

On the other hand, some gender-role assignment does occur in most families, not always to the detriment of the father nor to the greater benefit of the mother. In fact, family life is often more conducive to the gratification of adult males than of adult females, but too asymmetrical leanings towards the father can become highly dysfunctional for both the adult female and the children. Androgynous sharing of tasks seems to be a growing impetus in many healthy families known to us. A division of labor that is not so gender-based or uncomplimentary to females seems to work better than an old-fashioned, patriarchal arrangement, whereby only a female can scrub a toilet or milk a cow and only a male can chop wood or mow grass.

For their part, children take very naturally to androgynous work and play, only seriously questioning the gender propriety of different behaviors after they have reached about five years of age. Boys are much more attentive to what is appropriate for boys than are girls about what they ought to be doing as girls. Girls are more comfortable about their femaleness, from all appearances, even if they have husky builds, great vigor, and tomboy tastes. The main thing that a family does is to work out and formulate (subject to revisions again and again, naturally) the work load of housekeeping chores with no more or less attention being given to gender than that particular family must provide. When such decisions are not unfair or compulsive, they work best and endure longer.

Intimacy is a development in conjugal relations that has extensive conse-quences for the marital pair and for their preparation for parenthood. Sexuality ceases to be compulsive and becomes enveloped in relatedness. It is no longer so likely to subserve nonsexual purposes—power, performance, ego. The fertile couple spend hours together, dropping much of the fly-by-night, catch-as-catch-can quality of their sexual times with each other. What was mechanical becomes more natural, less excessive and forced. Many of the sectors of their lives become rather intertwined, encompassing more than the man-woman parts of relating to each other.

Some writers refer to this development in intimacy as a move into alloeroticism. Alloeroticism does not necessarily mean a great reduction in orgasmic frequency, for indeed it may increase, but means that a deeper love is shared between two persons. Their relationship has, if anything, become *more* eroticized because the nonsexual components have been transmuted into a shared existence—a living of one person for the other. Relatedness validates each person, something like the preadolescent chumship did. As Lord Kennet, writing as Wayland Young, stated in his book, *Eros Denied:*

> If the affection which may link a virgin boy and girl is love, what can we call the affection which may link a man and woman who live together, fuck together, come together, and have children? If the lesser is love, there is no name left for the greater. . . . (1964, p. 359)

When an adult male and female together establish true intimacy, they have made the ground on which parenthood can flourish, so they are ready for parenting. Often, they decide that they want a child.

Having a wanted child is a developmental milestone for the family's life cycle. The accidental child is always at risk of parental distortions, ranging from neglect and indifference to rejection, crazy identification patterns, role reversal, and so on. The wanted child is at a premium. In taking the developmental history of the child and of the marriage and family from the parent(s), we always have to inquire if the child was wanted and planned for.

If the child was unplanned, it is imperative to ask when the pregnancy was really endorsed and "cathected" by mother and by father. In general, the sooner a child was eagerly anticipated, the better for the health of child and family.

Dependency and then growing autonomy of the child present another crisis in family development. In a family for children, the parents are (parent is) equally delighted by a child who walks and talks as by a totally dependent, happy baby. The capability for accepting the child's growth, rolling with the child's punches, is an index of healthy parenting and family functioning. Once the child can stand alone ("stand on its own two feet") and talk (say "No"), the child is embarked on a journey towards enculturation and socialization that warms parents' hearts, because they foresee new ways of relating. Despite some negativism from the child, the parents welcome the child's growth in autonomous functioning, and the family is strengthened in proportion to the parental acceptance of the child's new behavior. Especially during the first five or six years, the child will continue to benefit from being in a family that will not push, but watch and wait and condone, a young child's moves toward a greater independence of will. The second year of life, in particular, will not be a time, if the family is for children, when the parents will try to break the child's will. Instead, parents will expectantly try to discern what way the child was meant to go and not impose any Big Lessons on the child until the child has presented the parent(s) with some of the child's own learning objectives and told them what the child's potential and wishes might be. Gardner Murphy (1958) characterized this:

> ... the parent will let the child tell him where his tastes, his loves, his demands upon life lie. The parent will supply restraints and disciplines primarily when the child is defeating his own ends, especially when the child is clearly showing, as most children do sooner or later, that he actually wants goals, order, and a sense of direction rather than chaos. But it will be (a parent's) first concern that the child live in the child's own idiom before he be asked to understand the idiom of others. (p. 317)

King Solomon's attitude that each child should be brought up in "a way that is her or his own" is the idea. Some antichild ideologies contend that this strenuous effort by a parent, to empathize with a child and to wait to see what inner nature is to unfold within the child, is only a lack of moral fiber. Or some ideologies may attempt to trivialize this outlook by calling it "permissiveness," but the soundness of the basic notion cannot be deprecated by its critics nor soft-pedaled by its proponents.

Growth in parental empathy is one of the hallmarks of a family for children. By empathy, we mean the ability imaginatively to take up the child's role, stand in the child's shoes, and see the world as the child sees it. Empathy is not a put-down, as sympathy, pride, and shame may be, but empathy puts oneself in the experienced world of the other—specifically, puts the parent, in imagination, in the child's world. Such imaginative concern goes beyond identifications, because, in empathy, self and other are interchanged for a time. At those times, genuine dialogue can occur and healing syntheses can be prefigured through a dialectic of giving and taking, exploring and learning.

Oddly, some parents balk at empathy as a concept. They have been children, so empathy should be relatively easy, at least in general terms of imagining the child's estate—how a child might think, feel, or do. Since parents who are able to do this role playing seldom have children with reactive disorders, child psychiatrists may see fewer empathic parents than a school teacher, for example. Still, among parents of child psychiatry patients, empathy is spread out from much to none. Since among those for whom empathy for the child is sparse or missing the children's problems are more serious, some credence can be given to the assertion that increasing empathy is a vital sign of effective family functioning for children. It is called for in every stage of child development and provided in the family for children.

Discipline becomes the rocks on which many parent-child relations crash, break up, and run aground, but in a family for children, discipline is as easy as Gardner Murphy depicted it. What emerges is a loving discipleship, not a fearful obedience. When rules are flexible and rule-makers have a heart, a happy outcome is guaranteed.

Deprivation of rewards and ignoring the child's misbehavior are more productive of changed behavior than physical punishment. In a family for children, physical force is among the last-resort measures and will never be used if it can possibly be avoided. If the family is honest and expressive of emotion, however, it may be that a parent will "lose it" and box a child's ears, even if the parent is firmly against such an action on grounds of principle (belief in nonviolence, regret that one was himself or herself beaten during childhood, along with a determination not to repeat the intergenerational cycle of violence, and so on). When such a slipup occurs and a child is struck by an irate parent, in a family for children the parent will apologize as soon as control is regained. Children, hearing an apology, will forgive easily in most instances. Many child advocacy groups, including the American Academy of Pediatrics, have taken stands against corporal punishment of children in the family, the schools, and psychiatric and correctional facilities for children. A group that has spearheaded the drive against corporal punishment is End Violence Against the Next Generation, with its headquarters at 977 Keeler Avenue, Berkeley, California 94708.

Acceptance of grandparents may be at the center of a true crisis, since it is fraught with strong emotions; it may be the focus of conflict between the spouses if there are two; it may be taxing for a single parent to achieve; and it may be impeded by the child or children who relish the alliance with grandparents against parents and enjoy wedging them apart. But in some fashion the parents come to terms with grandparents, a process aided by the grandparents' mellowed acceptance of parents, thereby permitting the older generation to have meaningful interactions with both the younger and the youngest generation. A child psychiatrist, Arthur Kornhaber (1986), depicted the intricacies of the parent-grandparent relationship in a family for children. Kornhaber's book gives a place of psychic importance to grandparents. Kornhaber is associated with the Foundation for Grandparenting, Box A, Jay, New York 12941, a group that aids grandparents to be better parents to their now-grown children and to give care to their grandchildren, too. Children and grandparents easily can become natural allies, forming a bridge that includes the parents, to the benefit of the child.

If young parents cannot "make peace" with their own progenitors, the odds are that something is amiss. Making peace does not mean capitulation to the authoritarian dictates of intransigent grandparents, but only that they are seen for what they are—potentially valuable figures in a child's resource network. In a family for children, the parents are not so abrasive that they would try to forbid the grandparents to function in the child's life. Neither parents nor grandparents own the children, so fighting over who has proprietorship is a bit silly, but both generations can give care, each different and special, to young children.

An acknowledged need for outer supports and interests for a family is a trait related to the acceptance of grandparents but inclusive of many others beside the parents' parents. Moral extensions of the family unit abounded in earlier times in the U.S.—an extended family household, youths who entered the labor force by moving to urban areas and boarding with urban-dwelling relatives and acquaintances, farming and farm home-demonstration agents, family reunions periodically held, churches and temples, granges, clubs, and neighborhood gatherings for picnics, festivals, dances.

By contrast, the contemporary family shows an overwhelming propensity for splitting off into separate households with only parents and children contained therein, a trend called "nucleation propensity" by demographers. Nucleated and sequestered, the family is made especially vulnerable during economic depressions, which are recurrent, and other family adversities such as illness, madness, death, all of which may be visited on a family. Cut off from others, the nucleated family is more readily cast adrift and unable to cope with ordinary and unusual crises. It is almost a truism that a family for children cannot retreat from participation in the wider society.

Parents who are compulsively family-centered, mistaking domesticity for bondage, and who have no "outside activities" with their agemates, are more easily victims of burnout, to the children's detriment, than parents who do have time for recreation and communication with nonfamily members. Adams et al. (1965) discovered that the parents of child psychiatry patients were more totally embedded in the family circle than the parents of nonclinical children, and were also more lacking in empathy for their offspring than were nonclinical parents.

At no time is the necessity for external supports more evident than when marital dissolution occurs. Until 1958, the main reason that a mother-only family arose was the death of the father, but today the main reason is the divorce of the parents, hurling the mother and children into poverty overnight. In a family for children, the parents are not as likely to divorce, because they acknowledge that although easy, no-fault divorce is handy, their concern to give care to the children does not permit their conjugal relations to stay in the spotlight. They become more tolerant of peccadillos in each other and find ways to get help for a marriage that has serious problems or is unproductive, without throwing their child-care functions into the wind. One in two marriages ends in divorce in the U.S.; children are rarely beneficiaries of a marital breakup. External supports help greatly, however, in alleviating the tragic effects of divorce.

In a free-market society, devoid of a general policy to support families, families have to fend for themselves in establishing supportive networks, thus doing on their own initiative what might be done as a matter of governmental policy. The family for children has many outreaching fingers into the larger community, participates in community activities such as voting, being active in voluntary community activities, and having a high index of social participation. In all those ways, the family builds a network of caring and concern that goes beyond its own front door. Children need their escape hatches, too, windows that reveal the great outdoors.

Emptying the nest is a critical but inevitable part of a family's story. The offspring are grown up enough to be released from the temporary guardianship in which their parents held them during their formative years. Now that they are formed, they leave home. The parental pair becomes a "childless" conjugal pair once again, cycling the family back to the situation of its beginnings before the conjugal nest was converted into a family with a child. In an earlier era, one of the parents often would have died by the time the nest was emptied, when the ages of the parents would be around 50, near the limits of the general life expectancy. Today, the procreative family lasts for a smaller proportion of the life span of its members, and parents grow older before dying. The procreative family today may not be the one-and-only arrangement for adults. Often the woman (erstwhile mother) lives far beyond 50 but many of her senescent years may be spent in widowhood or in establishing a new relationship with another man.

To consider elderly parents whose children have grown up and departed as bleak, lonely, and pathetic is not sensible. The life cycle and its developmental sequences through sickness and health made emptying of the nest, and for that matter, dying itself, as an understood and accepted part of living. There were many deeds and fantasies preparing them for an empty nest to come later. Besides, being human, the elderly acknowledge that the season for caregiving to children will end, but in imagination they can shift to being constructive grandparents and perhaps even become better friends to their children. It is ironic that in economic declines such as that of the past decade in the U.S., offspring, even in their late twenties and early thirties, return to the parental nest when marriages go on the rocks and find that, when homeless, their former caregivers can take them in and treat them as honored guests. But, even if the grown-up offspring leave for good and can retain separate dwellings, life for the elderly erstwhile caregivers has not ended but retains a lively quality because loving sustenance comes both from past experiences remembered and from present experiences savored.

In this section we have surveyed some of the changes occurring in a family for children. Our purpose is to make the point that even though a wholesome family's life is patterned and structured (not disorganized), there are numerous challenges to and changes in the structure; the family undergoes development and changes and its effectiveness derives from its being able to cope with changes as well as established patterns.

FUNCTIONS

This portion of the chapter addresses what a family is good for—for children, for adults, and for society—and closes with a consideration of family life's social context. A functional analysis of family life from the standpoint of adults and children who are in the family and from the society which is also in the family in a fundamental way should move us further in explaining what is done by a family for children.

For adults, the family's developing structures can be seen to function in the following four ways:

1. psychic security derived from companionship and interdependence
2. psychic security derived from parenting or caregiving to young people
3. sexual gratification with a relatively reliable partner
4. physical security from being in an economic unit that will attend to one's needs and wishes "in sickness and in health"

It should be pointed out that the mother-only family is less supplying of the first and third of the listed functions, by definition. Furthermore, it usually works out to be disadvantaged on the fourth function but that is an adversity that is not intrinsic to the mother-only family, for it does not happen in nations that give special supports to mother-only families. Hence, the two-parent family more readily functions in the four ways we have shown, but we caution the reader to refrain from facile overidealization of the two-parent family because our message is that a family that functions for children functions, regardless of its structural characteristics. Granted, the mother-only family can, but may not, disserve the mother yet serve the children.

Not all two-parent families provide either mother or father with affectionate companionship from an agemate, or sexual gratification with a fairly durable partner, or even economic security. If a two-parent family does provide those features, its chances of functioning better for adults are enhanced.

For children, or for a child, the family of orientation is an instrumentality for life itself, as we saw in Chapter 14. Being helpless and dependent, the child must have a caregiver who provides the child with all the sustenances, material and spiritual, that survival requires. Hence, the family's functions for a child are quite simply these two:

1. physical security as a nonproductive consumer
2. psychic security from a feeling of belonging and from ego identity

At birth, the child's animal survival needs are not object-directed or person-specific, but shortly the physical caregiver becomes a love object, and strong emotional cravings lead to attachments without which the child may also die. Bound up in the infant's attachments is a specific need for belonging with a specific person, and without the particular other, the infant does not have a sense of belonging but instead a feeling of alienation, distress, and dissatisfaction, a basic anxiety that deranges the life cycle so that the baby will not grow to realize his or her full human potential. Ultimately, as we have said, the dependency is lessened because the infant becomes more autonomous physically and emotionally. But a drive towards mutual dependence, towards relatedness or interdependence, is so set in motion that no human animal will ever be able to stand alone or wish to be that independent. Interdependence is what human beings crave, and they lessen their dependencies only because they become dependable to others, not independent of others. All those valuable lessons are learned by the fortunate child in growing up in a family for children.

For the larger community or society, the family also subserves certain functions, six of which we highlight: procreation, education, sexuality regulation, home economics, health delivery, social order, and control. Anthropologists have proclaimed for many decades that the family is where both gene pools and values come together and interfuse. The family is where human biology and human culture (which is also biologically important) meet. In particular, the class system of any society is distributed among its family groupings, so that class becomes embedded in the family, again determining survival chances of its members. Therefore, the reproductive function of the family is important and it assortatively assigns newborns to positions within the class system. Uncommonly immature and dependent, the human newborn must have an adult caregiver—the two make the irreducible family.

Education of the young is an important family function from the society's perspective. The procreative female is also an educative female as soon as she gives care and nurture to the newborn. Socialization and enculturation begin at the mother's breast and, even if later learning occurs in other relationship contexts, overtones and shadows of a mothering teacher will persist for the human being. The aspect of education emphasized by psychoanalysis is learning through identification, learning from the parental example, learning through modeling; but as we indicated in Chapter 2, many modalities of learning are accessible to be used by parent and child. Society owes a lot to parents who shape and train their children to be human.

The regulation and channeling of sexuality, something for which the human neonate is ready at birth, is done by the family for society. Lucky children not only see and receive love but also "hear others speak of love," as Rochefoucauld stated.

Most societies favor and most families in most societies still prepare the young for societally condoned sexuality—placing a premium on marital sexuality, not premarital or extramarital; outlawing incest and adultery; and setting up sanctions to discourage, even while making provision for some exceptions, fornication and mismating. It remains an interesting fact of family living that children are able to predict with great accuracy when they are five years old if they will have families by age 30. A taste for marriage and family is learned early and abides long.

Home economics demonstrates that the family is the basic consumption and income transfer vehicle for the economic institutions of the society. In preindustrial times the family was often the basic productive unit, too. As an economic unit the family is conservative of economic institutions, ever attempting to work within the established order so as to earn the funds to be transferred to the helpless, the ones who do not work and earn. As long as children are given care and have their economic needs of food, shelter, clothing, and health care met within the family, the society is safe and the family is safe from outside intervention. It is a trade-off with an economic base.

Health delivery in a nation with unsocialized medicine is left to the family, too. Health maintenance, prevention of disability and disorder, and care of the sick members are done by the family. The medical and dental bills are expected to be paid by the family, and the family is held accountable for seeing that medical neglect does not occur. Every family member learns some of the skills of practical nursing for family members who are ill, including those with mental disorders. Hence, health delivery is very much a family issue, done for society by the family, but not always done well because the number of malnourished children increases in the U.S. and the ranks of the poor are swollen mainly by children and women whose health is always imperiled when poverty exists.

Social order and control is a basic task of any society, and in ours the task is mainly handed over to the family. If either children or adults have any inclinations towards being docile, that usually gets materialized within the family, and if anyone is incorrigible within the family, they will be so outside. The family is not only a paramount training ground for parenting but also an intensive training camp for conformity—alas, sometimes for too automatic and ritualistic conformity.

The multitude of functions subserved by families for their members and for the larger community have been boiled down and simplified by a sociologist, Robert Weiss (1979), to these three tasks which must be completed by a workable family for children: income production and transfer, homemaking and home maintenance, and child care. That places even greater emphasis on the survival and maintenance functions of the family, spelling out in very practical terms what will be the earmarks of a family that works: economic subsistence, home maintenance, and child care.

DEFINITIONS OF A GOOD PARENT

Having surveyed the structures, developmental changes, and functions of a healthy family for children, we are now in a slightly better position to define what makes for a healthy and effective parent, a good parent, an "ordinary devoted parent" of a growing child. A good parent aids the family's effectiveness rather than detracting from it. A good parent is deserving of good children, which we seek to define in the next section of this chapter.

A good parent has a realistic perspective on his or her original family; as was indicated earlier, the parent can be accepting of the grandparents now. Total acceptance may be hard to attain, so we would say that the parent's own family of origin must have been reckoned with, seen through, and transcended in a compassionate spirit. That may be the first thing accomplished by a good parent.

A second attainment is to have enjoyed the conjugal pairing and to have put it into proper perspective, so that it does not sacrifice the children.

A third attainment is success in moving from dependency (relating to others as the sources of one's provisions) into dependability, so that one realizes his or her potential through service to others. The service persists throughout developmental crises, with the parent radiating security and empathy. That kind of parent has some valuable things to teach to the next generation.

A fourth attribute is the retention of a sense of selfhood that reaches beyond roles played, even the parental role. The confrontation of one's true self and respect for that true self are, in an older terminology, a blessing that a good parent shares with other human beings who know and accept themselves. Self-knowledge and selfhood are virtues going beyond parenthood, perhaps.

DEFINITIONS OF GOOD CHILDREN

If we are to undertake defining what good parents are, we need to try to do the same for children. A good child is an overall healthy and happy child whose parents' love shows in many aspects of the child's life. Among the more objective dimensions of healthy childhood are: 1) a growing competence that is validated not only by the parents who love their offspring, but also by persons who are not family—peers, teachers, neighbors, etc.; and 2) domestic and custodial stability, in which the child participates by being there with at least one adult who loves and protects the child. Two semiobjective dimensions of a child's growth towards health are: 1) increasing patterning in and incorporation of viable values, developing a conscience in a milieu where nihilism and absurdity are minimal; 2) an expansion in the range of love and compassion, from mother to other adults and children, until eventually, when a grown-up, the erstwhile child will have a benign disposition towards offspring and all children and, in a sense, all of humankind. Then there are two final characteristics that are entirely inner or subjective: 1) a favorable picture of oneself and enjoyment of bodily pleasures as good; 2) a residue of some unsocialized uniqueness to be added to one's feeling like all others who are human and certain others who are human: the joy of autonomy, creativity, spontaneity, and unprogrammed ecstasy free from adult intrusions; the right to play and do useless things for the sheer fun derived.

Good children, in short, are both individuated and interdependent. They can be cooperative on occasion, nonviolent, and learn to do some things for others.

FAMILY AND SOCIETY FOR CHILDREN?

Can a family serve children well? Can a society give any of its first-rate priorities to children? A family can serve children, we believe, although a great accumulation of evidence in child psychiatry is that many families are not fit for children. We also believe that all social institutions should be appraised (as Thomas Jefferson recommended in his prescription for periodic revolution) and modified so that their healthier impact on children can be secure.

Making social institutions, including the family, fit for children would necessitate radical transformations of American institutional life. The costs would be high; as examples, the schools would be well financed and more wholesome than daytime prisons, and the Air Force would have to hold bake sales to buy any new bombers. A program of personalized, genuine day care would be spread across all the residential settlements of America. A multitude of services for families would be in place. It is an interesting consideration.

Questions for Study and Action

1. List and describe each of the four subsystems that make up the family system.

2. Give a clear and succinct description of a family that shows each of the following characteristics and, in your description of each family's trait, explain what it means to a child in that family.
   (a) lack of stability
   (b) ill-defined roles for members

      (c) conflicted roles for members

      (d) abrogated generation boundaries

      (e) distorted perceptions vaguely expressed

      (f) rigidity or inflexibility

      (g) enmeshment

      (h) pseudomutuality

3. Show how a father-husband could be very disappointed and unhappy if he transferred attitudes he learned in his *original family* into his *procreative family.* Give examples of his attitudes towards father, mother, and a younger sibling.

4. Can you find as many as four facts that refute the authors' statement, "The family is a kind of erotic hotbed because both the generations are sexually attuned, ready, and able." At what age do penile erection and vaginal lubrication appear in boys and girls?

5. Distinguish between:
      (a) intimacy and lust
      (b) sexual desire and sexual-object preference
      (c) androgyny and high masculinity or femininity
      (d) phallic and alloerotic sentiments
      (e) core-gender identity and sex-role differentiation

6. Give three reasons that planned and wanted children are not "at risk" to the extent that unwanted, unplanned children are. To what pathological conditions are unwanted children made vulnerable?

7. Why is parental empathy the heartpiece of a happy, successful family? Define empathy and explain why it is crucial to realizing a parent's full potential.

8. Why has it been claimed that a family, like an individual person, has a life cycle? Explain some of the stages in the family's cycle: beginning, middle, and end.

9. At least 84 *different* types of families-with-children were found in Woodlawn, a black ghetto area in Chicago. Interview each of three persons known to you about his/her particular family and *who lives in it.* Are your friends' families as diversified as the ones in Woodlawn? Why?

10. What is the meaning of this truth: The U.S. is the only industrialized nation in the world with *children* making up a *majority* of those living *below the poverty level?* Which term would you prefer to describe this: *juvenilization of poverty* or *impoverishment of children?* What is the difference?

For Further Reading

Adams, P.L., Milner, J.R., & Schrepf, N.A. *Fatherless Children*. New York: Wiley Interscience, 1984.

Adams, P.L., Schwab, J.J., & Aponte, J.F. Authoritarian parents and disturbed children. *Am. J. Psychiatry*, 121(12):1162–1167, 1965.

Guidubaldi, J., & Perry, J.D. Divorce and mental health sequelae for children: A two-year follow-up of a nationwide sample. *J. Amer. Acad. of Child Psychiatry*, 24(5):531–537, 1985.

Hofling, C., & Lewis, J. (Eds.). *The Family: Evaluation and Treatment*. New York: Brunner/Mazel, 1980.

Kornhaber, A. *Between Parents and Grandparents*. New York: St. Martin's Press, 1986.

Murphy, G. *Human Potentialities*. New York: Basic Books, 1958.

U.S. Dept. of Commerce, Bureau of the Census. *1980 Census of Population and Housing (Supplementary Report). Provisional Estimates of Social, Economic, and Housing Characteristics, March 1982*. Washington, DC: U.S. Government Printing Office, 1982.

Walsh, F. (Ed.). *Normal Family Processes*. New York: Guilford, 1982.

Weiss, R.S. *Going It Alone*. New York: Basic Books, 1979.

Young, W. *Eros Denied*. New York: Grove, 1964.

IV

CRISIS NOW

Childhood is often portrayed as a continuous thread, with few surprises and shocks. Even writers on psychopathology during childhood seem to wind up making child- hood and children seem devoid of novelty, unperplexing, and unalarming. We do not share the view that childhood is blissful and contented, containing nothing new. Instead, we see many flukes and surprises for any adults who try to serve children.

Children are often unhappy and poorly served, even by the family institution, by school, by hospital, by court. Children are all too often victimized by the very adults on whom they should hope to rely for protection and security. In this section we deal more closely with emergencies that may bring startle to adults, including the child psychiatrist.

36

Emergencies

Psychiatric emergencies of children are fewer and often less dangerous than those of adults and adolescents. Nevertheless, four of these are potentially lethal: a) suicide; b) violence by others to the child, i.e., child abuse and neglect; c) violence by the child to others; and d) accidental poisoning. Child abuse and neglect are described separately in Chapters 27–30 but must also be considered emergencies.

SUICIDE

Suicide in children has been the stepchild of suicidology and of clinicians in general. The limelight has recently been taken by adolescent suicide, and most textbooks (even those dealing with children) tend to give insufficient attention to childhood suicide by dwelling instead on the current "epidemic" of adolescent suicides.

Even more so than in adult/adolescent suicide, there is an undetermined, but probably large, proportion of childhood lethal accidents that are in reality suicides but are not reported or even recognized as such. Many "accidental" poisonings are probably in this category, as are other "accidents." Some coroners actually refuse to record child suicides.

543

The *form* of suicide is different in children from that in older individuals, and is to some extent age-dependent, even within childhood. Younger children (preschoolers) have appropriately prelogical notions of lethality and will ingest safe substances (forbidden foods) to excess, or gulp down available toxic chemicals. Running into the street and into the path of vehicles is another measure. Older children will plan their acts, so strangulation, drowning, jumping off ledges, getting run over by cars, and poisoning with heating gas are measures that they employ.

The psychodynamic or motivational rationale of childhood suicide is that it is either a desperate attempt at discharge of vindictive aggression against close family members, usually parents, or of aggression against the self. In addition, the element of impulsivity is almost always present. Why do these children choose suicide? Most authors now believe that they learn to use suicide as a problem-solving means. Suicide has become a "language." Many suicidal children are found to have depressed, suicidal mothers.

CASE 36-1   Simon, aged eight years, was seen at the emergency room after ingesting an *overdose of his mother's supply of* alprazolam (Xanax). He came from a seemingly intact family. However, in the course of a family session, it became clear that *mother had had several episodes of depression*, with at least one *suicide attempt*, and that the maternal grandfather had died by *suicide*. The *relationship* between the parents was *strained*, and father had recently *lost* his *job* because of too many absences from his workplace due to *alcoholism*. The parents' treatment of Simon bordered on *child abuse;* the parents explained some of it on the basis of *Simon's difficult behavior: he had been diagnosed* as having *"minimal brain damage"* shortly before the present incident. Of late, the parents admitted that they had simply given up on Simon and *were paying little attention to him or his wishes*, while *punishing* him capriciously.

Comment. The child reacted to both an intolerable environment as well as his own feelings of rage and need to "get back at" his parents. He had learned that suicide could get things done for him by observing his depressed and suicidal mother. The physician who knows there is a family history of suicide, depression, legal difficulties, alcohol and drug abuse, and family violence will always be alert to serious depression in any boy like Simon.

As adults, we all (including clinicians) tend to forget how helpless a child can feel and, indeed, is. Although hurt by parents, the child may be quite realistically unable to "move mountains." A suicide attempt may be the only effective way to change an intolerable environment. The precipitating event may appear trivial—usually it is a slight or rejection—but in the context of severely disturbed family relationships and severely vitiated self-esteem, it can indeed be "the last straw."

CASE 36-2   Elaine was five years old when she started attending kindergarten. There she was *scolded by her teacher* for consistently ignoring the teacher's requests, orders, and admonitions; in short, all attempts to have her collaborate with the usual routine were unheeded. Elaine was a shy, yet *irritable, even irascible,* and *impulsive* child. Shortly after a scolding one day, Elaine was restrained in the nick of time by her older brother from *jumping* from her third floor apartment window into the street below. She explained that she was mad at everybody and that her mother and teacher were going to feel sorry for what they had done to her. Shortly thereafter, Elaine *swallowed* some of mother's cologne and tried *to eat* mother's makeup, but was quickly detected by one of mother's boyfriends and rushed to the emergency room.

Elaine was raised, together with her older brother, by her *single* mother. She had only a vague acquaintance with her father, who visited haphazardly. Mother made little effort to disguise her *rejection* of Elaine and her predilection for the older, more "independent" (i.e., less demanding) son. Elaine had also overheard mother's boyfriend *threaten suicide to prevent mother from terminating their relationship.* It was this man who took Elaine to the emergency room.

Comment. This case vignette illustrates a "disciplinary crisis" (i.e., school discipline) as the precipitating event—a relatively frequent finding. The important feature, however, was the rejection by mother, "priming" the child to react to the "last straw" with a desperate attempt to set matters right. Suicide had been imitated from mother's boyfriend who had used it as a powerful interpersonal tool.

PSYCHOPATHOLOGY

Much has been written about the child's concept of the finality of death. There is almost universal agreement that up to age four or five years, or roughly through the preschool years, normally intelligent children view death as reversible. Suicidal acts by preschoolers are, therefore, at least theoretically, not intended to be lethal, and one has the impression that imitation combined with impulsivity plays a major role when a suicide is completed. Yet this is not all that goes into early childhood suicide: these children do indeed find themselves hurting in a helpless position, with significant rejection visited upon them in various, sometimes covert, ways. It is a matter of conjecture as to how depressed these younger suicide attempters feel, given the difficulties of reliably diagnosing depression at that age. Perhaps we are witnessing in them the retroflexion of rage against themselves in an incomplete stage, since revenge against the rejecting parent is quite openly stated.

In school-aged children, depression is often more apparent. Some authors insist that school-aged and older children who attempt suicide are seriously disturbed in their object relationships. Unfortunately, depression or beginning schizophrenia very often go unrecognized and a suicide attempt may be their first undeniable indication.

Whenever severe affective or thought disorders are not in immediate evidence, death (and, by extension, suicide) means reversible separation. In the first- or second-grader, it assumes an overtly murderous character, with retaliation getting more prominent as the child gets older; finally, around age nine years, death assumes definitive, irreversible, forms in the child's mind.

Any psychiatric condition, or none at all, can underlie suicide. Depending on the study done, up to half of the suicidal children could not be diagnosed as suffering from any mental disorder.

TREATMENT

This can be viewed in two stages: the immediate and the long-term.

(a) Immediate

Obviously, the medical-surgical treatment of preserving life comes first. Acute psychiatric treatment—crisis intervention—should begin as soon as the patient's physical condition permits it. The clinician should make full use of the emotional impact, the "upsetting of the applecart," that the suicide attempt has produced on the family. The child's suicide attempt was, after all, aimed at "rattling the cage," at shaking up the family structure, so that changes can be made.

Experience has confirmed the logic of the obvious therapeutic conclusion: meet with the family immediately. Many families are ready to "spill it all out" at this stage, and fullest therapeutic use should be made of this, even though this means that the interview may last more than an hour. Other families are not so ready to talk, but must still be approached, although with reasonable delicacy.

The child himself or herself is usually quite willing to answer specific questions. These should be aimed in *two* main directions: *one* at the child's perception of his/her "inner" world (impulses, fantasies, wishes, anger, depression, etc.); the *other* at the "outer" world (i.e., family, school, peers) and the child's complaints about it and how it affects the "inner" world. Thus we try to elicit what conditions the child had tried to correct by attempting suicide.

From these approaches to both child and parents, the clinician must arrive at a preliminary decision about whether the child can be released to go home to the same environment, *or* hospitalized, and/or placed in a different home.

The question arises of what to do with the child who threatens suicide for what are, by all appearances, small frustrations. Some of these children are pampered, "spoiled," and at the same time sophisticated in the manipulative use of statements such as, "I wish I could die," or "I would be better off dead." The remarkable effect of these phrases on their parents serves as a reinforcer, so that these children make frequent use of them. The clinician has to distinguish between such "firing blanks" and the more substantial suicidal threats by discerning the overall clinical picture: Are there stresses on the child, however latent, that the child cannot cope with?

The important point to remember is to take *all* suicidal statements seriously, evaluate all of them conscientiously, and exclude as "nondangerous" only those for whom the intrapsychic and family situations are such that the child can be expected to continue living within their context, even if the present situation were to continue unaltered.

When to hospitalize depends on:

- the age of the child—the older, the more likely the need for hospitalization;
- the presence of depression;
- the extent of chaos in the family—the greater the chaos, the less availability of adults who can safeguard the child;
- the extent and intensity of violence, aggression, or hostility in the family, especially as it carries over into child abuse;
- the presence of depression and history of suicide in the family (positive family history of affective disorders).

The bottom line is: Is the child caught in an intolerable situation from which he or she sees no way out, except suicide?

Hospitalization rarely means a need to be on a locked or "secure" psychiatric ward. Child psychiatric hospital units are few and far between, are highly specialized and selective, and do not admit patients nearly quickly enough to be of use for acutely suicidal children. Therefore, it is necessary and quite feasible to make use of what is available—usually the pediatric floor of a general hospital. If the child is older, and/or severely depressed or violent, a psychiatric unit should be used. Obviously, the latter should be of a type that safeguards the child but does not expose him or her to danger from other patients.

(b) Long-term treatment

This belongs to the specialist and to specialized institutions. The child psychiatrist is the central figure but will be joined by members of a number of other disciplines, notably the social worker(s) from child-care social services agencies. It is interesting to note that a recent study found that the majority of suicidal children who had to be hospitalized were placed outside their original homes on discharge (Cohen-Sandler, Berman, & King, 1982).

Longer term work and follow-up with both the children themselves and the families are usually necessary. This decision should be left to the specialist.

It appears that no single type of psychiatric treatment is always more efficacious. The crucial ingredient is to establish a working relationship with the patient and his or her family as quickly as possible, and then do everything to maintain it. Although there is no particular "line" of questions required, we have found that a central question is: Does the child need protection, both against his or her own impulses and against an intolerable environment? Therefore, one approach in questioning would be: "Would you like to stay in the hospital (or special home, etc.) so that people can take care of you?" or, "Would you like to stay here while you, your parents, and we figure out who can best take care of you?" The first task, of course, is to make sure that the child has genuinely understood the questions. Any answer other than a clear "No!" should put the clinician on the alert. If the child cannot make up his or her mind, it is a mandate to the clinician seriously to consider hospitalizing the child. If the child indicates "Yes," however haltingly, it should be taken as a serious indication for hospitalization or for residential placement.

Generally, children do not present serious risks of suicide attempts while in the hospital. As in many crises, the hospital atmosphere has a stabilizing, indeed soothing, effect on the distressed child. The danger arises towards the anticipated end of hospitalization if the necessary changes have not been made. If the child realizes that the message of distress has not been understood and that the necessary changes will not occur once back at home, the child may need to "repeat the message."

CASE 36-3   Robby, aged eight years, had overdosed on his parents' whiskey and was hospitalized on the pediatric ward since he clearly indicated that his mother's alcoholism and father's frequent outbursts of abuse of mother were more than he could cope with. He was a "model patient" until he realized that the social worker, who was to arrange a temporary foster-home placement for him, was giving in to his father's wishes under the guise of giving the parents "a second chance." At that point, Robby became difficult to manage and was caught trying to snitch a container of pills at the nurses' station.

When Robby's therapist confronted him with this act, Robby started crying and stated that nobody took him seriously; he also remarked that *nobody loved him and nobody took care of him* since his grandmother had *died* a year earlier. She had taken care of him during his mother's frequent bouts of drunkenness and his father's long absences (father was a long-distance truck driver).

During the subsequent two weeks in the hospital, Robby made three more suicide attempts (all of which were fortunately intercepted by the staff), until the social worker announced that Robby would not be going to his parent's home. Follow-up a year later indicated that Robby was doing well in a foster home.

Comment. Although there was plenty for Robby to be sad about, he was not in a dead-end (i.e., completely hopeless) situation: he understood that the hospital staff was trying to help, and sensed that they were in a position to help (if they got the right message). His suicide attempts were expressions of extreme distress on the one hand, and desperate appeals to bring about relief from this distress on the other. Had the child not been hospitalized on a unit whose staff was alert to the dangers of suicide, and had the social worker not understood the message of urgently needed changes in the patient's environment, tragedy may have resulted after all.

Repeated suicidal attempts may also occur if the child has been removed from her or his original family and if the patient perceives or misperceives the foster home or other new environment as either perpetuating the same old pressures or creating new ones. This underscores the finding that suicide is a learned behavior, often used repeatedly to solve a variety of interpersonal problems. In that case, long-term psychotherapy is indicated. It may have to be started in a specialized, long-term child psychiatric hospital and to be continued in a residential center or in the psychiatrist's office.

The content of psychotherapy usually deals with the child's aggression and excessively harsh superego, as well as with more immediately practical issues such as exploring alternatives to suicide for problem solving. The specific type of intervention should be left to the specialist.

PROGNOSIS

Since environmental pressures play such an instrumental role in childhood suicide, it follows that prognosis will depend heavily on what changes the child's suicide attempts have leveraged within the child's immediate world.

CASE 36-4   Penelope was seven-and-a-half years old when she threatened suicide by writing several notes ("I love you") to her family members, including her grandmother. She subsequently tried to take mother's sleeping pills, but was caught in time. Both parents had been abused as children, were themselves reported once for child abuse (excessive spanking), and continued to discipline Penelope in the severest manner.

Following a series of family interviews, the parents started displaying more affection to the child and focusing on her achievements rather than her transgressions. Penelope became happier, and her self-accusatory explanations of her troubles almost ceased. The parents then discontinued treatment. Four months later, Penelope was seen at the emergency room having cut her wrists. The parents had reverted to their old ways. Penelope eventually was placed in a foster home.

Comment. The conditions that elicited Penelope's suicide attempts recurred, and with them Penelope's suicide attempts.

As suicide attempts by children often emerge in the context of severe family pathology, removal of the child becomes a necessity if other treatment approaches do not effect substantive changes sufficiently quickly and permanently. It follows that parental and family psychopathology constitute one set of prognostic determinants.

Another set is the individual psychopathology of the child. Depression with its feelings of helplessness and hopelessness has been given differing importance, since the diagnosis of depression in children is still not uniform (see Chapter 15, on childhood depression). Severe depression and schizophrenia should alert the clinician to the danger of recidivism. Yet the clinician must be *warned* that *absence* of depression and schizophrenia does *not* lessen the danger. Diagnoses such as Personality Disorders, Conduct Disorders, and Somatoform Disorders are no insurance at all against a poor prognosis, and if used pejoratively (such as "hysterical," "attention-getting," "manipulative") may actually contribute to the poorest prognosis—to successful suicide.

ACCIDENTAL POISONING

This is sometimes discussed as a separate child psychiatric emergency. In our opinion, it is part of the differential diagnosis of childhood suicide, the crucial goal being to rule out a "masked" suicide attempt, just as one would have to rule out suicide in other "accidents." For this latter reason, most accidental poisonings merit psychiatric evaluation along with the medical intervention that may be lifesaving.

VIOLENCE

Violence by children was practically unheard of two decades ago. It has become an increasingly frequent presenting complaint for psychiatric referral. When the parent is unable to deal with it, it becomes an emergency. Today, most violence by children is towards other children. Parricide is rare.

ETIOLOGY AND PATHOGENESIS

Etiology in most instances is multiple—a combination of factors within the child, his family, and the culture. We will list and discuss each of these factors in turn, remembering, however, that they never occur in isolation.

(a) Within the child

- temperamental/constitutional factors: high reactivity and poor adaptability to change (the classical "difficult child");
- attention deficit disorder: this is the main contributor to child violence because of its classical impulsivity and lack of judgment (deficient ego development—developmental lag). The syndrome is described in Chapter 21 and can occur developmentally or "de novo," following head trauma or central nervous system disease;
- severe neurotic conflicts rarely lead to aggression of such severity as to constitute a true emergency;
- functional childhood psychosis, unlike psychosis in adults, rarely causes violence per se. The same can be stated for toxic psychoses of children.

(b) Outside the child

Within the family, the most common scenario is that of "institutionalized violence" or violence as the family style: problems are settled by physical aggression, and the child learns from the parents' example. Wife beaters and child batterers produce violent offspring.

Another contributing family factor is parental *inability* to deal with aggression. Although this seems the opposite of family violence, psychodynamically it may be the other side of the same coin; the parents have to defend so heavily against their own aggression that they cannot modulate it and allow moderate amounts to be transformed into discipline.

Parental criminality is a direct and powerful influence, especially if it is of a violent crime career. Criminal and violent parents also tend to reward the same behavior in their children. This applies to noncriminal, but highly primitive, parents, too—parents who invariably seem to produce children with above-average aggression. Both mental illness and child abuse in the parents have been found to correlate significantly with childhood violence.

Outside the family, there is a larger violent culture surrounding the child. A powerful cultural influence, most particularly in terms of violence, is television as portrayer of the culture. Our view of TV's role now is corroborated by a number of studies in this country and abroad (Murray, 1980; Rothenberg, 1983).

An interesting conclusion from these studies, and one that is of practical value to the clinician, is that the more vulnerable the child to such violence-breeding influences, the more likely he or she is to be exposed to them. Thus, it has been stated that the psychosocial stressors accompanying poverty put a child at risk for both being involved in interpersonal violence and watching television violence.

CLINICAL DESCRIPTION

One amazing form of childhood violence comes out when children frighten adults and "hold them hostage." While this usually borders on the ridiculous, there have been instances where children have threatened and killed adults with firearms, not only to mug them but also to seek revenge. The adult "held hostage" or "locked in the bathroom" is usually a somewhat comically inadequate or severely neurotic mother (occasionally, father or grandparent) and the child "difficult" and/or hyperactive. The scene, as a rule, is harmless, yet tragically portrays the extreme lack of structure in the family.

Of yet greater danger is violence against younger siblings. Tragedies sometimes occur because of inadequate parental supervision of an impulsive, aggressive child. The most frequent example of a violent child is the hyperactive child (ADHD) reacting to a mixture of environmental permissiveness and overstimulation, the latter often in the form of aggression, extreme punitiveness, or taunting.

CASE 36-5   Three young male friends from the same neighborhood started engaging in *petty vandalism and stealing*. They subsequently "graduated" to dealing in marijuana. Their leader, Kevin, started *feeling that he could have anything he wanted*. His little gang *dominated the children* in the neighborhood. Until this happened, the boys, including Kevin (aged 11), had maintained a friendly relationship with a fatherly neighborhood storekeeper. One evening, Kevin wanted to buy cigarettes from the storekeeper who refused to sell them to him. Kevin threatened the old man, who, however, stood firm. As this happened in the presence of his two cohorts, Kevin's *standing in their eyes* was jeopardized. He went home, unlocked the cabinet where his stepfather kept his shotgun, loaded it, and went back to the store. Flanked by his friends, he pulled the trigger. Hit in the chest, the storekeeper collapsed and the three boys ran to Kevin's home. His friends were badly shaken, but Kevin *showed no remorse,* although he took elaborate measures to *hide* the gun in the basement.

In the police and court proceedings, Kevin continued to try to *manipulate* to his advantage whatever circumstances he could, *covertly* and sometimes *overtly supported* by his parents. They especially kept projecting much of the blame and responsibility onto Kevin's companions.

By the time this tragedy happened, *Kevin's parents had given up on him.* Kevin's mother had divorced his father four years earlier after years of his *sadistic abuse, both of her and of Kevin*. The father was subsequently jailed for *rape*. Mother then married an *ineffectual* man given to solitary pursuits and displaying *paranoid* thinking. He had a past history of *psychiatric hospitalization*. Kevin had been diagnosed as suffering from *Attention–Deficit Hyperactivity Disorder* and was being treated on and off, but the parents did not follow through with their appointments. Mother became involved in a career of her own, and both parents chose to *turn their backs on Kevin's behavior*, except to *react episodically and inconsistently* with verbal harangues. On those occasions, stepfather would close off the disputes by *physical threats*.

Comment. This sort of tragedy is usually the culmination of a number of factors; in this case they include:

1. *Organic (developmental and genetic)*—Attention–Deficit Hyperactivity Disorder and a family history of criminality;
2. *Environmental*—abuse, followed by the example of a paranoid parent lacking adequate influence on the patient;
3. *Sociocultural*—the opportunity for gratification (in money and power) beyond what an immature person could tolerate; and finally, perhaps,
4. *Toxic*—since Kevin was not only trading in marijuana, but using it as well, the toxic influence of the drug played a facilitating role.

TREATMENT

We shall address emergency intervention and short-term treatment only, since long-term treatment is a multifaceted and often multidisciplinary approach, varying with the individual "mix" of etiological factors.

Emergency intervention aims primarily at establishing safety. The child has to be calmed and so do the parents, especially if the child is young. In most instances, this presents little difficulty. The danger stems from the possibility of accidental harm to anyone, and parental overreaction and underreaction have to be dealt with so that common sense prevails again.

As soon as the immediate situation is under control, treatment must be individualized according to the child's and, especially, the parents' psychopathology. This is in the purview of the specialist only.

We would like to emphasize short-term hospitalization of the preschool- and school-aged child as an effective mode of crisis intervention. As mentioned previously, this is done on the pediatric or general ward, and the child can be released after two to three days, during which time the parents can collect their wits and a preliminary decision can be reached on whether the child can return to his or her original home or will need to be placed in a foster home.

Patently dangerous children (i.e., those who use weapons or dangerous tools) should be hospitalized in a specialized psychiatric unit. The same applies to firesetters, although the vast majority of the latter present little danger of further firesetting once in a psychiatric institution. Psychiatric institutionalization is a must if the violent child is found to be psychotic.

SCHOOL PHOBIA

School refusal is considered an emergency because early intervention carries with it a high degree of reversibility, decreasing as the condition is allowed to continue and to become a way of life. It has been described in Chapter 16.

ACUTE UNCOMPLICATED BEREAVEMENT (V62.82)

CLINICAL DESCRIPTION

Death of a parent, sibling, or other close family member often results in childhood behavioral difficulties that reflect a variety of defensive or coping mechanisms. Sudden, unexpected death of a loved person is tantamount to massive psychological trauma in a child. Death that is expected, and that eventuated slowly, is handled differently and will be discussed elsewhere. Hyper-activity with various degrees and forms of aggressiveness is the most frequent clinical picture. Neurotic disorders, notably separation anxiety (often manifested as school phobia), psychosomatic disorders, and manifestations of regression are other expressions of bereavement in children.

CASE 36-6   Timmy, aged seven years, became *aggressive, destructive,* and *impervious to discipline* within two weeks following the death of his maternal grandfather. This was noticed both at home and at school where he had *not* had major difficulties previously.

Timmy *had not* cried much at the funeral, although he had been very close to grandfather. In fact, grandfather had largely filled the role of father for Timmy, especially since father (who had divorced mother four years earlier) had shown little interest in Timmy.

Although aggressive, obnoxious, and *ostensibly fearless* during the day, Timmy became *fearful* and *"whiney"* at night. There was a scene every evening as Timmy insisted on *sleeping in mother's bed.* Concerned that neither she nor Timmy would get enough sleep, mother invariably *yielded* to Timmy's demands. Even so, she could barely overcome Timmy's *reluctance* to go onto the school bus in the morning. He *cried* and clung to her, but once on the bus, he became the "scourge of the entire bus." Moreover, mother herself was in a state of *mourning* for her father, on whom she had been quite dependent.

Comment. More often than not, children do not express grief verbally but express it in behavior and with "neurotic" mechanisms. The patient here showed phobic (separation anxiety at night and in the morning) and counterphobic (defiant and fearless of authority) mechanisms as well as regression.

We often see the sequence of phenomena originally described by John Bowlby for parental loss: protest, despair, detachment. The child's hyperactivity and aggressiveness occur in the stage of protest. Loss of previous interests and activity emerges in the stage of "despair" and "no longer caring," but also "looking for new attachments," and is the final stage.

We attribute much importance to correct understanding and handling of children's grieving because the prognosis is markedly improved with early intervention. Delayed grief is pathological in children as in adults and is even more easily missed in children. Mourning must be done.

TREATMENT

Treatment must not only promote appropriate expressions of grief but also, specifically in children, look, almost simultaneously, to provide for the bereaved child's dependency needs. In the last analysis, the child will ask primarily: "Will I be taken care of?"

Emergency intervention, therefore, must address both the child's reactions and the environment. The child may be stunned and confused by sudden death, and the physician should allow for expression of both grief and anger for being abandoned. The child may wonder, "How did this happen?" and, "Why did this happen to me?" The former question should be answered in a simple, explanatory way; the latter, with exploration of the child's magical thoughts—the idea, perhaps conviction, that his negative, aggressive thoughts and wishes have brought about the death. A simple, definitive statement that the child's own wishes did not cause the death is often effective, especially when given by an authoritative person during the height of the crisis when everything is "fresh," "on the surface," and ready to be cognitively mastered, fueled by the energy of the acute stress and upset.

The second part of the emergency treatment, dealing with the environment, addresses the question: "Who will take care of the child?" A single, grieving, surviving parent may be too grief-stricken to be of much help himself or herself, and incapable, in that state, of arranging for outside help. The professional should step in here. It is of interest that the Chicago Institute of

Psychoanalysis endeavors to give crisis help to bereaved children and parents in that city, thus acknowledging that a grief crisis can benefit from some specialized assistance.

ACUTE MASSIVE TRAUMA

We include here both physical and mental trauma. The two are often combined. Physical trauma results not only from natural (floods, tornadoes, etc.) and man-made (car, aircraft, etc.) disasters, but also from abuse and serious illness. Psychological trauma again comprises all forms of child abuse, terrorism, and the effects of serious mental or physical illness in the family.

Although there are some symptoms, or rather, clusters and arrangements of symptoms, that are specific to each of the above, children's reactions to acute massive trauma bear a common core syndrome. This basic core will be described here. Likewise, in the emergency treatment, we shall attempt to offer a basic formula. The reader can then adapt this formula to the knowledge gained from the respective specific sections in this book (especially the chapters on child abuse).

CLINICAL DESCRIPTION

First, the definition of what constitutes massive trauma has to be established: this has to be done specifically for childhood, and, in addition to the DSM-III-R categorization that it be "outside the range of usual human experience," it has to be specifically threatening to a child's view of his or her world. Usually, this means a loss of, or threat of loss of, the usual basic support systems in the child's life.

The basic symptoms are the child's suffering from:

- anxiety
- depression and guilt
- regressive phenomena, especially excessive dependence or excessive aggressiveness
- poor concentration and poor schoolwork
- psychosomatic complaints
- most characteristic startle reactions when perceiving similar stimuli, or flashback reactions without an external precipitating event (in other words, intrusion of the traumatic theme into consciousness)

The child's reaction will depend on the age of the child (the older the child, the more preexisting pathology plays a role), on the nature of the trauma (loss of or separation from parents and siblings is worst) and, of course, on the availability of support systems following the trauma (parents, siblings, or peer group).

CASE 36-7   Sheldon was six years old when he was assaulted by a neighbor-hood *dog*. Following emergency treatment for the injuries, he appeared physically headed for *recovery* from the wounds. However, he almost immediately developed *nightmares,* complained of *stomach aches,* could *not pay attention in school,* and would *panic* at *any scene evoking the potential of attack,* predatory behavior, wild animals, and, of course, dogs themselves. He would also *startle without apparent precipitating event or cause.* He also started *wetting his bed* at night again.

Comment. This case highlights the fact that the stressor is specific for the child and his developmental age. The patient's reactions were quite similar to what another child may have shown following a plane crash, natural disaster, or a kidnapping or terrorist attack. Since Sheldon was not separated from his parents and nothing had happened to his parents, there were no symptoms of depression or guilt.

We would expect these symptoms to affect the child's overall character development much less than the much more pervasively damaging stress of child abuse and, especially, sexual abuse.

TREATMENT

The goal of emergency intervention is to prevent the "burying" of the traumatic experience before mastery can have occurred.

The immediate treatment is crisis intervention, i.e., psychological support is marshalled and directed to the point of greatest trauma. For instance, if the parents are missing, emotional warmth and support are immediately provided, especially when the child is young. If large environmental upheavals have been part of the trauma (such as loud explosions, etc.), appropriate reassurances are given.

It should be borne in mind that whenever possible, the child should be with his family, as this is his/her "natural security blanket." The most important part of any post-traumatic treatment is the "reenactment" of the trauma. This is now considered a "must" to prevent chronic anxiety. Basic child psychiatric techniques are especially valid here: forced confrontation is to be avoided, but the "dissociative" approach (i.e., where the child relates his/her reactions in a "third person") is as helpful here as in the longer term psychotherapies. The goal is not "catharsis", i.e., the "discharge" of "locked-up" emotions; rather, what needs to be achieved is for the child to detoxify and get a "handle" on the traumatic event. The child then attains a sense of understanding (in age-appropriate terms) of what happened, his/her role in the event (especially the lack of any guilt or responsibility on the child's part for the catastrophe), and the reassertion of the child's self-image and self-esteem. Finally, the child is helped to find ways to deal with the reality of the aftermath.

PROGNOSIS

This depends on the premorbid or pretraumatic psychological adjustment and emotional stability of the child and his or her family. As a general rule, the more stable and adaptable and the less ambivalent the intrafamilial relationships had been, the better the prognosis. In addition, a more adaptable and flexible basic temperament of the child will also make for a better prognosis.

However, the nature of the massive trauma and subsequent interventions will also play an important part. Thus, natural events are generally handled better, and competent and sensitive post-traumatic help will go a long way to improve the prognosis.

For treatment and prognosis of Post-traumatic Stress Disorder (PTSD), the reader is referred to the fuller description in Chapter 17.

Questions for Study and Action

1. Write out a list of *"Physician's Orders"* for Penelope's (Case 36-4) care in the hospital. First, give *general maintenance orders* (where to admit her, diet, ambulation, suicide precautions, etc.); then *diagnostic orders* (lab work needed, psychological and other consultations to be sought); and then *therapeutic orders* (include medications, crisis psychotherapy for Penelope and any others in her family who need it). Is that a sane method of proceeding? What else should be included?

2. Describe in detail the crisis intervention therapy required for Penelope and her parents. Specify how long the crisis will be expected to last. Also, what public agencies need notification when suicide has been attempted? What does the law say about suicide?

3. If Kevin (Case 36-5) had been certified to be tried as an adult, what sort of developmental assessment would be required by a psychiatrist engaged by Kevin's defense attorney? Why have so many more minors been certified to be tried as adults *since 1980*? What does the trial and punishment of juveniles as adults say about the changing status of children in this country since 1980?

4. Explain how a bereaved child, manifesting anxiety and restlessness, shows us afresh that children need to be supplied with security by the adults who care for them—that children consume, while adults must provide, security.

5. Explain to a professional colleague and peer how *crisis theory* presents a special instance of *homeostatic systems theory* applied to the child's family. Who are or were:

Ludwig von Bertalanffy, Erich Lindemann, Lydia Rappaport, James Grier Miller, Walter B. Cannon, and Lawrence J. Henderson?

6. Why do some critics contend that systems theory (or equilibrium theory) is basically conservative, ruling out the chance that real change (or radical change) can occur?

7. Why is "accidental death mimicking suicide" a high risk in pubertal boys who masturbate while having a plastic bag over their heads and inhaling nitrite? What other examples of probable accidents that result in self-inflicted death do you know of?

8. Review what specifics of family history make depression the likely diagnosis in a child with aberrant behavior. What makes for a positive family history of affective disorder?

9. Why has one polemicist stated the following: "After all, it is parental competency or incompetency that determines whether a mentally ill child needs to be hospitalized."

10. What is meant by the following assertion: "School refusal—school phobia—is the most frequent emergency in child psychiatry"?

For Further Reading

Carlson, G.A., & Cantwell, D.P. Suicidal behavior and depression in children and adolescents. *J. Amer. Acad. of Child Psychiatry*, 21:361, 1982.

Cohen-Sandler, R., Berman, A.L., & King, R.A. A follow-up study of hospitalized suicidal children. *J. Amer. Acad. of Child Psychiatry*, 21:398, 1982.

Murray, J.P. *Television and Youth: 25 Years of Research and Controversy.* Boys Town, NE: Boys Town Center for the Study of Youth Development, 1980.

Pfeffer, C.R. Suicidal behavior of children: A review with implications for research and practice. *Am. J. Psychiatry*, 138:154–159, 1981.

Rothenberg, M.B. The role of television in shaping the attitudes of children. *J. Amer. Acad. of Child Psychiatry*, 22:86–87, 1983.

Shafii, M., Carrigan, S., Whittinghill, J.R., & Derrick, A. Psychological autopsy of completed suicide in children and adolescents. *Am. J. Psychiatry*, 142:1061, 1985.

Terr, L.C. Psychic trauma in children: Observations following the Chowchilla school-bus kidnapping. *Am. J. Psychiatry*, 138:14–19, 1981.

V

CHILD PSYCHIATRY, SIMILAR BUT DIFFERENT

Up to now we have dwelled on clinical issues, a focus that we do not wish to depart from at any point in this book. But we do wish now to move our presentation a little beyond psychopathology and treatment.

In this final part of Beginning Child Psychiatry, *we turn to some professional matters concerning the field of child psychiatry: what it is and is not; to what fields it shows correspondences and continuities; what it takes to be a member of this rather young medical specialty; and what some of its promise and hope might be. This is a part of the book that looks at some guild concerns but, we hope, in not too parochial or self-serving a manner.*

Only one chapter makes up this part, The Profession of Child Psychiatry. By reading this chapter the beginner should have a more secure grasp of what this exciting profession has to offer. Although we do not include any cases in this part, we do urge you to answer the questions and do further reading to enhance your learning.

37

The Profession of Child Psychiatry

This chapter surveys child psychiatry's drawing on general medicine and pediatrics *(clinical sciences)*, on the *basic biological sciences* of neuroscience, pharmacology, genetics, and ethology, and on the *pure and applied biosocial or behavioral sciences* of clinical psychology, social work, psychiatric epidemiology and systems science—all contributing to the unique body of theory, research, and clinical study that give child psychiatry a very special identity as a biomedical specialty and a biosocial discipline, both as science and art.

CLINICAL SCIENCES

All of the scientifically grounded healing arts derive from *medicine*, a mainstream parceled out today into Internal Medicine, Family Practice, Pediatrics, Obstetrics and Gynecology, Psychiatry, Surgery, and a host of derivatives from those parent disciplines. The medical graduate today, thanks to the good offices two or three generations ago of the American Medical Association in setting up standards for medical schools, has had at least a light-touch acquaintance with a number of clinical departments and the bodies of theory and practice with which such departments work. Graduates of any approved medical school know the same things, more or less, and that gives each M.D. a standard minimum of theoretical

knowledge, practical skills, and know-how which is a uniform intellectual product hardly matched by any other academic degree holders.

Many of the clinical skills (much of the medical knowledge, too) that we have
alluded to and relied on in this book are derived from the rich traditions of
general medicine: inspection-percussion-auscultation-palpation in the physical
examination; taking the history of the present illness, of previous ills and
injuries in the systems review, of the family's experiences with physical and
mental disorders, of the patient's daily living habits and problems in work and
love and friendly sociability, and so on. As we gather and validate our observations of the patient, begin to plan the diagnostic workup, consider the differential
diagnosis, and begin planning a rational treatment, we are, in child psychiatry,
using the core clinical skills of general medicine. They are old but very sound.
The mental (status) examination, too, derives from the codified practices of
general medicine: how the patient presents herself or himself; the overall
behavior; the speech; intellectual powers; memory; judgment; and all the rest of
a good depiction of a human being who may be (or may be becoming) *a case
of a disorder.*

It sounds impersonal when a physician says that (s)he cannot cope with a
human person in all the fullness of that marvelous being but must press forward
only to see if that person *embodies caseness.* But as compassionate teachers and
scientific healers, we need to keep the patient's *problems* in full view. Granted, we
protect ourselves through some distancing from the full humanity of our
patients and permit ourselves to look at their disorders, admittedly only a small
part of the patients. The distancing that we do as dedicated healing professionals
also protects and shields our patients, something wise Hippocrates of Cos
advised us to do. As a result, the professional relationship is less sticky, not so
ambivalent, not so steeped in love and hate, not a part of our human longing to
attach to others and to be with others in warm, moist, and sexy ways, or else to
reject others and repudiate contact. Neither we nor our patients can keep
sensible bearings if we do not maintain a professional relationship between
doctor and patient—objective but not devoid of interest, empathy, and compassion.
In a word, incorporating medical ethics is a vital part of being a doctor, i.e., a
lenient but persistent and democratic teacher and a scientific healer.

Scientific medicine appears to some of its critics to have become overly
technical—a morass of apparatuses, technology, laboratory studies, and highly
impersonal, almost dehumanized, cost-to-benefit accounting. Yet contemporary
internists proclaim that their "cognitive skills" are vital, referring to the doctor–
patient interaction and to their teaching about illness, health, health maintenance,
and disease prevention that that interaction subsumes. Pediatrics, now a sister
discipline, but originally child psychiatry's parent discipline, assuredly makes
great allowances for the interpersonal factor—at least, that is the case with

general clinical pediatrics, if not always with the finely delineated subspecialties within pediatrics.

Pediatrics, from which child psychiatry (pedopsychiatry) descended, shares with child psychiatry much of the social history of the past two centuries. Both pediatrics and child psychiatry concentrate their work on growing, developing organisms; that concentration on dependent (unproductive) youths would never have been possible without the work of numerous revolutionaries and reformers who were advocates for the child's health, welfare, and education. Public health measures have advanced greatly during the past century so that more children can survive; that certainly has created a facilitating environment for pediatrics and many other child-oriented disciplines. The exploitation of children's labor in mills, mines, and fields has been outlawed (really, only since 1946) and now more children are set free to learn and to play, being healthier at the same time, even in countries with unsocialized medicine.

Advances and discoveries within pediatrics itself have had enormous impact on the health and welfare of children. Just consider the inroads made against infectious diseases, nutritional disorders, endocrine, congenital and genetic disorders, neoplasms, and others, many of which were attained because of the expansion of pediatric research, theory, and practice. Truly, the field of pediatrics helped to spawn the field of child psychiatry. Evidences of this kinship/heritage can be seen in the Appendix.

There is a fun side to the relationship between pediatrics and child psychiatry today and we shall allude to that briefly. Physicians in both specialties seem to be more playfully childlike than other medical specialists. They laugh, often at one another's jokes. Both specialties are remarkably congenial to accepting women in their ranks. Furthermore, both fields are economically deprived, at least in medical schools, relative to other departments in the "academic medical jungle," and both pediatricians and child psychiatrists quip that "children are a very soft constituency." Yet, reputedly, there are differences too. For one thing, pediatricians are said to be shorter in stature than child psychiatrists, whatever that anthropometry may portend. For another item, it is claimed that pediatricians idealize childhood in general, whatever that may be, as a happy era in the life cycle, whereas child psychiatrists see childhood in general as an unhappy chamber of horrors. Further, it is stated by some observers that while pediatrics desexualizes child and family, child psychiatry does not do so!

When child psychiatry became a certifying medical specialty in 1959, after some deliberation and negotiation, it evolved that the specialty board for certifying competence in child psychiatry would be under auspices of the American Board of Psychiatry and Neurology (ABPN) and not the American Board of Pediatrics. The psychiatrists had more political clout at that time (and now), but in deference to the American Board of Pediatrics, one representative of Pediatrics was to be a member of the Committee on Certification in Child Psychiatry. That situation persists, regarding certification of specialists in child psychiatry.

In many medical schools today, child psychiatry and pediatrics are close and continuous collaborators, a morally enriching arrangement. The American Academy of Pediatrics and the American Academy of Child and Adolescent Psychiatry hold joint and overlapping national meetings frequently and cooperate in many projects of mutual concern. In a few universities, a recent trial undertaking of joint training programs (a triple-board experiment) will enable a person with two years of pediatric residency to obtain one-and-a-half years of a special general psychiatry residency, followed by another 18 months of child and adolescent psychiatry—whereupon the seasoned graduate of the five-year programs can obtain board certifications in Pediatrics, Psychiatry, and Child Psychiatry. In most places, however, the total years of training required for all three boards still remains at a minimum of six-and-a-half years, a full one-and-a-half years beyond the total time taken in the experimental triple-board project.

BASIC BIOLOGICAL SCIENCES

Child psychiatry has intellectual roots in many of the basic biomedical sciences, a fact that is often a surprise to nonmedical colleagues in the mental health professions. From the numerous biomedical disciplines, we select here for a brief consideration the neurosciences, pharmacology, genetics, and ethology, the last one sometimes known as behavioral biology.

The neurosciences, fortunately, have begun to "come together" in the last decade or two, for before then they were splintered into neuroanatomy, neurochemistry, neurophysiology, neuropathology, and so on, often the orphan children of academic departments of neurology, medicine, or neurosurgery. Oddly, what seems to have been the vanguard and impetus to the surge forward of a generic neuroscience has been an offshoot of neurochemistry, namely, neuroendocrinology. Even 30 years ago the paradigm (or metaphor) to depict nerve action was that of electric current conducted as if down a wire, although the catecholamines were known and epinephrine and norepinephrine were regarded as hormonal secretions of the adrenals, embryologically of sympathetic neural origin. Gradually, neural hormones have taken over in neuroscience. Today, the "thrust" is on hypothalamus, pituitary and all the target organs of the pituitary, on dopamine as a norepinephrine precursor, on acetylcholine, serotonin and a growing list of transmitters and blockers of transmission. The current paradigm is of a complex chemical chain of action, including GABA and a number of amino acids, polypeptides, and opioid peptides in brain and cord. Since peptides are so numerous in the nerve endings in the GI tract, some brain research has been confounded in the search for those substances in the brain. Also, the rhythmic periodicity (circadian rhythms) of secretions makes random sampling of no value.

The situation today has become one in which research into neurohumors provides most promise to our understanding of many mental disorders of children. So it might be said that our optimism can be directed in particular to neuroendocrinology as our current basic biological science in child psychiatry. The study of neurohumors has been intimately connected to neuropsycho-pharmacology, to which we turn now for brief exposition.

Psychopharmacology had little to offer child psychiatry until there began to be demonstrated, by neuroscience, the sites and mechanisms of various drugs' actions on the neurohumors: amphetamines as central stimulants (like the monoamines) and also as anorexic agents; the neuroleptics acting diversely but perhaps mainly as dopamine antagonists; the antidepressants having adrenergic and anticholinergic impacts on the central nervous system where they block receptor reuptake of indoleamines and catecholamines; the anxiolytics and antihistamines hydroxyzine and diphenhydramine blocking acetylcholine's muscarinic action in the brain and also blocking H-1 histamine receptors. A firm part of preparing any drug for consumption by children nowadays is to know and document its adverse effects, safety, efficacy, affect on brain chemicals and receptors, and its mechanism of action at the neurohumoral sites.

General psychiatry has been more eager to accept mind-altering drugs than has child psychiatry. Child psychiatrists have a reluctance to employ drugs with children, a reticence being based on both a resistance to change from a traditional one-method treatment (read, individual psychotherapy) and a legitimate concern for altering brain functions in younger and still growing human beings. Nonetheless, more and more child psychiatrists are now rushing to be open-minded and partake of what has been called the third revolution in psychiatry, community mental health, with its reliance on psychopharmacotherapeutic agents (see Chapter 2).

Genetics, too, is a basic biological science for child psychiatry, especially for the primary and secondary prevention of Axis II conditions like Autism, Mental Retardation, and other Developmental Disorders (see Chapters 22 and 26). Discovery of fragile X-chromosomes in some autistic and mentally retarded children has spurred a vigorous diagnostic technology that serves better any preventive efforts: amniocentesis, fetal biopsy, tissue culture, DNA restriction endonuclease, and others. Down's syndrome can be detected in utero as can other gender-related chromosomal aberrations. Pediatric geneticists are valued consultants to child psychiatrists.

Many genetic disorders of childhood, including many *genogenic* mental disorders, are not well understood and employ weak evidence that they are genetically transmitted at all. Faith helps when child psychiatrists, as some do, contend that heredity is king. Those who say that Tourette's, Developmental Reading Disorder, ADHD, alcohol and drug abuse, Depression, Conduct Disorders, Functional Enuresis, and Obsessive Compulsive Disorder "must be" genogenic lean on flimsy reeds for their data base. Such equivocal findings as a high familial incidence, higher incidence in first-degree relatives than in more distant kin, higher concordance in identical twins than fraternal twins than in sibs, higher incidences in adopted-away offspring than would be expected by chance alone —all of those are taken as proofs when in reality they are only circumstantial or suggestive evidence. Proof of the "genogenicity" of a mental disorder comes only when the gene-chromosome pattern that is connected with the disorder has been demonstrated and the genome mapped. It is feasible to expect sounder genetic work to be done by geneticists in the future and that can only be a boon to children everywhere.

Ethology or behavioral biology is another basic science for child psychiatry. The substance of ethological research (Konrad Lorenz with geese, Tinbergen with birds, and von Frisch with bees) fascinates the child psychiatrist because, after all, (s)he is a general biologist, but when Lorenz transposes his sound findings about the behavior of a goose to human behavior, the child psychiatrist may wish to cry out, "Stop! Enough already!" The ethological *approach, methods, concepts, theories,* and *techniques* can be applied to children and their parents to good effect, but crossing the species-lines with generalizations about specific behavior becomes a bit silly.

Ethologists themselves, unlike their self-proclaimed descendants who popularize some of the findings of ethologists (Ardery, Farb, Tiger) or sociobiologists who reinterpret ethology to support social Darwinist views, espouse extreme caution about carry-over of observed behavior from chickens or river geese to mammals and to man. The anthropologist Weston La Barre (1954) wrote a book, *The Human Animal,* that largely avoided the trap. Interestingly, a popular TV talk-show host, Phil Donahue (1985) wrote a book by the same title which shuns rather well the trap of overgeneralizing on nonhuman animal behavior to explain humankind.

The sound ethological point remains to be stressed that our bodies, with both phylogenetic and ontogenetic programming, are always with us until we die and that even our elaboration of varied cultures, languages, religions, etc., have a biological significance and basis. Only to our peril do we neglect or deny our animal, mammalian, and human essence.

When the ethologist has compared species that are closer to humans (e.g., Harlow's monkeys' attachment behavior to wire and cloth "mothers"), the analogies seem less farfetched but, even so, the monkey is not human. More importantly, the human baby is not a monkey, neither rhesus nor macaque.

Meticulous observation of behavior, describing the behavior observed, recording and analyzing behavior are all hallmarks of the ethological methods useful in child psychiatry. Yet another ethological application in child psychiatry is the use of evolutionary theory to enlighten behavioral observations made on the young of a nonhuman species and then to take the generalizations thus derived to formulate hypotheses about the behavior of young human animals. When those hypotheses are tested, whether they get confirmed or disconfirmed, something new has been learned about the young human animal as an individual or in small groups.

The matter of human aggression and warfare does not seem to be well explained by ethologists who observe large male cats, lions, and tigers. Those lower animals are depicted as viciously battling over territory or hierarchy. But some ethologists take their cat-deductions, based on pecking order in chickens originally, transfer those deductions to human animals, and soon make unfounded guesses and analogies regarding Hiroshima, Nagasaki, and the terror of an escalating cold war. Psychiatry, too, pales in accounting for human violence. Some ethologists, such as Peter Klopfer of Duke University, seem sounder as they depict human intraspecific violence as "a cultural artifact"; or Robert A. Hinde, who hit the mark in writing:

> Human capacities for cognitive functioning, for communication by verbal language, and for the generation and maintenance of cultural diversity, introduce dimensions of complexity simply not present in the animal world. (Hinde, 1985, p. 119)

BEHAVIORAL OR BIOSOCIAL SCIENCES

When H.S. Sullivan depicted psychiatry as the study of interpersonal relations, he considered psychiatry itself to be a biosocial science. Other biosocial sciences that stand alongside psychiatry and child psychiatry are psychology, sociology, anthropology, political science, home economics, social work, family studies, medical sociology, psychiatric epidemiology, social stratification theory, social history, and general systems science. Each of these fields can bring fresh perspectives and insights to child psychiatrists when they are studied seriously or learned through reading and academic collegiality.

People who learn or practice child psychiatry on university campuses that permit interaction with humanists, social scientists, educators, engineers, natural scientists, and technologists attest to the derived richness of having access to numerous disciplines. Child psychiatry is not a simple, one-track field.

We want to highlight four of these biosocial disciplines as basic to child psychiatry: social work, clinical child psychology, psychiatric epidemiology, and systems science. Without firm knowledge of these, the child psychiatrist may be hampered.

Social work applies many of the "pure" social sciences in its theory and practice and, together with psychology and child psychiatry, is one of the trio of child mental health fields that sometimes are jokingly called "The Holy Trinity of Child Psychiatry." Recently, social work has loosened its curriculum considerably and, unfortunately, has lost form at the very same time that economic adversities have set in, so that many social workers currently find themselves unequipped for available jobs. The core skills needed of a social worker in a child psychiatry setting are: individual casework, group work, and community organization. Today many child psychiatric social workers are most adept at individual casework and family casework and know comparatively less about group work with children or community organization. Yet most social workers are effective repositories of information about community agencies (for health, education, and welfare), and child psychiatrists feel happy to learn from and collaborate with child psychiatric social workers.

Rooted in movements for social criticism and social reformation, social work still imbues many of its students with a deep sense of respect for human difference, for human life, and for saner social institutions. When those passions are aligned with child and family advocacy, or patient advocacy, they make the social worker a highly valued teaching and clinical colleague of the child psychiatrist.

Clinical child psychology is a vital biosocial science for child psychiatry. Lawrence Kubie and others have regretted that this field "joined" child psychiatry prematurely, for they feel its scientific and clinical gains to date would have grown further had clinical child psychology stood longer as as unadulterated, independent field. To give a countervailing statement, one has to ask, "What would child psychiatry have done without it?"

The very history of the field shows its having served as a basic biosocial or behavioral science for child psychiatry. Its origins in academic departments of psychology have kept it close to a research and experimental focus; even when the person who has had strong research-scientist training moves into clinical settings, there persists in the clinical child psychologist a strong spirit of inquiry, critique, and questioning. That skeptical spirit and research know-how bring valuable assets to the clinical scholar: capability in research design, methods, and techniques (the latter including knowledge of statistics and ways of interpreting data that are amassed).

From the days of Binet and Simon and their junior colleague, Jean Piaget, clinical psychologists have worked on perfecting intelligence testing so that the tests are valid and reliable. These tests offer all who study children some very important information about learning capabilities that are in some ways biologically given, but also subject to coarctation and diminution by environmental conditions and experiences such as rejection, poverty, mental disorder, and disvaluing of intellectual attainments. In practical terms, the IQ tests are important for child psychiatry's diagnostic and prognostic work. This has very conspicuously been the case in work done by Michael Rutter and others for the World Health Organization, who proposed that intellectual level be made a separate diagnostic axis. DSM-III and DSM-III-R did not heed their admonitions, but at a future date the IQ of the child being diagnosed may be consigned to a separate axis. The intelligence quotient is important.

Other psychological testing has been well standardized and has proven clinically useful too. Projective testing (Rorschach, TAT, CAT, Michigan Pictures, Sentence Completion, Word Association, and so on) aids therapeutic planning and management in child psychiatry. Neuropsychological testing batteries also aid in educational planning for neurally impaired children. Psychoeducational testing aids greatly in individualized educational planning for any child with a mental disorder, but still more so if the child has specific learning disorders, specific developmental disorders, perceptual motor difficulties, problems in visual-motor integration, and so forth. Knowing the child's academic capacities is important. One handy thing is the ready availability of psychological testing not only for the child patient but also for the family—parents and sibs—because the clinical psychologist has expertise with all ages before specializing in work with children.

Psychiatric epidemiology brings numerous concepts, methods, and skills as well as a body of information and theory to underpin child psychiatry. Much of psychiatric genetics is epidemiological in approach (family studies) and virtually all of our information and enlightened perspective about incidence, morbidity, mortality, natural history, and prevalence of mental disorders have been derived from ("lifted from") epidemiology.

Social psychiatry is not an easy term to define and explain but in the form of epidemiology, social psychiatry becomes crystal clear. Hence, in delineating and explicating risk factors for childhood mental disorders, epidemiology has made invaluable additions to child psychiatry's grasp on the psychosocial etiology of children's mental ills. The landmarks in child psychiatric epidemiology research have been erected by several child psychiatrists who employed epidemiological approaches and methods. Michael Rutter, David Shaffer, Benjamin Pasamanick, Sheppard Kellam, David R. Offord, and Felton S. Earls are all cases in point: child psychiatrists doing important epidemiological research. Although his predoctoral training was in sociology, Charles E. Holzer of UTMB-Galveston has commenced research into the epidemiology of mental disorders in households on Galveston Island, using the general survey technique. The novelty is that Holzer included households with children and administered standardized, structured, diagnostic instruments to children, too.

Clinical child psychiatrists for years might have known—impressionistically and anecdotally—for example, how ravaging poverty, sexism, marital discord, and racism could be as stressors precipitating mental disorder; however, it is the epidemiologist who draws a representative sample of people on whom hypotheses are tested out, and etiological nexuses are claried by means of such case control studies. The epidemiologist unabashedly enters the community to make excellent comparisons of prevalence in nonclinical as well as clinical populations and brings considerable illumination to those whose conclusions are based solely on their work with clinical populations, that is, with individual patients. Etiology in child psychiatry may not have to remain so indefinite and speculative if epidemiology is made more available. Whereas today we "punt" and try not to leave out genogenic, chemogenic, histogenic, and sociogenic causes, our inclusiveness hardly elucidates our knowledge or conceals our basic ignorance. Epidemiology can help us particularly with any and all of the reactive disorders: stress disorders, responses to disasters and terror, reactive psychoses, and adjustment disorders.

Systems science is the fourth discipline in the behavioral/biosocial sciences group that has great relevance for child psychiatry and will be discussed briefly now. Crisis–intervention as a treatment strategy is based on general systems and crisis theory, and that is but one practical illustration of child psychiatry's indebtedness to systems science. There are several other examples.

The psychologist and general psychiatrist James Grier Miller is a foremost proponent of systems science in application to the subject matter of psychiatry. His work of many years culminated with the 1978 publication of his monumental *Living Systems,* applying a mechanistic paradigm of explanation of occurrences at the seven levels of cell, organ, organism, group, organization, society, and supranational system. At each of the seven hierarchical levels, there are largely open systems that process—through "inputs, throughputs, and outputs"—various kinds of matter and/or energy and/or information. For individuals and small groups, such as children and families, the subsystems processing information are most relevant for organism and group.

Systems science has enlightened one of the major trends in family group psychotherapy by concentrating on communication styles and patterns that emerge and change as that mode of therapy is applied in the family group. The jargon of transducers, channel and net, decoder, associator, memory, decider, encoder, and output transducer may become a bit difficult, but it is logical and does give a unified approach. Salvador Minuchin's structural family group therapy draws on systems science. Also, the approach of Lyman Wynne and, to an extent, that of Bateson, Jackson, and Satir (strategic family group therapy) adopt systems concepts and apply them clinically, mainly by identifying and altering communication patterns intrafamilially. When communication changes, the personal and familial systems are also altered.

Another worthwhile body of theory and practice has arisen out of systems science: health services research. The notion of assessing a community's needs as a prelude to starting up new service programs is certainly more rational than leaving such matters to guesswork, to flying "by the seat of our pants," and to the sometimes cruel and wasteful turnings of the "free market." If national priorities are ever deflected from war preparations to human services, then needs assessment and health services research, including evaluation research, will be important for child psychiatric services delivery.

CHILD PSYCHIATRY

Child psychiatry, thus, is a field that plays a part in the combined and holistic enterprise of understanding young children with and without mental disorders. Naturally, the pathological is of more direct concern, but it is forever risky to generalize about sick children without simultaneously comparing them to well ones. In its tasks, child psychiatry is interactive with at least the following: medicine, pediatrics, neuroscience, pharmacology, genetics, ethology, social work, child psychology, psychiatric epidemiology, and systems science.

How then can we define child psychiatry since we know that it has biological, biomedical, and biosocial roots? It is a multidisciplinary field that for training purposes utilizes team work for a more effective educational curriculum. The team is not always the most efficient way to deliver mental health services to children and families, but for efficient teaching of young child psychiatrists the team approach is unexcelled. The team consists of basic biological scientists, child psychiatrists, child clinical psychologists, and psychiatric social workers in most training programs. Not always integral to the "inner family" of disciplines aforementioned but often placed in other departments are other medical specialists, particularly in general pediatrics and pediatric-genetics; child development researchers; communication disorders specialists; epidemiologists; medical humanists, medical and social historians, experts in women's studies or family studies; lawyers and child advocates; and others.

Still, *training in child psychiatry* is not unfocused or diluted. A national curriculum has been devised and adopted as a standard by most approved training sites. The resident in training learns child and adolescent development, psychopathology, psychobiology, therapies in various modalities, community organization, and consultation.

Persons who hold M.D. (or D.O.) degrees are acceptable applicants into approved child psychiatry residency training programs. The first post-M.D. year, PGY-1, is spent in an internship equivalent, usually with something between four months and 12 months in a primary practice field such as family medicine, internal medicine, pediatrics, or (more rarely) obstetrics and gynecology. PGY-2 is, for most people, their first year of full-time learning of general psychiatry, followed by PGY-3 in general psychiatry. Since four years are needed for certification in general psychiatry, and the first year of fellowship in child psychiatry suffices to fulfill that requirement, most people do their PGY-4 in child psychiatry (counting it both ways, i.e., for general and child psychiatry) and then PGY-5 in child psychiatry will complete their formal postdoctoral specialty training as child psychiatrists. Some elect to do four postdoctoral years (PGY-1 to PGY-4) in general psychiatry before embarking on PGY-5 and PGY-6 in child psychiatry. In some programs, child psychiatry may be completed earlier, e.g., in PGY-2 and PGY-3. The training period is a lengthy one; even for those who take an accelerated option, it requires five years after obtaining the M.D. degree. There is a lot to be learned about children and families and society. The training is done with national standards and guidelines but with little cramping of the individual program or its training director.

Other standardizing, optimizing, and qualifying bodies do oversee each program, notably the LCGME's (Liaison Council on Graduate Medical Education) residency review group. Periodically, an on-site visit is made to each training program by a representative of LCGME, every three to five years, for a candid look at the functioning program. If the reviewing group have questions, they may dispatch a Specialist Site Visitor to visit the questioned program for a deeper look. Moreover, the Committee on Child Psychiatry of the American Board of Psychiatry and Neurology, Inc., promulgates "Essentials of Training in Child Psychiatry" to assure that minimum clinical expertise will be engendered in each trainee, monitored, and tested. As a result of these essentials and minimums, and descriptions of a good program, there can be national standards, resulting in specialty board candidates' being simultaneously both a heterogeneous group and a group with some uniformity of knowledge and skills, when they go to take specialty board examinations.

The *board examinations* themselves are unusually forthright and not anxiety-producing for most candidates. (Some people would fluster and sputter if asked to repeat the letters of the alphabet, of course.) A written exam, using the examiners as a criterion group, is given, and oral clinical examinations that deal with varied ages of children and adolescents, plus an exam on community and interprofessional consulting and relationships. The clinical examinations strive to assess clinical competences in interviewing, attentive observation of actual children for psychiatric data (on tapes, brief clinical vignettes, or live patients), the approach that a candidate shows to a diagnostic workup, differential diagnosis, and treatment planning. Within a two-day period the examinations are over and the failure rate is not astoundingly high. Those who pass the exam are then certified in one of the newest of medical specialties, child and adolescent psychiatry. Exams may thereupon be over for the diplomate, but the profession of child psychiatry is one of lifelong learning and accountability to patients and to the profession, as well as to the larger community.

Many child psychiatrists go primarily into private clinical practice, but not exclusively so. Surveys show repeatedly that private practitioners in the field of child psychiatry do consultations to child-caring agencies, exercise privileges in local hospitals, and devote time to teaching, research, continuing education, and learning. Few child psychiatrists do full-time research, unfortunately, even in medical schools. Full-time teaching occupies a minority. Work in state hospitals, public clinics, and public administration occupies a good number, but fewer than those who are in private practice.

Professional organizations to which child psychiatrists belong are, to name some examples:

1. The American Academy of Child and Adolescent Psychiatry, with 3616 Wisconsin Avenue, NW, Washington, DC 20016 being its headquarters' location. The Academy has student members and various categories of membership available to people who do a considerable portion of their work as child psychiatrists. The annual meetings of the Academy carry CME credits and are productive meetings, where interested persons can learn and have reunions. The *Journal of the American Academy of Child and Adolescent Psychiatry* provides informative reading of what is being done scientifically in child psychiatry and related disciplines.

2. The American Association of Psychiatric Services for Children (AAPSC) is a smaller organization than the Academy because clinics and agencies are its members, not individuals. It is more clinically focused than the Academy. AAPSC is multidisciplinary in its clinical membership and publishes a *Newsletter* and an official journal, *Child Psychiatry and Human Development.* Its national office is at 1001 Connecticut Avenue, NW, Suite 800, Washington, DC 20036.

3. The American Orthopsychiatric Association is a multidisciplinary mental health organization that was founded by child psychiatrists and others in 1924. Early on, its concerns were principally child psychiatry and development. Today, however, with a broadened membership that includes educators, nurses, art/speech/music/occupational and other therapists, as well as gerontologists, city planners, and others, "Ortho" has a lessened interest in child psychiatric issues at its annual meetings. The membership of Ortho from all disciplines is concentrated in the North and Northeast of the U.S. and some large cities in other geographic areas. The national office of the American Orthopsychiatric Association is at 19 West 44th Street, Suite 1616, New York, New York 10036.

4. The American Psychiatric Association (APA) is the professional association for all psychiatrists. Since child psychiatrists are certified in general psychiatry, then in child psychiatry, most child psychiatrists opt to join APA and/or attend its meetings. The APA had a longstanding Committee on Child Psychiatry that has now been broadened and upgraded within APA to a formal *Council* on Children, Adolescents and Their Families. Interesting and timely topics have

been addressed well by that Council in position papers and official actions of the APA. The national office of APA is at 1400 K Street, NW, Washington, DC 20005. The *official journal* of the APA is the *American Journal of Psychiatry*.

Four other organizations having membership by invitation, or for specially trained persons, engage child psychiatrists in active membership and leadership: the American College of Psychiatrists, the Group for the Advancement of Psychiatry, the American Academy of Psychoanalysis, and the American Psychoanalytic Association. A section of Child Analysis of the American Psychoanalytic Association is available for child psychiatrists who have had both psychoanalytic and child-analytic training in psychoanalytic institutes approved by the American Psychoanalytic Association.

Child psychiatry, consequently, is a medical subspecialty ("superspecialty," some would argue) concerned with helping (through scientific expertise) young people who have problems in behavior, affects, and thinking. Child psychiatrists are bound by medical ethics and incorporate the identity of physicians without derogating their colleagues from nonmedical backgrounds. Arrogance, hubris, and self-serving seem inevitably to plague many professionals but child psychiatrists do not proudly nurture such hubris whenever it appears in their midst. The physician identity means that a child psychiatrist strives to be a scientific healer, a teacher of health principles, and a citizen advocate on behalf of all children and their needs.

Questions for Study and Action

1. What are the main differences in training and expertise *between* a child psychiatrist and:
    (a) a behavioral pediatrician?
    (b) a social pediatrician?
    (c) a child-clinical psychologist?
    (d) a child psychoanalyst?
    (e) a child-psychiatric social worker
    (f) a child-psychiatric nurse specialist?
    (g) a general psychiatrist?

2. Point out both the fallacy and merit in the following statement about what kind of person should be recruited into child psychiatry: "Demonstrated past success in both the biosocial and biomedical sciences is a good credential for the aspiring child psychiatrist, because nothing succeeds like success. Even our predecessors in

absurd paradox, the ancient alchemists, asserted while working with lead, 'To get gold you must begin with gold.' Nonetheless, earnest industriousness is not enough. . . . What is meant to be unearthed in the applicant is the soul of a poet."

3. How could prior training as an entomologist help someone to be an excellent child psychiatrist? Explain fully, emphasizing skills not informational content.

4. Interview three child psychiatrists to see what proportion of their average work week is devoted to teaching, research, reading and learning, individual consultation, family consultation, hospital work, work in community child-care agencies, and other professional activities. What do they do for recreation?

5. Child psychiatry began in the United States in juvenile court-attached child guidance clinics. Today, if you were a juvenile court judge, list six situations in which you could utilize the services of a child psychiatrist.

6. Imagine that you are a child psychiatrist who consults with a family services agency, and describe what you might do as:
   (a) a patient-oriented consultant (i.e., about cases)
   (b) a consultant oriented to the agency staff itself
   (c) a systems-oriented consultant

7. If you directed a training program for child psychiatry residents or fellows, what would you cover in a seminar on "Psychobiology of Childhood"? Design five modules for learning psychobiology.

8. Briefly describe eight fields that are basic sciences for child psychiatry.

9. What arguments, pro and con, can you give on this topic: "Child psychiatry deserves separate departmental status in schools of medicine."

10. How would you train child psychiatry residents in research design, methodology, and techniques? Would you rely mostly on the individual tutorial, small group, or lecture in facilitating their learning? Give a quick outline of the curriculum you would plan to enhance their aptitudes for scientific research.

For Further Reading

Adams, P.L. The influence of new information from social sciences on concepts, practice and research in child psychiatry. *J. Amer. Acad. of Child Psychiatry*, 21:533–542, 1982.

Donahue, P. *The Human Animal.* New York: Simon & Schuster, 1985.

Earls, F. *Studies of Children*. Part of a series, *Monographs in Psychosocial Epidemiology*. New York: Prodist, 1980.

Goldman, J., L'Engle Stein, C., & Guerry, S. *Psychological Methods of Child Assessment*. New York: Brunner/Mazel, 1983.

Herskowitz, J., & Rosman, N.P. *Pediatrics, Neurology and Psychiatry—Common Ground*. New York: Macmillan, 1982.

Hinde, R.A. Ethology in relation to psychiatry. In M. Shepherd (Ed.), *Handbook of Psychiatry, Vol. 5: The Scientific Foundations of Psychiatry*. Cambridge, MA: University Press, 1985, pp. 119-133.

Klopfer, P.H. Aggression and its evolution. *Psychiatry & Soc. Sci. Behavior*, 3:2-7, 1969.

La Barre, W. *The Human Animal*. Chicago: University of Chicago Press, 1954.

Lorenz, K. *Evolution and the Modification of Behavior*. Chicago: University of Chicago Press, 1956.

Miller, J.G. *Living Systems*. New York: McGraw-Hill, 1978.

Rapoport, J.L., & Ismond, D.R. Biological research in child psychiatry. *J. Amer. Acad. of Child Psychiatry*, 21:543-548, 1982.

Smith, D.W. *Recognizable Patterns of Human Malformations*. Philadelphia: W.B. Saunders, 1982.

Wilner, J.R. Psychopharmacology in childhood disorders. *Psychiat. Clin. N. Amer.*, 7:831-843, 1984.

Afterword

Child psychiatry has been designated as the medical specialty showing the most severe shortage. We hope that our efforts to make the field interesting and attractive for the beginner will contribute something towards undoing the scarcity of specialists in child psychiatry. Committed and well-trained people are sorely needed.

The practice of child psychiatry as a clinical specialty or as a research discipline is a choice that holds promise of a career of service to underserved youthful humanity and, as a consequence, holds some rewards that are intrinsically gratifying to a service-oriented person; to the inquisitive scholar it will be a specialty that is at the forefront of scientific challenge and payoff, too. Amidst scarcity, small contributions—when they are sound and have met the canons of logic and the test of having empirical basis—can have an effect far beyond the individual investigator's usual reach.

We end this work with the hope that some of our enthusiasm for the field of child psychiatry has not been kept hidden from our readers.

Appendix

SELECTED CHRONOLOGY FOR CHILD PSYCHIATRY TO 1970

The following Selected Chronology has been designed to show the interplay during history between physicians, psychologists, educators, child advocates, and moralists. Our idea is that out of those diverse strains have come the body of attitudes and information that have created the post-1970 discipline of child psychiatry.

Students who have already used the Chronology have reported to us that, after a first reading, it is a good idea to go through it again, marking all the educators, then all the medical thinkers, then the social reformers and moralists, and then the academic psychologists, for in that way the interrelationships of the separate threads become more vivid.

B.C.

5000	Earliest cities were built in Mesopotamia.
3000	Chief deities still included Mother Goddess in Sumeria, Egypt, Phoenicia, and Scandinavia, but patriarchal religions began to gain ascendancy in Indo-Europe.
1000	Pantheistic Brahminism and Atmanism developed in India, teaching identity of self, transmigration of soul, and caste system.
c.950	King Solomon advocated, "Educate a child in a way that is his own." First written statement of maxim, "Follow children, not theory."
630	Zoroaster was born.
604	Lao-tse, founder of Taoism, was born.
538	Siddhartha Gautama, aged 35 years, found enlightenment at Buddh Gaya, near Benares. Originator of Buddhism.
460	Hippocrates of Cos, Father of Medicine, was born (died in 377 B.C.).
431	Empedocles advanced the idea of four humors: blood (sanguine). bile (choleric), black bile (melancholia), and phlegm (phlegmatic)—basis of perennial views on temperament as a biological given.
429	Hippocrates emphasized the importance of child nutrition and recognized the deleterious effects of malnutrition and dehydration on young children.
339	Socrates was condemned to death (drinking poison, hemlock) for spreading unconventional ideas that influenced youth to impiety.

165   Judah Maccabee and his brothers retook Jerusalem from the Syrians and made one day's worth of oil burn for eight days—basis for Hanukkah, Feast of Dedication celebrated in December by Jewish children.

7   An infant named Joshua (Jesus) was born at Bethlehem to a Jewish woman married to a carpenter—later to found a movement preaching brotherly love, a purely spiritual kingdom, and shifting emphasis of Judeo-Christian views on deity from father to son.

A.D.

29   Jesus was crucified in Jerusalem, having attacked the privileged, rich, and powerful and sided with the poor, underprivileged, and weak—including children. Followers anticipated end of the world and their messiah's return.

30   Celsus, a Roman physician, stated: "I am of the opinion that the art of medicine ought to be rational."

431   Cult of the Virgin Mary began to spread, viewing her as the mother of God, a countervailing influence within male-exalting established Christianity.

501   Susruta medical book, an Indian classic, was compiled.

598   First English school was founded at Canterbury.

610   A new religion (no less patriarchal than Jewish and Christian ones) began to be preached in secret by Mohammed, a 41-year-old Arab camel driver and caravan leader.

629   Mohammed returned to Mecca with the Koran, warning of the approach of the last days.

970   Abud al-Daula founded, in Baghdad, a hospital with interns and externs, a nursing service, and an elaborate pharmacy.

994–1064   Ali ibn-Hazm, forerunning Freud and Sullivan, wrote that "no one is moved to act, or resolves to speak a single word, who does not hope by means of this action or word to release anxiety from his spirit."

1021   Epidemics of St. Vitus's dance (chorea) swept Europe—the victims called on St. Vitus, a third-century child martyr.

1030   Avicenna (Abu Sina), Arab physician, in *Canon of Medicine,* described these five stages of childhood: infancy (before walking), babyhood (walking unsteady, teeth form), childhood (walking and dentition, before "pollution"), puberty (hair and pollution), and youth (until body growth ceases). He also emphasized the moral character of children's caretakers.

1080   Constantine the African, now in the guise of a monk at Monte Cassino's Benedictine monastery and school, who formerly studied medicine and magic in Babylon, translated Galen and Avicenna into Latin.

1212   Benedictine medical school at Salerno (founded in the 9th century) drew on Arabic, Jewish, Latin, and Greek medical teaching, employed some women physicians on its faculty, dissected pigs, adopted Arabic dietetics, and did not observe Christian dogmas very strictly.

1212	Children's Crusade, a summertime religious movement that enlisted some 50,000 children aiming to conquer Muslim-held Palestine by love instead of force. In coastal European cities the Christian merchants arranged to transport them not to Palestine but to North Africa, where they were sold into slavery.
1472	Paolo Bagellardo, an Italian physician, wrote the first pediatric text in Latin, published in Padua.
1473	Bartholomaeus Metlinger wrote the second pediatric text, 27 pages long, in German, in Augsburg.
1483	Cornelius Roelin (Roelants), a Belgian, authored the third pediatric incunabulum.
1524	Martin Luther urged education for children in public school, advocated literacy for the German public; he completed first German translation of Bible in 1534.
1526	Juan Vives, a Spaniard working in France, advocated courteous treatment, enlightenment, and instruction for all the poor and insane.
1545	Thomas Phayre wrote *Boke on Children*, the first pediatric text in English.
1580	Michel de Montaigne in his *Essais* called attention to the rights of the child to be a child and not a miniature adult.
1601	The English Poor Law was passed during Elizabeth I's reign; it established the virtue of child labor in law for the next three centuries.
1602	Felix Plater (1536–1614), anatomist in Basel, classified 23 mental diseases in *Praxis Medica* (1602–8), the first medical textbook published in the 17th century that dealt with psychiatry, but said that mental disorders were the Devil's handiwork and not results of natural causes.
1616	Paracelsus discovered cretinism in Switzerland (no sea waters).
1618	Johann Amos Comenius, a Moravian leader, in *School of Infancy* described types of education suitable for the child's first six years.
1622	Richard Baddeley wrote about a "Boy of Bilson" who was thought to be possessed, but proved to be feigning madness. No one investigated why the boy did what he did.
1628	John Earle, in *Microcosmographie,* saw the child as angelic, "the best copy of Adam before he tasted of Eve or the apple."
1632	St. Vincent de Paul founded the Maison de St. Lazare in Paris to humanize care of amentia and dementia patients.
1637	Mary Dyer was delivered of an anencephalic infant and ostracized; she was later executed (in 1660) as a Quaker on Boston Common.
1654	Comenius published the first picture book for children in Nuremberg.
1672	Thomas Willis, an anatomist and iatrochemist, described some children who "passed into obtuseness and hebetude during adolescence."
1676	Thomas Sydenham (1624–1689), father of epidemiology and "the English Hippocrates," in *Observationes Medicae* differentiated between St. Vitus's

dance ("Sydenham's Chorea") and hysteria, demonstrating that the latter affected men and children, not solely women.

1689   John Locke—back in England from exile—made a distinction between mental retardation and insanity, and advocated education.

1689   R. Morton described the anorexia syndrome as "nervous consumption."

1714   Bernard de Mandeville, in *Fable of the Bees,* extolled parents' requiring obedient bowing down of children.

1716   Von Pernau stated that behavior as well as morphology is species specific.

1748   William Cadogan published a pamphlet advocating breast feeding.

1755   George Baker wrote of sibling rivalry, "It is possible to see an infant weaken and languish most wretchedly from this emotion as if from wasting disease."

1762   Rousseau wrote *Emile;* he advocated education for children.

1762   Des Réaumur pointed out that behavior may precede organ development (goats butt before they have horns). Some see this as a milestone in behavioral biology.

1774   Johann Heinrich Pestalozzi wrote on how adjustment integrates physical, intellectual, and moral factors. He also observed and kept a diary of his own child, and emphasized direct observation of children—knowing the child.

1784   Valentin Haüy established the first school for the blind in Paris.

1784   Perière taught deaf mutes to communicate.

1787   Dietrich Tiedemann kept the first careful journal record of a child's growth.

1790   Condorcet, French revolutionary, wrote *The Admission of Women to Full Citizenship.*

1791   Philippe Pinel advocated moral treatment of the insane (children were still not involved).

1792   Mary Wollstonecraft (the poet Shelley's mother-in-law) wrote *Vindication of the Rights of Women.*

1796   Edward Jenner first scratched lymph from cowpox pustule into the skin of James Phipps, an eight-year-old, who then resisted smallpox.

1796   Charles Caldwell published the first U.S. monograph on pediatrics, a dissertation required of him as a medical graduate of the University of Pennsylvania.

1798   Jean Itard treated Victor, the wild boy of Aveyron, at Paris's Institution for the Deaf and Dumb.

c. 1800   Johann Peter Frank (1745–1821) first urged attention to social pediatrics —school hygiene, state's responsibility for child health, and medical care for bastards, orphans, and fostered infants.

1807   James Parkinson (of palsy fame) warned parents against both overindulgence and inconsistency in disciplining their infants.

1809	John Haslam's textbook described an autistic five-year-old admitted to Bethlem Asylum ("bedlam") in 1799.
1812	Benjamin Rush made perhaps the first reference to insanity in children in his book; he, himself, had a psychotic son.
1817	Henry Holland, writing on pellagra, compared adult mental disorder to childhood cognition.
1817	Rev. Thomas Gallaudet set up a program to educate the deaf in his Connecticut parish.
1825	First "day nursery" established in U.S. by Robert Owen, New Harmony, Indiana.
1828	Caspar Hauser, *homo ferus*, appeared on the streets of Nuremberg.
1829	Perkins Institution for the Blind was founded in Boston.
1830	Bronson Alcott, who kept Puritan behavioral records on his daughters, published them.
1832	Amariah Brigham, a founder of the APA, wrote that "insane" adults, especially mothers, predispose children to having mental disorders.
1834	Louis Braille (1809–52), blind since age three, invented raised point system of writing and music.
1837	Friedrich Froebel opened the first kindergarten in the village of Blankenburg, Thuringia.
1837	Edouard Séguin, a Christian socialist, established a school for idiots in Paris; he wrote a treatise on the treatment of idiots in 1846.
1838	Jean Étienne Dominique Esquirol differentiated the mentally defective from the psychotic child, attempted to classify insanity into age groups, and saw insanity as having an emotional basis.
1840	J. Guggenbuhl, C.M. Seagert, and J. Conolly opened schools for the retarded in Switzerland, Germany, and England, respectively.
1842	Massachusetts was the first state to limit working hours to 10 hours daily for children under 12 years of age.
1844	*American Journal of Insanity* (forerunner of *American Journal of Psychiatry*) began; not until 1890 did a single article deal with children.
1845	Wilhelm Griesinger, the first ego psychiatrist, advised educational treatment of disordered children and described both mania and melancholia in children.
1847	Charles West published the pediatric classic, *Lectures on Diseases of Children*, in London.
1848	K. Marx and F. Engels wrote *The Communist Manifesto*.
1848	Edouard Séguin wrote the first textbook on mental retardation.
1848 (or 50)	Samuel Ridley Howe established the first state school (Massachusetts) for the retarded in the U.S. under Séguin's influence.
1852	Paul Siogvolk called for "The Rights of Children" in *Knickerbocker*, USA.

1853   Children's Aid Society was founded to aid New York's homeless and destitute children.

1854   Charles West (London) wrote on the higher incidence of moral insanity in children and urged pediatricians to be aware of childhood mental disorders.

1856   Le Paulmier wrote a thesis on nervous afflictions in childhood.

1857   Benedict A. Morel wrote on the theory of degeneration—mental retardation due to family degeneration, originated term *démence précoce.*

1858   Daniel Schreber, a pediatrician, wrote a brainwashing manual which paralleled the later psychotic symptoms of one son, a famous Judge Schreber.

1859   Charles Darwin wrote *Origin of Species;* publication was delayed to honor his wife's concern about ostracism and a bad reputation.

1860   Abraham Jacobi founded the first American pediatric clinic in New York City. He was also an ardent advocate of breast feeding.

1860   Elizabeth Peabody established the first U.S., English-speaking kindergarten in Boston.

1860   Wilhelm Griesinger proposed the concept of psychogenic causality in mental subnormality—he was called by some the first ego psychiatrist.

1867   Henry Maudsley first attempted to classify childhood psychopathology. He wrote on seven types of insanity in early life and believed all had an organic materialistic base: "larvated epilepsy."

1868   W.W. Gull described anorexia nervosa as a picture like tuberculous consumption.

1870   A case of child abuse was resolved by a landmark decision to include children under a cruelty-to-animals law in N.Y. State. This was the first law in U.S. to "interfere" with parental ownership of children.

1871   Ewald Hecker described pubertal psychosis, *Hebephrenie.*

1871   Charles Darwin published *The Expression of the Emotions in Man and Animals,* citing child as well as adult examples in text and photos.

1874   Karl Ludwig Kahlbaum described *Katatonie.*

1875   Francis W. Parker, called the father of progressive education by John Dewey, began education for child development in the curriculum of Quincy, Massachusetts, schools.

1877   Charles Darwin published "A Biographical Sketch of an Infant," in *Mind.* Wilhelm Preyer, as a result of Darwin's work, made direct observations and wrote a book called *The Mind of a Child* (English version in 1888).

1880   G. Stanley Hall sent out his questionnaire about normal behavior of young persons.

1881   Wilhelm Preyer's *Die Seele des Kindes* was published—careful observation of neonatal reflexes and their fate.

1884	Friedrich Engels (Marx collaborator) wrote *The Origin of the Family, Private Property and the State.*
1884	*The Archives of Pediatrics* was first published.
1885	Georges Gilles de la Tourette first described compulsive tics with copro-lalia.
1887	Herrmann Emminghaus wrote on psychic disturbances of childhood, divided psychoses into those due to physical causes and those due to psychosocial conditions. He called for separate diagnostic schemes for adult and child.
1887	Annie Sullivan, teacher from the Perkins Institution, began teaching Helen Keller to communicate.
1888	William Morris wrote, "Children have as much need for a revolution as the proletariat have."
1888	Abraham Jacobi became head of the pediatric section of the AMA.
1889	Children's Charter became law in Britain, allowing state intervention into family oppression and allowing children to testify against parents.
1890	Charles Edward Spitzka stated that 25% of all mental disorders in U.S. children were due to masturbation.
1890	John M. Keating's *Cyclopedia* had four chapters on childhood psycho-pathology. These included hysteria and insanity.
1890	Nils wrote on hysteria in children.
1891	G. Stanley Hall published a journal called *Pedagogical Seminary*, the first journal in child psychology, emphasizing studying normal child development.
1892	Kate Douglas Wiggin's *Children's Rights* was published—parents must make sacrifices and serve their children's changing needs, allowing a child to have own world.
1893	Millicent W. Shinn's *Notes on the Development of a Child* was published—pre-Gesell study of early childhood behavior.
1893	Lillian Wald, reformer, made her Visiting Nurses' Service the basis of Henry Street Settlement, New York City.
1894	J. Séglas at Salpêtrière said obsessions might occur before puberty.
1894	Illinois Society of Child Study was founded.
1895	James Scully stated that play reveals the mental processes in a child.
1896	Freud first used the term *psychoanalysis*, having recognized in 1895 the value of free association over hypnosis.
1898	National Federation of Day Nurseries first met.
1899	Marcel Manheimer wrote *Mental Difficulties of Childhood.*
1899	Jane Addams and Ellen Starr founded Hull House, Chicago.
1899	John Dewey published *The School and Society.*

1899	Illinois and Colorado passed a law for the establishment of Juvenile Courts.
1900	Ellen Key, a noted feminist, predicted the 20th century would be "the century of the child," since women would earlier have achieved equal rights.
1900	1.7 million U.S. children under 16 years old were employed in paying occupations.
1900	S. Freud's *The Interpretation of Dreams* was published.
1901	First U.S. housing code was adopted for City of New York, where most tenements had no windows.
1904	National Child Labor Committee was formed to press for protective legislation (ultimately) requiring schooling of all children to take them out of mills, mines, and fields.
1904	Ivan Pavlov was given the Nobel Prize for work on conditional reflexes.
1905	Freud published three essays on his theory of sexuality, one being devoted to childhood sexuality (including oral and anal with genital).
1905	Benjamin Knox Rachford, head of pediatrics at Cincinnati General Hospital, wrote *The Neurotic Disorders of Childhood*.
1905	Alfred Binet published with Théodore Simon tests of intelligence to use with French schoolchildren.
1905	Santé de Sanctis described "dementia praecocissimo catatonica" in young retardates.
1906	Massachusetts was the first state to require medical exams for all school pupils.
1906	Lightner Witmer, University of Pennsylvania, had the first clinic for children. He coined the terms *clinical psychology* (1896) and *psychological clinic*.
1906	Following Upton Sinclair's novel, *The Jungle*, the first food and drugs act was passed.
1906	John Spargo's *The Bitter Cry of the Children* was published: "Capital(ism) has neither morals nor ideals" and calls out greedily for children.
1907	Maria Montessori, the first woman physician graduated from the University of Rome (1894), set up her Casa dei Bambini in Rome's San Lorenzo slums, applying educational strategies used earlier only with retarded children. She fled Mussolini in 1934.
1907	Lightner Witmer published a journal called *Psychological Clinics*.
1907	Adler, Freud, Steckel, Rank, Ferenczi, Jung, Abraham, and Eitingon formed the first Psychoanalytic Society in Vienna.
1908	Binet test was first used in the United States.
1908	Clifford Beers wrote *A Mind that Found Itself*.
1908	Theodor Heller, Austrian educator, described children who, normal

until three or four years old, began deterioration and regression: "dementia infantilis."

1908	Archibald Garrod described alcaptonuria (first known inborn error of metabolism).
1908	Water was first chlorinated in the U.S.
1909	William Healy established the Chicago Psychopathic Institute to serve the Juvenile Court.
1909	Clifford Beers formed the National Committee on Mental Hygiene with Adolf Meyer and others.
1909	The first White House Conference on Children (T. Roosevelt) was held.
1909	Freud published his paper on the treatment of "Little Hans," who was Herbert Graf, the son of Max Graf.
1909	Freud, Jung, and Meyer were guests of G. Stanley Hall for a congress held at Clark University, Worcester, Massachusetts.
1909	National Association for Advancement of Colored People was organized by 47 whites and 6 blacks.
1910	The first college psychiatrist was appointed at Princeton, a Dr. Patton.
1910	The Woodcraft Indians (Ernest Thompson-Seton) and the Sons of Daniel Boone (Dan C. Beard) merged to form Boy Scouts of America.
1911	Having left Freud's group and set up a "Free Psychoanalytic Society," Adler founded the Society for Individual Psychology.
1912	A children's clinic in Boston's Psychopathic Hospital was established by Ernest E. Southard; he first used the multidisciplinary approach and coined the term *social psychiatry*.
1912	Children's Bureau was established in the U.S. government.
1912	The Campfire Girls and Girl Scouts were separately formed this year.
1913	The Louisville Child Guidance Clinic was founded; also the Phipps Clinic in Baltimore began accepting children as patients.
1913	D.H. Lawrence completed *Sons and Lovers,* a novel of the mother–son bonding.
1914	Wilhelm Stern—*Psychology of Early Childhood*—added theory to empirical study.
1914	Homer Lane (an American) founded Little Commonwealth, a self-governing community for 40–50 delinquent children in Dorset, England.
1915	William Healy's book, *The Individual Delinquent,* was published.
1915	The libido theory of Freud was published.
1915	Pellagra was shown to have dietary cause in corn meal, fatback meat, and molasses (three Ms).
1916	Owen-Keating Act was passed, forbidding interstate shipment of goods manufactured by children under 14, or under 16 if children worked more than 8 hours per day.

1916	Montana sent pacifist Jeanette Rankin to Washington as the first Congresswoman ever in U.S.
1916	Bernard Glueck set up the first orthopsychiatry team (three disciplines) in the Westchester County Welfare Department, New York.
1916	Lewis M. Terman at Stanford University revised the Simon-Binet and introduced the term *IQ*.
1917	The Judge Baker Guidance Clinic was established in Boston by William Healy, M.D., and Augusta Bronner, Ph.D., his wife.
1918	Education Act in Britain made school attendance compulsory and forbade children to be employed for wages during school hours.
1918	August Aichhorn established his home for wayward boys in Vienna.
1919	Hermine Hug-Hellmuth treated a child using play therapy.
1919	Melanie Klein started treatment of children.
1920	Anton S. Makarenko organized The Gorky Colony for rehabilitation of homeless and delinquent children (Besprizornije) after the Soviet revolution.
1920	Freud's structural theory of the mind was published.
1920	Child Welfare League of America was formed.
1920	Lightner Witmer at Penn State described Don, a three-year-old with a "fear psychosis."
1921	The Commonwealth Fund held a conference on juvenile delinquency.
1921	The Habit Clinic in Boston was established by Douglas Thom.
1921	A.S. Neill founded Summerhill in Leiston, Suffolk, a free and self-governing school.
1922	Alfred Adler established the first child guidance clinic in Vienna (grew to a total of 30 by 1933).
1922	Several U.S. child guidance clinics were established on a pilot or demonstration basis by the Commonwealth Fund.
1922	Congressional laws *against* child labor were invalidated by the U.S. Supreme Court, until 1936–41.
1922	Clarence Darrow published his book, *Crime, Its Causes and Treatment*.
1923	The phallic phase was defined as a libidinal substage of the Oedipal phase.
1923	Tetanus toxoid was developed at the Pasteur Institute by Gaston Ramon, a French bacteriologist.
1923	Children's psychiatric service was started at Bellevue Hospital, New York.
1923	The Children's Clinic was started at Allentown, Pennsylvania, State Hospital.
1923	Jean Piaget's book, *The Language and Thought of the Child*, was published.
1924	Susan Isaacs founded Malting House School, England, for preschoolers.

1924	American Orthopsychiatric Association was formed: multidisciplinary.
1924	Otto Rank's book, *The Trauma of Human Birth*, was published, giving paramountcy to the mother in the child's mental life, and so was attacked by the patriarchal Freudians.
1925	*Wayward Youth* was published by Aichhorn (English trans. 1935).
1926	Mississippi became the last American state to provide universal public schooling.
1926	Peckham Pioneer Health Centre began in England—for families, totally nonauthoritarian (1926-39, 1946-51).
1926	A. Homburger published a book on childhood psychopathology in Germany.
1926	The term *encopresis* was first employed by S. Weissenberg as a parallel to *enuresis*.
1927	Institute for Child Guidance was founded in New York City: Lawson G. Lowrey, Director; David M. Levy, Chief of Staff.
1929	Richard Hughes's book, *The Innocent Voyage (High Wind in Jamaica)*, was published—about not so innocent children seized by pirates.
1930	Child psychiatry services were established at Johns Hopkins University.
1930	*American Journal of Orthopsychiatry* publication commenced.
1930	Susan Isaacs' book, *Intellectual Growth in Young Children*, began a running debate with Jean Piaget.
1930	Katherine M. Banham-Bridges published "A Genetic Theory of the Emotions," tracing emotional development in infants.
1930	International Congress on Mental Hygiene was held in Washington, D.C.
1931	Third White House Conference on children was held.
1932	Melanie Klein published her method of child psychoanalysis.
1932	Howard Potter defined infantile schizophrenia at the APA meeting.
1933	Publication of *Dynamics of Therapy in a Controlled Relationship*, the first book on child therapy, by Jessie Taft, a Rankian psychologist who taught in the Pennsylvania School of Social Welfare.
1933	The term *child psychiatry* was first used.
1934	A. Folling—PKU elucidated as causing one form of mental retardation.
1934	Josef Stalin decreed that children in the U.S.S.R. over 12 years of age would be punished as adults, e.g., eight years in a labor camp for stealing potatoes or grain.
1935	The first U.S. textbook on child psychiatry was published by Leo Kanner.
1935	Attention deficit with hyperkinesis was described in postencephalitic patients (E.D. Bond and L.H. Smith).
1936	Congress passed the Fair Labor Standards Act, restricting labor under age 16; upheld by the Supreme Court in 1941.

1937	The first congress on child psychiatry was held in Paris.
1938	Louise Despert differentiated acute schizophrenic disorder (in young people) from that of insidious onset.
1938	David Levy advocated release therapy, a focused play therapy.
1939	Abram Kardiner published the first of studies of "culture and personality," using a combination of projective system and reality system (Rorschach responses, myths, ideology, child rearing and economic practices) to derive a "basic personality" for a given culture.
1940	Karl Landsteiner and Alexander S. Wiener discovered Rh factor in blood.
1940s	Therapeutic milieu came into use in U.S.; German doctors aided in research/extermination (Loesung) of thousands of "defective" children in Europe.
1940	Publication of *The Heart Is a Lonely Hunter,* by Carson Smith McCullers—a novel of spiritual isolation in early adolescence.
1941	Olive Kendon founded Children's House in the slums of Manchester, England—run by children, not adults.
1941	Charles Bradley reported four cases of "schizophrenia in childhood."
1941	Adelaide Johnson and coworkers coined the term *school phobia.*
1942	Ives Hendricks proposed that mastery of environment is an instinctual drive separate from Eros and Thanatos.
1942	William Henry Beveridge in Britain proposed cradle-to-grave social security program.
1942	Publication of the second book on child therapy by Frederick Allen, Philadelphia Child Guidance Clinic, also a Rankian.
1942	By Executive Order 9066, F.D. Roosevelt interned 110,000 Japanese-Americans in concentration camps.
1943	Leo Kanner described infantile autism in 11 children—8 boys, 3 girls.
1943	Flanders Dunbar popularized the term *psychosomatic.*
1943	Samuel R. Slavson started working with therapy groups of children.
1943	Arnold L. Gesell and Frances Ilg's book, *The Infant and Child in the Culture of Today,* urged autonomy for the infant.
1944	Bruno Bettelheim established an orthogenic school in Chicago.
1944	Anne Frank and family, after two years in hiding, were betrayed in Amsterdam to the Gestapo and shipped to Auschwitz.
1945	Heinz Hartmann and Ernst Kris published on ego's conflict-free sphere.
1945	Penicillin (discovered 1928) and streptomycin were made available commercially.
1946	NIMH was established by the Mental Health Act.

1946	Group for the Advancement of Psychiatry was established under the Menningers' leadership to shake up APA stodginess.
1946	Jean Piaget's book, *Play, Dreams and Imitation in Childhood*, was published.
1946	UNICEF was founded.
1946	Benjamin Spock's *Pocket Book of Baby and Child Care* appeared.
1946	John Caffey, a pediatric radiologist, reported an interesting radiological syndrome of multiple long-bone fractures along with subdural hematomas in children—there was no mention that it is parent-induced.
1947	Virginia Axline described child therapy using the methods of Carl Rogers.
1947	Lauretta Bender (wife of Paul Schilder) wrote on early-onset schizophrenia and stated it was a form of "embryonal lag" encephalopathy appearing in pseudoretarded, pseudoneurotic, and pseudopsychopathic forms.
1947	A.A. Strauss and H. Werner described Minimal Brain Damage; Strauss and L. Lehtinen's book appeared in 1950.
1948	A. Bergman and S. Escalona wrote on the "stimulus barrier."
1948	World Health Organization was established in Geneva under the auspices of the United Nations.
1948	13 essential vitamins had now been isolated, with several synthesized.
1949	American Association of Psychiatric Clinics for Children (AAPCC) was founded as a standard-setting group.
1949	Melitta Sperling described a psychosomatic type of object relationship.
1949	Beata Rank described the atypical child; Margaret Mahler the child with symbiotic psychosis; and William Goldfarb childhood schizophrenia: organic and nonorganic.
1950	Papal Bull of Pius XII promulgated the assumption of the Virgin Mary, united with Son and Godhead—status was given to mother alongside father and son.
1950	Franz Alexander postulated specific conflict for specific physical symptoms.
1950	Meprobamate (an addicting ataraxic) was synthesized, inaugurating the era of the tranquilizers.
1952	James Robertson's film "A Two-Year-Old Goes to Hospital" came out.
1952	Margaret S. Mahler further described symbiotic psychosis.
1952	Salk's hypodermic vaccine against poliomyelitis was tested in this year when 50,000 were stricken by polio in U.S.
1952	DSM-II was published with a few categories of children's disorders.
1954	Fritz Redl and David Wineman published *Controls from Within: Techniques for the Treatment of the Aggressive Child*.

1954	Rudolf Ekstein and Robert Wallerstein wrote on the ego of the border-line child and also on object constancy in psychosis.
1954	Chlorpromazine was first marketed in the U.S.
1956	Konrad Lorenz's book, *Evolution and the Modification of Behavior,* was published.
1956	Paul Goodman's *Growing Up Absurd* appeared.
1958	American Academy of Child Psychiatry was formed, membership by invitation.
1958	A. Mirsky described increased pepsinogen blood levels and oral longings in patients with peptic ulcers.
1958–61	Nathan Ackerman explicated family therapy.
1959–66	Lee Robins was conducting her work on sociopaths *(Deviant Children Grown Up,* 1966).
1959	Therese Benedek proposed *parenthood* as a further stage in libidinal development.
1959	American Board of Psychiatry and Neurology, Inc., established a sub-specialty Committee on Certification in Child Psychiatry.
1960	C.H. Kempe spelled out the Battered Child Syndrome as parent-induced.
1960	Michael Duane headed Risinghill School in London, which became a community center for the families.
1961	Over 300 infants whose mothers took Thalidomide were born with phocomelia in West Germany.
1963	U.S. Children's Bureau first took a stand that day care benefitted both children and "families."
1963	Community Mental Health Centers Act was passed.
1963	Sylvia Ashton-Warner's *Teacher* was published.
1963	The American Psychological Association formed a section on clinical child psychology.
1963	Bernard Rimland, father of an autistic son, wrote on organicity of the reticular activating system in autism.
1965	Konrad Lorenz's book, *Evolution and the Modification of Behavior,* was published in English, University of Chicago.
1965	The Joint Commission on Mental Health of Children was established, supporting child advocacy.
1965	The term *community child psychiatry* was first used.
1965–66	The American Academy of Child Psychiatry opened membership to all trained child psychiatrists and began to grow in influence.
1966	Group for the Advancement of Psychiatry, Committee on Child Psychiatry, published *Psychopathological Disorders in Childhood.*

1966   The John F. Enders measles vaccine (produced in 1962) began to be
        used.

1967   John McDermott and Stuart Finch described autoimmunological fac-
        tors in ulcerative colitis.

1967   The Gault decision by the Supreme Court first gave constitutional
        protection to children who were arrested and brought to court.

1968   The American Association of Psychiatric Services for Children became
        the new name of AAPCC (1949).

1970   Jean Piaget's book, *The Principles of Genetic Epistemology,* was published.

Index

597